MOLECULAR PATHOLOGY LIBRARY SERIES

Philip T. Cagle, MD, Series Editor

For other titles published in this series, go to
www.springer.com/series/7723

Molecular Pathology of Endocrine Diseases

Edited by

Jennifer L. Hunt
Massachusetts General Hospital, Boston, MA, USA

Springer

Editor
Jennifer L. Hunt
Massachusetts General Hospital
Boston, MA
USA

ISBN 978-1-4419-1706-5 e-ISBN 978-1-4419-1707-2
DOI 10.1007/978-1-4419-1707-2
Springer New York Dordrecht Heidelberg London

Library of Congress Control Number: 2010921196

Printed on acid-free paper

Springer is part of Springer Science+Business Media (www.springer.com)

Series Preface

The past two decades have seen an ever accelerating growth in knowledge about molecular pathology of human diseases, which received a large boost with the sequencing of the human genome in 2003. Molecular diagnostics, molecular targeted therapy, and genetic therapy are now routine in many medical centers. The molecular field now impacts every field in medicine, whether clinical research or routine patient care. There is a great need for basic researchers to understand the potential clinical implications of their research whereas private practice clinicians of all types (general internal medicine and internal medicine specialists, medical oncologists, radiation oncologists, surgeons, pediatricians, family practitioners), clinical investigators, pathologists and medical laboratory directors, and radiologists require a basic understanding of the fundamentals of molecular pathogenesis, diagnosis, and treatment for their patients.

Traditional textbooks in molecular biology deal with basic science and are not readily applicable to the medical setting. Most medical textbooks that include a mention of molecular pathology in the clinical setting are limited in scope and assume that the reader already has a working knowledge of the basic science of molecular biology. Other texts emphasize technology and testing procedures without integrating the clinical perspective. There is an urgent need for a text that fills the gap between basic science books and clinical practice.

In the *Molecular Pathology Library* series, the basic science and the technology is integrated with the medical perspective and clinical application. Each book in the series is divided according to neoplastic and non-neoplastic diseases for each of the organ systems traditionally associated with medical subspecialties.

Each book in the series is organized to provide specific application of molecular pathology to the pathogenesis, diagnosis, and treatment of neoplastic and non-neoplastic diseases specific to each organ system. These broad section topics are broken down into succinct chapters to cover a very specific disease entity. The chapters are written by established authorities on the specific topic from academic centers around the world. In one book, diverse subjects are included that the reader would have to pursue from multiple sources in order to have a clear understanding of the molecular pathogenesis, diagnosis, and treatment of specific diseases. Attempting to hunt for the full information from basic concept to specific applications for a disease from varied sources is time-consuming and frustrating. By providing this quick and user-friendly reference, understanding and application of this rapidly growing field is made more accessible to both expert and generalist alike.

As books that bridge the gap between basic science and clinical understanding and practice, the *Molecular Pathology Library Series* serves the basic scientist, the clinical researcher, and the practicing physician or other health care provider who require more understanding of the application of basic research to patient care, from "bench to bedside." This series is unique and an invaluable resource to those who need to know about molecular pathology from a clinical, disease-oriented perspective. These books will be indispensable to physicians and health care providers in multiple disciplines as noted above, to residents and fellows in these multiple disciplines as well as their teaching institutions, and to researchers who increasingly must justify the clinical implications of their research.

Houston, TX — Philip T. Cagle

Contents

Section 3 Parathyroid Diseases

Section 4 Pituitary Diseases

Section 5 Adrenal Diseases

Section 6 Pancreatic Neuroendocrine Tumors

Section 7 Other Neuroendocrine Lesions

Contributors

Zubair W. Baloch, MD, PhD
Professor, Pathology and Laboratory Medicine, University of Pennsylvania Medical Center, Philadelphia, PA, USA

Christine B. Warren Baran, BA
Cleveland Clinic Lerner College of Medicine of Case Western Reserve University, Cleveland, OH, USA

Ahmed S. Bedeir, MD
Pathologist, Department of Pathology, Caris Diagnostics, Phoenix, AZ, USA

Eren Berber, MD
Staff Surgeon, Division of Endocrine Surgery, Endocrine and Metabolism Institute, Cleveland Clinic, Cleveland, OH, USA

Steven D. Billings, MD
Co-Section Head, Departments of Anatomic Pathology and Dermatology, Cleveland Clinic Foundation, Cleveland, OH, USA

Philip T. Cagle, MD
Weill Medical College of Cornell University, New York, NY, USA
The Methodist Hospital, Houston, TX, USA

Sally E. Carty, MD
Professor of Surgery, Section of Endocrine Surgery, Department of Surgery, University of Pittsburgh School of Medicine, Pittsburgh, PA, USA

Simion Chiosea, MD
Assistant Professor, Department of Pathology, University of Pittsburg Medical Center, Pittsburgh, PA, USA

Sanja Dacic, MD, PhD
Associate Professor of Pathology, Department of Pathology, University of Pittsburgh, Pittsburgh, PA, USA

Ronald R. de Krijger, MD, PhD
Professor, Department of Pathology, Erasmus Medical Center, University Medical Center Rotterdam, Rotterdam, The Netherlands

Ronald A. DeLellis, MD
Professor, Department of Pathology, Alpert Medical School, Brown University, Providence, RI, USA
Pathologist in Chief, Rhode Island Hospital, Providence, RI, USA

Dima L. Diab, MD
Clinical Fellow, Diabetes, and Metabolism, Department of Endocrinology, Cleveland Clinic, Cleveland, OH, USA

Lori A. Erickson, MD
Associate Professor, Department of Laboratory Medicine and Pathology, Mayo Clinic, Rochester, MN, USA

Amir H. Hamrahian, MD
Staff, Diabetes, and Metabolism, Department of Endocrinology, Cleveland Clinic, Cleveland, OH, USA

Adrian M. Harvey, MD, MEd, MSC
Clinical Assistant Professor of Surgery and Oncology, Endocrine Surgeon, Department of Surgery, Foothills Medical Center, Calgary, AB, Canada

Eric Hsi, MD
Section Head, Hematopathology, Department of Clinical Pathology, Cleveland Clinic, Cleveland, OH USA

Jennifer L. Hunt, MD, MEd
Associate Chief of Pathology, Director of Quality and Safety, Associate Professor of Pathology, Department of Pathology, Harvard Medical School, Massachusetts General Hospital, Boston, MA, USA

Ashraf Khan, MD, FRCPath
Professor of Pathology; Director of Surgical Pathology, Department of Pathology, UMass Memorial Medical Center, University of Massachusetts Medical School, Worcester, MA, USA

Alyssa M. Krasinskas, MD
Associate Professor of Pathology, Department of Pathology, University of Pittsburgh Medical Center, Pittsburgh, PA, USA

Todd G. Kroll, MD, PhD
Department of Pathology, Loyola University Medical Center, Chicago, IL, USA

Shih-Fan Kuan, MD, PhD
Associate Professor, Department of Pathology, University of Pittsburgh Medical Centers, Pittsburgh, PA, USA

Virginia A. LiVolsi, MD
Professor, Department of Pathology and Laboratory Medicine, University of Pennsylvania, Philadelphia PA, USA

Ricardo V. Lloyd, MD, PhD
Professor, Department of Pathology, Mayo Clinic, Rochester, MN, USA

Anne Marie McNicol, BSc, MBChB, MD, MRCP(UK), FRCPGlas, FRCPath
Professor, Department of Molecular and Cellular Pathology, UQ Centre for Clinical Research, The Royal Brisbane and Women's Hospital, Brisbane, Australia

Mira Milas, MD
Staff; Endocrinology and Metabolism Institute Director, The Thyroid Center Associate Professor of Surgery, Department of Endocrine Surgery, The Cleveland Clinic, Cleveland, OH, USA

Jamie C. Mitchell, MD
Staff Surgeon, Department of Endocrine Surgery, The Cleveland Clinic, Cleveland, OH, USA

Melissa Peck Piliang, MD
Associate Staff, Departments of Dermatology and Anatomic Pathology, Cleveland Clinic Foundation, Cleveland, OH, USA

Richard A. Prayson, MD
Section Head, Neuropathology; Professor, Department of Anatomic Pathology, Cleveland Clinic Foundation, Cleveland, OH, USA

Raja R. Seethala, MD
Assistant Professor of Pathology and Otolaryngology, Department of Pathology, University of Pittsburgh Medical Center, Pittsburgh, PA, USA

Allan Siperstein, MD
Chair, Professor of Surgery, Department of Endocrine Surgery, Cleveland Clinic, Surgery Institute, Cleveland, OH, USA

Michael T. Stang, MD
Assistant Professor of Surgery, Section of Endocrine Surgery, Division of Surgical Oncology, Department of Surgery, University of Pittsburgh Medical Center, VA Pittsburg Healthcare System, Pittsburgh, PA, USA

Edward B. Stelow, MD
Assistant Professor, Department of Pathology, University of Virginia, Charlottesville, VA, USA

Lawrence Tsao, MD
Staff, Department of Pathology and Laboratory Medicine Institute, Cleveland Clinic, Cleveland, OH, USA

Francien H. van Nederveen, MD
Department of Pathology, Erasmus Medical Center, Rotterdam, The Netherlands

Otto Walter, MD
Surgical Pathology Fellow, Department of Pathology, UMass Memorial Medical Center, Worcester, MA, USA

Sigrid Wayne, MD
Fellow, Department of Pathology, University of Pittsburgh Medical Center, Pittsburgh, PA, USA

Section 1
General Endocrine Molecular Pathology

1 Molecular Oncogenesis

Jennifer L. Hunt

Introduction

Oncogenesis in all organ systems is generally considered to be an extremely complex process, with poorly understood etiology and drivers. There is substantial evidence that much of carcinogenesis is driven by changes at the molecular level, at the DNA, RNA, or the protein expression level. New evidence also suggests that alterations in small RNA molecules (microRNA) can contribute to carcinogenesis, though this process is incompletely understood. Finally, environmental, nutritional, and external factors are almost certainly linked to carcinogenesis in some organ systems. It is precisely because of the complexity in all of these widely divergent drivers of carcinogenesis that we continue to search for the causes of cancer in most organ systems.

It is important to classify carcinomas based on one fundamental feature before any attempt at understanding the underlying etiology can be made. Tumors that are sporadic and tumors that are hereditary must be differentiated from one another. Though the genes involved may have overlapping profiles, in the sporadic case the alterations occur in terminally differentiated cells and in the hereditary case, the primary genetic events are inherited at the germline level. In many cases, carcinogenesis and the molecular pathways that lead to tumors are more clearly delineated in hereditary tumors. In sporadic tumors, the pathways tend to be highly complex and involve many different molecular events.

In nonhereditary, sporadic tumors and hyperplasias, a number of factors can be causally related to the pathology. The genetic causes will be extensively discussed in the following chapters for each endocrine organ system and individual tumor types. But, it is also important to consider other factors, such as environmental, nutritional, and external factors. For example, an important driver of thyroid disease in certain unique patient populations is exposure to radiation. The link between tumorigenesis and exposure to radiation link has been best studied in the population of individuals who were exposed to nuclear fall out after the Chernobyl disaster, which occurred in northern Ukraine in 1986.[3] In most studies, a significant increase in thyroid cancer was identified in the years following the exposure.[31,36] This included thyroid cancers occurring in young children, and thyroid cancers with a much more aggressive clinical course.[23] The molecular alterations in these patients are different from sporadic thyroid tumors.[9,24]

Though the source of radiation and the mechanisms are different from those seen in nuclear disasters, external beam radiation has also been linked to thyroid cancer. In past decades, radiation was used to treat banal disease, such as acne, thymus enlargement, and tinea. Patients who were exposed to this radiation were found to be at risk for future development of thyroid cancer, particularly when dosages were relatively low, and the radiation occurred during childhood and early adolescence.[29] Interestingly, the molecular analysis of these tumors indicates that they are more similar to the tumors in Chernobyl patients than to sporadic tumors.[2,4,6]

Despite all these potential contributors to carcinogenesis, one of the most important drivers of tumors remains alterations in tumor associated genes, in particular tumor suppressor genes (TSGs) and oncogenes. These are discussed in detail in this chapter, along with some of the more typical assays that are used to detect mutations and alterations in these tumor genes.

Tumor Suppressor Genes

Tumorigenesis through the inactivation of tumor suppressor genes was first postulated by Dr. Alfred George Knudson in the early 1970s, in seminal work with retinoblastoma.[21,22] Knudson elegantly showed that hereditary retinoblastoma and sporadic tumors had similar molecular mechanisms and involved the retinoblastoma gene. His theory, which is now known as *Knudson's Hypothesis*, predicted that both copies of the retinoblastoma gene needed to harbor mutations for tumorigenesis to occur.

Normal cells have two functional copies of each wild-type (nonmutated) tumor suppressor gene, one inherited from each parent. In the process of tumorigenesis, one copy of the

J.L. Hunt (ed.), *Molecular Pathology of Endocrine Diseases,* Molecular Pathology Library 3,
DOI 10.1007/978-1-4419-1707-2_1, © Springer Science+Business Media, LLC 2010

TABLE 1.1. Common tumor suppressor genes, their chromosomal location, function, and any associated inherited syndromes.

Tumor suppressor gene	Chromosomal location	Function	Inherited syndromes
P53	17p13	Cell cycle regulation, apoptosis	Li–Fraumeni syndrome
RB1	13q13	Cell cycle regulation	Retinoblastoma
WT1	11p13	Transcriptional regulation	Wilm's tumor
NF1	17q11.2	Catalysis of RAS inactivation	Neurofibromatosis type 1
NF2	22q12.2	Linkage of cell membrane to cytoskeleton	Neurofibromatosis type 2
APC	5q21	Signaling through adhesion molecules	Familial adenomatosis polyposis
DCC	18q21.3	Transmembrane receptor	
BRCA1	17q21	Repair double strand breaks	Familial breast cancer
BRCA2	13q12.3	Repair double strand breaks	Familial breast cancer
MSH2	2p22–p21	DNA mismatch repair	Mismatch repair syndromes
MLH1	3p21.3	DNA mismatch repair	Mismatch repair syndromes
VHL	3p26–p25	Regulation of transcription elongation	Von Hippel Lindau syndrome
PTEN	10q23	Regulated cell survival	Cowden syndrome

TSG develops an inactivating mutation. This first mutation is often a point mutation or small deletion mutation, and this is termed the first genetic hit. This first hit can occur spontaneously, or it can be inherited in cancer syndromes that make patients susceptible to specific tumors. Alone, the first mutation is not tumorigenic and usually has no ramifications for cell function, because the second copy of the TSG is still functioning. This is why tumor suppressor genes are also referred to as "recessive genes" – they require both copies to be mutated in order for loss of function.[25] The second genetic hit affects the second copy of the TSG, and this may be due to point mutations or more commonly, larger deletion mutations. It is uncommon for cells to have two large deletion mutations (biallelic deletion), because these would be considered to be lethal for the cell.[19] The cells that harbor these two mutated copies of the TSG have a loss of function of the TSG activity, and this is how carcinogenesis is thought to be stimulated.

One of the most famous illustrations of Knudson's hypothesis is the Vogelstein model of familial colon cancer progression.[8,37] In this classic example, germline mutations in the APC gene (chromosome 5q21) occur in patients affected by Familial Adenomatous Polyposis as the first hit, and somatic mutations (usually deletions) in the second copy of the APC gene represent the second hit. With both copies of the gene functionally lost, colon cancer progression occurs. The colon adenoma to carcinoma pathway is probably one of the best studied examples of tumorigenesis via the tumor suppressor pathway. Some of the most common tumor suppressor genes are listed in Table 1.1.

Assays Used to Detect Tumor Suppressor Gene Mutations

DNA Polymorphisms

A large percentage of the genetic code is redundant, with only a small amount of DNA being unique from person to person.[10,27] The differences in the genetic code are predominantly due to variable regions, called "polymorphisms." There are several different types of variable areas within the genetic code. The most common and most utilized for genetic testing are the short tandem repeats (STR) and the single nucleotide polymorphisms (snp). STRs are short redundant nucleotide sequences that vary from 2 to 7 base pairs in length that are repeated for a variable number of times. Polymorphisms have different levels of variability that are highly population dependent. When an individual has inherited two copies of the polymorphism that are different from one another, the two copies of the polymorphism can be discriminated from each other by PCR-based assays.

Being able to test for polymorphisms has great value for determining identify, which is used particularly in the area of forensic testing and paternity testing.[5,12,13,18,28,33,34] But, polymorphisms are also used in diagnostic testing in anatomic pathology as well, especially for loss of heterozygosity (LOH) and microsatellite instability testing.

Detecting Loss of Heterozygosity

Loss of heterozygosity (LOH) analysis relies upon our ability to discriminate between the two inherited copies of a particular gene. Unfortunately, the coding regions of our genes are usually highly conserved through evolution and are therefore identical in sequence on each of the two alleles that we have inherited (one maternal allele and one paternal allele). To do this type of assessment, molecular techniques utilize the polymorphisms in the genome that are in close proximity to genes of interest.

PCR is used in an LOH analysis, with primers that flank the polymorphism. In an informative person at that locus, the PCR amplicons will have different lengths, since they have two copies of the gene that have different numbers of repeat units. PCR products of different sizes will migrate at different speeds during electrophoresis. In normal cells, if we analyze an STR locus in an informative patient, we expect that there will be two differently sized PCR products of approximately the same amount, one from each chromosomal copy of the gene. In tumor cells, there may be deletion mutations present, which will alter the ratio of the PCR product amount from the two different PCR products. When one copy of the STR is lost, there will be only one PCR product, or the genotype will appear to be homozygous at that locus. Because the normal was originally heterozygous, we label this situation as "loss of heterozygosity."

A ratio of the amount of PCR product present for the two alleles can be obtained from capillary electrophoresis electropherograms as the ratio of the peak heights for the two products. If one is using gel based electrophoresis, this assessment is by visual inspection – if one band is less than 50% the intensity of the second band, this is indicative of loss. The calculation to determine if there is true loss of genetic material should include a comparison of the tumor allele ratio to that of the normal allele ratio. This will help to account for variability in PCR for the two alleles that might be secondary to the size of the PCR products or other variables that affect amplification efficiency.[32]

Oncogenes

Proto-oncogenes are nonmutated genes that, when mutated, stimulate carcinogenesis through activation. When mutated, these genes are designated as oncogenes. Oncogenes are referred to as dominant genes, because only one copy of the gene needs to be mutated to lead to overexpression or activation. Examples of some oncogenes are given in Table 1.2.

A variety of mutational events can transform a proto-oncogene to an oncogene, including point mutations, translocations, amplifications, and deletions. Because most of these mutations will be activating mutations, the protein product of the oncogene is often overexpressed because of the mutation. This protein product may be detectable by immunohistochemistry (IHC) or overabundant mRNA may be able to be detected by molecular techniques as well. However, overexpression of an oncogene protein product by IHC alone does not imply that there is a genomic mutation, since epigenetic mechanisms can also be responsible for protein overexpression.

In surgical pathology, some of the most common oncogene tests are those for translocations, amplifications, and point mutations. Though translocations were first described in sarcomas and hematologic malignancies, solid tumors are now being described with novel translocations as well. These translocations, for the most part, involve an oncogene partner that is juxtaposed next to an activating gene. The oncogene is then aberrantly activated in the tumor cells. Some common translocations in different types of tumors are listed in Table 1.3.

Amplifications are also now becoming common targets for assessment at the molecular level. There are several genes that have amplifications in specific tumor types that have prognostic or even therapeutic value, with *HER2/neu* in breast cancer and *EGFR* in several tumor types being the classic examples.[30,35,38,39]

Finally, assays for point mutations are increasing in clinical importance because of the association between some oncogene point mutations and potential drug targets. *CKIT* mutations in gastrointestinal stromal tumors and *EGFR* mutations in lung cancer were among the first tumor mutational assays that were proposed to have real significance in selecting targeted therapies.[1,11,14,15,20] As targeted therapies are introduced into the market place, it is likely that molecular analysis will continue to increase in importance. These targeted drugs are expensive and can have significant side effects, making the demand for companion diagnostic testing even higher to avoid the risks of uninformed treatment of patients who may not even respond to a particular drug. Assessing for additional acquired point mutations during tumor treatment will also likely become an important application of molecular technology. Many of the tumors being treated with targeted therapies are at risk for developing secondary mutations that will confer a resistance to the drug treatment.[7,14,26]

Assays Used to Detect Oncogene Mutations

Detecting Translocations

Reverse-transcription and polymerase chain reaction (RT-PCR) has long been considered to be the gold standard as the most powerful assay to detect translocations. In this assay, mRNA is extracted from the tissue and subjected to reverse transcription to yield cDNA. The cDNA is then amplified using PCR. The primers are carefully selected to amplify

Table 1.2. Common oncogenes, their chromosomal location, tumors that commonly harbor mutations in the gene, and any associated hereditary syndrome.

Oncogene	Chromosomal location	Tumor	Inherited syndromes
RET	10q11.2	Medullary thyroid carcinoma	MEN syndromes
N-RAS	1p13	Breast	
K-RAS	12p12.1	Pancreatic cancer	
H-RAS	11p15.5	Bladder cancer	
MET	7q31	Renal cell carcinoma	
CDK4	12q14	Sarcomas	
ERBB2/NEU	7q12–q21	Breast, ovarian, gastric, and colon cancer	
MYC	8q24.12	Many cancers	
ATM	11q22.3	Ataxia Telangiectasia	ATM
C-KIT	4q12	Gastrointestinal stromal tumors	

TABLE 1.3. Examples of tumors that harbor translocations.

Tumor	Molecular mutations	Location
ALL	MLL–AF-4	t(4:11)
	BCR–ABL	t(9;22)
	ELA–PBX	t(1;19)
	TEL–AML1	t(12;21)
	MYC–IgH	t(8;14)
Alveolar rhabdomyosarcoma	PAX3–FKHR	t(2;13)
	PAX7–FKHR	t(1;13)
AML-M2	ETO–AML1	t(8;21)
AML-M3	PML–RARA	t(15;17)
AML-M4eo	CBFB–MYH11	t(16;16) inv
Mantle cell lymphoma	BCL1–IgH	t(11;14)
Burkitt's lymphoma	IgH–MYC	t(8;14)
	IgK–MYC	t(2;8)
	IgL–MYC	t(8;22)
Clear cell sarcoma	EWS–ATF1	t(12;22)
CML	BCR–ABL	t(9;22)
Dermatofibrosarcoma protuberans	COL1A1–PDGF	t(17;22)
Desmoplastic small round cell tumor	EWS–WT1	t(11;22)
Ewing's sarcoma	EWS–FLI1	t(11;22)
	EWS–ERG	t(21;22)
	EWS–ETV1	t(7;22)
Extraskeletal myxoid	EWS–CHN	t(9;22)
chrondrosarcoma	RBP56	t(9;17)
Fibrosarcoma	ETV6–NTRK3	t(12;15)
Follicular lymphoma	BCL2–IGH	t(14;18)
Follicular thyroid carcinoma	PPARγ–PAX8	t(2;3)
Large cell lymphoma	BCL6–IgH	t(3;14)
	IgH–BCL8	t(14;15)
Marginal zone lymphoma	API2–MALT1	t(11;18)
Myxoid/round cell	TLS–CHOP	t(12;16)
liposarcoma	EWS–CHOP	t(2;22)
	EWS–CHOP	t(12;22;20)
Papillary thyroid carcinoma	RET–PTC	Rearrangement on 10q11.2
Synovial sarcoma	SYT–SSX1 or SYT–SSX2	t(x;18)

abnormal fusions across two different genes. Although RT-PCR is still considered to be the most sensitive and specific tool to assess for translocations, it is not the most practical approach in the clinical diagnostic laboratory, mainly because working with mRNA from tissue is complicated by the lability of the nucleic acids. Though mRNA can be extracted from paraffin embedded samples, for example, it is not of high quality and has generally undergone significant degradation.[16] Therefore, unless fresh or frozen tissue is available, it is often preferable to utilize a different approach.

Translocations can be detected in paraffin embedded tissues by using fluorescent in situ hybridization (FISH) based assays. Two different approaches are possible, fusion probes or break-apart probes. The choice of which type of probe sets to use will depend largely on the type of translocations, the consistency of the partner genes, and the availability of commercial probes.

In fusion probe detection, dual color probes, or chromosome specific paints, are used to localize each chromosome involved in the translocation. After hybridization, abnormal apposition of the two probes, which are normally distant to one another, indicates the presence of a translocation. Because the cells can be fragmented or cut in several planes or overlapping in paraffin embedded tissues, the signals for the two gene partners can be entirely or partially absent or can also be artificially overlapping each other. Therefore, a minimum number of cells must be examined before a definitive call is made about the presence of the translocation; this cutoff should be established in each laboratory that does the assay as part of the validation process.

In break-apart probe systems, the two probes are localized to the same gene, but flank the area that is typically a known break point. This system is preferable for translocations that have one consistent gene partner and a variety of other potential partners. In normal cells, the two signals are next to one another and overlapping. In cells that harbor a translocation, the two signals are separated, as they are now located on two different chromosomes secondary to the translocation.

Detecting Amplifications

FISH can also be used very effectively to detect gene amplifications. In this type of assay, a region specific probe is used in combination with a second probe for the chromosome in general. For example, to assess for EGFR amplification, there will be a probe for the EGFR gene and a second probe for chromosome 7 to be used as a comparison. By assessing both the copy number of the gene and the number of chromosomes present, one is able to resolve whether there is true gene amplification as opposed to polyploidy.

Detecting Point Mutations

The detection of point mutations in specific genes in the practice of anatomic pathology has been long complicated by several key issues. First, the DNA that can be obtained from paraffin embedded tissues is degraded, as compared to that obtained from fresh tissues.[16] Even though the DNA is degraded, most assays can be successfully implemented with careful planning. PCR-based assays should be designed with short PCR products (ideally under 200 basepairs) to account for the DNA fragmentation that is caused by formaldehyde.[16] Second, samples from tumors are notoriously heterogeneous. They contain not only tumor cells, but stromal cells, inflammatory cells, areas of potential necrosis. These tissue factors will also affect the sensitivity of any given assay. To address the heterogeneity of tissues, many tumor assays utilize microdissection to first obtain a relatively pure tumor sample.[17]

There are a number of excellent approaches that can be used to detect point mutations in oncogenes. The most traditional approach is conventional gene sequencing. Most assays of this type combine an initial PCR reaction for the specific area of interest (i.e., the exons that most commonly harbor mutations) with subsequent sequencing reactions. Although sequencing used to use radioactivity for the analysis, advanced sequencers are now available that are rapid, cost-effective, and use other detection technology that does not harbor the same risks as radioactivity. One typical approach is to use capillary electrophoresis machines to analyze the products from the sequencing reaction. Abnormal peaks represent mutant basepairs, and these are usually easily recognized in tumor samples.

The most significant problem that arises with gene sequencing is one of sensitivity. The assay will only detect a mutant allele when the cells that harbor it represent approximately 20% or more of the initial tumor sample. Therefore, tumor purity becomes a very important issue to address before using traditional gene sequencing. Other approaches, including pyrosequencing and allele specific PCR, have better sensitivities and are able to detect mutant that is present in the 1–2% range.

References

1. Antonescu CR. Targeted therapies in gastrointestinal stromal tumors. *Semin Diagn Pathol*. 2008;25:295–303.
2. Assaad A, Voeghtly L, Hunt JL. Thyroidectomies from patients with history of therapeutic radiation during childhood and adolescence have a unique mutational profile. *Mod Pathol*. 2008;21:1176–1182.
3. Bogdanova TI, Zurnadzhy LY, Greenebaum E, et al. A cohort study of thyroid cancer and other thyroid diseases after the Chornobyl accident: pathology analysis of thyroid cancer cases in Ukraine detected during the first screening (1998–2000). *Cancer*. 2006;107:2559–2566.
4. Bounacer A, Wicker R, Caillou B, et al. High prevalence of activating ret proto-oncogene rearrangements, in thyroid tumors from patients who had received external radiation. *Oncogene*. 1997;15:1263–1273.
5. Cohen J. Genes and behavior make an appearance in the O. J. trial. *Science*. 1995;268:22–23.
6. Collins BJ, Schneider AB, Prinz RA, Xu X. Low frequency of BRAF mutations in adult patients with papillary thyroid cancers following childhood radiation exposure. *Thyroid*. 2006;16:61–66.
7. Engelman JA, Janne PA. Mechanisms of acquired resistance to epidermal growth factor receptor tyrosine kinase inhibitors in non-small cell lung cancer. *Clin Cancer Res*. 2008;14: 2895–2899.
8. Fearon ER, Hamilton SR, Vogelstein B. Clonal analysis of human colorectal tumors. *Science*. 1987;238:193–197.
9. Fugazzola L, Pierotti MA, Vigano E, Pacini F, Vorontsova TV, Bongarzone I. Molecular and biochemical analysis of RET/PTC4, a novel oncogenic rearrangement between RET and ELE1 genes, in a post-Chernobyl papillary thyroid cancer. *Oncogene*. 1996;13:1093–1097.
10. Fujiyama A, Watanabe H, Toyoda A, et al. Construction and analysis of a human-chimpanzee comparative clone map. *Science*. 2002;295:131–134.
11. Fukui T, Ohe Y, Tsuta K, et al. Prospective study of the accuracy of EGFR mutational analysis by high-resolution melting analysis in small samples obtained from patients with non-small cell lung cancer. *Clin Cancer Res*. 2008;14:4751–4757.
12. Georgiou M, Hatzaki A, Koutselinis A. Identification of an alleged offender of murder by VNTR analysis: case report. *Am J Forensic Med Pathol*. 2000;21:162–165.
13. Grubwieser P, Zimmermann B, Niederstatter H, Pavlic M, Steinlechner M, Parson W. Evaluation of an extended set of 15 candidate STR loci for paternity and kinship analysis in an Austrian population sample. *Int J Legal Med*. 2007;121(2):85–89.
14. Heinrich MC, Maki RG, Corless CL, et al. Primary and secondary kinase genotypes correlate with the biological and clinical activity of sunitinib in imatinib-resistant gastrointestinal stromal tumor. *J Clin Oncol*. 2008;26:5352–5359.
15. Heinrich MC, Owzar K, Corless CL, et al. Correlation of kinase genotype and clinical outcome in the North American Intergroup Phase III Trial of imatinib mesylate for treatment of advanced gastrointestinal stromal tumor: CALGB 150105 Study by Cancer and Leukemia Group B and Southwest Oncology Group. *J Clin Oncol*. 2008;26:5360–5367.
16. Hunt JL. Molecular pathology in anatomic pathology practice: a review of basic principles. *Arch Pathol Lab Med*. 2008;132: 248–260.
17. Hunt JL, Finkelstein SD. Microdissection techniques for molecular testing in surgical pathology. *Arch Pathol Lab Med*. 2004;128:1372–1378.
18. Hunt JL, Swalsky P, Sasatomi E, Niehouse L, Bakker A, Finkelstein SD. A microdissection and molecular genotyping assay to confirm the identity of tissue floaters in paraffin-embedded tissue blocks. *Arch Pathol Lab Med*. 2003;127:213–217.
19. Iwasa Y, Michor F, Komarova NL, Nowak MA. Population genetics of tumor suppressor genes. *J Theor Biol*. 2005;233: 15–23.
20. Judson IR. Prognosis, imatinib dose, and benefit of sunitinib in GIST: knowing the genotype. *J Clin Oncol*. 2008;26:5322–5325.
21. Knudson AG Jr. Genetics and the etiology of childhood cancer. *Pediatr Res*. 1976;10:513–517.
22. Knudson AG Jr, Strong LC. Mutation and cancer: a model for Wilms' tumor of the kidney. *J Natl Cancer Inst*. 1972;48:313–324.
23. Nikiforov Y, Gnepp DR. Pediatric thyroid cancer after the Chernobyl disaster. Pathomorphologic study of 84 cases (1991–1992) from the Republic of Belarus. *Cancer*. 1994;74:748–766.
24. Nikiforov YE, Rowland JM, Bove KE, Monforte-Munoz H, Fagin JA. Distinct pattern of ret oncogene rearrangements in morphological variants of radiation-induced and sporadic thyroid papillary carcinomas in children. *Cancer Res*. 1997;57: 1690–1694.
25. Payne SR, Kemp CJ. Tumor suppressor genetics. *Carcinogenesis*. 2005;26:2031–2045.
26. Rubin BP, Duensing A. Mechanisms of resistance to small molecule kinase inhibition in the treatment of solid tumors. *Lab Invest*. 2006;86:981–986.
27. Sakaki Y, Watanabe H, Taylor T, et al. Human versus chimpanzee chromosome-wide sequence comparison and its evolutionary implication. *Cold Spring Harb Symp Quant Biol*. 2003;68: 455–460.
28. Sanchez JJ, Phillips C, Borsting C, et al. A multiplex assay with 52 single nucleotide polymorphisms for human identification. *Electrophoresis*. 2006;27:1713–1724.
29. Schlumberger M, Cailleux AF, Suarez HG, de Vathaire F. Irradiation and second cancers. The thyroid as a case in point. *C R Acad Sci III*. 1999;322:205–213.

30. Sequist LV, Joshi VA, Janne PA, et al. Epidermal growth factor receptor mutation testing in the care of lung cancer patients. *Clin Cancer Res.* 2006;12:4403s–4408s.
31. Shakhtarin VV, Tsyb AF, Stepanenko VF, Orlov MY, Kopecky KJ, Davis S. Iodine deficiency, radiation dose, and the risk of thyroid cancer among children and adolescents in the Bryansk region of Russia following the Chernobyl power station accident. *Int J Epidemiol.* 2003;32:584–591.
32. Slebos RJ, Umbach DM, Sommer CA, Horner GA, Choi JY, Taylor JA. Analytical and statistical methods to evaluate microsatellite allelic imbalance in small amounts of DNA. *Lab Invest.* 2004;84:649–657.
33. Staiti N, Di Martino D, Saravo L. A novel approach in personal identification from tissue samples undergone different processes through STR typing. *Forensic Sci Int.* 2004;146 Suppl: S171–S173.
34. Sweet DJ, Sweet CH. DNA analysis of dental pulp to link incinerated remains of homicide victim to crime scene. *J Forensic Sci.* 1995;40:310–314.
35. Toth J, Egervari K, Klekner A, et al. Analysis of EGFR gene amplification. Protein over-expression and tyrosine kinase domain mutation in recurrent glioblastoma. *Pathol Oncol Res.* 2009;15(2):225–229.
36. Tuttle RM, Becker DV. The Chernobyl accident and its consequences: update at the millennium. *Semin Nucl Med.* 2000;30:133–140.
37. Vogelstein B, Fearon ER, Hamilton SR, et al. Genetic alterations during colorectal-tumor development. *N Engl J Med.* 1988;319:525–532.
38. Wolff AC, Hammond ME, Schwartz JN, et al. American Society of Clinical Oncology/College of American Pathologists guideline recommendations for human epidermal growth factor receptor 2 testing in breast cancer. *J Clin Oncol.* 2007;25: 118–145.
39. Yatabe Y, Takahashi T, Mitsudomi T. Epidermal growth factor receptor gene amplification is acquired in association with tumor progression of EGFR-mutated lung cancer. *Cancer Res.* 2008;68:2106–2111.

2 Systematic Autoimmune Diseases

Sigrid Wayne

Introduction

Autoimmunity is defined as an immune response directed against a self-antigen – an antigen of host origin, within host tissue. Autoimmunity encompasses nonpathologic, naturally occurring immune responses, such as cold autoantibodies to red blood cell antigens, as well as pathologic conditions caused by the autoimmune response: i.e., *autoimmune disease*. Any component of the immune system may be involved in autoimmunity, including the innate immune system, B-cell responses, and T-cell responses.

Autoimmune diseases may be classified by the scope of organ involvement as either localized or systemic. Localized autoimmune diseases are characterized by an immune attack restricted to a specific organ or tissue, for example type I diabetes mellitus, Hashimoto's thyroiditis, Addison's disease, and lymphocytic hypophysitis. In some forms of localized autoimmune disease, although the targeted self-antigen is limited, the consequences of the tissue damage may be systemic, for example, type I diabetes mellitus. By contrast, the targeted self-antigen in systemic autoimmune diseases, tends to be more widely distributed, leading to widespread tissue damage: for example, systemic lupus erythematosus (SLE) and vasculitis. It thus follows that endocrine organ involvement by autoimmune disease may be localized (Hashimoto's, Grave's, Addison's, etc.) or can be part of a systemic process when the organ contains the targeted self-antigen.

Understanding of the etiologic factors of autoimmune disease, both genetic and environmental, is increasing. The genetic component of autoimmune diseases tends to be multigenic. In addition to genes linked to specific diseases (to be discussed in the sections that follow), several genes have been implicated as general risk factors for autoimmunity (Table 2.1).[1–4] There is accumulating evidence that vitamin D deficiency may be an environmental factor predisposing to autoimmune disease; vitamin D normally participates in T helper and dendritic cell function.[5,6] Prolactin has a role in the immunoregulation as well; prolactin promotes B-cell proliferation and immunoglobulin production in response to antigen, and inhibits apoptosis and negative selection of autoreactive B-cells.[6,7] Hyperprolactinemia may confer a general risk for the development of autoimmune disease. An additional possible risk factor for autoimmune disease is microchimerism – the presence of non-self stem cells or their progeny within an individual, most commonly derived from transplacental trafficking of stem cells during pregnancy. Persistent microchimerism over years may elevate the risk for autoimmune disease.[8]

This chapter will review systemic autoimmune disease focusing on the molecular/genetic aspects (when known), and endocrine organ manifestations.

Systemic Lupus Erythematosus

Systemic lupus erythrematosus (SLE) is the quintessential systemic autoimmune disease, notable for the heterogeneity in clinical presentation and course. The annual incidence of SLE ranges from 1.9 to 5.6 per 100,000,[9] and, as is true for most autoimmune diseases, predominantly affects females of reproductive age. While any organ may be involved, the most common clinical scenario includes constitutional symptoms, and skin, musculoskeletal, and hematologic manifestations.

The spectrum of disease in SLE is an expression of the ubiquity of the target antigens: DNA/protein complexes, RNA/protein complexes, and cell membrane and intracellular molecules. Tissue damage is mediated primarily by pathogenic autoantibodies and immune complex deposition, although a role for direct tissue toxicity by T-cells may also contribute.[10]

Both environmental and genetic factors are implicated in the etiology of SLE. Environmental factors include UV light, infection, drugs, and (female) gender.

J.L. Hunt (ed.), *Molecular Pathology of Endocrine Diseases,* Molecular Pathology Library 3,
DOI 10.1007/978-1-4419-1707-2_2, © Springer Science+Business Media, LLC 2010

TABLE 2.1. Systemic autoimmune disease: general susceptibility genes for autoimmune disease.[1–4]

Gene	Name	Location	Function	Disease associations
HLA region	Human leukocyte antigen	6p21.3	Antigen presentation; immune regulation	Specific haplotypes associated with different ADs (see text)
CTLA-4	Cytotoxic T-lymphocyte associated antigen-4	2q33	Expressed on activated T-cells; down regulates T-cell function	Animal models: SLE, MS, IDDM Human disease: SLE, IDDM
FCRL3	Fc receptor-like 3	1q22–q22	Role in early B-cell maturation, activation	SLE, RA, AITD
PTPN22	Protein tyrosine phosphatase, non-receptor, type 22	1p13	Lymphoid tyrosine phosphatase	SLE, IDDM, RA, AITD
PDCD1	Programmed cell death 1	2q37	Inhibition of T-cell proliferation and cytokine production	SLE, RA

AD autoimmune disease; *SLE* systemic lupus erythematosus; *MS* multiple sclerosis; *IDDM* insulin dependent diabetes mellitus; *RA* rheumatoid arthritis; *AITD* autoimmune thyroid disease.

Clinical Features

The diagnosis of SLE is based on a combination of clinical and laboratory features. Clinical features are manifold; the following represent the more common manifestations and are used to identify patients for clinical studies[11]:

- Skin disorder: malar rash, discoid rash, photosensitivity
- Oral ulcers
- Arthritis
- Serositis: pleuritis, pericarditis, effusions
- Renal disorder: proteinuria, cellular casts
- Neurologic disorder: seizures, psychosis
- Hematologic disorder: cytopenias
- Immunologic disorder: false positive serologic test for syphilis, positive lupus erythematosus cell preparation, anti-Smith (Sm) nuclear antigen
- Antinuclear antibody

Vasculitis, presumably due to antiphospholipid antibodies, anti-endothelial cell antibodies, and anti-double stranded (ds)-DNA antibodies, may also occur.[12]

Laboratory studies useful in the diagnosis of SLE include cell counts to assess for cytopenias, urinalysis to detect glomerular disease, and serology. Autoantibodies assayed, with a range of sensitivity and specificity, are directed against nuclear antigens (ANA), ds-DNA, Sm, ribonucleoprotein (RNP), Ro, La, phospholipids, and ribosomal P.

Pathogenesis

The key initiating event in SLE appears to be the release of self-antigen in a susceptible individual. As suggested by murine studies, the pathogenesis can be summarized by the following "antinucleosome to anti-ds-DNA hypothesis." External factors such as UV light, infection, drugs, and dietary factors may cause the release of self-antigen either by direct cellular injury or by indirect injury mediated by an immune response to exogenous antigens. Cellular injury culminating in apoptosis releases nuclear antigens within nucleosomes, triggering the formation of anti-DNA/protein antibodies. With maturation and somatic mutation some of these initial anti-DNA/protein antibodies evolve into autoantibodies with anti-single stranded (ss)-DNA and anti-ds-DNA specificity.[10]

As noted, these events must occur in the background of a susceptible individual; "susceptibility" encompasses genetic and hormonal factors, which result in multiple derangements of the immune system:

- Hyperactivated B-cells
  - Increased numbers of B-cells
  - Abnormal B-cell responses to activating signals
  - Impaired apoptosis of autoreactive B-cells
  - Increased levels of B-cell promoting cytokines: interleukin (IL)-10, IL-6
- Hyperactivated T-cells
  - Change in ratio of helper to suppressor/natural killer (NK) cells (skewed towards helper T-cells)
  - Abnormal activation
  - Accelerated apoptosis
  - Increased levels of T-cell promoting cytokines: IL-2, sIL-2R, interferon (IFN)-γ
- Abnormalities of monocytes and macrophages
  - Defective processing of immune complexes
  - Increased secretion of IFN-γ
- Abnormalities of immunoregulation
  - Possible defective immune tolerance
  - Inadequate clearing of immune complexes

These alterations create an environment with increased release of autoantigens, increased responsiveness to autoantigens with autoantibody production, decreased down-regulation of the immune response, and impaired clearance of antigen–antibody complexes.

Genetics

A genetic predisposition for SLE is evidenced by a 58% concordance rate of disease in monozygotic twins (a tenfold increase compared to dizygotic twins), as well as an eightfold increased risk for SLE in first degree relatives of an affected individual.[10] Several susceptibility genes have been identified (Table 2.2).

HLA genes, particularly class II (DR, DQ, DP) and class III (complement components C2 and C4), have been found to be associated with SLE.[10] HLA-DR2 and DR3 confer a relative risk of developing SLE of 2–3 across diverse ethnic groups, while different extended HLA haplotypes predispose

TABLE 2.2. Systemic autoimmune disease: susceptibility genes for SLE.[10]

Gene	Name	Location	Function	Disease associations
HLA region	Human leukocyte antigen	6p21.3	Antigen presentation; immune regulation	Specific extended haplotypes associated with SLE in different ethnic groups
C2, C4	Complement components 2 and 4	6p21.3	Complement cascade; deficiency impairs clearance of apoptotic bodies	Deficiency associated with high risk for SLE
C1q	Complement component 1, q subcomponent	1p36.3–p34.1	Complement cascade; deficiency impairs clearance of apoptotic bodies	Deficiency associated with high risk for SLE
C1r	Complement component 1, r subcomponent	12p13	Complement cascade; deficiency impairs clearance of apoptotic bodies	Deficiency associated with high risk for SLE
C1-INH	Complement component 1 inhibitor	11q11–q13.1	Complement cascade; deficiency impairs clearance of apoptotic bodies	Deficiency associated with high risk for SLE
FcγRIIA	Cell surface Fc-receptor	1q21–q23	Binds Fc portion of Ig; clearance of immune complexes	Certain polymorphisms predispose to SLE
FcγRIIIA	Cell surface Fc-receptor	1q23	Binds Fc portion of Ig; clearance of immune complexes	Certain polymorphisms predispose to SLE
IL-10	Interleukin-10	1q31–q32	Stimulates B-cell activation, proliferation, differentiation, and Ig production	Promoter polymorphisms enhance IL-10 production
MBL	Mannose binding lectin	10q11.2–q21	Activates complement cascade	Polymorphisms in promoter and exon 1 associated with SLE
PDCD1	Programmed cell death 1	2q37	Inhibition of T-cell proliferation and cytokine production	Intronic SNP associated with SLE in Europeans and Mexicans

Ig immunoglobulin; *SNP* single nucleotide polymorphism.

to disease in different ethnic groups, and to different spectra of clinical manifestations. Amino acid sequences in disease associated class II proteins appear to enhance autoantibody production. Deficiencies of HLA class III complement components C2 and C4, as well as of non-HLA complement components C1q, C1r, and C1-inhibitor (INH) impart a high risk for SLE. Such deficiencies impair clearance of apoptotic bodies, increasing exposure to self-antigens.[10]

Clearance of immune complexes is impaired by certain polymorphisms of white blood cell surface Fc-receptors; these include polymorphisms of genes encoding the FcγIIA and FcγIIIA receptors (FCGR2A, FCGR3A).[10]

Certain promoter polymorphisms in the IL-10 gene have also been linked to SLE. As noted previously, serum levels of IL-10, a cytokine that stimulates B-cell activation, proliferation, differentiation, and immunoglobulin (Ig) production are elevated in SLE. These promoter polymorphisms appear to enhance IL-10 production.[10]

Linkage analysis studies have identified three additional chromosomal regions linked to SLE: 1q41–43, 4p16–15, and 16q12–13. The gene poly(ADP-ribose) polymerase, encoding an enzyme involved in apoptosis-associated DNA repair is a candidate gene within the chromosome 1 locus. On chromosome 16 is the candidate gene nucleotide-binding oligomerization domain containing 2 (NOD2), encoding a protein involved in monocyte interaction with bacteria. Variants of NOD2 are associated with Crohn's disease.[10]

Endocrine Organ Involvement

Autoantibodies may arise in SLE that react with antigens within endocrine organs. The thyroid is the endocrine organ most commonly affected; antithyroid antibodies, including anti-thyroglobulin and anti-microsomal antibodies, are detectable in up to 35% of SLE patients. Hypothyroidism, usually clinically silent, is present in 6–15%,[9,13–18] a rate higher than the normal population. Euthyroid sick syndrome is seen in up to 15%.[15]

Abnormalities in pituitary hormone levels have been identified in SLE, including elevated follicle stimulating hormone, luteinizing hormone, and prolactin, compared to normal controls.[19,20] It is unclear whether this finding represents a hormonal milieu that predisposes to SLE or results from the disease.

Endocrine organs may also theoretically be affected by the vasculitis that occurs in SLE.

Sarcoidosis

Sarcoidosis is a systemic inflammatory disease featuring noncaseating granulomas in multiple organ systems, most commonly in the lungs and intrathoracic lymph nodes. The etiology is unknown, but evidence points to an exuberant T-cell mediated immune response to an antigenic stimulus. As in SLE, exogenous triggers including infectious agents and occupational exposures are suspected to initiate the inflammatory cycle in genetically predisposed individuals.[11,21]

Clinical Features

Sarcoidosis may affect almost any organ, with presentation depending on the pattern of involvement. It is not unusual for the diagnosis to result from work up of incidental chest radiographic abnormalities in an asymptomatic patient. Commonly involved organs include the lungs, lymph nodes, skin, heart, eye, and nervous system. Biopsy, most commonly of the lung, intrathoracic lymph nodes, and skin, with demonstration of noncaseating granulomas and exclusion of other causes of granulomata, remains the gold standard for the diagnosis of sarcoidosis.[11] Angiotensin converting enzyme (ACE) levels and T lymphocyte subsets in bronchoalveolar lavage fluid are adjunctive studies. The extent and course of disease may be monitored by serial imaging.

Pathogenesis

The proximate cause of sarcoidosis is unknown. Granulomas in tissue result from a predominantly T helper cell mediated immune response leading to release of cytokines such as IFN-γ, IL-2, and tumor necrosis factor (TNF)-α, and recruitment of macrophages. The antigen triggering the initial response is unknown, but a variety of infectious agents and occupational/environmental exposures have been implicated.[11,21] An autoimmune component may be operational in the maintenance of the immune response.

Genetics

The existence of a "genetically predisposed" state is suggested by familial clustering of sarcoidosis as well as by increased incidence of disease in monozygotic compared to dizygotic twins. Weak associations have been identified with several genes. HLA-DRB1*15 and HLA-DQB1*0602 are linked to more chronic forms of disease, while HLA-DRB1*03 and HLA-DQB1*0201 are associated with a milder form of disease.[21] Polymorphisms in transporter associated with antigen-processing (TAP) genes 1 and 2, encoding transporters essential in antigen processing for MHC-I antigen presentation, have been identified in British and Polish sarcoidosis patients. Disease associated polymorphisms have also been found in genes encoding inflammatory mediators such as the TNF-α promoter, ACE gene, IL-1α, complement receptor 1, and chemokine receptor genes.[21]

Endocrine Organ Involvement

Endocrine organ involvement in sarcoidosis may result from granulomatous infiltration or autoimmune mechanisms.[18]

Granulomatous infiltration is the cause of hypothalamic–pituitary sarcoid, with diabetes insipidus representing the most frequent clinical manifestation. Other manifestations include syndrome of inappropriate antidiuretic hormone (SIADH), hyperprolactinemia, hypothyroidism, hypoadrenalism, growth hormone deficiency, and morbid obesity.[22–25] Sarcoid granulomas may rarely involve the thyroid, resulting in hypothyroidism, cold nodules, and, uncommonly, hyperthyroidism.[22,26–28] The adrenal is also a rare site for granulomatous infiltration, which may result in primary adrenal insufficiency.[22]

Endocrine involvement in sarcoidosis associated with autoimmunity has been reported in 19.2% of patients, based on serologic evidence,[18,22,29] with autoimmune thyroid disease (Graves and autoimmune thyroiditis), Addison's disease, and polyglandular autoimmune syndrome type II occurring more frequently than in the general population.[22,30]

Additionally, suppression of parathyroid function may follow the hypercalcemia seen in 5–10% of sarcoidosis patients. Hypercalcemia appears to be caused by elevated levels of 1,25-dihydroxyvitamin D3 and parathyroid-hormone related protein generated by sarcoid granulomas.[22]

Sjogren's Syndrome

Sjogren's syndrome is a common systemic disorder characterized by xerostomia and xerophthalmia secondary to autoimmune injury to exocrine glands. Half of Sjogren's syndrome cases are primary, while the remainder are secondary: associated with another autoimmune connective tissue disorder. The prevalence has been reported as 0.5–5%, with 90% of cases occurring in women in midlife.[10]

Clinical Features

Autoimmune destruction of salivary and lacrimal glands is responsible for the predominant clinical manifestations of xerostomia and xerophthalmia with associated sequelae such as photophobia, redness, ocular fatigue/pain, infection, dental caries, and intraoral candidiasis.[10] Additional xeroses include dry sinonasal mucosa, vaginal dryness, dry skin, and decreased sweat volume. Sjogren's syndrome is associated with systemic symptoms such as musculoskeletal (arthralgias, myalgias), cutaneous (dry skin, purpura, vasculitis), gastrointestinal (esophageal dysmotility, pancreatitis, hepatitis), renal (renal tubular acidosis, interstitial nephritis), neurologic (neuropathy, central nervous system disease), and hematologic (leukopenia, anemia, lymphoma). Diagnosis hinges on the presence of xeroses accompanied by either autoantibodies or a positive minor salivary gland biopsy demonstrating a quantitatively appropriate mononuclear inflammatory infiltrate with glandular damage.[10]

Pathogenesis

The autoimmune attack on exocrine glandular epithelium is hypothesized to be triggered in a genetically susceptible individual by an emotional or physiologic stress or an epitheliotropic virus, such as Epstein–Barr virus (EBV), that activates the epithelium. Because epithelial cells express MHC class I and II molecules as well as CD80 and CD81, they are capable of acting as antigen presenting cells and activating T-cells. Lymphocytes may thus be recruited and activated, launching a cycle of epithelial damage via apoptosis, release/presentation of autoantigens, and further immune attack. This process is mediated by proinflammatory cytokines IL-1β, TNF-α, IL-2, and IL-6.[10,31]

Within salivary glands, the lymphocytic infiltrate is predominantly T-cell; however, a B-cell contribution exists as well: foci of predominantly IgA expressing plasma cells and occasional germinal centers may be noted. Several different autoantibodies may be identified in Sjogren's syndrome patients, and may contribute to epithelial destruction. Antibodies to ribonuclear proteins Ro (SS-A) and La (SS-B) are present in75 and 40% of patients respectively. Additional autoantibodies may target fodrin (a cytoskeletal protein) and muscarinic M3 receptor.[10]

An additional mechanism of glandular damage is suggested by the presence of matrix degrading metalloproteinases within salivary glands in Sjogren's syndrome patients.[10]

Genetics

Familial clustering and twin studies suggest a genetic component to Sjogren's syndrome. Polymorphisms with the HLA DRB1/DQA1/DQB1 haplotype correlate with susceptibility to Sjogren's syndrome in different ethnic groups, with clinical features, and with production of autoantibodies. Also linked to Sjogren's syndrome are TAPs and TNF alleles on chromosome 6, as well as the IL-10 promoter region and glutathione transferase M1 on chromosome 1.[10]

Endocrine Organ Involvement

Sjogren's syndrome is strongly associated with autoimmune thyroid disease. Thyroid disease, is more common in Sjogren's syndrome patients than controls (30% versus 4%),[32,33] and may precede or follow the diagnosis of Sjogren's syndrome..[10,31,32] Antibodies to thyroid antigens – thyroid peroxidase, thyroglobulin, T3, T4 – are frequently identified.[18] Clinically, such patients usually present with Hashimoto's thyroiditis, although Graves disease may occasionally result, with concordant histologic findings.

Systemic Sclerosis

Systemic sclerosis (scleroderma) is a connective tissue disorder of unknown etiology manifesting as thickening and fibrosis of the skin, internal organs, and blood vessels. The incidence is 18–20 per million per year, affecting predominantly women, with onset typically between 30 and 50 years. Systemic sclerosis occurs worldwide and affects all racial groups.[10]

Clinical Features

Approximately 70% of patients initially present with symptoms of systemic sclerosis related vasculopathy: Raynaud's phenomenon – changes in skin color (blue, white, red) in fingers, toes, ears, and nose due to vasospasm/relaxation triggered by cold or emotional stress. With disease progression, the skin becomes thickened, taut, and indurated. The extent of skin involvement distinguishes clinical subgroups with varying prognosis. Involvement of the heart, lungs, gastrointestinal tract, and kidney by fibrosis or injury secondary to vasculopathy contributes most prominently to morbidity and mortality in systemic sclerosis.[10]

Pathogenesis

Alterations in fibroblasts and extracellular matrix are the immediate cause of disease. Fibroblasts are hyperproliferative, hypersecretory, and resistant to apoptosis. Both the structure of the collagen produced and its degradation are normal. Evidence strongly supports that the generalized fibrosis of systemic sclerosis is a secondary phenomenon; however, the proximate cause is unknown. Autoantibodies, including nonspecific ANAs, anticentromere antibodies (seen in 50–96% of patients with limited disease), and anti-DNA topoisomerase I (Scl70-70) antibodies (seen in 20–40% of patients), have been identified in systemic sclerosis patients. There is also evidence of T-cell activation and turnover. The significance of these immune abnormalities, the role of proinflammatory and fibroblast stimulating cytokines, and whether they are a cause or an effect of the disease are unclear.[10]

Histopathologic findings in affected skin include an increase in hyalinized collagen within the reticular dermis and subcutis and a mononuclear perivascular and interstitial inflammatory infiltrate. Small arteries and microvasculature exhibit lumen reduction by a collagenous hyperplasia of the intima.[10]

Genetics

Based on rare reports of familial clustering and disease concordance in identical twins higher than accounted for by chance, a genetic component of the disease appears likely. Linkage with HLA-A1, -B8, and -DR3 haplotypes has been established.[10]

Endocrine Involvement

Hypothyroidism is identified in up to 25% of systemic sclerosis patients; it is often occult. Fibrosis of the thyroid gland, found in 14% of unselected systemic sclerosis patients at autopsy, is the most likely mechanism of thyroid hypofunction. Lymphocytic infiltration of the gland and antithyroid antibodies are uncommon.[10,34–37] A case of hypoparathyroidism due to parathyroid fibrosis has been reported.[38]

Rheumatoid Arthritis

Rheumatoid arthritis (RA) is a systemic autoimmune disorder in which synovial tissue is the target, although constitutional symptoms, and multiorgan manifestations are also common. Disease prevalence is 0.5–1% of adults, affecting women twice as often as men and increasing in prevalence with age. Distribution is worldwide. Smoking, coffee consumption, and silica exposure are risk factors for disease, while estrogen use is protective.[11]

Clinical Findings

Most patients with RA present with complaints of joint pain, stiffness, and/or swelling of gradual onset and involving multiple joints – typically the small joints of the hands and toes. Involvement of the proximal interphalangeal and metacarpophalangeal hand joints and metatarsophalangeal toe joints, with sparing of the distal interphalangeal joints is characteristic. Constitutional symptoms are often present. With disease progression, larger joints may be affected, and loss of function and deformity result. On exam the involved joints are warm and swollen.[11]

Extra-articular RA may have numerous manifestations. In the skin, rheumatoid nodules and pyoderma gangrenosum may be seen. Cardiac involvement may present as pericarditis, valve disease, and premature atherosclerosis. Interstitial lung disease, pleural effusions, and bronchiolitis obliterans may occur. Neurologic involvement may take the form of entrapment neuropathy, cervical myelopathy, and mononeuritis simplex. Anemia, thrombocytosis, lymphadenopathy, and Felty's syndrome may be present. The kidney may develop amyloidosis. Ocular disease may occur. RA associated vasculitis may be identified in any organ system.[11]

Autoantibodies are frequently present in RA. Approximately 80% have rheumatoid factor (RF), an antibody specific to IgG, while 70% have anti-cyclic citrullinated peptide (CCP) antibodies. ANAs and anti-neutrophil cytoplasm antibodies may be detected in up to 30% of patients.[11]

Pathogenesis

The etiology of RA is unknown. Similar to other systemic autoimmune diseases, it is postulated that in a genetically susceptible individual, external triggers set into a motion a cycle of cellular injury, autoantigen exposure, and immune response. Proposed triggers are many, including microbial antigens and smoking. Both cellular and humoral immune responses appear critical in perpetuating the cycle. Activated T helper cells are prominent in synovial tissue. The role of autoantibodies such as RF and anti-CCP is unclear; however, their presence is correlated with more aggressive disease.[11]

The attack on the synovium eventuates in proliferative synovitis with an infiltrate of lymphocytes and plasma cells, forming a pannus that covers the articular surface and erodes and infiltrates the underlying cartilage and bone.

Genetics

The contribution of genetic factors to development of RA is significant. Concordance rates in twins are 15–20% for monozygotic and 5% for dizygotic. HLA-D4, specifically polymorphisms of the amino acid sequence of the third hypervariable region on the DRβ1 chain, are strongly associated with RA. This amino acid sequence has been termed the "shared epitope" or "at-risk allele" and correlates with more aggressive disease. Another susceptibility gene has identified as a polymorphism in the intracellular protein tyrosine phosphatase nonreceptor 22 (*PTPN22*).[11]

Endocrine Organ Involvement

Thyroid gland involvement is common in RA patients, manifesting as hypothyroidism, hyperthyroidism, or nodular goiter in up to 34% of patients.[39] Thyroid disease is primarily autoimmune in pathogenesis; antithyroid antibodies including anti-thyroperoxidase and anti-thyroglobulin, occur with greater frequency in patients than in controls.[18,37,39–43]

Idiopathic Inflammatory Myopathies

The idiopathic inflammatory myopathies encompasses a diverse group of muscle diseases characterized by proximal muscle weakness and nonsuppurative inflammation of skeletal muscle. Included under this rubric are polymyositis (PM) and dermatomyositis (DM), as well as myositis associated with malignancy or collagen vascular disease, and inclusion body myositis.[10]

Clinical Features

The prevalence of idiopathic inflammatory myopathies ranges from 0.5 to 9.3 cases per million. Women are affected more frequently than men. In the United States, African-Americans have the highest rate of disease. Onset of muscle weakness is typically insidious, with a bimodal age of onset: 10–15 years old in children, and 45–60 years old in adults.[10]

Criteria for the diagnosis of PM are proximal muscle weakness, elevated serum levels of skeletal muscle derived enzymes (creatine kinase, aldolase, lactate dehydrogenase, aspartate aminotransferase, alanine aminotransferase), electromyographic evidence of myopathy, and skeletal muscle inflammation on biopsy. Weakness most commonly first presents in the shoulder and pelvic muscle girdles. The addition of a skin rash to these criteria allows for the diagnosis of DM; skin involvement is variable between patients and over the disease course. Constitutional symptoms and involvement of other organ systems (cardiac: conduction abnormalities, cardiomyopathy, congestive heart failure; pulmonary: interstitial fibrosis) may occur.[10]

Numerous autoantibodies are associated with PM and DM, some of which are specific for myositis, while other may be present but are nonspecific. Among the specific antigens are several aminoacyl-transfer RNA (tRNA) synthetases, the most common of which is anti-histidyl-tRNA (anti-Jo-1). Individual patients express only one myositis specific autoantibody, and autoantibodies correlate with clinical subsets/prognosis.[10]

Pathogenesis

Evidence suggests that the idiopathic inflammatory myopathies are autoimmune processes initiated by exogenous triggers in a genetically predisposed individual. Seasonal variation in disease onset, and animal models lend support to the hypothesis that viruses are the exogenous triggers.

The histologic changes seen on muscle biopsy are nonspecific. In PM, fiber necrosis and regeneration with an endomysial mononuclear inflammatory infiltrate is classic. In DM, perivascular inflammation is prominent. These morphologic differences correlate with differences in pathogenesis. Although autoantibodies are present in PM and DM, PM appears to result from antigen-directed cell-mediated cytotoxicity. The lymphocytes surrounding and invading muscle fibers in PM are predominantly oligoclonal CD8+ cytotoxic T-cells, and muscle fibers exhibit increased surface expression of HLA class I molecules. T-cell-muscle fiber adhesion is enhanced by intercellular adhesion molecule-1 (ICAM-1) on fibers and complementary adhesion molecule, lymphocyte function associated antigen-1, on lymphocytes. Cell death results by an unknown mechanism; apoptosis has not been demonstrated.[10]

Humoral immune mechanisms appear to be operational in DM, with CD4+ T-cells mediating B-cell production of autoantibodies, which, with complement, cause damage to perimysial vasculature.[10]

Genetics

Familial clustering suggests a genetic component to the idiopathic inflammatory myopathies, although no specific genetic marker has been uncovered. HLA B8, HLA-DR3, AND HLA-DRW52 are strongly associated with adult and pediatric PM and DM. Greater prevalence of the TNF-α-308A allele is seen in Caucasian PM/DM patients.[10]

Endocrine Organ Involvement

Endocrine organ involvement in PM/DM has not been systematically documented, although several case reports have identified an association of PM or DM with autoimmune thyroid disease, manifesting as hypo- or hyperthyroidism.[18,44–48]

Mixed Connective Tissue Disease

Mixed connective tissue disease (MCTD) is a systemic autoimmune disease that can be viewed as an overlap syndrome encompassing features of SLE, scleroderma, and PM/DM. Whether MCTD represents a distinct clinical entity remains an unresolved debate. Epidemiology is similar to other autoimmune connective tissue diseases.

Clinical Features

Features of SLE, scleroderma, and PM/DM often present metachronously, over the course of several years. Diverse organ involvement is typical, notably involving the skin and mucous membranes, joints, muscle, lungs, heart, GI tract, blood vessels, hematologic system, and kidney. Constitutional symptoms are common as well.[10]

Diagnosis rests on the symptom profile in the presence of high titer autoantibody against a ribonuclease-sensitive extractable nuclear antigen, U1 RNP, corresponding to a speckled pattern ANA. Anti-endothelial antibodies are also frequently identified, and correlate with pulmonary disease and spontaneous abortion.[10]

Pathogenesis

Pathogenic models revolve around the mechanism of exposure of U1 RNP to the immune system. U1 RNP is a uridine rich RNA particle that participates in messenger RNA splicing.[49,50] As such, it is a nuclear antigen, normally sequestered from the immune system. The central pathogenic role of U1 RNP is supported by development of MCTD-like lung disease in mice immunized with portions of the U1 RNP antigen.[49] In human disease, viral infection has been suggested as a trigger of apoptotic release of nuclear antigens; molecular mimicry with viral antigens may also contribute to the autoimmune response.[50,51]

Genetics

A subset of MCTD patients with erosive arthritis exhibits an increased frequency of HLA-DR4.[52] An increased frequency of immunoglobulin allotypes Gm1.3 and 3 has been reported in paticnts.[53]

Endocrine Organ Involvement

Autoimmune thyroid disease is particularly common in MCTD patients: Hashimoto's thyroiditis is 556-fold and Graves disease is 76-fold more common in MCTD than in the general population.[17,54]

Vasculits

Systemic vasculitis encompasses approximately 20 types of primary vasculitis (classified by the caliber of vessel affected), as well as several types of secondary vasculitis (associated with other disease processes such as connective tissue disease, malignancy, and infection). All are united by the presence of destructive inflammation of blood vessels. A detailed discussion of each type of vasculitis is beyond the scope of this chapter; this section will focus on common themes in clinical features, pathogenesis (when known), and histologic findings of the primary vasculitides (Table 2.3).[10,11,55]

TABLE 2.3. Systemic autoimmune disease: clinicopathologic features of selected vasculitides.[10,11,55]

Type of vasculitis	Predominant vessel size	Sites involved	Pathogenesis	Histologic features
Takayasu's arteritis	Large	Aorta and major branches; pulmonary arteries	Cytotoxic T-cell attack on smooth muscle cells	Granulomatous vasculitis with GC; fibrosis
Giant cell arteritis	Large	Branches of aorta and carotids	CD4+ T-cell response to UK antigen; granuloma formation	Granulomatous vasculitis with GC
Cogan's syndrome	Large	Eyes, audiovestibular system	UK; aberrant T-cell response?	Mixed inflammation; occasional granulomas
Behçet's disease	Large	Orogenital mucosa, eye, skin	Inflammatory cascade initiated by UK trigger; immune complex mediated?	LCV
Polyarteritis nodosa	Medium	Skin, peripheral nerves, GI tract, other viscera	Immune complex mediated (HBV infection)	Necrotizing vasculitis with mixed inflammation
Buerger's disease	Medium	Arteries and veins in distal extremities	UK; anti-endothelial Abs and ANCAs have been identified	Neutrophilic, lymphocytic vasculitis with thromboses and microabcesses
Kawasaki's disease	Medium	Oral mucosa, skin, lymphadenopathy, heart	UK; superantigen causing generalized immune system activation?	Segmental necrosis with prominent neutrophilic infiltrate and karyorrhexis
Cutaneous leukocytoclastic vasculitis	Small	Skin, joints	Immune complex mediated	LCV with occasional eosinophils
Henoch–Schönlein purpura	Small	Skin, joints, GI tract, kidneys	Immune complex mediated (IgA); commonly follows upper respiratory infection	LCV with lymphocytes and eosinophils
Essential cryoglobulinemia	Small	Skin, joints, kidneys, lungs, peripheral nerves	Immune complex mediated (HCV infection)	LCV
Wegener's granulomatosis	Small	Upper and lower respiratory tract, kidneys, skin, eyes	ANCA mediated	Necrotizing, granulomatous vasculitis; mixed inflammation
Microscopic polyangiitis	Small	Kidneys, lungs, joints, skin	ANCA mediated	Necrotizing glomerulonephritis, LCV
Churg–Strauss syndrome	Small	Upper and lower respiratory tract, heart, peripheral nerves	ANCA mediated; associated with atopy	Necrotizing, granulomatous vasculitis; mixed inflammation with prominent eosinophils

GC giant cells; *UK* unknown; *LCV* leukocytoclastic vasculitis; *ANCA* anti-neutrophil cytoplasm antibody; *Abs* antibodies.

Clinical Features

There is considerable variation in the epidemiologic profiles of the different vasculitides, including age predominantly affected, and geographic prevalence. Apart from a link between smoking and Buerger's disease, and smoking and giant cell arteritis in women, no environmental or occupational risk factors have been identified.[10,11]

Although most vasculitides have a predilection to involve specific organs, and the constellation of presenting features correlates with the profile of organ involvement, vasculitides share certain features. These include constitutional symptoms such as fever, weight loss, rash, and elevated acute phase reactants. Lesions of vasculitis are typically painful, and patients will report pain corresponding to the involved organs. Multiorgan involvement is the rule.[10,11]

The differential diagnosis is extensive, and diagnosis of vasculitis rests on biopsy of affected tissue.

Pathogenesis

The etiology of most forms of vasculitis is unknown. While united by the histologic finding of destructive inflammation of blood vessels, the destruction is not in all cases due to an autoimmune attack on blood vessel antigens.

Varying pathogenic models have been postulated in several types of vasculitis. In large vessel vasculitides, the adventitial layer appears to be the initial target of the pathologic process, and becomes inundated with activated T-cells. For example, in Takayasu's arteritis, cytotoxic CD8+ T-cells contribute to the damage of smooth muscle cells via perforin and granzyme B. By contrast, the T-cells in giant cell arteritis appear to be predominantly CD4+ cells, which are attracted by an as yet unknown adventitial antigen; a neoantigen generated by an infectious agent or by aging has been suggested. IFN-γ secretion promotes granuloma formation, with subsequent necrosis and elastic lamina destruction.[10]

Medium and small vessel vasculitides present additional pathogenic mechanisms[10,11]:

- Superantigens, which are microbial derived proteins that can stimulate large populations of T-cells via binding of class II MHC molecules outside the antigen-binding groove, are implicated in Kawasaki's disease.
- Viral infection may be associated with immune complex-mediated vascular injury due to the deposition of antibody–viral antigen complexes in vessels. Such a mechanism appears to underly most cases of polyarteritis nodosa, associated with hepatitis B (HBV) infection, and mixed cryoglobulinemia, associated with hepatitis C (HCV) infection.
- Three types of vasculitis, Wegener's granulomatosis, microscopic polyangiitis, and Churg–Strauss syndrome, are associated with anti-neutrophil cytoplasm antibodies (ANCAs) – antibodies directed against antigens within the primary granules of neutrophils and monocytes. The targets of the most common ANCAs are proteinase 3 (PR3) and myeloperoxidase (MPO). Surface expression of these antigens is abnormally elevated early in the disease process, and binding of ANCAs triggers granulocyte activation and release of reactive oxygen species, granule contents, and lysosomal enzymes, all of which effect endothelial injury.[56] This process is promoted by cytokines and CD4+ T-cells.
- A variety of infectious agents have been proposed to be triggers of vasculitis. Possible pathogenic mechanisms include molecular mimicry–microbes sharing epitopes with vessel walls; bystander injury due to widespread inflammation leading to exposure of autoantigens; and generation of neoantigens via the interaction between microbe and vessel molecules.[57]
- Antiendothelial antibodies have been identified within the sera of vasculitis patients in in vitro assays. While in vitro endothelial injury has been demonstrated, the significance of these autoantibodies in vivo is unknown.

On biopsy, there may be histologic overlap among the varying subtypes of vasculitis, depending on the type and the stage of disease. Most commonly a mixed inflammatory infiltrate is seen, although specific morphologic features may dominate the picture (see Table 2.3).

Genetics

Behçet's disease has been linked to HLA-B51, which is present in 80% of Asian patients.[10] Familial occurrence of giant cell arteritis has been reported, and 60% of patients have HLA-DRB1*04 variants that share a common sequence in the B1 molecule.[10]

Endocrine Organ Involvement

While none of the vasculitides appear to target endocrine organs, these organs may occasionally be affected. An increased rate of hypothyroidism and higher frequency of antithyroid antibodies have been reported in patients with giant cell arteritis,[58] however a multicenter case-control study failed to confirm a significant difference from the control population.[59] Rare cases of multinodular goiter associated with giant cell arteritis of the thyroid arteries have been reported.[60]

Rare cases of pituitary involvement have been reported in patients with vasculitis including Wegener's granulomatosis, Takayasu's disease, Behçet's disease, and Cogan's syndrome.[61–64]

Isolated occurrences of pheochromocytoma in Behçet's disease have been noted.[65,66]

Summary

Systemic autoimmune diseases share a proximate etiology of an immune attack on self-antigens. In most cases, the trigger of this attack is unknown. Mounting evidence suggests that autoimmune diseases result from a complex interaction of environmental and other unknown factors in a genetically predisposed individual. Genetic predisposition is complex as well, with polymorphisms in multiple genes, most commonly related to immune function, imparting variably increased susceptibility to disease.

References

1. Chistiakov DA, Chistiakov AP. Is FCRL3 a new general autoimmunity gene? *Hum Immunol.* 2007;68:375–383.
2. Kristiansen OP, Larsen ZM, Pociot F. CTLA-4 in autoimmune diseases – a general susceptibility gene to autoimmunity? *Genes Immun.* 2000;1:170–184.
3. Vang T, Miletic AV, Arimura Y, Tautz L, Rickert RC, Mustelin T. Protein tyrosine phosphatases in autoimmunity. *Annu Rev Immunol.* 2008;26:29–55.
4. Merriman TR, Pearce SH. Genetic progress towards the molecular basis of common autoimmunity. *Discov Med.* 2006;6:40–45.
5. Cantorna MT, Mahon BD. Mounting evidence for vitamin D as an environmental factor affecting autoimmune disease prevalence. *Exp Biol Med (Maywood).* 2004;229:1136–1142.
6. Orbach H, Zandman-Goddard G, Amital H, et al. Novel biomarkers in autoimmune diseases: prolactin, ferritin, vitamin D, and TPA levels in autoimmune diseases. *Ann N Y Acad Sci.* 2007;1109:385–400.
7. Orbach H, Shoenfeld Y. Hyperprolactinemia and autoimmune diseases. *Autoimmun Rev.* 2007;6:537–542.
8. Sarkar K, Miller FW. Possible roles and determinants of microchimerism in autoimmune and other disorders. *Autoimmun Rev.* 2004;3:454–463.
9. Benseler SM, Silverman ED. Systemic lupus erythematosus. *Rheum Dis Clin North Am.* 2007;33:471–498, vi.
10. Harris E, Budd RC, Genovese MC, Firestein GS, Sargent JS, Sledge CB. *Kelley's Textbook of Rheumatology.* 7th ed. Philadelphia, PA: Elsevier; 2005.
11. Goldman L, Ausiello D. *Cecil Medicine.* 23rd ed. Philadelphia, PA: Elsevier; 2008.
12. Cieslik P, Hrycek A, Klucinski P. Vasculopathy and vasculitis in systemic lupus erythematosus. *Pol Arch Med Wewn.* 2008;118:57–63.
13. Vianna JL, Haga HJ, Asherson RA, Swana G, Hughes GR. A prospective evaluation of antithyroid antibody prevalence in 100 patients with systemic lupus erythematosus. *J Rheumatol.* 1991;18:1193–1195.
14. Pyne D, Isenberg DA. Autoimmune thyroid disease in systemic lupus erythematosus. *Ann Rheum Dis.* 2002;61:70–72.
15. Miller FW, Moore GF, Weintraub BD, Steinberg AD. Prevalence of thyroid disease and abnormal thyroid function test results in patients with systemic lupus erythematosus. *Arthritis Rheum.* 1987;30:1124–1131.
16. Magaro M, Zoli A, Altomonte L, et al. The association of silent thyroiditis with active systemic lupus erythematosus. *Clin Exp Rheumatol.* 1992;10:67–70.
17. Arnaout MA, Nasrallah NS, el-Khateeb MS. Prevalence of abnormal thyroid function tests in connective tissue disease. *Scand J Rheumatol.* 1994;23:128–132.
18. Szyper-Kravitz M, Marai I, Shoenfeld Y. Coexistence of thyroid autoimmunity with other autoimmune diseases: friend or foe? Additional aspects on the mosaic of autoimmunity. *Autoimmunity.* 2005;38:247–255.
19. Li J, May W, McMurray RW. Pituitary hormones and systemic lupus erythematosus. *Arthritis Rheum.* 2005;52:3701–3712.
20. Jara LJ, Vera-Lastra O, Miranda JM, Alcala M, Alvarez-Nemegyei J. Prolactin in human systemic lupus erythematosus. *Lupus.* 2001;10:748–756.
21. Mason RJ, Broaddus VC, Murray JF, Nadel JA. *Murray & Nadel's Textbook of Respiratory Medicine.* 4th ed. Philadelphia, PA: Elsevier; 2005.
22. Porter N, Beynon HL, Randeva HS. Endocrine and reproductive manifestations of sarcoidosis. *QJM.* 2003;96:553–561.
23. Bell NH. Endocrine complications of sarcoidosis. *Endocrinol Metab Clin North Am.* 1991;20:645–654.
24. Tabuena RP, Nagai S, Handa T, et al. Diabetes insipidus from neurosarcoidosis: long-term follow-up for more than eight years. *Intern Med.* 2004;43:960–966.
25. Miyoshi T, Otsuka F, Takeda M, et al. An elderly patient with sarcoidosis manifesting panhypopituitarism with central diabetes insipidus. *Endocr J.* 2007;54:425–430.
26. Papi G, Briganti F, Artioli F, et al. Sarcoidosis of the thyroid gland associated with hyperthyroidism: review of the literature and report of two peculiar cases. *J Endocrinol Invest.* 2006;29:834–839.
27. Ozkan Z, Oncel M, Kurt N, et al. Sarcoidosis presenting as cold thyroid nodules: report of two cases. *Surg Today.* 2005;35:770–773.
28. Cabibi D, Di Vita G, La Spada E, Tripodo C, Patti R, Montalto G. Thyroid sarcoidosis as a unique localization. *Thyroid.* 2006;16:1175–1177.
29. Rodriguez MC, Rani D, Faas FH. Unusual clinical course of Graves' thyrotoxicosis and concomitant sarcoidosis: case report and review of literature. *Endocr Pract.* 2007;13:159–163.
30. Antonelli A, Fazzi P, Fallahi P, Ferrari SM, Ferrannini E. Prevalence of hypothyroidism and Graves disease in sarcoidosis. *Chest.* 2006;130:526–532.
31. Mitsias DI, Kapsogeorgou EK, Moutsopoulos HM. Sjogren's syndrome: why autoimmune epithelitis? *Oral Dis.* 2006;12:523–532.
32. D'Arbonneau F, Ansart S, Le Berre R, Dueymes M, Youinou P, Pennec YL. Thyroid dysfunction in primary Sjogren's syndrome: a long-term followup study. *Arthritis Rheum.* 2003;49:804–809.
33. Jara LJ, Navarro C, Brito-Zeron Mdel P, Garcia-Carrasco M, Escarcega RO, Ramos-Casals M. Thyroid disease in Sjogren's syndrome. *Clin Rheumatol.* 2007;26:1601–1606.
34. Antonelli A, Ferri C, Fallahi P, et al. Clinical and subclinical autoimmune thyroid disorders in systemic sclerosis. *Eur J Endocrinol.* 2007;156:431–437.
35. Marasini B, Ferrari PA, Solaro N, Selmi C. Thyroid dysfunction in women with systemic sclerosis. *Ann N Y Acad Sci.* 2007;1108:305–311.
36. Kahl LE, Medsger TA Jr, Klein I. Prospective evaluation of thyroid function in patients with systemic sclerosis (scleroderma). *J Rheumatol.* 1986;13:103–107.
37. Innocencio RM, Romaldini JH, Ward LS. Thyroid autoantibodies in autoimmune diseases. *Medicina (B Aires).* 2004;64:227–230.
38. Sentochnik DE, Hoffman GS. Hypoparathyroidism due to progressive systemic sclerosis. *J Rheumatol.* 1988;15:711–713.
39. Walker DJ, Griffiths M, Griffiths ID. Occurrence of autoimmune diseases and autoantibodies in multicase rheumatoid arthritis families. *Ann Rheum Dis.* 1986;45:323–326.
40. Caron P, Lassoued S, Dromer C, Oksman F, Fournie A. Prevalence of thyroid abnormalities in patients with rheumatoid arthritis. *Thyroidology.* 1992;4:99–102.

41. Andonopoulos AP, Siambi V, Makri M, Christofidou M, Markou C, Vagenakis AG. Thyroid function and immune profile in rheumatoid arthritis. A controlled study. *Clin Rheumatol.* 1996;15:599–603.
42. Atzeni F, Doria A, Ghirardello A, et al. Anti-thyroid antibodies and thyroid dysfunction in rheumatoid arthritis: prevalence and clinical value. *Autoimmunity.* 2008;41:111–115.
43. Michou L, Rat AC, Lasbleiz S, Bardin T, Cornelis F. Prevalence and distribution of autoimmune diseases in 368 rheumatoid arthritis families. *J Rheumatol.* 2008;35:790–796.
44. Stevanato F, Martinello F, Pesce R, Terribile IV, Saia A, Trevisan CP. A case of polymyositis in autoimmune thyroiditis with hyperthyroidism. *Riv Neurol.* 1991;61:17–19.
45. Araki K, Minami Y, Ueda Y, Kashima K. A case of polymyositis associated with chronic thyroiditis presenting as hyperthyroidism. *Jpn J Med.* 1990;29:46–51.
46. Sakata S, Fuwa Y, Goshima E, et al. A case of Graves' disease associated with polymyositis. *J Endocrinol Invest.* 1989;12: 837–840.
47. Gamsky TE, Chan MK. Coexistent dermatomyositis and autoimmune thyroiditis. *West J Med.* 1988;148:213–214.
48. Kato H, Uyeki Y, Kitajima Y, Yaoita H. A case of dermatomyositis and Hashimoto's thyroiditis. *J Dermatol.* 1988;15:273–275.
49. Greidinger EL, Zang Y, Jaimes K, et al. A murine model of mixed connective tissue disease induced with U1 small nuclear RNP autoantigen. *Arthritis Rheum.* 2006;54:661–669.
50. Venables PJ. Mixed connective tissue disease. *Lupus.* 2006;15: 132–137.
51. Keith MP, Moratz C, Tsokos GC. Anti-RNP immunity: implications for tissue injury and the pathogenesis of connective tissue disease. *Autoimmun Rev.* 2007;6:232–236.
52. Hoffman RW, Greidinger EL. Mixed connective tissue disease. *Curr Opin Rheumatol.* 2000;12:386–390.
53. Black CM, Maddison PJ, Welsh KI, Bernstein R, Woodrow JC, Pereira RS. HLA and immunoglobulin allotypes in mixed connective tissue disease. *Arthritis Rheum.* 1988;31:131–134.
54. Biro E, Szekanecz Z, Czirjak L, et al. Association of systemic and thyroid autoimmune diseases. *Clin Rheumatol.* 2006;25:240–245.
55. Mazlumzadeh M, Matteson EL. Cogan's syndrome: an audiovestibular, ocular, and systemic autoimmune disease. *Rheum Dis Clin North Am.* 2007;33:855–874, vii-viii.
56. Ozaki S. ANCA-associated vasculitis: diagnostic and therapeutic strategy. *Allergol Int.* 2007;56:87–96.
57. Yang YH, Chuang YH, Wang LC, Huang HY, Gershwin ME, Chiang BL. The immunobiology of Henoch-Schonlein purpura. *Autoimmun Rev.* 2008;7:179–184.
58. Bowness P, Shotliff K, Middlemiss A, Myles AB. Prevalence of hypothyroidism in patients with polymyalgia rheumatica and giant cell arteritis. *Br J Rheumatol.* 1991;30:349–351.
59. Duhaut P, Bornet H, Pinede L, et al. Giant cell arteritis and thyroid dysfunction: multicentre case-control study. The Groupe de Recherche sur l'Arteritea Cellules Geantes. *BMJ.* 1999;318:434–435.
60. Granel B, Serratrice J, Chaudier B, et al. Multinodular goitre with giant cell vasculitis of thyroid arteries in a woman with temporal arteritis. *Ann Rheum Dis.* 2001;60:811–812.
61. Kanatani M, Nakamura R, Kurokawa K, et al. Hypopituitarism associated with Cogan's syndrome; high-dose glucocorticoid therapy reverses pituitary swelling. *Jpn J Med.* 1991;30:164–169.
62. Toth M, Szabo P, Racz K, et al. Granulomatous hypophysitis associated with Takayasu's disease. *Clin Endocrinol (Oxf).* 1996;45:499–503.
63. Yong TY, Li JY, Amato L, et al. Pituitary involvement in Wegener's granulomatosis. *Pituitary.* 2008;11:77–84.
64. Jin-No M, Fujii T, Jin-No Y, Kamiya Y, Okada M, Kawaguchi M. Central diabetes insipidus with Behcet's disease. *Intern Med.* 1999;38:995–999.
65. Bethea L, Khan S. Behcet's disease and pheochromocytoma. *J S C Med Assoc.* 1999;95:295–298.
66. Oishi S, Koga B, Sasaki M, Umeda T, Sato T. Pheochromocytoma associated with Behcet's disease. *Jpn J Clin Oncol.* 1989;19: 283–286.

3
MicroRNAs in Endocrine Diseases

Simion Chiosea

Introduction

MicroRNAs are noncoding single-stranded 18- to 24-nt long RNAs that regulate diverse cellular processes, including cell death and proliferation.[1] Production and function of microRNA requires a set of proteins.[2]

Less than 2% of the human genome is translated into protein, yet more than 40% of the genome is transcribed into RNA, that is into noncoding RNA.[3] Transporting RNA (t-RNA) is probably the best-known example of a noncoding RNA. A more recently described species of noncoding RNAs, such as short interfering RNA (siRNA) and microRNA, are involved in regulation of gene expression through complementary interaction with 3′ untranslated region (UTR) of target messenger RNA (mRNA). MicroRNA and siRNA are quite distinct (Table 3.1) and no connection between microRNAs and siRNAs was made until 2001, when Dicer, the enzyme that converts long double stranded RNA into siRNAs, was discovered to convert precursor microRNAs into mature microRNAs.[4]

Many microRNA genes are mapped to intergenic areas and are expressed independently.[5] About two thirds of microRNAs are encoded in clusters of two to three microRNA genes and are transcribed as polycistrons showing similar expression patterns.[2,6] High sequence homology and concordant expression pattern of microRNA-221 and microRNA-222 in papillary thyroid carcinoma (PTC) (see below) are most likely due to their clustering on X chromosome.[6] Finally, about a quarter of microRNA genes are hosted within introns. Some of the latter microRNAs follow a recently described alternative pathway of microRNA maturation, in which a subset of debranched introns have structure of precursor microRNA allowing them to enter microRNA-processing pathway without Drosha-mediated cleavage.[7,8]

Differential expression of microRNA is described in severals types of human endocrine neoplasms, including thyroid carcinomas (PTC,[9–11] anaplastic thyroid carcinoma, ATC,[12] follicular thyroid carcinoma, FTC,[13]) and pituitary adenoma, PA.[14,15]

The list of miR with known cancer gene targets continues to grow: let-7 negatively regulates *Ras*,[16] microRNA-221 and microRNA-222 down-regulate kit receptor[17] and p27(Kip1) protein, a key player in cell cycle control,[18] and microRNA-16-1 and microRNA-15a repress *Bcl-2*.[19]

MicroRNA and Neoplasms of Thyroid Gland

Currently, most of the effort is directed to more common sporadic thyroid neoplasms derived from follicular epithelial cells (i.e., PTC, follicular carcinomas, follicular adenomas, and ATC).

Our present knowledge of microRNA abnormalities in follicular cell derived thyroid carcinomas is based on several studies of 70 benign thyroid tissue samples and benign fine needle aspiration biopsies (FNAB) and about 180 samples of thyroid neoplasms (including eight FNA samples "suspicious for carcinoma") (Tables 3.2 and 3.3). When clinical information is available, it appears that a very heterogeneous group of thyroid carcinomas was studied. For instance, analyses of PTC routinely include various histological variants, pathological stages T1 through T4a, cases with and without metastases to lymph nodes, etc.[9,11] The set of PTC examined by Tetzlaff et al, is somewhat more uniform/homogenous, with classic variants only being included.[11] In that study, the microRNA signatures was apparently unique to PTC. However, it might be too early to assume that all PTCs will exhibit the same microRNA profile independently of patients' age, gender, or mutational status.

On a more technical note, although most of microRNA profiling and validation was done on fresh frozen tissue, the utility of formalin-fixed paraffin embedded tissue has also been convincingly demonstrated.[11,12] All studies used total RNA and arrays with probes up to 245 human microRNAs. For a summary of differentially expressed and validated microRNAs see Table 3.3.

J.L. Hunt (ed.), *Molecular Pathology of Endocrine Diseases,* Molecular Pathology Library 3,
DOI 10.1007/978-1-4419-1707-2_3, © Springer Science+Business Media, LLC 2010

TABLE 3.1. Distinctive features of MicroRNA and siRNA.

	MicroRNA	siRNA
Target	Regulate hundreds or more of endogenous genes per microRNA	Few targets, usually exogenous (i.e., viral)
Effect	Number of microRNAs that are bound to the target mRNA determines the degree of translational inhibition	Degradation of cognate mRNA
Processing and products	MicroRNA is generated from one arm of the stem-loop to yield a single-stranded RNA[a]	Two complementary siRNAs in equal abundance, both functionally potent
Origin	Endogenous gene	Long dsRNA, exogenous
Potential application	Diagnostic and therapeutic	Therapeutic

[a]Mature microRNA entering RNA Induced Silencing Complex (RISC) is single-stranded.

TABLE 3.2. Thyroid samples and microRNA profiling.

Reference	Tissue type	Normal thyroid samples, *n*	Thyroid cancer types[b]	Neoplastic samples (including samples used for validation), *n*
9[a]	Frozen	26	PTC	20
10	Frozen	10[c]	PTC	69; FNA "suspicious for cancer," 8
			FA	8
11	FFPE	20[d]	PTC	20[e]
13	Frozen	4	FTC	17
			FA	12
12	Frozen/FFPE	10	ATC	30
			PTC	At least 3

FTC follicular thyroid carcinoma; *FA* follicular adenoma; *PTC* papillary thyroid carcinoma; *ATC* anaplastic thyroid carcinoma; *FNAB* fine needle aspiration biopsy; *MNG* multinodular goiter, *FFPE* formalin fixed paraffin embedded tissue.

[a]135 samples of FFPE PTC were not included in microRNA profiling.

[b]Outlines thyroid cancer types compared to each other as part of limited validation panel.

[c]Unspecified number of benign FNAB.

[d]Unlike other studies, PTC was compared to its histologic mimic, i.e., hyperplastic/colloidal nodules of MNG.

[e]All PTC of classic variant.

The following issues are raised by currently available results and practical necessities of diagnostic pathology (Tables 3.2 and 3.3):

1. At present, no single study directly and comprehensively compared microRNA expression across all major types of thyroid carcinomas. Only limited comparative analysis of follicular carcinomas to follicular adenomas and anaplastic thyroid carcinomas to papillary thyroid carcinomas was performed as part of validation panels (Table 3.3). At first glance, "unique microRNA signatures" characterize PTC, follicular carcinomas, and anaplastic thyroid carcinomas. However, there remain several caveats. For instance, microRNA downregulation as a general trend initially seemed to be restricted to anaplastic thyroid carcinoma. Now, it is described in histologically benign tissue of multinodular goiter (MNG). Ironically, it is the same microRNA-30a-5p, among others, that now appears to be downregulated in both anaplastic carcinoma and multinodular goiter.[11,12] Furthermore, all three studies of microRNA expression in PTC, highlighted microRNA-222 as microRNA that is consistently upregulated, when compared to normal thyroid tissue and hyperplastic/colloid nodules of MNG. However, microRNA-222 appears to be upregulated 1.98-fold ($p = 0.0212$) in ATC.[12] Since microRNA-222 upregulation of 1.98-fold was less than arbitrary cutoff of twofold change used by authors, it was not included in validation experiments. Of note, microRNA-222 and microRNA-221, the two microRNAs most consistently upregulated in PTC (Table 3.3), are both clustered on chromosome X and show concordant expression patterns.[6] In light of this fact, the mechanism of isolated microRNA-221 upregulation in histologically benign thyroid tissue warrants further investigation before it can be reliably included in a clinical test.[9,11]
2. In everyday practice, hyperplastic/colloid nodules are being sampled by FNAB to rule out thyroid malignancy. These nodules may be diagnostically challenging when they are solitary. When they are multiple, meaningful clinical surveillance is very difficult. Evaluation of microRNA

TABLE 3.3. Quantitative MicroRNA abnormalities and thyroid carcinomas.

Reference	Thyroid cancer type	MicroRNA deregulation: Up-regulation, >2-fold, microRNA	MicroRNA deregulation: Down-regulation, >2-fold, microRNA	Successfully validated microRNA and method
10	PTC	221, 222, 213, 220, and 181b	None	NB: 221, 222, 181b; RT-PCR: pre-miR-221, -222, -181b (up-regulated in 7/8 FNABs)
9	PTC	221, 222, 146, 21, 181a, 220, 155	None	NB: 221, 146b; RT-PCR: 221, 222, 146b
11	PTC vs. MNG	221, 222, 21, 31, 172, 213, 223, 181b, 34a	345, 292as, 300, 218	RT-PCR: 21, 31, 221, 222
13	FTC vs. FA	192, 197, 328, 346	None	RT-PCR: 197 and 346
12	ATC	None	30d, 125b, 26a, 30a-5p	NB and RT-PCR: 30d, 125b, 26a, 30a-5p; ISH: 30d

FTC follicular thyroid carcinoma; *FA* follicular adenoma; *PTC* papillary thyroid carcinoma; *ATC* anaplastic thyroid carcinoma; *FNAB* fine needle aspiration biopsy; *MNG* multinodular goiter; *FFPE* formalin fixed paraffin embedded tissue; *NB* northern blot; *ISH* in situ hybridization; *pre-miR* precursor microRNA.

profiles in thyroid carcinomas and their benign histological mimics appears to be a potentially practical approach. Currently, with the exception of work by Tetzlaff et al, the general trend is to compare thyroid neoplasms to grossly unremarkable thyroid tissue – situation where routine cytological or histological evaluation remains a "gold standard" diagnostic approach.[11]

3. Finally, microRNA profiling still needs additional validation, where the profiling is done on a well-characterized set of thyroid neoplasms controlled for time-proven histological and genetic prognosticators (e.g., pathologic stage, age, gender, BRAF, RAS, and ret/PTC1 and ret/PTC3 mutational status).

Papillary Thyroid Carcinoma, C-KIT, p27Kip1, and MicroRNA-221/222 Cluster

C-Kit is a tyrosine kinase receptor involved in cell differentiation and growth. Reduced C-kit levels in PTCs were reported more than a decade ago.[20] It is apparent now, that *C-kit* mRNA is targeted by microRNA-221 and -222.[17] Furthermore, He et al showed that downregulation of Kit protein correlated with strong overexpression of microRNA-221, microRNA-222, and microRNA-146b. Sequencing of microRNA-221 and microRNA-222 binding domains in *KIT* 3′-UTR revealed 3169G→A single nucleotide polymorphism (SNP) within microRNA-221 and microRNA-222 recognition sites. Heterozygosity for 3169G→A leads to modification in microRNA:target messenger RNA duplex conformation and decrease in efficiency of microRNA mediated *C-kit* translational inhibition. These results illustrate how changes in microRNA target genes influence its responses to microRNA.[9] Of note, microRNA-221 overexpression in PTC cell line (NPA) boosted cell proliferation with more than twofold increase in number of colonies. When microRNA-221 was blocked in NPA cells, approximately 20% decrease in cell numbers was noticed 96 h after microRNA-221 antisense oligonucleotide transfection.[10]

Another direct consequence of microRNA-221/222 cluster upregulation is reduced level of p27(Kip1) protein and progression to the S phase of cell cycle.[18]

MicroRNA and Papillary Thyroid Carcinoma Cell Lines with RET/PTC and BRAF^{V600E} Mutation

Genetically, PTCs feature abnormalities in RET/PTC-RAS-BRAF pathway.[21] Limited studies of microRNA profile in cell lines harboring ret/PTC1 rearrangement [Nthy-ori 3-1 transfected with ret/PTC 1 and TPC-1] and normal thyroid cell lines revealed significant upregulation of four microRNAs (128a, 128b, 139, and 200a) and downregulation of another four microRNAs (154, 181a, 302b, 302c).[22]

Two cell lines containing BRAF^{V600E} point mutation [Nthy-oriBRAF and KAT-10] featured dramatic upregulation of microRNA-200a, microRNA-200b, and microRNA-141 with downregulation of microRNA-127, microRNA-130a, and microRNA-144 when compared to normal thyroid cell lines N-thy-ori 3-1.[23]

Since none of the studies summarized in Tables 3.2 and 3.3, characterized mutational status of their PTC cases, it is difficult to extrapolate/compare microRNA abnormalities described in these three cell lines to clinical specimens. None of the microRNAs highlighted by studies of clinical samples was differentially expressed in cell lines with known mutations. However, one could still suggest the possibility of correlation between microRNA profiles and ret/PTC and/or BRAF mutations.

MicroRNA and Pituitary Adenoma

Comprehensive microRNA profiling has revealed a set of 24 microRNAs capable to differentiating 15 functioning and 17 nonfunctioning pituitary adenomas from five normal pituitary glands.[14] Furthermore, microRNA signatures appeared to suggest the hormone-secreting profile of PA.

Moreover, microRNA-15a and microRNA-16-1 expression in pituitary adenomas secreting growth hormone and prolactin is about 70% lower than in nonneoplastic pituitary tissue. The downregulation of microRNA-15a and microRNA-16-1 correlates with increase of *RARS* mRNA (arginyl-tRNA synthetase), which leads to decrease in p43 secretion, a cytokine involved in angiogenesis and inflammation.[24]

References

1. Hwang HW, Mendell JT. MicroRNAs in cell proliferation, cell death, and tumorigenesis. *Br J Cancer*. 2006;94(6):776–780.
2. Bartel DP. MicroRNAs: genomics, biogenesis, mechanism, and function. *Cell*. 2004;116:281–297.
3. Matera AG, Terns RM, Terns MP. Non-coding RNAs: lessons from the small nuclear and small nucleolar RNAs. *Nat Rev Mol Cell Biol*. 2007;8:209–220.
4. Hutvagner G, McLachlan J, Pasquinelli AE, Balint E, Tuschl T, Zamore PD. A cellular function for the RNA-interference enzyme Dicer in the maturation of the let-7 small temporal RNA. *Science*. 2001;293:834–838.
5. Rodriguez A, Griffiths-Jones S, Ashurst JL, Bradley A. Identification of mammalian microRNA host genes and transcription units. *Genome Res*. 2004;14:1902–1910.
6. Altuvia Y, Landgraf P, Lithwick G, et al. Clustering and conservation patterns of human microRNAs. *Nucleic Acids Res*. 2005;33:2697–2706.
7. Okamura K, Hagen JW, Duan H, Tyler DM, Lai EC. The mirtron pathway generates microRNA-class regulatory RNAs in Drosophila. *Cell*. 2007;130:89–100.
8. Ruby JG, Jan CH, Bartel DP. Intronic microRNA precursors that bypass Drosha processing. *Nature*. 2007;448:83–86.
9. He H, Jazdzewski K, Li W, et al. The role of microRNA genes in papillary thyroid carcinoma. *Proc Natl Acad Sci USA*. 2005;102:19075–19080.

10. Pallante P, Visone R, Ferracin M, et al. MicroRNA deregulation in human thyroid papillary carcinomas. *Endocr Relat Cancer.* 2006;13:497–508.
11. Tetzlaff MT, Liu A, Xu X, et al. Differential expression of miRNAs in papillary thyroid carcinoma compared to multinodular goiter using formalin fixed paraffin embedded tissues. *Endocr Pathol.* 2007;18:163–173.
12. Visone R, Pallante P, Vecchione A, et al. Specific microRNAs are downregulated in human thyroid anaplastic carcinomas. *Oncogene.* 2007;26:7590–7595.
13. Weber F, Teresi RE, Broelsch CE, Frilling A, Eng C. A limited set of human MicroRNA is deregulated in follicular thyroid carcinoma. *J Clin Endocrinol Metab.* 2006;91:3584–3591.
14. Bottoni A, Zatelli MC, Ferracin M, et al. Identification of differentially expressed microRNAs by microarray: a possible role for microRNA genes in pituitary adenomas. *J Cell Physiol.* 2007;210:370–377.
15. Bottoni A, Piccin D, Tagliati F, Luchin A, Zatelli MC, degli Uberti C. miR-15a and miR-16-1 down-regulation in pituitary adenomas. *J Cell Physiol.* 2005;204:280–285.
16. Johnson SM, Grosshans H, Shingara J, et al. RAS is regulated by the let-7 microRNA family. *Cell.* 2005;120:635–647.
17. Felli N, Fontana L, Pelosi E, et al. MicroRNAs 221 and 222 inhibit normal erythropoiesis and erythroleukemic cell growth via kit receptor down-modulation. *Proc Natl Acad Sci USA.* 2005;102: 18081–18086.
18. Visone R, Russo L, Pallante P, et al. MicroRNAs (miR)-221 and miR-222, both overexpressed in human thyroid papillary carcinomas, regulate p27Kip1 protein levels and cell cycle. *Endocr Relat Cancer.* 2007;14:791–798.
19. Cimmino A, Calin GA, Fabbri M, et al. miR-15 and miR-16 induce apoptosis by targeting BCL2. *Proc Natl Acad Sci USA.* 2005;102: 13944–13949.
20. Natali PG, Berlingieri MT, Nicotra MR, et al. Transformation of thyroid epithelium is associated with loss of c-kit receptor. *Cancer Res.* 1995;55:1787–1791.
21. Hunt J. Understanding the genotype of follicular thyroid tumors. *Endocr Pathol.* 2005;16:311–321.
22. Cahill S, Smyth P, Finn SP, et al. Effect of ret/PTC 1 rearrangement on transcription and post-transcriptional regulation in a papillary thyroid carcinoma model. *Mol Cancer.* 2006;5:70.
23. Cahill S, Smyth P, Denning K, et al. Effect of BRAFV600E mutation on transcription and post-transcriptional regulation in a papillary thyroid carcinoma model. *Mol Cancer.* 2007; 6:21.
24. Ko YG, Park H, Kim T, et al. A cofactor of tRNA synthetase, p43, is secreted to up-regulate proinflammatory genes. *J Biol Chem.* 2001;276:23028–23033.

Section 2
Thyroid Diseases

4 Clinical Detection and Treatment of Thyroid Diseases

Jamie C. Mitchell and Mira Milas

Introduction

While thyroid cancer is relatively rare overall, accounting for less than 1% of all human malignancies, it is the most common endocrine malignancy, comprising nearly 90% of all endocrine cancers.[1] The vast majority are well-differentiated cancers derived from follicular epithelium and most of these are papillary carcinomas (PTC). Prognosis is generally favorable, with only 1,500 thyroid cancer-related deaths per year,[2] and a 10-year survival of greater than 90%. However, the incidence of PTC has been on the rise during recent years, perhaps due to increased rates of detection with the almost ubiquitous use of imaging studies with ever-increasing sensitivity.[3,4]

The traditional diagnosis of thyroid cancer relies on the use of ultrasound-guided fine needle aspiration biopsy (FNA) of thyroid nodules, which in most situations yields a sensitivity of approximately 94%.[5] Treatment then includes surgical resection followed by radioactive iodine ablation therapy, and subsequent TSH suppressive therapy for confirmed cases of thyroid cancer. Despite the excellent outcomes for most patients using this regimen, intense research continues to be conducted into novel forms of therapy for thyroid cancer. These studies are focused on several clinical situations, where traditional therapy has failed. For example, up to 20% of patients with well-differentiated thyroid cancer will experience a recurrence of their disease following traditional therapy. As many as 5% of these patients will have tumors that undergo high grade transformation resulting in tumors with more aggressive growth, metastatic spread, and loss of the ability to take up iodine. These features render the tumors unresponsive to traditional therapy.[6–8] Poorly differentiated and anaplastic thyroid cancers also do not respond to conventional chemotherapy or external beam radiation.[9] Novel therapies to treat these patients are needed.

Medullary thyroid cancers (MTC) which are derived from parafollicular C-cells, also tend to be more aggressive than well-differentiated follicular cancers and do not take up radioactive iodine. There are few therapeutic options for patients with medullary carcinoma who have advanced disease or distant metastases.

A final area of intense research concerning thyroid cancer relates to improving the ability to diagnose cancer preoperatively. FNA is often able to identify papillary thyroid cancers pre-operatively, at rates approaching 95% in most situations. However, when cytologic analysis reveals a hypercellular follicular lesion, FNA cannot distinguish between benign follicular lesions and follicular carcinoma since capsular or vascular invasion can only be confirmed by histologic analysis. As the risk of malignancy in this setting is 20%, many patients with a pre-operative diagnosis of follicular lesion will undergo surgery and have histologically confirmed benign disease.

With the completion of the human genome project, a powerful new set of tools is emerging for researchers to tackle such problems. With advancing insights into the molecular pathogenesis of thyroid malignancies, potential targets for the development of novel therapies and diagnostic modalities are being revealed (Figure 4.1). This chapter focuses on how these new molecular techniques are being utilized in the management of thyroid cancer.

Follicular-Derived Carcinoma

There have been two approaches in utilizing molecular techniques to improve the accuracy of preoperative diagnosis of follicular thyroid cancer. The first is to examine known genetic alterations (discussed in Chap. 7) and gene expression patterns associated with thyroid cancer in FNA specimens. The other is to use a peripheral blood assay to predict and then follow the progression of thyroid carcinoma.

J.L. Hunt (ed.), *Molecular Pathology of Endocrine Diseases*, Molecular Pathology Library 3,
DOI 10.1007/978-1-4419-1707-2_4, © Springer Science+Business Media, LLC 2010

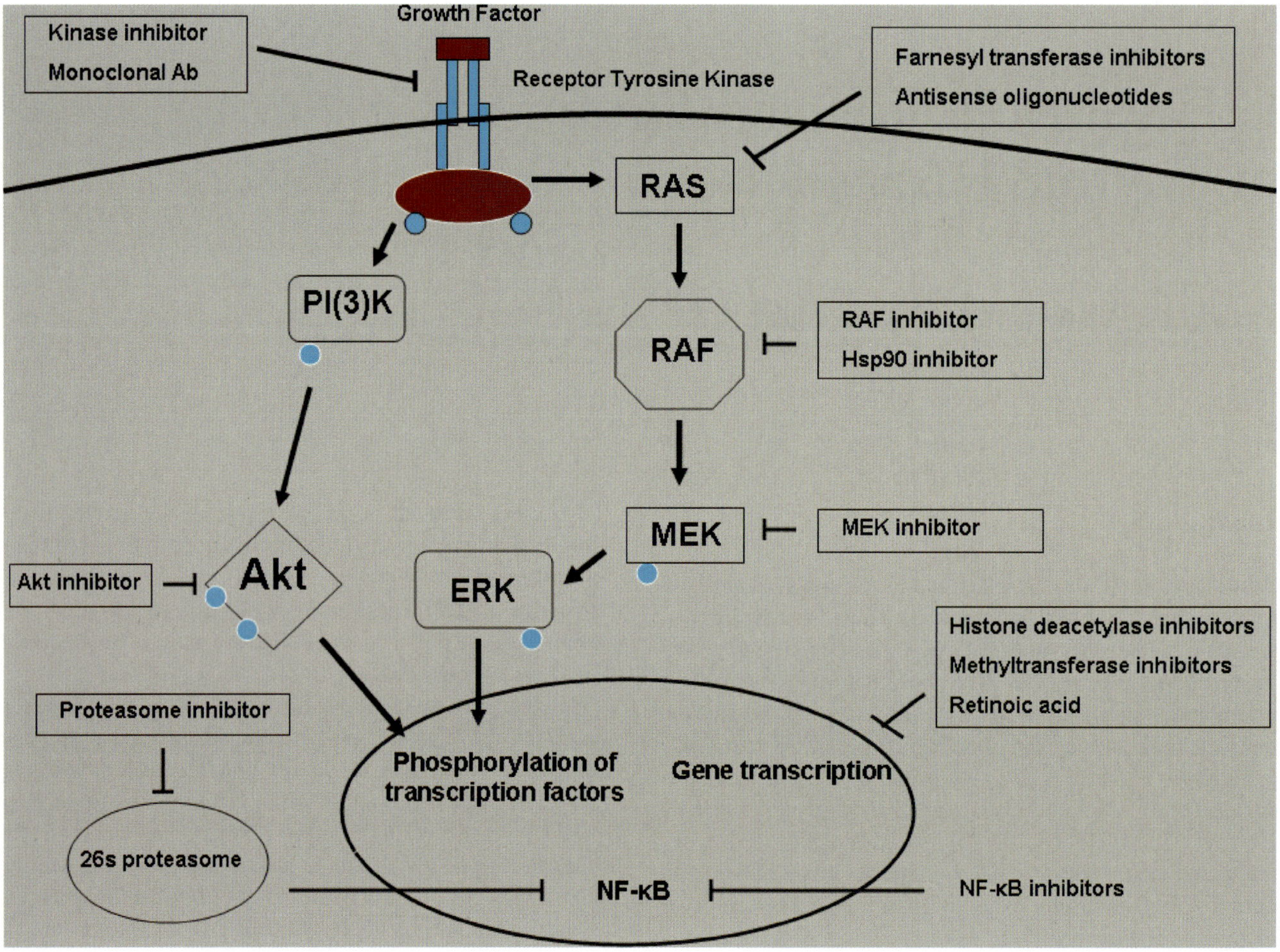

FIG. 4.1. Molecular targets involved in thyroid cancer pathogenesis.

Differential Diagnosis Through Molecular Testing

Gene Profiling for Diagnosis

While the above studies have focused on investigating the ability of molecular markers known to be associated with thyroid cancer to distinguish between benign and malignant lesions through RT-PCR or immunocytochemical analysis of cytology specimens, another group of researchers have attempted to tackle the same problem using a different approach. As mentioned previously, the completion of the human genome project in 2003 provided researchers with a powerful new tool with which to answer these questions. New technologies emerged to allow researchers to utilize the wealth of information waiting to be discovered in the 3,000,000,000 base pairs and 25,000 genes contained in the human genome. One important technology to emerge has been the use cDNA microarrays. This is a powerful method for quantitative analysis of cancer-specific gene expression associated with the pathology or altered biology of cancer cells,[10] where tissue samples are applied to a gene chip containing every gene in the human genome. Sophisticated software allows quantification of the expression of each of these genes, allowing comparison of expression patterns of thousands of genes in hundreds of tumors in a relatively short time-period.

Several authors have published reports showing that sets of genes of various sizes can accurately separate thyroid lesions into predictable categories. Weber and colleagues identified three genes, cyclin D2, prostate differentiation factor, and protein convertase 2, which classified follicular lesions into benign and malignant groups with 100% sensitivity and 95% specificity.[11] Rosen et al showed that a six-gene combination accurately distinguished between benign and malignant thyroid lesions with 75% sensitivity and 100% specificity.[12] Other groups use all differentially expressed genes determined using microarray analysis to separate lesions into benign and malignant groups, such as Barden and colleagues who used 105 differentially expressed genes in follicular adenomas and carcinomas to cluster unknown thyroid lesions into benign and malignant groups with 100% accuracy.[13] Several other groups have reported similarly promising results suggesting that this technology will likely have a role in the management of thyroid lesions in the future.[14,56] Several obstacles remain, however, such as standardizing the assays, as there is variability in the gene chips, the software, and the primers utilized in this process. Additionally, microarray analysis is not currently readily available in most centers, and therefore the clinical applicability of this technology will require more uniform access.

Several other markers are undergoing early stage testing for their potential utility in the management of thyroid cancer. Examples include the well-described fusion gene of paired box-8 (PAX8)/peroxisome proliferator-activated receptor (PPAR)-γ thought to be involved in the pathogenesis of follicular thyroid cancers,[15] the gene for IgG Fc binding protein which in early studies has been found to be differentially expressed in follicular cancers and adenomas,[16] and the tumor suppressor gene PTEN which has been shown to be involved in the pathogenesis of follicular thyroid tumors associated with Cowden's syndrome.[17] These studies have generated a great deal of excitement as researchers close in on a possible solution to the diagnostic dilemma concerning the cytologic diagnosis of certain thyroid lesions. The results of ongoing research in this area will be required to bring this promise to clinical fruition. Table 4.1 summarizes markers being examined for the improved diagnosis of thyroid lesions preoperatively.

Peripheral Blood Assays for Diagnosis

In addition to analyzing molecular markers in FNA specimens, researchers have looked at thyroid-specific markers in the peripheral blood as a means of diagnosing thyroid cancer. Using RT-PCR to detect and amplify thyroid-specific genes in the peripheral circulation, several targets have been identified to detect thyroid carcinoma, including thyroglobulin (Tg), thyroid peroxidase, thyrotropin (TSH) receptor, and the sodium/iodide symporter.[18–21] The most extensively studied gene has been Tg, and this has been studied primarily for its use in the follow up of differentiated thyroid cancer following thyroidectomy and T4 suppressive therapy, particularly in the setting of present anti-Tg antibodies.[22,23] However, there have been conflicting results concerning its ability to detect thyroid cancer, with some studies detecting this marker in healthy subjects, and others failing to detect it in patients with known metastatic disease, raising doubts about its clinical utility.[24,25]

A peripheral blood marker which has shown promise in the preoperative diagnosis of thyroid cancer has been TSHR-mRNA. Chia and colleagues showed that this marker had potential utility in distinguishing benign from malignant follicular neoplasms, correctly predicting 71% of follicular lesions diagnosed by cytology. They additionally showed a direct relationship between peripheral TSH-mRNA levels and extent of disease. While studies are ongoing, this marker has promise as an adjunct to the preoperative diagnosis of follicular thyroid lesions as well as in the follow up of differentiated thyroid cancer.[26]

Treatment and Molecular Targets

In addition to advances in the diagnosis of thyroid lesions, there has been a great deal of research into providing new and better therapies for thyroid cancers that do not respond to traditional treatment options. Up to 30% of differentiated thyroid cancers do not respond to traditional radioactive iodine or standard chemo-radiotherapy regimens. Similarly, advanced medullary thyroid cancers with distant metastases is a challenge to treat, as they do not respond to the traditional adjuvant therapies available, and they are obviously not responsive to radio-active iodine. Consequently, there has been much research directed at seeking alternative therapies using molecular markers as targets. Such therapeutic strategies include the use of kinase inhibitors, redifferentiation therapy, and gene therapy. Table 4.2 summarizes potential targets for novel therapeutic agents in the treatment of thyroid cancer.

TABLE 4.1. Molecular targets being investigated to differentiate benign and malignant thyroid lesions pre-operatively.

Marker	Method of analysis
Galectin-3	Immunocytochemistry
CD44	Immunocytochemistry, RT-PCR
Telomerase	TRAP assay, RT-PCR
HMGI(Y) protein	RT-PCR, immunocytochemistry
COX-2	RT-PCR
HBME-1	Immunocytochemistry
TSHR mRNA	RT-PCR of peripheral blood
Genetic profiling	Microarray analysis

RT-PCR reverse transcriptase-polymerase chain reaction; *TRAP* telomerase repeat amplification protocol; *HMGI(Y)* high mobility group 1 (Y); *COX-2* cyclooxygenase-2; *HBME-1* Hector Battifora mesothelial cell; *TSHR mRNA* thyrotropin receptor messenger ribonucleic acid.

TABLE 4.2. Potential molecular targets for therapy in thyroid cancer.

Drug	Target
Kinase inhibitors	
Sorafenib (BAY-43-9006)	BRAF, VEGFR, RET, PDGFR
Axitinib (AG-013736)	VEGFR, c-KIT, PDGFR
Motesanib (AMG-706)	VEGFR, c-KIT, PDGFR, RET
Sunitinib	VEGFR, PDGFR, FLT-3
NVP-AEE788	VGFR, EGFR
XL-184	VEGFR, c-MET
Gefitinib (Iressa)	EGFR
Vandetanib (ZD6474, Zactima)	VEGFR, EGFR, RET
Imatinib (Gleevec)	c-KIT, PDGF, Bcr-Abl, RET
Other therapeutic agents	
Celecoxib	COX-2
Irinotecan	Topoisomerase
Bortezomib (PS-341)	26S proteasome, NF-κB
17-AAG	Hsp90
Combrestatin A4 (CA4P)	Tubulin
Rosiglitazone	PPAR-γ agonist
KP372-1	Akt
SAHA	Histone deacetylase
Depsipeptide (FK288)	Histone deacetylase
Sodium butyrate	DNA methyltransferase
Retinoic Acids	Nuclear receptors

Gene Therapy

The strategy of most gene therapy approaches is to introduce an exogenous gene designed specifically to manipulate tumor cells to render them more susceptible to localization and destruction. Several areas of study employing gene therapy are underway, but most are in early stages using in vitro and in vivo animal models. The following section will summarize the areas of gene therapy undergoing active investigation.

Corrective Gene Therapy

Corrective gene therapy aims to restore normal function to a gene which has been deleted or harbors a mutation; typically, these targets are tumor suppressor genes. p53, which is involved in DNA repair and apoptosis, has been shown to be involved in thyroid dedifferentiation in a high percentage of poorly differentiated thyroid cancers.[27] Early studies have shown that introduction of wild-type p53 into thyroid cells harboring a mutated p53 gene results in re-emergence of a more differentiated phenotype, measured primarily by the presence of thyroid peroxidases, thyroglobulin, and the sodium/iodide symporter.[28,29]

Immunomodulatory Gene Therapy

This method of gene therapy introduces genes that enhance or induce the host immune system to respond to the presence of malignant cells. While many tumor cells express tumor-specific antigens, they develop mechanisms to evade the host immune system. The cytokine interleukin 2 (IL-2) activates natural killer (NK) cells and other effector cells, thereby upregulating both specific and nonspecific immunity.[30] Several published reports have shown this approach to be feasible. Using a BALB/c mouse model of medullary thyroid cancer, the authors showed tumors engineered to secrete high levels of IL-2 exhibited significant inhibition of growth.[31] Additionally, tumor cells containing the IL-2 gene were injected into tumor-free mice without any subsequent growth, suggesting long-term immunity.

Cytoreductive Gene Therapy

Cytoreductive gene therapy employs the strategy of introducing novel genes which cause tumor cell death, or facilitate the use of selective cytotoxic agents against tumor cells. Typically, a gene which encodes for an enzyme is introduced into tumor cells. This enzyme activates a non-toxic prodrug, which will then attack only those cells with the enzyme and spare healthy cells. One study showed that the herpes simplex virus thymidine kinase and the prodrug gancyclovir resulted in dose-dependent death in two thyroid cancer cell lines.[32] Gancyclovir, a nucleotide analog that is preferentially phosphorylated by the HSV thymidine kinase, competes with normal nucleotides during replication and consequently inhibits cell propagation.

Gene Silencing

This technique employs the use of antisense RNA segments that bind to specific genes, usually oncogenes, and inhibit their expression. C-myc is a proto-oncogene that encodes for a nuclear protein involved in cell proliferation. It has been shown to be constitutively expressed in thyroid cancers, and that the use of antisense RNA to silence this gene may lead to tumor growth inhibition.[33]

Redifferentiation Therapy

Dedifferentiated thyroid cancers lose the ability to concentrate iodine and cease to express TSH receptors, thus rendering them impervious to standard radioiodine and TSH suppressive therapy. Redifferentiation therapy attempts to induce the reversal of these changes in tumor cells to make them susceptible once again to standard therapy.

Retinoic Acids

Retinoic acids are the biologically active metabolites of vitamin A. These have been used in several human cancers, with the greatest effects being seen with certain types of leukemia.[34] Several in vitro studies showed retinoic acid inhibited growth and the ability of thyroid cells to metastasize. They also stimulated thyroid specific functions, such as expression of the sodium-iodide symporter and increased iodine uptake. These results led to clinical trials in patients who had unresectable dedifferentiated thyroid cancer with no iodine uptake. Radioiodine uptake increased in 40% of patients; there was reduction of tumor size in 11%, and 31% showed no further growth.[35]

Deoxyribonucleic Acid Methyltransferase Inhibitors

Promoter methylation is a common mechanism of regulation of gene expression. Methylation prevents transcription from occurring, in effect turning the gene off until required by the cell. Many thyroid cancers have been shown to contain a high degree of methylation. Methylation is likely to be involved in the loss of the sodium-iodide symporter function in carcinomas, which is responsible for preventing iodide uptake by cancer cells.[36] Published reports have shown using in vitro and in vivo models of thyroid cancer that the use of the demethylating agents sodium butyrate and 5-azacytidine inhibit tumor growth and cause dedifferentiated thyroid cancer cells to regain the ability to take up iodide.[37,38]

Histone Deacetylase Inhibitors

Histones are nuclear proteins that are involved in the condensing of DNA into chromatin. Histone deacetylation is required to unfold DNA, allowing access of promoter regions for gene transcription. Inhibitors of histone deacetylation, such as depsipeptide (FK288), have been shown to increase the expression of the sodium-iodide symporter and iodide uptake in poorly differentiated and undifferentiated thyroid cancer cells.[39]

There are phase II human trials of recurrent or metastatic thyroid cancer currently underway for depsipeptide.

Suberoylanalide hydroxamic acid (SAHA) is another histone deacetylase that has been studied in the treatment of thyroid cancer. Preclinical studies with anaplastic and poorly differentiated thyroid cancers showed growth arrest and induction of apoptosis with this agent. Phase I study results of 73 patients, six of whom had thyroid cancer, showed one patient with a partial response, two patients with disease stabilization, and one patient with increased uptake of radioiodide in metastases.[40]

Tyrosine Kinase Inhibitors

An area of intense research in the treatment of thyroid cancer is in the use of tyrosine kinase inhibitors. Receptor tyrosine kinases are the most commonly overexpressed receptors in thyroid cancers. Consequently, these have become natural targets for novel directed therapies in these cancers. The following section will summarize the status of this area of research.

Angiogenesis Inhibitors

Angiogenesis is the development of new blood vessels which, in part, allows tumors to grow. Angiogenesis is a complex process with multiple factors that are recently beginning to be elucidated. One protein which has become the focus of research in many types of cancer is vascular endothelial growth factor (VEGF). This protein is a tyrosine kinase which stimulates neovascularization by binding to VEGF receptors on endothelial cells.[41] VEGF has been shown to be upregulated in thyroid cancers. Several inhibitors of VEGF have been developed, and many of these have been studied in the treatment of thyroid cancer.

Sorafenib

Sorafenib is a multitarget inhibitor which binds to both the VEGF and BRAF tyrosine kinase receptors. This has been evaluated in the treatment of thyroid cancer in a phase II trial, where 19 patients with metastatic, iodine-resistant papillary thyroid cancer were treated. Five patients manifested a partial response to therapy, and eight others had no disease progression. Median duration of response was 14.2 months with a median time to progression of greater than 4 months (4 days to 14 months). Evaluation of tumor tissues showed treatment with sorafenib caused reduction of pERK, downstream target of VEGFR and BRAF, and pAKT, downstream of VEGFR.[42] This drug currently is approved for the treatment of renal cell cancer and hepatocellular carcinoma.

Axitinib

Axitinib (AG-013736) is an inhibitor of VEGFR-1, 2 & 3. Sixty patients with metastatic or unresectable thyroid cancer were evaluated with this drug in a single arm multicenter clinical trial. All patients had cancers refractory to radioiodine therapy, or were not suitable candidates for this treatment for other reasons. Most patients had differentiated thyroid cancer, with two having anaplastic cancer. 18 patients had partial responses and 30 had stable disease, with a median progression free survival that had not been reached at 273 days of follow up. Therapy with this drug was generally well tolerated at a dose of 5 mg twice a day.

Motesanib

AMG 706 (Motesanib) is another drug that inhibits several tyrosine kinases, including VEGFR, PDGFR, c-Kit, and RET. This was evaluated in a phase II trial of patients with advanced differentiated or medullary thyroid cancer, with patients receiving daily doses until disease progression occurred or toxicity became unacceptable. Of the 93 patients with advanced differentiated disease, 12% had a partial response and 69% had stable disease. Of the 83 patients with sporadic or hereditary MTC, two had partial responses and 43 had stable disease for longer than 6 months. Toxicity included diarrhea and hypertension, and was generally well tolerated.

Sunitinib

Sunitinib is an orally administered tyrosine kinase inhibitor with activity against VEGFR, platelet derived growth factor receptor (PDGFR), and fms-related tyrosine kinase 3 (FLT-3). There is a phase II trials of this drug currently underway. Other VEGF receptors such as NVP-AEE788 and PTK787/ZK222584, have shown promise in animal models or in vitro models, but have yet to undergo human trials.[43] XL-184, which inhibits multiple tyrosine kinases such as VEGFR and c-MET is currently undergoing phase I/II trials of several tumor types, including thyroid cancer. Results of phase I trials showed partial responses in three of seven patients with MTC.

Other Targets of Signaling Pathways

Gefitinib

This is another tyrosine kinase inhibitor which targets epidermal growth factor receptor (EGFR). This has been shown to be expressed on malignant thyroid cells and has been associated with a worse prognosis in differentiated thyroid cancers. A phase II trial of patients with radioiodine resistant thyroid cancer showed no objective response using RECIST criteria, but there was reduction in tumor size in 32% of patients, and 12% of patients showed no progression of disease after 1 year. Overall survival was 17.5 months.

Celecoxib

COX-2 has been shown to be upregulated by two oncogenes associated with thyroid cancer, RET/PTC1 and 2. Celecoxib, a COX-2 inhibitor, seemed a possible target for directed therapy, but showed poor results in a phase II study of patients with metastatic differentiated thyroid cancer.[44]

KP372-1

The PI3K/Akt signaling pathway is involved in cell proliferation and growth and has been recognized as being involved in cancer pathogenesis. Inhibiting this signaling pathway with the Akt inhibitor KP372-1 has been shown to induce apoptosis in thyroid cancer cells in preclinical studies.

Medullary Thyroid Cancer

Medullary thyroid cancer has been associated with rearrangements in the RET protooncogene, another receptor tyrosine kinase. Inhibitors of this kinase have been studied as new therapies for advanced cases of MTC unable to be cured surgically.

Vandetanib

ZD6474 (Vandetanib, Zactima), is an anilinoquinazoline compound which inhibits VEGFR2 & 3, EGFR, and RET tyrosine kinases. A single arm phase II trial of 30 patients showed a 17% partial response rate, and a 50% stable disease rate. Calcitonin levels were decreased by at least 50% in 23 patients. These results have led to an international phase II trial comparing this drug with placebo. Additionally, sorafenib, motesanib, sunitinib and axitinib have all been evaluated in the treatment of MTC with varying results.

Imatinib

Imatinib (Gleevec) is a tyrosine kinase inhibitor with activity against several kinases, including c-KIT, PDGF, Bcr-Abl, and RET. More commonly known for its treatment of GI stromal tumors, it has also undergone phase II trials for the treatment of MTC. Unfortunately, 15 patients with disseminated disease showed no objective responses, although four patients had stable disease over 24 months. Three patients had to discontinue treatment because of side effects.[45] There is also a phase II trial ongoing for the treatment of anaplastic thyroid cancer, although early results show limited efficacy.[46] Several of these tyrosine kinase inhibitors with activity against multiple kinases are being looked at as possible therapeutic options for both follicular cancers and MTC.

Anti-CEA Monoclonal Antibodies

In addition to calcitonin, 70–90% of MTC's express carcinoembryonic antigen (CEA) on their surface. Researchers have tried to exploit this as a means of directing targeted therapy at advanced MTC. A group of researchers published results of a study examining the use of ^{90}Y-labeled human anti-CEA monoclonal antibodies to treat advanced MTC in a phase I trial. Of 15 patients treated with this in combination with doxorubicin, partial responses were seen in three, with one patient exhibiting a 68% reduction in local and hepatic metastatic disease. While the overall therapeutic response was modest, the authors concluded that this may be a therapeutic option in selected patients, particularly those with more limited, earlier stage disease.[47]

Topoisomerase Inhibitors

The topoisomerase inhibitor irinotecan has been shown to have inhibitory effects on MTC alone or in combination with other agents such as cetuximab and CEP-751 in preclinical studies. There is a phase II clinical trial of irinotecan for the treatment of MTC ongoing.

Proteasome Inhibitors

The proteasome is a 26S protein involved in proteolysis, and has been shown to represent the primary degradation pathway for proteins involved in the regulation of cell proliferation, survival, and apoptosis. Proteins targeted for degradation undergo modification by the covalent addition of the low molecular weight polypeptide ubiquitin, after which the proteasome complex recognizes the protein and degrades it. Regulation of the proteasome has been found to be involved in many pathologic processes, including the pathogenesis of malignant transformation (Figure 4.2).

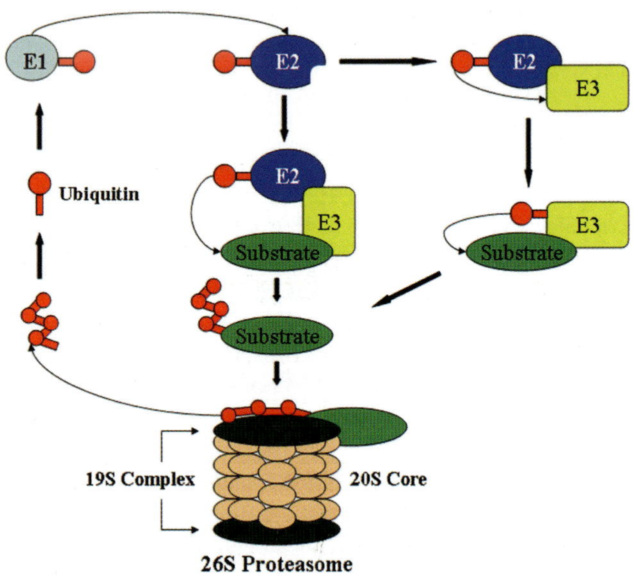

FIG. 4.2. Schematic of the 26S proteasome. Proteins targeted for degradation are polyubiquitinated by the actions of three key enzymes, E1, E2, and E3. Ubiquitinated proteins are recognized by the proteasome, funneled through the 20S core, and degraded by proteolysis.

Bortezomib (PS-341) is a proteasome inhibitor which has been approved for use in the treatment of progressive multiple myeloma.[48] A large scale phase II trial is currently underway examining its efficacy in the treatment of a variety of other tumors.[49] Early studies have also been published examining its potential role in the treatment of MTC and anaplastic thyroid cancer. One group has shown that treatment with bortezomib induced apoptosis of MTC cells in vitro. Another published study reports the induction of significant apoptosis of anaplastic thyroid cancer cells at doses achieved in the clinical setting.[50]

NF-κB

NF-κB is a transcription factor known to be a central activator of antiapoptotic cascades, and felt to play a key role in cancer pathogenesis. Inhibitory factors called IκB prevent NF-κB action, but phosphorylation of these inhibitory factors leads to ubiquitination and degradation by the 26S proteasome. Early in vitro and in vivo experiments have shown that treatment with nonspecific NF-κB inhibitors results in massive apoptosis of thyroid cancer cells, and deserves additional investigation.[51]

Other Targets in Thyroid Cancer

Hsp90 Inhibitors

Hsp90 is a chaperone that stabilizes growth factor receptors and molecules involved in cell signaling. Inhibition of this protein leads to downregulation of signaling pathways involved in cell proliferation and growth, such as MAPK. 17-Allylamino-17-demethoxygeldanamycin (17-AAG) is the first Hsp90 inhibitor to enter into clinical studies. Early studies have shown that treatment with 17-AAG increased radioiodide accumulation in thyroid cancer cells.[52] Currently, there is a phase II trial of 17-AAG in advanced thyroid cancer.

Combrestatin A4

Combrestatin A4 (CA4P) is a tubulin binding protein that has been shown to have direct antineoplastic activity against thyroid cancer cells. Studies in mouse models of anaplastic thyroid cancer (ATC) showed significantly lower tumor sizes in treated mice.[53] A phase I clinical trial showed a durable response in one patient with ATC,[54] and a phase II trial is underway currently.

PPAR-γ Agonists

This protein is involved in the regulation of cellular growth and differentiation, and is thought to be involved in thyroid cancer pathogenesis. Preclinical studies have shown growth inhibition and induction of apoptosis in papillary thyroid cancer cell lines after treatment with the PPAR-γ agonists rosiglitazone and troglitazone.[55] A clinical trial of rosiglitazone in the treatment of advanced or metastatic thyroid cancer is currently underway. Table 4.3 summarizes the status of current clinical trials for novel treatment methods for thyroid cancer.

The wealth of ongoing research has yielded promising results in the development of new diagnostic and treatment modalities in the management of thyroid cancer. It is a very exciting time in the field of thyroid oncology, and the possibility that some of these new modalities could soon be added to our armamentarium in the management of thyroid cancer seems tantalizingly close. The dedication of the many talented scientists involved in the ongoing studies in this area will hopefully transform these promising results into clinical reality in the near future.

TABLE 4.3. Current clinical trials for thyroid cancer.

Agent	Target	Status
Sorafenib	RET, BRAF, VEGFR	Recruiting for phase II trial in patients with advanced ATC and metastatic MTC
Imatinib	c-KIT, PDGF, Bcr-Abl, RET	Recruiting for phase II trial of patients with ATC, and phase I/II trial in combination with other chemotherapeutic agents of patients with MTC
Axitinib	VEGFR, c-KIT, PDGF	Recruiting for phase II trial of patients with ^{131}I-refractory metastatic or locally unresectable differentiated thyroid cancer
Motesanib	VEGFR, PDGFR, RET	Recruiting for phase II trial in patients with advanced differentiated or MTC
Sunitinib	VEGFR, PDGFR, FLT-3	Recruiting for phase II trial in patients with ^{131}I-refractory advanced differentiated or MTC
Gefitinib	EGFR	Recruiting for phase II trial of patients with ^{131}I-resistant thyroid cancers
Vandetanib	VEGFR, EGFR, RET	Recruiting for phase II trial of patients with metastatic or locally advanced MTC
Irinotecan	Topoisomerase	Recruiting for phase II trial of patients with metastatic MTC
Bortezomib	26S proteasome	Recruiting for phase II trial of patients with metastatic papillary or follicular carcinoma
Combrestatin A4	Tubulin	Recruiting for phase II trial of patients with advanced ATC
17-AAG	Hsp90	Recruiting for phase II trial of patients with advanced MTC or differentiated thyroid cancer
Rosiglitazone	PPAR-γ	Recruiting for pilot study of patients with advanced differentiated thyroid cancer
FK228	Histone deacetylase	Recruiting for phase II study of patients with ^{131}I-refractory metastatic non-medullary thyroid cancer

References

1. Correa P, Chen VW. Endocrine gland cancer. *Cancer*. 1995; 75(1 Suppl):338–352.
2. Jemal A, Siegel R, Ward E, Murray T, Xu J, Thun MJ. Cancer statistics, 2007. *CA Cancer J Clin*. 2007;57(1):43–66.
3. Colonna M, Guizard AV, Schvartz C, et al. A time trend analysis of papillary and follicular cancers as a function of tumour size: a study of data from six cancer registries in France (1983–2000). *Eur J Cancer*. 2007;43(5):891–900.
4. Mitchell J, Parangi S. The thyroid incidentaloma: an increasingly frequent consequence of radiologic imaging. *Semin Ultrasound CT MR*. 2005;26(1):37–46.
5. Nunez C, Mendelsohn G. Fine-needle aspiration and needle biopsy of the thyroid gland. *Pathol Annu*. 1989;24(Pt 1):161–198.
6. Mazzaferri EL, Massoll N. Management of papillary and follicular (differentiated) thyroid cancer: new paradigms using recombinant human thyrotropin. *Endocr Relat Cancer*. 2002;9(4):227–247.
7. Schlumberger MJ. Papillary and follicular thyroid carcinoma. *N Engl J Med*. 1998;338(5):297–306.
8. Coelho SM, de Carvalho DP, Vaisman M. New perspectives on the treatment of differentiated thyroid cancer. *Arq Bras Endocrinol Metabol*. 2007;51(4):612–624.
9. Haugen BR. Management of the patient with progressive radioiodine non-responsive disease. *Semin Surg Oncol*. 1999;16(1):34–41.
10. Yano Y, Uematsu N, Yashiro T, et al. Gene expression profiling identifies platelet-derived growth factor as a diagnostic molecular marker for papillary thyroid carcinoma. *Clin Cancer Res*. 2004;10(6):2035–2043.
11. Weber F, Shen L, Aldred MA, et al. Genetic classification of benign and malignant thyroid follicular neoplasia based on a three-gene combination. *J Clin Endocrinol Metab*. 2005;90(5): 2512–2521.
12. Rosen J, He M, Umbricht C, et al. A six-gene model for differentiating benign from malignant thyroid tumors on the basis of gene expression. *Surgery*. 2005;138(6):1050-1056. discussion 1056–1057.
13. Barden CB, Shister KW, Zhu B, et al. Classification of follicular thyroid tumors by molecular signature: results of gene profiling. *Clin Cancer Res*. 2003;9(5):1792–1800.
14. Huang Y, Prasad M, Lemon WJ, et al. Gene expression in papillary thyroid carcinoma reveals highly consistent profiles. *Proc Natl Acad Sci USA*. 2001;98(26):15044–15049.
15. Reddi HV, McIver B, Grebe SK, Eberhardt NL. The paired box-8/ peroxisome proliferator-activated receptor-gamma oncogene in thyroid tumorigenesis. *Endocrinology*. 2007;148(3):932–935.
16. O'Donovan N, Fischer A, Abdo EM, et al. Differential expression of IgG Fc binding protein (FcgammaBP) in human normal thyroid tissue, thyroid adenomas and thyroid carcinomas. *J Endocrinol*. 2002;174(3):517–524.
17. Gimm O, Perren A, Weng LP, et al. Differential nuclear and cytoplasmic expression of PTEN in normal thyroid tissue, and benign and malignant epithelial thyroid tumors. *Am J Pathol*. 2000;156(5):1693–1700.
18. Ringel MD, Ladenson PW, Levine MA. Molecular diagnosis of residual and recurrent thyroid cancer by amplification of thyroglobulin messenger ribonucleic acid in peripheral blood. *J Clin Endocrinol Metab*. 1998;83(12):4435–4442.
19. Tallini G, Ghossein RA, Emanuel J, et al. Detection of thyroglobulin, thyroid peroxidase, and RET/PTC1 mRNA transcripts in the peripheral blood of patients with thyroid disease. *J Clin Oncol*. 1998;16(3):1158–1166.
20. Biscolla RP, Cerutti JM, Maciel RM. Detection of recurrent thyroid cancer by sensitive nested reverse transcription-polymerase chain reaction of thyroglobulin and sodium/iodide symporter messenger ribonucleic acid transcripts in peripheral blood. *J Clin Endocrinol Metab*. 2000;85(10):3623–3627.
21. Chinnappa P, Taguba L, Arciaga R, et al. Detection of thyrotropin-receptor messenger ribonucleic acid (mRNA) and thyroglobulin mRNA transcripts in peripheral blood of patients with thyroid disease: sensitive and specific markers for thyroid cancer. *J Clin Endocrinol Metab*. 2004;89(8):3705–3709.
22. Savagner F, Rodien P, Reynier P, Rohmer V, Bigorgne JC, Malthiery Y. Analysis of Tg transcripts by real-time RT-PCR in the blood of thyroid cancer patients. *J Clin Endocrinol Metab*. 2002;87(2):635–639.
23. Ringel MD, Balducci-Silano PL, Anderson JS, et al. Quantitative reverse transcription-polymerase chain reaction of circulating thyroglobulin messenger ribonucleic acid for monitoring patients with thyroid carcinoma. *J Clin Endocrinol Metab*. 1999;84(11):4037–4042.
24. Bojunga J, Roddiger S, Stanisch M, et al. Molecular detection of thyroglobulin mRNA transcripts in peripheral blood of patients with thyroid disease by RT-PCR. *Br J Cancer*. 2000;82(10):1650–1655.
25. Bugalho MJ, Domingues RS, Pinto AC, et al. Detection of thyroglobulin mRNA transcripts in peripheral blood of individuals with and without thyroid glands: evidence for thyroglobulin expression by blood cells. *Eur J Endocrinol*. 2001;145(4):409–413.
26. Chia SY, Milas M, Reddy SK, et al. Thyroid-stimulating hormone receptor messenger ribonucleic acid measurement in blood as a marker for circulating thyroid cancer cells and its role in the preoperative diagnosis of thyroid cancer. *J Clin Endocrinol Metab*. 2007;92(2):468–475.
27. Fagin JA, Matsuo K, Karmakar A, Chen DL, Tang SH, Koeffler HP. High prevalence of mutations of the p53 gene in poorly differentiated human thyroid carcinomas. *J Clin Invest*. 1993;91(1):179–184.
28. Battista S, Martelli ML, Fedele M, et al. A mutated p53 gene alters thyroid cell differentiation. *Oncogene*. 1995;11(10):2029–2037.
29. Fagin JA, Tang SH, Zeki K, Di Lauro R, Fusco A, Gonsky R. Reexpression of thyroid peroxidase in a derivative of an undifferentiated thyroid carcinoma cell line by introduction of wild-type p53. *Cancer Res*. 1996;56(4):765–771.
30. Nanni P, Forni G, Lollini PL. Cytokine gene therapy: hopes and pitfalls. *Ann Oncol*. 1999;10(3):261–266.
31. Zhang R, Baunoch D, DeGroot LJ. Genetic immunotherapy for medullary thyroid carcinoma: destruction of tumors in mice by in vivo delivery of adenoviral vector transducing the murine interleukin-2 gene. *Thyroid*. 1998;8(12):1137–1146.
32. Nishihara E, Nagayama Y, Mawatari F, et al. Retrovirus-mediated herpes simplex virus thymidine kinase gene transduction renders human thyroid carcinoma cell lines sensitive to ganciclovir and radiation in vitro and in vivo. *Endocrinology*. 1997;138(11):4577–4583.
33. Cerutti J, Trapasso F, Battaglia C, et al. Block of c-myc expression by antisense oligonucleotides inhibits proliferation of human thyroid carcinoma cell lines. *Clin Cancer Res*. 1996;2(1):119–126.

34. Chomienne C, Fenaux P, Degos L. Retinoid differentiation therapy in promyelocytic leukemia. *FASEB J*. 1996;10(9):1025–1030.
35. Grunwald F, Menzel C, Bender H, et al. Redifferentiation therapy-induced radioiodine uptake in thyroid cancer. *J Nucl Med*. 1998;39(11):1903–1906.
36. de Capoa A, Grappelli C, Volpino P, et al. Nuclear methylation levels in normal and cancerous thyroid cells. *Anticancer Res*. 2004;24(3a):1495–1500.
37. Venkataraman GM, Yatin M, Marcinek R, Ain KB. Restoration of iodide uptake in dedifferentiated thyroid carcinoma: relationship to human Na+/I-symporter gene methylation status. *J Clin Endocrinol Metab*. 1999;84(7):2449–2457.
38. Massart C, Denais A, Gibassier J. Effect of all-trans retinoic acid and sodium butyrate in vitro and in vivo on thyroid carcinoma xenografts. *Anticancer Drugs*. 2006;17(5):559–563.
39. Furuya F, Shimura H, Suzuki H, et al. Histone deacetylase inhibitors restore radioiodide uptake and retention in poorly differentiated and anaplastic thyroid cancer cells by expression of the sodium/iodide symporter thyroperoxidase and thyroglobulin. *Endocrinology*. 2004;145(6):2865–2875.
40. Kelly WK, O'Connor OA, Krug LM, et al. Phase I study of an oral histone deacetylase inhibitor, suberoylanilide hydroxamic acid, in patients with advanced cancer. *J Clin Oncol*. 2005;23(17): 3923–3931.
41. Folkman J. Tumor angiogenesis: therapeutic implications. *N Engl J Med*. 1971;285(21):1182–1186.
42. Gupta-Abramson V, Troxel AB, Nellore A, et al. Phase II trial of sorafenib in advanced thyroid cancer. *J Clin Oncol*. 2008;26(29):4714–4719.
43. Kundra P, Burman KD. Thyroid cancer molecular signaling pathways and use of targeted therapy. *Endocrinol Metab Clin North Am*. 2007;36(3):839–853, viii.
44. Mrozek E, Kloos RT, Ringel MD, et al. Phase II study of celecoxib in metastatic differentiated thyroid carcinoma. *J Clin Endocrinol Metab*. 2006;91(6):2201–2204.
45. de Groot JW, Zonnenberg BA, van Ufford-Mannesse PQ, et al. A phase II trial of imatinib therapy for metastatic medullary thyroid carcinoma. *J Clin Endocrinol Metab*. 2007;92(9): 3466–3469.
46. Dziba JM, Ain KB. Imatinib mesylate (gleevec; STI571) monotherapy is ineffective in suppressing human anaplastic thyroid carcinoma cell growth in vitro. *J Clin Endocrinol Metab*. 2004;89(5):2127–2135.
47. Sharkey RM, Hajjar G, Yeldell D, et al. A phase I trial combining high-dose 90Y-labeled humanized anti-CEA monoclonal antibody with doxorubicin and peripheral blood stem cell rescue in advanced medullary thyroid cancer. *J Nucl Med*. 2005;46(4):620–633.
48. Kane RC, Bross PF, Farrell AT, Pazdur R. Velcade: U.S. FDA approval for the treatment of multiple myeloma progressing on prior therapy. *Oncologist*. 2003;8(6):508–513.
49. Montagut C, Rovira A, Albanell J. The proteasome: a novel target for anticancer therapy. *Clin Transl Oncol*. 2006;8(5): 313–317.
50. Conticello C, Adamo L, Giuffrida R, et al. Proteasome inhibitors synergize with tumor necrosis factor-related apoptosis-induced ligand to induce anaplastic thyroid carcinoma cell death. *J Clin Endocrinol Metab*. 2007;92(5):1938–1942.
51. Namba H, Saenko V, Yamashita S. Nuclear factor-kB in thyroid carcinogenesis and progression: a novel therapeutic target for advanced thyroid cancer. *Arq Bras Endocrinol Metabol*. 2007;51(5):843–851.
52. Marsee DK, Venkateswaran A, Tao H, et al. Inhibition of heat shock protein 90, a novel RET/PTC1-associated protein, increases radioiodide accumulation in thyroid cells. *J Biol Chem*. 2004;279(42):43990–43997.
53. Dziba JM, Marcinek R, Venkataraman G, Robinson JA, Ain KB. Combretastatin A4 phosphate has primary antineoplastic activity against human anaplastic thyroid carcinoma cell lines and xenograft tumors. *Thyroid*. 2002;12(12):1063–1070.
54. Dowlati A, Robertson K, Cooney M, et al. A phase I pharmacokinetic and translational study of the novel vascular targeting agent combretastatin a-4 phosphate on a single-dose intravenous schedule in patients with advanced cancer. *Cancer Res*. 2002;62(12):3408–3416.
55. Ohta K, Endo T, Haraguchi K, Hershman JM, Onaya T. Ligands for peroxisome proliferator-activated receptor gamma inhibit growth and induce apoptosis of human papillary thyroid carcinoma cells. *J Clin Endocrinol Metab*. 2001;86(5): 2170–2177.
56. Mazzanti C, Zeiger MA, Costouros NG, et al. Using gene expression profiling to differentiate benign versus malignant thyroid tumors. *Cancer Res*. 2004;64(8):2898–2903.

5 Autoimmune Thyroid Diseases

Ashraf Khan and Otto Walter

Introduction

The discovery in 1956 that Hashimoto's thyroiditis is an autoimmune disease spelled the end of the concept of horror autotoxicus and introduced the reality of human autoimmunity. Soon after, Graves' disease was discovered to be directly caused by a serum factor, subsequently identified as an autoantibody. These diseases have served as invaluable models for the understanding of the organ specific autoimmunity. While Graves' disease and Hashimoto's thyroiditis are the two most common autoimmune thyroid diseases, autoimmune etiology has been also implicated in other forms of thyroiditides like Riedel's, postpartum, silent and focal lymphocytic thyroiditis.

Graves' Disease

Graves' disease is characterized by diffuse hyperplasia of the thyroid gland, thyrotoxicosis due to excessive thyroid hormone synthesis, and the presence of thyroid-associated autoantibodies in the serum.

Historical Background

As early as the fifth century BC, the ancient Greeks described the combination of goiter, exophthalmos, and palpitations which is the known constellation of symptoms in patients with Graves' disease.[1] In 1786, Parry[2] was the first to recognize and describe a group of patients with a combination of symptoms including rapid heart beat, goiter, and sometimes exophthalmos. These findings were, however, published only in 1825 after Parry's death by his son in an obscure book.[3] Later Robert Graves, in 1835, and Carl Basedow, in 1840, also described a group of patients with symptoms similar to those described by Parry.[4] The continental European doctors being unaware of Graves' description, called it Basedow's disease, and this term is still used by some in Europe.[4] Both Parry and Graves thought that these symptoms were a result of a cardiac disease, and even after Basedow's report the goiter was not considered of much importance.[4] In the 1860s after the description of cases with nervousness by Charcot, the cardiac origin gave way to a neurologic etiology, a belief that was dominant for the rest of the nineteenth century.[4] By the late nineteenth century, with the introduction of thyroidectomies, it was observed that the removal of goiters improved nervousness in patients who survived surgery. This fact was supported by other observations in the 1890s, when too much thyroid extract led to nervousness and weight loss, symptoms similar to Graves' disease. This discovery gave way to the thyroid origin of what is now universally known as Graves' disease.[4] The autoimmune origin was established only in 1957.

Clinical Features

Graves' disease is seen mostly in women, with a female-to-male ratio of 8:1. The most common age of presentation is in the third or the fourth decade.[5] Patients usually present with a characteristic clinical triad of diffuse enlargement of the thyroid (goiter), thyrotoxicosis with associated cardiovascular symptoms and ocular changes. The third component, localized infiltrative dermopathy (pretibial myxedema) is seen only in selected cases.

The most common clinical symptoms and signs include nervousness, excessive sweating, heat intolerance, palpitations, fatigue, tachycardia, muscle wasting, weight loss, diffuse goiter, tremors, and eye changes.[5]

Pathogenesis

The hallmark of GD is the production of TSH receptor stimulating autoantibodies. Other secondary autoantigens include thyroid peroxidase, thyroglobulin, and the sodium/iodide cotransporter[6,7] can be also detected. The TSH receptor-stimulating antibody is specific to Graves' disease.[8] It functions like TSH, activates the adenyl cyclase-cAMP and protein kinase C-phosphoinositide signal transduction pathways,[9] leading to increased synthesis and release of thyroid hormone and hyperplasia of thyroid follicular cells. T cells,

J.L. Hunt (ed.), *Molecular Pathology of Endocrine Diseases*, Molecular Pathology Library 3,
DOI 10.1007/978-1-4419-1707-2_5, © Springer Science+Business Media, LLC 2010

predominantly T helper (CD4) cells of both H1 and H2 subtypes, constitute the majority of the intrathyroidal lymphocytes in Graves' disease. Other minor cell populations include T suppressor (CD8) lymphocytes, B lymphocytes, and plasma cells.

What initiates the autoimmune reaction in Graves' disease is not entirely clear. Possible mechanisms include molecular mimicry or cross-reactivity between infectious agents and thyroid proteins. Such similarity was detected between *Yersinia enterocolitica* antigens and the TSH receptor.[10] There is no evidence however, that either *Yersinia* or viral infection causes Graves' disease. Other mechanisms suggested for the initiation of the immune reaction in Graves' disease include direct induction of major histocompatibility complex (MHC) class II molecule expression such as HLA-DR on the surface of thyrocytes as a result of viral infection. Thus, the thyroid follicular cells may act themselves as antigen-presenting cells, presenting their own antigens, generating production of thyroid autoantibodies.[11] Risk factors of Graves' disease include genetic susceptibility such as HLA-B8, HLA-DR3 in Caucasians; HLA-DR5 in Japanese; HLA-DR9 in Chinese; HL-b13 and DR5/8 in Koreans[12]; polymorphism of CD 40 and CTLA-4 genes affecting the T helper cell function (reviewed in ref. [13]) infections, stress, sex steroids, pregnancy and the postpartum period, cigarette smoking, and iodine.[6,14]

Pathology of Graves's Disease

The gross and microscopic appearance of the thyroid gland in Graves' disease varies with preoperative treatment. In general, grossly the thyroid gland shows mild to moderate diffuse symmetrical enlargement with a smooth surface (Figure 5.1). The gland has a softer consistency than the normal thyroid and sectioning reveals a fleshy red-brown cut surface. Histological examination (Figure 5.2a–d) shows markedly hyperplastic follicles with sometimes irregular jagged contours, lined by tall columnar cells. The decreased amount of colloid may appear pale and depleted, with scalloping observed at the periphery. The thyrocytes may show epithelial hyperplasia with papillary and pseudopapillary formations. This latter feature together with the presence nuclear chromatin clearing and rare foci of calcifications mimicking psammoma bodies should not be mistaken for papillary carcinoma. The important distinguishing feature in Graves' disease is the diffuse presence of these changes throughout the gland, along with the presence of round, basally placed nuclei, and the absence of other nuclear changes of papillary carcinoma.[1] Additional histological features in Graves' disease include a variable degree of lymphocytic infiltrate of the stroma. The interstitial lymphoid cells are predominantly of T-helper (CD4) subtype that aid in the production of antibodies of the B cells.[15,16] Preoperative medical treatment may alter the characteristic histologic picture in Graves' disease: larger follicles filled with colloid or atrophied follicles with Hürthle cell metaplasia can be found mimicking Hashimoto's thyroiditis.[17,18] Iodine therapy can diminish hyperplasia resulting in almost normal appearing gland. Radioactive iodine may cause follicular disruption and atrophy with associated Hürthle cell metaplasia, fibrosis, and cellular and nuclear pleomorphism.[19] Propylthiouracil therapy may increase hyperplasia.

Thyroid Nodules and Cancer in Graves' Disease

Thyroid nodules are a common clinical problem in the general population, but the prevalence of palpable thyroid nodules in Graves' disease is increased by more than threefold when compared to the general population.[20] Whereas the prevalence of palpable thyroid nodule is 3.2–4.7% in iodine-

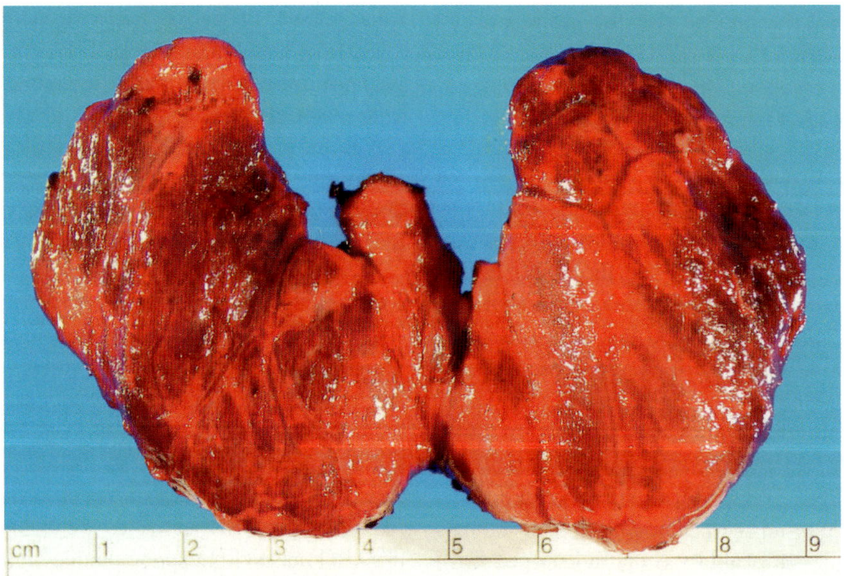

FIG. 5.1. Gross picture of a thyroidectomy specimen from a patient with Graves' disease.

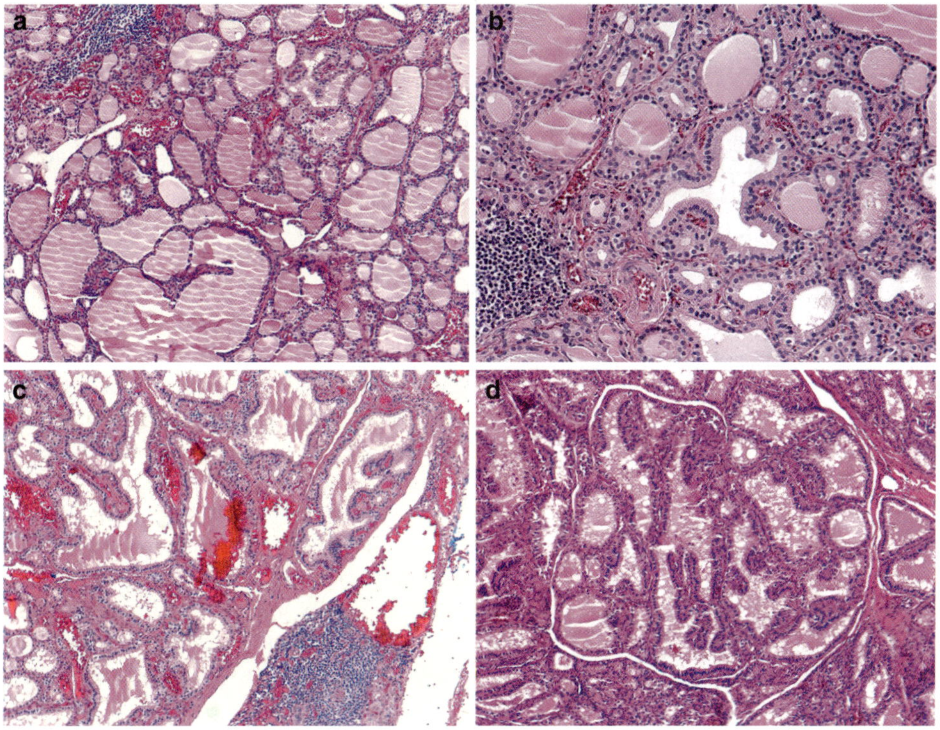

FIG. 5.2. Graves' disease; (**a**) hyperplastic thyroid follicles with irregular outlines and lymphocytic infiltrate (40×), (**b**) follicles lined by tall columnar thyrocytes (200×), (**c**) thyroid follicles with depleted colloid and peripheral scalloping of the colloid (100×), (**d**) thyroid follicles with multiple pseudo-papillary epithelial hyperplasia.

sufficient areas,[21] in one large multi-institution study the prevalence of palpable thyroid nodules in patients with hyperthyroidism was 15.8%.[22] Other studies have reported similar results.[18,20,23] The prevalence of cancer in Graves' disease has been reported to range from 0 to 9.8%, while in Graves' disease patients with palpable nodules the prevalence increased, ranging from 5.8 to 45.8%.[20] In a study that included 325 patients with Graves' disease, Stocker et al found papillary thyroid carcinoma in 1.85% of all these patients, in 15.2% of these patients with cold nodules on scintiscan; in 25% of these patients with palpable nodules, and in 27.3% of those undergoing surgery.[24] Thus, it seems that thyroid scintigraphy is an important preliminary investigation in the evaluation of Graves' disease patients, and the high prevalence of thyroid cancer in those patients with cold nodules and palpable nodules warrants further diagnostic evaluation including a fine needle aspiration biopsy. Thyroid cancer arising in the background of Graves' disease is thought to be of a more aggressive phenotype when compared to that in euthyroid patients. The patients may present with nodal and distant metastases, bilateral and multicentric tumors with invasive growth.[25–28] This, however, has not been supported by some other studies.[23,29–31] It is interesting to hypothesize if the anti-TSH receptor-stimulating antibodies may stimulate the thyroid cancer cells for an early metastatic growth in the same way as TSH stimulates growth of tumor cells expressing TSH receptor.[20]

Hashimoto's Thyroiditis

Historical Background

In 1912, H. Hashimoto described four cases goiter for which he called "struma lymphomatosa" (lymphomatous goiter).[32] All patients were females with goiter and the characteristic histological changes of lymphocytic thyroiditis which soon became known as Hashimoto's thyroiditis (HT). The autoimmune nature of this disease was established in 1956, when Roitt et al detected autoantibodies against thyroglobulin in patients with HT.[33] One year later, Trotter et al in 1957 identified a second antigen in the microsomal fraction of thyroid homogenates, which proved to be thyroid peroxidase (TPO).[34]

Clinical Features

Hashimoto's thyroiditis most frequently affects middle-aged women, though it is also the most common cause of sporadic goiter in children. It is the most common cause of hypothyroidism in areas of the world, where iodine levels are sufficient. Patients may present with hypothyroidism, goiter or both. Widespread use of thyroid function tests have also identified many cases of Hashimoto's thyroiditis with subclinical hypothyroidism characterized with positive anti-TPO and antithyroglobulin antibodies in the serum associated with high TSH and normal T4.[35] The goiter, when present, is firm and often lobulated, which may be mistaken for a multinodular goiter or carcinoma. Hashimoto's thyroiditis presenting as goitrous hypothyroidism has been found to be associated with HLA-D3 and HLA-D5.[36] It may also coexist with other autoimmune diseases including pernicious anemia, diabetes mellitus, Sjögren's syndrome, chronic hepatitis, adrenal insufficiency, and Graves' disease. There appears to be a familial predisposition for the development of Hashimoto's thyroiditis: up to 5% first-degree relatives of patients with Hashimoto's thyroiditis may have positive antithyroid antibodies in their serum.[36–38] There is also a high prevalence of autoimmune thyroid disease in patients with Down's syndrome, familial Alzheimer's disease, and Turner's syndrome.[39–43]

Pathogenesis of Hashimoto's Thyroiditis

Hashimoto's thyroiditis is a thyroid-specific autoimmune disorder, in which both humoral and cellular immune mechanisms play a role. The inflammatory process is initiated by the activation of thyroid-specific CD4 positive T helper cells.[44] The cause of the activation is not entirely clear; both viral and bacterial infections have been implicated,[45–47] but there are no conclusive supporting data. Another hypothesis implies that thyrocytes express HLA-DR antigen and become antigen-presenting cells, thereby exposing the thyroid cellular proteins to the CD4 T helper cells, which initiates the formation of autoantibodies against the thyroid autoantigens.[48–51] Thyroglobulin autoantibodies are prevalent in HT; high titers of anti-Tg IgG can be found in >80% of HT patients,[52] furthermore 94% of the Tg positive patients also have antibodies to TPO.[53] Anti-TPO antibodies are complement fixing and thus directly cytotoxic for thyrocytes.[54] Blocking anti-TSHR antibodies were detected in 10% of HT patients.[55] There is limited evidence that these effects play a major role in the destructive mechanisms of HT.

In addition to the pathway of thyroid cell injury, an alternative pathway involving cytotoxic T (CD8) cells and apoptosis has been more recently proposed.[56–66] It has been shown that a significant population of intrathyroidal lymphocytes in Hashimoto's thyroiditis are of CD8 phenotype having a cytotoxic/suppressor activity (reviewed in refs. [56,67]). Some studies have shown that follicular cells from tissue samples of Hashimoto's thyroiditis exhibit strong staining for the death receptor Fas and Fas ligand (FasL), together with a high apoptotic rate as compared normal controls.[68,69] Bcl-2 inhibits apoptosis; immunohistochemical studies have shown a decreased expression of Bcl-2 in thyroid follicles from Hashimoto's thyroiditis patients compared to normal controls and also in patients with Graves' disease. Furthermore, interfollicular lymphocytes exhibit weak staining for FasL and strong expression of bcl-2.[64,68,70] These data suggest that in patients with Hashimoto's thyroiditis, the thyrocytes undergo apoptosis by upregulation of Fas and FasL and downregulation of bcl-2, which is independent of the antibody-mediated thyroid cell injury.

Pathology of Hashimoto's Thyroiditis

The thyroid gland in Hashimoto's thyroiditis is symmetrically enlarged and has a pale pink to yellow, lobulated cut surface. The accentuation of the lobulations may make the gland appear nodular on gross examination. Characteristic histologic features of Hashimoto's thyroiditis include atrophy of the thyroid follicles with oncocytic (Hürthle cell) metaplasia of the follicular epithelium and abundant lymphoplasmacytic infiltrate with lymphoid follicles including germinal centers (Figure 5.3a–d). In addition, there may be varying degrees of fibrosis and foci of squamous metaplasia associated within the atrophic follicles. The peri-thyroidal lymph nodes are generally enlarged and show evidence of reactive lymphoid hyperplasia. The milieu of lymphocytic inflammation and regenerative hyperplasia results in increased risk of thyroid carcinoma and lymphoma. In some cases, there may be aggregates of oncocytic cells forming partially encapsulated hyperplastic nodules.[1] The oncocytic cells may show nuclear enlargement and cytologic atypia. The follicular cells may show clearing of the nuclear chromatin and grooves, which may be mistaken for papillary carcinoma.[1,71–73] Therefore, strict histologic criteria should be followed in making the diagnosis of papillary carcinoma in the background of Hashimoto's thyroiditis.[1] On immunohistochemistry, the lymphocytic population is composed of a mixture of B and T cells (Figure 5.4a–b). The T cells are predominantly activated CD4+ helper cells with evidence of HLADRII expression.[36,49] In addition, there are also CD8+ cytotoxic/suppressor T cells, B cells, and plasma cells.[36] As mentioned earlier, the CD8+ cells are thought to play a role in Fas-FasL-mediated thyroid follicular cell apoptosis and cytotoxicity. The plasma cells show reactivity with immunoglobulin γ (IgG), α (IgA) and μ (IgM) heavy chains and both κ and λ light chains. Immunohistochemistry may also be useful in differentiating a dense lymphoid infiltrate of Hashimoto's thyroiditis from lymphoma, which may arise in the background of Hashimoto's thyroiditis. The lymphoid infiltrate in Hashimoto's thyroiditis is polyclonal as described previously and lacks evidence of light chain restriction on κ or λ. Additional molecular studies and flow cytometry may sometimes be useful in difficult cases.

Histologic Variants of Hashimoto's Thyroiditis

In addition to the classic form of Hashimoto's thyroiditis, many variants have been described, including the following.

Fibrous Variant

This comprises approx 10% of the cases and is usually seen in elderly patients who present with markedly enlarged goiter and hypothyroidism.[74,75] On gross examination, the gland has a firm consistency due to a marked degree of fibrosis. Microscopically, there is extensive atrophy of the

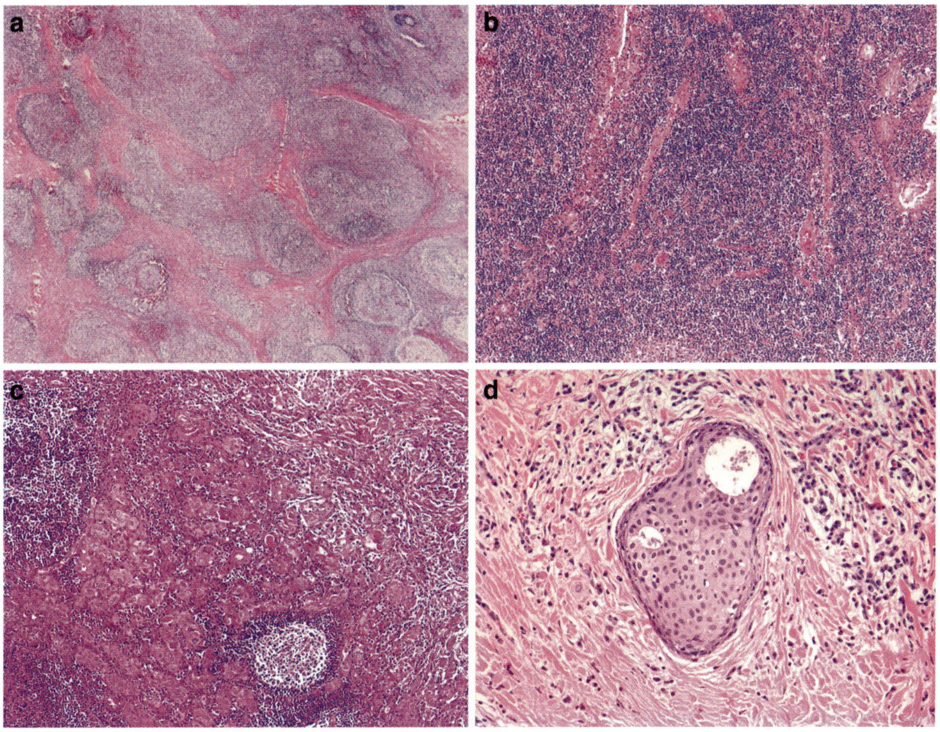

FIG. 5.3. Hashimoto's thyroiditis, (**a**) advanced disease with prominent lymphocytic infiltrate, fibrous septae and atrophic follicles (20×), (**b**) lymphocytic infiltrate and atrophic thyroid follicles (40×), (**c**) oncocytic or Hürtle cell metaplasia with a lymphoid follicle (100×), and (**d**) thyroid follicles with squamous metaplasia (400×).

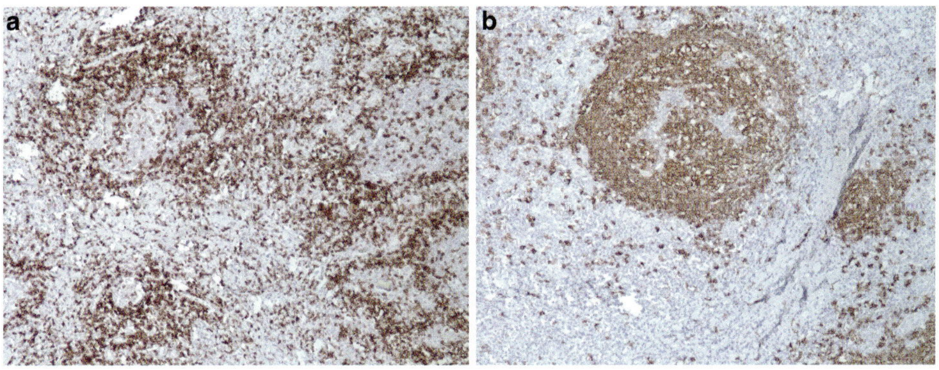

FIG. 5.4. Hashimoto's thyroiditis with (**a**) diffuse lymphocytic infiltrate including T lymphocytes (CD3 positive) and (**b**) B lymphocytes with lymphoid follicles (CD20 positive), immunoperoxidase staining.

thyroid follicles with diffuse fibrosis (Figure 5.5a–b), which in some areas has a keloid-like appearance. This fibrotic process is confined within the thyroid capsule, which is an important feature to distinguish it from Riedel's thyroiditis. In Riedel's thyroiditis, there is involvement of the surrounding structures such as muscles, nerves, and sometimes the parathyroid glands by the fibrotic process. Other features that help to differentiate are the lack of vasculitis or myointimal proliferation, which can be seen in Riedel's thyroiditis. Squamous metaplasia may be seen within the follicles. Foci of the classic form of Hashimoto's thyroiditis with lymphoplasmacytic infiltrate and oncocytic metaplasia may also be seen.

Fibrous Atrophy Variant

This is also referred to as idiopathic myxedema and is characterized by a very small (2–5 g in weight) fibrotic thyroid gland, which is often barely identifiable on gross examination.[71] There is widespread destruction of the thyroid parenchyma with replacement by fibrous stroma. The histological features are similar to the fibrous variant of

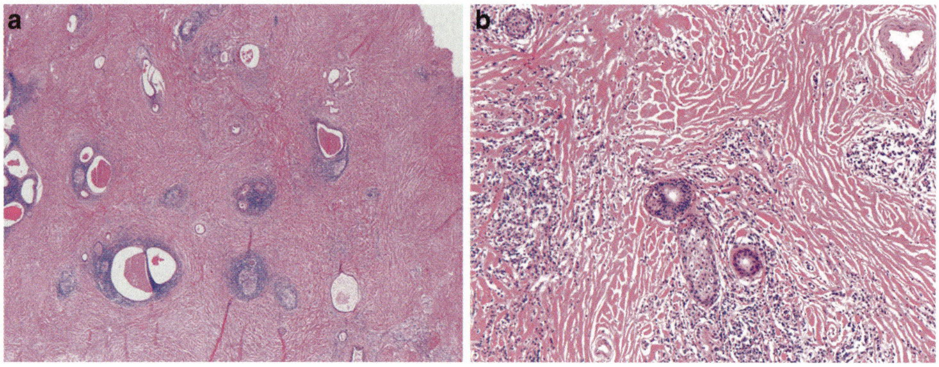

FIG. 5.5. Hashimoto's thyroiditis fibrosing variant, (**a**) dense fibrosis with atrophic follicles some showing squamous metaplasia (20×), (**b**) fibrosing variant with thick collagen fibers (200×).

Hashimoto's thyroiditis, the only difference being a much smaller gland.[5]

Juvenile Variant

This is a form chronic lymphocytic thyroiditis seen in younger patients and is often associated with hyperthyroidism, with later progression to hypothyroidism. The follicular atrophy and oncocytic metaplasia is focal and hyperplastic changes may be in the thyroid follicles.[71]

Other Forms of Thyroiditides

Riedel's Thyroiditis

Riedel's thyroiditis is a rare disorder causing hypothyroidism due to the destruction of the thyroid gland and its replacement by fibrous tissue. This extensive fibrotic process extends into the extrathyroidal tissues of the neck and therefore this entity has sometimes been referred to as *invasive fibrous thyroiditis.*[76] The clinical presenting features include a rapidly enlarging hard neck mass causing compression of the trachea and esophagus mimicking carcinoma.[77] Hypocalcemia due to hypoparathyroidism may sometimes be present because of the fibrous destruction of parathyroid.[78]

The etiology of Riedel's thyroiditis is not known; autoimmune inflammation has been suggested because of the lymphoplasmacytic infiltrate in the thyroid and the presence of thyroid autoantibodies reported in patients with Riedel's thyroiditis.[78] In view of the extensive fibrosis, Riedel's thyroiditis is also considered to be part of disseminated idiopathic fibrosing disorders, which include retroperitoneal and mediastinal fibrosis. These latter disorders have been found to be associated with or may develop after the diagnosis of Riedel's thyroiditis.[79]

The thyroid gland in Riedel's thyroiditis is enlarged with a hard consistency because of extensive asymmetrical fibrosis. This has been often referred to as "woody thyroid." The fibrosis often extends into the extrathyroidal soft tissues. On the cut surface, the gland is tan gray in color with loss of normal lobulations.[5] Microscopy reveals replacement of the normal thyroid parenchyma by dense sclerotic and acellular fibrous tissue. In addition, a mixed inflammatory infiltrate comprising mainly lymphocytes and plasma cells with few neutrophils and eosinophils may be seen. Vascular changes in the form of intimal proliferation and thrombosis may also be seen. In longstanding cases, the specimen may sometimes contain only dense sclerotic fibrous tissue with no residual thyroid follicles, making a diagnosis of Riedel's thyroiditis in the absence of thyroid tissue difficult. In these cases, a clinicopathological correlation is essential to make the diagnosis of Riedel's thyroiditis.

The differential diagnosis of Riedel's thyroiditis includes a fibrosing variant of Hashimoto's thyroiditis (see discussed above) and anaplastic carcinoma. Although this distinction can be more easily made on thyroidectomy specimens, small biopsies may sometimes pose a problem. Riedel's thyroiditis is distinguished from a paucicellular variant of anaplastic carcinoma by the absence of nuclear pleomorphism, atypia, and mitoses which are usually seen in the latter.[5]

Postpartum Thyroiditis

Postpartum thyroiditis is a rare autoimmune disorder characterized by transient hyperthyroidism followed by persistent hypothyroidism associated with lymphocytic infiltrate in the thyroid occurring within the first year after delivery.[78,80] It occurs up to 10% of the women in the US. It has been regarded as a variant of Hashimoto's thyroiditis.[81] The autoimmune etiology of postpartum thyroiditis has been supported by the finding of a more common prevalence of the disease among women with HLA-DR3, DR4, or DR5 phenotypes, which is similar to that seen in Hashimoto's thyroiditis. In addition, postpartum thyroiditis is seen associated with thyroid autoimmune disorders such as type I diabetes mellitus, Graves' disease, and primary autoimmune hypothyroidism.[80] Postpartum thyroiditis occurs most commonly in women with positive antithyroid peroxidase antibody in early pregnancy; the titers decline during pregnancy and then rapidly rise again after delivery.[80] The thyroid gland may be slightly diffusely enlarged and histology shows lymphocytic infiltrate associated with some follicular disruption and focal hyperplasia.[5]

Silent Thyroiditis

This form of thyroiditis has also been referred to as *atypical subacute thyroiditis*, *painless thyroiditis*, *chronic lymphocytic thyroiditis*, and *transient hyperthyroidism with lymphocytic thyroiditis*.[5] It shares abnormal thyroid function with subacute (de Quervain's) thyroiditis including transiently elevated blood levels of T4 and T3 associated with low radioactive iodine uptake. However, in contrast to the pain and tenderness seen in de Quervain's thyroiditis, patients present with a painless thyroid enlargement.[8] The etiology of silent thyroiditis is uncertain, both autoimmune and viral etiology has been proposed.[82] On gross examination, there is slight diffuse enlargement of the thyroid gland. Microscopy shows preservation of the lobular architecture with a varying degree of lymphocytic infiltrate and associated follicular destruction. Oncocytic change may be seen but is uncommon.

Focal Lymphocytic Thyroiditis

This is mostly an incidental finding discovered in either surgically removed thyroid or at autopsy and is characterized by a focal lymphocytic infiltrate with preservation of normal lobular architecture and no significant alteration of thyroid functions. It is seen in 5–20% of adult autopsies, mostly in elderly women.[5] On gross examination, no specific changes can be seen. Microscopy reveals preservation of the follicular architecture with foci of lymphocytic infiltrate, which may be associated with germinal center formation in the interfollicular region. Focal lymphocytic thyroiditis may be seen associated with multinodular goiter and thyroid tumors.[5]

References

1. Baloch ZW, LiVolsi VA. Pathology of the thyroid gland. In: LiVolsi VA, Asa SL, eds. *Endocrine Pathology*. New York: Churchill Livingstone; 2002:61–88.
2. Murray D. The thyroid gland. In: Kalman K, Asa S, eds. *Functional Endocrine Pathology*. Oxford, UK: Blackwell; 1998:295–380.
3. Parry C. Collections from the Unpublished Medical Writings of the Late Caleb Hillier Parry. Diseases of the Heart. Enlargement of the Thyroid Gland in connection with Enlargement or Palpitation of the Heart. *London Underwoods Fleet-Street*. 1825:111–129.
4. Sawin C. The heritage of the thyroid. In: Braverman LE, Utiger RD, eds. *Werenr and Ingbar's the Thyroid: A Fundamental and Clinical Text*. Philadelphia: Lippincott Williams & Wilkins; 2000:3–6.
5. Lloyd R, Douglas B, Young W. Thyroid gland. In: Lloyd R, Douglas B, Young W, eds. *Atlas of Nontumor Pathology: Endocrine Diseases*. Washington, DC: Armed Forces Institute of Pathology; 2002:91–169.
6. Davies T. The pathogenesis of Graves' disease. In: Braverman LE, Utiger RD, eds. *Werner and Ingbar's the Thyroid: A Fundamental and Clinical Text*. Philadelphia: Lippincott-Raven; 1996:525–536.
7. Dai G, Levy O, Carrasco N. Cloning and characterization of the thyroid iodide transporter. *Nature*. 1996;379:458.
8. Daniels GH. Atypical subacute thyroiditis: preliminary observations. *Thyroid*. 2001;11:691–695.
9. Uyttersprot N, Allgeier A, Baptist M, et al. The cAMP in thyroid: from the TSH receptor to mitogenesis and tumorigenesis. *Adv Second Messenger Phosphoprotein Res*. 1997;31:125–140.
10. Burch HB, Nagy EV, Lukes YG, Cai WY, Wartofsky L, Burman KD. Nucleotide and amino acid homology between the human thyrotropin receptor and the HIV-1 Nef protein: identification and functional analysis. *Biochem Biophys Res Commun*. 1991;181:498–505.
11. Londei M, Lamb JR, Bottazzo GF, Feldmann M. Epithelial cells expressing aberrant MHC class II determinants can present antigen to cloned human T cells. *Nature*. 1984;312:639–641.
12. McLachlan SM, Rapoport B. Genetic factors in thyroid disease. In: Braverman LE, Utiger RD, eds. *Werner and Ingbar's the Thyroid: A Fundamental and Clinical Text*. 8th ed. Philadelphia: Lippincott Williams & Wilkins; 2000:474–487.
13. Jacobson EM, Tomer Y. The CD40, CTLA-4, thyroglobulin, TSH receptor, and PTPN22 gene quintet and its contribution to thyroid autoimmunity: back to the future. *J Autoimmun*. 2007;28:85–98.
14. Rose NR, Bonita R, Burek CL. Iodine: an environmental trigger of thyroiditis. *Autoimmun Rev*. 2002;1:97–103.
15. Burman KD, Baker JR Jr. Immune mechanisms in Graves' disease. *Endocr Rev*. 1985;6:183–232.
16. Paschke R, Schuppert F, Taton M, Velu T. Intrathyroidal cytokine gene expression profiles in autoimmune thyroiditis. *J Endocrinol*. 1994;141:309–315.
17. Chang DC, Wheeler MH, Woodcock JP, et al. The effect of preoperative Lugol's iodine on thyroid blood flow in patients with Graves' hyperthyroidism. *Surgery*. 1987;102:1055–1061.
18. Carnell NE, Valente WA. Thyroid nodules in Graves' disease: classification, characterization, and response to treatment. *Thyroid*. 1998;8:647–652.
19. McNicol A, Lewis P. The endocrine system. In: Lewis P, Symmers WE, eds. *Systemic Pathology*, vol. 1. 3rd ed. Edinburgh: Churchill Livingstone; 1996:131–185.
20. Belfiore A, Russo D, Vigneri R, Filetti S. Graves' disease, thyroid nodules and thyroid cancer. *Clin Endocrinol*. 2001;55:711–718.
21. Vander JB, Gaston EA, Dawber TR. The significance of nontoxic thyroid nodules. Final report of a 15-year study of the incidence of thyroid malignancy. *Ann Intern Med*. 1968;69:537–540.
22. Dobyns BM, Sheline GE, Workman JB, Tompkins EA, McConahey WM, Becker DV. Malignant and benign neoplasms of the thyroid in patients treated for hyperthyroidism: a report of the cooperative thyrotoxicosis therapy follow-up study. *J Clin Endocrinol Metab*. 1974;38:976–998.
23. Pacini F, Elisei R, Di Coscio GC, et al. Thyroid carcinoma in thyrotoxic patients treated by surgery. *J Endocrinol Invest*. 1988;11:107–112.
24. Stocker DJ, Foster SS, Solomon BL, Shriver CD, Burch HB. Thyroid cancer yield in patients with Graves' disease selected for surgery on the basis of cold scintiscan defects. *Thyroid*. 2002;12:305–311.

25. Ozaki O, Ito K, Kobayashi K, Toshima K, Iwasaki H, Yashiro T. Thyroid carcinoma in Graves' disease. *World J Surg*. 1990;14:437–440.
26. Belfiore A, Garofalo MR, Giuffrida D, et al. Increased aggressiveness of thyroid cancer in patients with Graves' disease. *J Clin Endocrinol Metab*. 1990;70:830–835.
27. Mazzaferri EL. Thyroid cancer and Graves' disease. *J Clin Endocrinol Metab*. 1990;70:826-829.
28. Behar R, Arganini M, Wu TC, et al. Graves' disease and thyroid cancer. *Surgery*. 1986;100:1121–1127.
29. Shapiro SJ, Friedman NB, Perzik SL, Catz B. Incidence of thyroid carcinoma in Graves' disease. *Cancer*. 1970;26:1261–1270.
30. Edmonds CJ, Tellez M. Hyperthyroidism and thyroid cancer. *Clin Endocrinol*. 1988;28:253–259.
31. Hales IB. Does Graves' disease or thyrotoxicosis affect the prognosis of thyroid cancer. *J Clin Endocrinol Metab*. 1992;75: 886–889.
32. Hashimoto H. Notes on lymphomatic thyroid changes (struma lymphomatosa). *Arch Klin Chirur*. 1912;97:219.
33. Roitt IM, Doniach D, Campbell PN, Hudson RV. Autoantibodies in Hashimoto's disease (lymphadenoid goitre). *Lancet*. 1956;2:820–821.
34. Trotter W, Belyavin G, Wadhams A. Precipitating and complement- fixing antibodies in Hashimoto's disease. *Proc R Soc Med*. 1957;50:961.
35. Weetman A. Chronic autoimmune thyroiditis. In: Braverman LE, Utiger RD, eds. *Werner and Ingbar's the Thyroid: A Fundamental and Clinical Text*. 8th ed. Philadelphia: Lippincott Williams & Wilkins; 2000:721–732.
36. del Prete GF. Cytolytic T lymphocytes with natural killer activity in thyroid infiltrate of patients with Hashimoto's thyroiditis: analysis at clonal level. *J Clin Endocrinol Metab*. 1986;62:52–57.
37. Burman P. Thyroid autoimmunity in patients on long term therapy with leukocyte-derived interferon. *J Clin Endocrinol Metab*. 1986;63:1086–1090.
38. Chopra IJ, Solomon DH, Chopra U, Yoshihara E, Terasaki PI, Smith F. Abnormalities in thyroid function in relatives of patients with Graves' disease and Hashimoto's thyroiditis: lack of correlation with inheritance of HLA-B8. *J Clin Endocrinol Metab*. 1977;45:45–54.
39. Doniach D, Bottazzo GF, Russell RC. Goitrous autoimmune thyroiditis (Hashimoto's disease). *Clin Endocrinol Metab*. 1979;8:63–80.
40. Ewins DL, Rossor MN, Butler J, Rogues PK, Mullen MJ, McGregor AM. Association between autoimmune thyroid disease and Familial Alzheimers disease. *Clin Endocrinol*. 1991;35:93–96.
41. Kennedy RL, Jones TH, Cuckle HS. Down's syndrome and the thyroid. *Clin Endocrinol*. 1992;37:471–476.
42. Shalitin S, Phillip M. Autoimmune thyroiditis in infants with Down's syndrome. *J Pediatr Endocrinol Metab*. 2002;15:649–652.
43. Roitt IM, Doniach D. A reassessment of studies on the aggregation of thyroid autoimmunity in families of thyroiditis patients. *Clin Exp Immunol*. 1967;2:727.
44. Weetman AP. Autoimmune thyroid disease: further developments in our understanding. *Endocr Rev*. 1994;15:788–830.
45. Tomer Y. Infection, thyroid disease, and autoimmunity. *Endocr Rev*. 1993;14:107–120.
46. Valtonen VV, Ruutu P, Varis K, Ranki M, Malkamaki M, Makela PH. Serological evidence for the role of bacterial infections in the pathogenesis of thyroid diseases. *Acta Med Scand*. 1986;219:105–111.
47. Dayan CM, Daniels GH. Chronic autoimmune thyroiditis. *N Engl J Med*. 1996;335:99.
48. Hanafusa T, Pujol-Borrell R, Chiovato L, Russell RC, Doniach D, Bottazzo GF. Aberrant expression of HLA-DR antigen on thyrocytes in Graves' disease: relevance for autoimmunity. *Lancet*. 1983;2:1111–1115.
49. Lloyd RV, Johnson TL, Blaivas M, Sisson JC, Wilson BS. Detection of HLA-DR antigens in paraffin-embedded thyroid epithelial cells with a monoclonal antibody. *Am J Pathol*. 1985;120:106.
50. Tamai H. Resistance to autoimmune thyroid disease is associated with HLA-DQ. *J Clin Endocrinol Metab*. 1994;78:94–97.
51. Yu M, Xu M, Savas L, Khan A. Discordant expression of Ii and HLA-DR in thyrocytes: a possible pathogenetic factor in Hashimoto's thyroiditis. *Endocr Pathol*. 1998;9:201–208.
52. Gentile F, Conte M, Formisano S. Thyroglobulin as an autoantigen: what can we learn about immunopathogenicity from the correlation of antigenic properties with protein structure? *Immunology*. 2004;112:13–25.
53. Tozzoli R, Villalta D, Kodermaz G, Bagnasco M, Tonutti E, Bizzaro N. Autoantibody profiling of patients with autoimmune thyroid disease using a new multiplexed immunoassay method. *Clin Chem Lab Med*. 2006;44:837.
54. Chiovato L. Antibodies producing complement-mediated thyroid cytotoxicity in patients with atrophic or goitrous autoimmune thyroiditis. *J Clin Endocrinol Metab*. 1993;77:1700–1705.
55. Tamaki H. Low prevalence of thyrotropin receptor antibody in primary hypothyroidism in Japan. *J Clin Endocrinol Metab*. 1990;71:1382–1386.
56. Bermann M. Differential autoantibody responses to thyroid peroxidase in patients with Graves' disease and Hashimoto's thyroiditis. *J Clin Endocrinol Metab*. 1993;77:1098–1101.
57. Giordano C, Stassi G, De Maria R, et al. Potential involvement of Fas and its ligand in the pathogenesis of Hashimoto's thyroiditis. *Science*. 1997;275:960–963.
58. Williams N. Autoimmunity: thyroid disease – A case of cell suicide? *Science*. 1997;275:926.
59. Arscott PL, Baker JR. Apoptosis and thyroiditis. *Clin Immunol Immunopathol*. 1998;87:207–217.
60. Palazzo FF, Hammond LJ, Goode AW, Mirakian R. Death of the autoimmune thyrocyte: is it pushed or does it jump? *Thyroid*. 2000;10:561–572.
61. Andrikoula M, Tsatsoulis A. The role of Fas-mediated apoptosis in thyroid disease. *Eur J Endocrinol*. 2001;144:561.
62. Lin JD. The role of apoptosis in autoimmune thyroid disorders and thyroid cancer. *BMJ*. 2001;322:1525–1527.
63. Stassi G, De Maria R. Autoimmune thyroid disease: new models of cell death in autoimmunity. *Nat Rev Immunol*. 2002;2:195–204.
64. Mitsiades N, Poulaki V, Mitsiades CS, Koutras DA, Chrousos GP. Apoptosis induced by FasL and TRAIL/Apo2L in the pathogenesis of thyroid diseases. *Trends Endocrinol Metab*. 2001;12:384–390.
65. Eguchi K. Apoptosis in autoimmune diseases. *Intern Med*. 2001;40:275–284.
66. Phelps E, Wu P, Bretz J, Baker JR. Thyroid cell apoptosis a new understanding of thyroid autoimmunity. *Endocrinol Metab Clin North Am*. 2000;29:375–388.
67. DeGroot LJ. The causes of autoimmune thyroid disease. *Endocr Rev*. 1989;10:537–562.
68. Hammond LJ, Lowdell MW, Cerrano PG, Goode AW, Bottazzo GF, Mirakian R. Analysis of apoptosis in relation to tissue

destruction associated with Hashimoto's autoimmune thyroiditis. *J Pathol.* 1997;182:138–144.
69. Stassi G, Todaro M, Bucchieri F, et al. Fas/Fas ligand-driven T cell apoptosis as a consequence of ineffective thyroid immunoprivilege in Hashimoto's thyroiditis. *J Immunol.* 1999;162:263–267.
70. Jiang Z, Savas L, Patwardhan NA, Wuu J, Khan A. Frequency and distribution of DNA fragmentation in Hashimoto's thyroiditis and development of papillary thyroid carcinoma. *Endocr Pathol.* 1999;10:137–144.
71. Livolsi VA. *Surgical Pathology of the Thyroid.* Philadelphia: Saunders; 1990.
72. Rosai J, Carcangiu ML, DeLellis RA. *Tumors of the Thyroid Gland-Atlas of Tumor Pathology.* Washington: Armed Forces Institute of Pathology; 1990.
73. Berho M, Suster S. Clear nuclear changes in Hashimoto's thyroiditis. A clinicopathologic study of 12 cases. *Ann Clin Lab Sci.* 1995;25:513–521.
74. Harach HR, Williams ED. Fibrous thyroiditis-an immunopathological study. *Histopathology.* 1983;7:739–751.
75. Katz SM, Vickery AL Jr. The fibrous variant of Hashimoto's thyroiditis. *Hum Pathol.* 1974;5:161–170.
76. Singer P. Primary hypothyroidism due to other causes. In: Braverman LE, Utiger RD, eds. *Werner and Ingbar's the Thyroid: A Fundamental and Clinical Text.* 8th ed. Philadelphia: Lippincott Williams & Wilkins; 2000:755–761.
77. De Lange WE, Freling NJM, Molenaar WM, Doorenbos H. Invasive fibrous thyroiditis (Riedel's struma): a manifestation of multifocal fibrosclerosis? A case report with review of the literature. *Q J Med.* 1989;72:709–717.
78. Best TB, Munro RE, Burwell S, Volpe R. Riedel's thyroiditis associated with Hashimoto's thyroiditis, hypoparathyroidism, and retroperitoneal fibrosis. *J Endocrinol Invest.* 1991;14: 767–772.
79. Hay ID. Thyroiditis: a clinical update. *Mayo Clin Proc.* 1985;60:836–843.
80. Roti E, Uberti E. Post-partum thyroiditis – A clinical update. *Eur J Endocrinol.* 2002;146:275–279.
81. Stagnaro-Green A. Postpartum thyroiditis: prevalence, etiology, and clinical implications. *Thyroid Today.* 1993; 16:1–11.
82. Volpe R. Is silent thyroiditis an autoimmune disease? *Arch Intern Med.* 1988;148:1907–1908.

6
Benign Nodular Thyroid Disease

Jennifer L. Hunt

Introduction

Benign nodular disease of the thyroid gland is exceedingly common in most of the world. In fact, some estimates have suggested that up to 70% of the population in the United States will have thyroid nodules detectable by ultrasound. The diagnostic categories for benign nodular thyroids include both multinodular disease and dominant single nodules, which can be of neoplastic or nonneoplastic origin. The benign nodular thyroid diseases are discussed in this chapter, along with the relevant molecular pathogenesis.

Sporadic Multinodular Goiter

Goiter is defined as diffuse or nodular enlargement of the thyroid gland. Goiter can have a variety of different etiologies, but importantly it should not be related to inflammatory processes. Multinodular goiter remains most common in endemic areas, where the disease is strongly associated with iodine deficiency in these selected geographic areas.[4] Endemic goiter that develops secondary to iodine insufficiency should affect both genders equally, but in most studies women are more susceptible than men, and there are still familial tendencies for the disease to occur.[4] This suggests that there are multiple factors, both environmental and genetic that contribute to the development of goiter. In nonendemic regions, goiter is much more common in women and the prevalence can still be relatively high, ranging between 0.4 and 5%.[4] The treatment for symptomatic goiter in particular generally remains surgical, with either a subtotal or total thyroidectomy.[31,41,43]

Goiter is often accompanied by one or more dominant nodules, which have been traditionally considered to be nonneoplastic nodules. At the histologic level, nodules arising in goiter can have a variety of different appearances. These nodules are usually not fully encapsulated, though they can have fibrosis within the nodule or around the periphery. The growth pattern within the lesion is nearly identical to that in the surrounding thyroid gland. This includes variably sized follicles, some of which are quite large and expanded by colloid. Reactive changes are common, including hemorrhage, cystic degeneration, and hemosiderin laden macrophage deposition. The terminology used for histologically documented nonneoplastic nodules in goiter is "dominant hyperplastic nodule."

Because of their multiplicity, the absence of a capsule, and the generally macro-follicular growth pattern, nodules in goiter were originally thought to be nonneoplastic and thus nonclonal. However, in several elegant studies which examined the clonality of these lesions using X-inactivation, (HUMARA assay) it has been shown that at least some nodules in multinodular goiter are clonal.[1,8,18,28] Follicular adenomas have always been thought to be clonal proliferations, and this has also been shown to be true at the molecular level, through analysis of somatic mutations in oncogenes, loss of heterozygosity analysis of tumors suppressor genes, and through X-inactivation studies.[1,11,16,29,39]

Hereditary Causes of Goiter

Hereditary, familial, or clustering within families who demonstrate multinodular goiter has been described and been studied for years, but relatively few gene candidates have been proposed. This is likely because goiter, like most other complex diseases, is polygenic. There are both environmental and genetic contributions to goiter as well. The purely genetic contribution is best illustrated through careful twin studies. In epidemiological analysis of monozygotic and dizygotic twin pairs, the genetic contribution to development of goiter has been estimated at 82%.[4]

Several gene candidates have been proposed to be associated with the development of goiter. The thyroglobulin gene (chromosome 8), multinodular goiter gene (MNG1, chromosome 14), TSH-receptor (chromosome 14q13), the Na^+/I^- symporter gene (NIS, chromosome 19p13.2–p12), and Gs alpha subunit gene (chromosome 20q13.2) have all been implicated for potential genetic contributions to goiter.[3,7,12,30,32]

J.L. Hunt (ed.), *Molecular Pathology of Endocrine Diseases*, Molecular Pathology Library 3,
DOI 10.1007/978-1-4419-1707-2_6, © Springer Science+Business Media, LLC 2010

Congenital Hypothyroidism

Congenital hypothyroidism is a condition that can have clinically devastating consequences if it goes unrecognized. But, newborn screening programs have greatly reduced the ramifications of this condition. Congenital hypothyroidism has both genetic and nongenetic contributions. It can also be a temporary condition caused by maternal factors, such as antibodies or drugs that cross the placenta and affect the newborn.

The presentation of a newborn with congenital hypothyroidism includes post-maturity, large posterior fontanel, and various forms of thyroid dysgenesis.[21] The dysgenesis can include agenesis, ectopic glands, or hypoplastic glands, or they can have enlarged thyroid glands.

Congenital hypothyroidism is a heterogeneous disorder with many potential genetic alterations. Defects in the pathways involved in thyroid hormone synthesis, storage, secretion, or utilization are more common and are referred to as primary hypothyroidism.[9,14,33] Defects at the pituitary or hypothalamic level that lead to congenital hypothyroidism, termed central hypothyroidism, are extremely rare.[9] Most cases are considered to be sporadic, with maximal estimates of 15% of cases being hereditary.[21] In the inherited cases, the inheritance patterns vary with the genetic mutations, but include autosomal dominant, recessive, and X-linked possibilities.[14]

Mutations have been described in many different genes, including the TSH receptor, the thyrotropin receptor, the Na^+/I^- symporter gene, and many other genes in the thyroid hormone pathways.[14,21] Several specific transcription factors have also been implicated in both the sporadic and hereditary forms of thyroid dysgenesis. These include PAX8 (chromosome 2q12–q14), TTF1 (NKX2.1, chromosome 14q13), and TTF2 (FOXE1, chromosome 9q22).[33] TTF2 germline mutations are responsible for the thyroid dysgenesis syndrome Bamforth–Lazarus syndrome.[33] Mutations in the pendrin gene (SLC26A4, chromosome 7q31) are responsible for the Pendred syndrome, which includes sensorineural hearing defects and goiter and iodine organification defects.[24,33]

Thyroid goiter is generally seen in patients with dyshormonogenesis. These thyroids have a unique histologic appearance, with bizarre atypical cells and abnormal architecture. Dyshormongenic goiter is generally seen in patients with defects in the steps leading to synthesis of thyroid hormone. The genes most commonly implicated are the thyroperoxidase, thyroglobulin, Na^+/I^- symporter gene, and the NADPH oxidases (such as thyroid oxidase-2, THOX2).[9]

Follicular Adenoma

Perhaps, the most common neoplastic condition of the thyroid is a benign follicular adenoma.[26] The typical follicular adenoma will be an encapsulated lesion with a follicular growth pattern. These tumors can also have oncocytic changes, in which case they may be referred to as "Hürthle cell adenoma." The lesion should have a reasonably complete capsule, though it may be variably thick and thin. Several other clues to the diagnosis of a neoplasm include the following: the nodule follicles should be different from the thyroid parenchyma outside of the nodule, and the thyroid follicles are often compressed and flattened on the outside of the nodule. Importantly, the cells are bland and remain small and round. They are essentially identical to thyroid follicular cells in the background thyroid gland. The cells in adenomas can also have Hurthle or oncocytic differentiation.

Thyroid follicular adenomas have been extensively studied at the molecular level. One of the first oncogenes discovered in the thyroid gland was the *RAS* gene, which is part of the RAS-RAF-MEK-MAPK pathway.[23] Follicular adenomas have been long known to harbor mutations in all three *RAS* genes, *H-RAS*, *K-RAS*, and *N-RAS*.[11,19,27] The *RAS* mutations are thought to be early mutations in the follicular neoplasia pathway, and therefore testing for *RAS* mutations has have never had a strong diagnostic role.[29]

Tumor suppressor gene alterations have been described in both benign and malignant follicular derived tumors. The genes involved are diverse and encompass a spectrum of common tumor suppressor genes. However, it has been shown in several studies that the rate of tumor suppressor gene loss of heterozygosity alterations in follicular adenomas is significantly lower than that seen in follicular carcinoma.[16,36,38] This is particularly true when adenomas are compared to follicular carcinomas with poor clinical outcome and higher grade histologic features.[17] In several CGH-based studies, follicular adenomas and follicular carcinomas did not have a vastly different profile of losses and gains, and these changes did not appear to be consistent from tumor to tumor.[5,37] One study did separate out cases diagnosed as aneuploid "fetal adenoma," which appeared to have a very consistent molecular profile that included gains of chromosomes 4, 5,7, 12, 14, 16, and 17 and losses of chromosomes 2, 11, and 15.[5]

Several studies have examined gene expression profiling to determine whether the expression patterns can differentiate between benign and malignant follicular tumors. Recent evidence does indicate that the profiles are different.[6,45] Despite the fact that there is an attempt to narrow the genes to a limited set of the most informative,[44] the clinical implications of these findings are still unclear, as the technique remains expensive and difficult to perform for routine tumor classification.

Papillary Hyperplastic Nodules

Some adenomas, or even benign hyperplastic nodules, can have an exuberant papillary growth pattern.[25] These lesions are often clinically found to be "hot" or toxic thyroid nodules. They tend to be particularly common in younger women.[2,10,20] They have been alternatively termed "papillary hyperplastic nodules" or follicular adenomas with papillary growth.

The striking feature in these lesions is a marked papillary growth pattern. But, in all of these lesions, the most critical diagnostic clue is the absence of nuclear features of papillary carcinoma. The nuclei tend to be small, dark, and basally located in the cells.[25] Other softer signs include edema and follicles within the papillary cores and the fact that the papillae are quite organized and tend to all point toward the center of the lesion. These are very important lesions to recognize, so that a misdiagnosis of carcinoma is not made.

Interesting molecular findings have been described in papillary hyperplastic nodules. More than half of these hyperfunctional nodules, both in a background of goiter and in the setting of solitary nodules, have been shown to harbor clonal mutations in the TSH-receptor.[12,13,15,22,34,35,40,42] These tumors do not appear to harbor mutations in the RAS genes.[32]

References

1. Apel RL, Ezzat S, Bapat BV, Pan N, LiVolsi VA, Asa SL. Clonality of thyroid nodules in sporadic goiter. *Diagn Mol Pathol*. 1995;4:113–121.
2. Baloch ZW, LiVolsi VA. Cytologic and architectural mimics of papillary thyroid carcinoma. Diagnostic challenges in fine-needle aspiration and surgical pathology specimens. *Am J Clin Pathol*. 2006;125 Suppl:S135–S144.
3. Bignell GR, Canzian F, Shayeghi M, et al. Familial nontoxic multinodular thyroid goiter locus maps to chromosome 14q but does not account for familial nonmedullary thyroid cancer. *Am J Hum Genet*. 1997;61:1123–1130.
4. Brix TH, Hegedus L. Genetic and environmental factors in the aetiology of simple goitre. *Ann Med*. 2000;32:153–156.
5. Castro P, Eknaes M, Teixeira MR, et al. Adenomas and follicular carcinomas of the thyroid display two major patterns of chromosomal changes. *J Pathol*. 2005;206:305–311.
6. Denning KM, Smyth PC, Cahill SF, et al. A molecular expression signature distinguishing follicular lesions in thyroid carcinoma using preamplification RT-PCR in archival samples. *Mod Pathol*. 2007;20:1095–1102.
7. Derrien C, Sonnet E, Gicquel I, et al. Non-hyperfunctioning nodules from multinodular goiters: a minor role in pathogenesis for somatic activating mutations in the TSH-receptor and Gsalpha subunit genes. *J Endocrinol Invest*. 2001;24:321–325.
8. Derwahl M. Molecular aspects of the pathogenesis of nodular goiters, thyroid nodules and adenomas. *Exp Clin Endocrinol Diabetes*. 1996;104(Suppl 4):32–35.
9. Djemli A, Van Vliet G, Delvin EE. Congenital hypothyroidism: from paracelsus to molecular diagnosis. *Clin Biochem*. 2006;39:511–518.
10. Drut R. Aspiration cytology of papillary hyperplastic thyroid nodule. *Arch Pathol Lab Med*. 2002;126:1156. author reply 1156–1157.
11. Ezzat S, Zheng L, Kolenda J, Safarian A, Freeman JL, Asa SL. Prevalence of activating ras mutations in morphologically characterized thyroid nodules. *Thyroid*. 1996;6:409–416.
12. Gabriel EM, Bergert ER, Grant CS, van Heerden JA, Thompson GB, Morris JC. Germline polymorphism of codon 727 of human thyroid-stimulating hormone receptor is associated with toxic multinodular goiter. *J Clin Endocrinol Metab*. 1999;84:3328–3335.
13. Gozu H, Avsar M, Bircan R, et al. Mutations in the thyrotropin receptor signal transduction pathway in the hyperfunctioning thyroid nodules from multinodular goiters: a study in the Turkish population. *Endocr J*. 2005;52:577–585.
14. Gruters A, Krude H, Biebermann H. Molecular genetic defects in congenital hypothyroidism. *Eur J Endocrinol*. 2004;151 (Suppl 3):U39–U44.
15. Holzapfel HP, Fuhrer D, Wonerow P, Weinland G, Scherbaum WA, Paschke R. Identification of constitutively activating somatic thyrotropin receptor mutations in a subset of toxic multinodular goiters. *J Clin Endocrinol Metab*. 1997;82: 4229–4233.
16. Hunt JL, Livolsi VA, Baloch ZW, et al. A novel microdissection and genotyping of follicular-derived thyroid tumors to predict aggressiveness. *Hum Pathol*. 2003;34:375–380.
17. Hunt JL, Yim JH, Carty SE. Fractional allelic loss of tumor suppressor genes identifies malignancy and predicts clinical outcome in follicular thyroid tumors. *Thyroid*. 2006;16:643–649.
18. Iliszko M, Kuzniacka A, Lachinski A, Babinska M, Kobierska-Gulida G, Limon J. Karyotypic characterization of 64 nonmalignant thyroid goiters. *Cancer Genet Cytogenet*. 2005;161: 178–180.
19. Karga H, Lee JK, Vickery AL Jr, Thor A, Gaz RD, Jameson JL. Ras oncogene mutations in benign and malignant thyroid neoplasms. *J Clin Endocrinol Metab*. 1991;73:832–836.
20. Khurana KK, Baloch ZW, LiVolsi VA. Aspiration cytology of pediatric solitary papillary hyperplastic thyroid nodule. *Arch Pathol Lab Med*. 2001;125:1575–1578.
21. Kratzsch J, Pulzer F. Thyroid gland development and defects. *Best Pract Res Clin Endocrinol Metab*. 2008;22:57–75.
22. Krohn K, Paschke R. Somatic mutations in thyroid nodular disease. *Mol Genet Metab*. 2002;75:202–208.
23. Lemoine NR, Mayall ES, Wyllie FS, et al. High frequency of ras oncogene activation in all stages of human thyroid tumorigenesis. *Oncogene*. 1989;4:159–164.
24. Lofrano-Porto A, Barra GB, Nascimento PP, et al. Pendred syndrome in a large consanguineous Brazilian family caused by a homozygous mutation in the SLC26A4 gene. *Arq Bras Endocrinol Metabol*. 2008;52:1296–1303.
25. Mai KT, Landry DC, Thomas J, et al. Follicular adenoma with papillary architecture: a lesion mimicking papillary thyroid carcinoma. *Histopathology*. 2001;39:25–32.
26. Mazzaferri EL. Solitary thyroid nodule. 1. Clinical characteristics. *Postgrad Med*. 1981;70:98–103.
27. Namba H, Gutman RA, Matsuo K, Alvarez A, Fagin JA. H-ras protooncogene mutations in human thyroid neoplasms. *J Clin Endocrinol Metab*. 1990;71:223–229.
28. Namba H, Matsuo K, Fagin JA. Clonal composition of benign and malignant human thyroid tumors. *J Clin Invest*. 1990;86: 120–125.
29. Namba H, Rubin SA, Fagin JA. Point mutations of ras oncogenes are an early event in thyroid tumorigenesis. *Mol Endocrinol*. 1990;4:1474–1479.
30. Neumann S, Willgerodt H, Ackermann F, et al. Linkage of familial euthyroid goiter to the multinodular goiter-1 locus and exclusion of the candidate genes thyroglobulin, thyroperoxidase, and Na+/I-symporter. *J Clin Endocrinol Metab*. 1999;84:3750–3756.
31. Olson SE, Starling J, Chen H. Symptomatic benign multinodular goiter: unilateral or bilateral thyroidectomy? *Surgery*. 2007;142:458–461. discussion 461–462.

32. Palos-Paz F, Perez-Guerra O, Cameselle-Teijeiro J, et al. Prevalence of mutations in TSHR, GNAS, PRKAR1A and RAS genes in a large series of toxic thyroid adenomas from Galicia, an iodine-deficient area in NW Spain. *Eur J Endocrinol.* 2008;159:623–631.
33. Park SM, Chatterjee VK. Genetics of congenital hypothyroidism. *J Med Genet.* 2005;42:379–389.
34. Paschke R. Constitutively activating TSH receptor mutations as the cause of toxic thyroid adenoma, multinodular toxic goiter and autosomal dominant non autoimmune hyperthyroidism. *Exp Clin Endocrinol Diabetes.* 1996;104:129–132.
35. Polak M. Hyperfunctioning thyroid adenoma and activating mutations in the TSH receptor gene. *Arch Med Res.* 1999;30: 510–513.
36. Rodrigues-Serpa A, Catarino A, Soares J. Loss of heterozygosity in follicular and papillary thyroid carcinomas. *Cancer Genet Cytogenet.* 2003;141:26–31.
37. Roque L, Rodrigues R, Pinto A, Moura-Nunes V, Soares J. Chromosome imbalances in thyroid follicular neoplasms: a comparison between follicular adenomas and carcinomas. *Genes Chromosomes Cancer.* 2003;36:292–302.
38. Sarquis MS, Weber F, Shen L, et al. High frequency of loss of heterozygosity in imprinted, compared with nonimprinted, genomic regions in follicular thyroid carcinomas and atypical adenomas. *J Clin Endocrinol Metab.* 2006;91: 262–269.
39. Satta MA, Nanni S, Della Casa S, Pontecorvi A. Molecular biology of thyroid neoplasms. *Rays.* 2000;25:151–161.
40. Sykiotis GP, Sgourou A, Papachatzopoulou A, et al. A somatic mutation in the thyrotropin receptor gene in a patient with an autonomous nodule within a multinodular goiter. *Hormones (Athens).* 2002;1:42–46.
41. Tezelman S, Borucu I, Senyurek Giles Y, Tunca F, Terzioglu T. The change in surgical practice from subtotal to near-total or total thyroidectomy in the treatment of patients with benign multinodular goiter. *World J Surg.* 2009;33(3):400–405.
42. Tonacchera M, Chiovato L, Pinchera A, et al. Hyperfunctioning thyroid nodules in toxic multinodular goiter share activating thyrotropin receptor mutations with solitary toxic adenoma. *J Clin Endocrinol Metab.* 1998;83:492–498.
43. Vaiman M, Nagibin A, Hagag P, Buyankin A, Olevson J, Shlamkovich N. Subtotal and near total versus total thyroidectomy for the management of multinodular goiter. *World J Surg.* 2008;32:1546–1551.
44. Weber F, Shen L, Aldred MA, et al. Genetic classification of benign and malignant thyroid follicular neoplasia based on a three-gene combination. *J Clin Endocrinol Metab.* 2005;90: 2512–2521.
45. Zhao J, Leonard C, Gemsenjager E, Heitz PU, Moch H, Odermatt B. Differentiation of human follicular thyroid adenomas from carcinomas by gene expression profiling. *Oncol Rep.* 2008;19:329–337.

7
Fine Needle Aspiration: Present and Future

Zubair W. Baloch and Virginia A. LiVolsi

Introduction

Thyroid nodules are common and they affect up to 7% of US population; they are often seen in women and the majority are benign. Fine-needle aspiration (FNA) is considered an essential tool in providing a rational approach to the clinical management of thyroid nodules. The results of FNA can determine whether a thyroid nodule should be followed clinically or undergo surgical excision.[1,2]

FNA Indications, Procedure, Specimen, and Classification

Every patient with a palpable thyroid nodule is a candidate for fine needle aspiration (FNA) and should undergo further evaluation to determine if an FNA is required. Thyroid nodules measuring at least 1.0 cm in dimension may be palpable, and these detectable lesions are considered to be clinically significant. However, some thyroid nodules measuring >1.0 cm may not be readily palpated because of their location in the thyroid gland.[2] Non-palpable nodules are generally discovered during radiologic examination of the head and neck for nonthyroidal lesions. Thyroid nodules can be biopsied by palpation and under ultrasound guidance; the latter is becoming the method of choice since it provides precise information regarding the location, size, and structure (solid vs. cystic) of the nodule and is more effective to obtain adequate samples for cytologic interpretation.[3]

Thyroid FNA specimens are usually prepared as air-dried smears for staining with Romanowsky (Diff-Quik®, Wright-Geimsa, Wright stains) and as alcohol fixed smears for Papanicolaou stains. Additional sample can be prepared as liquid based preparation or as a cellblock.[1]

Thyroid FNA specimens are usually classified by employing a tiered system that contains between three and six diagnostic categories. Several classification schemes have been proposed by various individual authors based on their personal/institutional experiences or by clinical organizations including Papanicolaou Society, American Thyroid Association, and American Association of Clinical Endocrinologist and special committees[1,2,4,5] (Table 7.1).

Cytomorphology of Thyroid Lesions

Nodular Goiter

The term goiter encompasses both nodular and diffuse enlargement of the thyroid, and it clinically can be divided into toxic and nontoxic variants based on the clinical symptoms and thyroid function tests (hypothyroid, euthyroid, or hyperthyroid).[6,7]

The cytology specimen features from a goiterous nodule depend somewhat upon the preparation method, but generally include copious watery colloid and small, round to oval shaped follicular cells with dark nuclei. The follicular cells are arranged in monolayer sheets, groups with follicle formation or as single cells.[8,9] The cytoplasm is usually scant in follicular cells and can show numerous, small blue-black granules (lysosomes containing hemosiderin and lipofuscin pigments).[9] Macrophages are usually present and their number depends upon the presence or absence of degenerative changes or a cystic component.[9,10] (Figure 7.1) The aspirates from a hyperplastic/adenomatoid nodule tend to be more cellular and contain an admixture of follicular cells and oncocytic cells arranged in monolayer sheets in a background of watery colloid and macrophages.[9–11]

Diffuse Toxic Goiter (Graves' Disease)

The patients with Graves' disease (GD) usually do not undergo FNA, except when they have solitary hypofunctioning (cold) nodules on radioiodine scan in the typical background of hyperfunctioning tissue. The specimens from GD are usually cellular, with features similar to hyperplastic goiter, but they also can contain lymphocytes and oncocytic cells. Although these FNAs can occasionally display focal nuclear chromatin clearing and rare intranuclear grooves, the other diagnostic nuclear features of papillary carcinoma are not observed.[12–15]

J.L. Hunt (ed.), *Molecular Pathology of Endocrine Diseases*, Molecular Pathology Library 3,
DOI 10.1007/978-1-4419-1707-2_7, © Springer Science+Business Media, LLC 2010

TABLE 7.1. Thyroid FNA classification schemes.

Papanicolaou Society of Cytopathology Task Force on Standards of Practice – 1997[4]	1. Inadequate/unsatisfactory 2. Benign 3. Atypical cells present 4. Suspicious for malignancy 5. Malignant
Diagnostic Terminology Scheme Proposed by American Thyroid Association (2006)[2]	1. Inadequate 2. Malignant 3. Indeterminate • Suspect for neoplasia • Suspect for carcinoma 4. Benign
Diagnostic Terminology Scheme Proposed by American Association of Clinical Endocrinologists & Associazione Medici Endocrinologi – 2006[5]	1. Benign 2. Malignant or suspicious 3. Follicular neoplasia 4. Nondiagnostic or ultrasound suspicious
NCI Thyroid FNA Consensus Conference – 2007[1]	1. Benign 2. Atypia of undetermined significance / Follicular lesion of undetermined significance 3. Neoplasm (follicular or Hurthle) / Suspicious for neoplasm (follicular or Hurthle) 4. Suspicious for malignancy 5. Malignant 6. Nondiagnostic

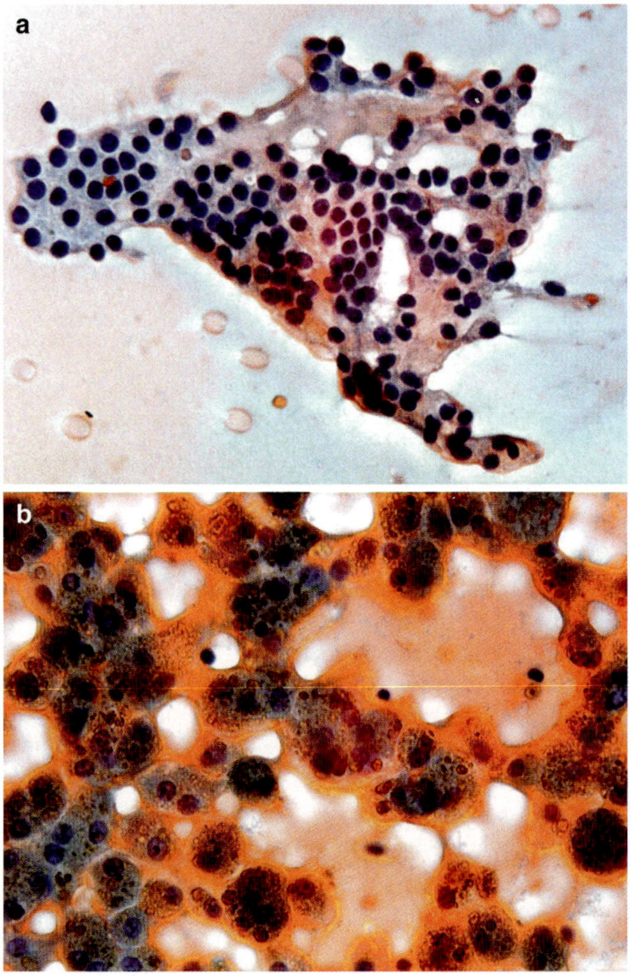

FIG. 7.1. FNA specimen of a goiterous nodule showing benign appearing follicular cells with *small dark nuclei* arranged in loosely cohesive group ((**a**) Papanicolaou stained alcohol fixed smear, 40×) and hemosiderin laden macrophages ((**b**) Papanicolaou stained alcohol fixed smear, 60×).

Autoimmune Thyroiditis

The FNA is usually performed in patients with chronic lymphocytic thyroiditis who present with distinct nodules.[16–18] The specimens from such cases usually contain Hurthle cells, follicular cells, lymphocytes, and few plasma cells in a background of scant colloid.

The lymphocytes are usually seen in the background, percolating between cell groups and in some cases one may see an intact lymphoid follicle. The Hurthle cells and follicular cells can display nuclear atypia, including chromatin clearing and nuclear grooves. The potentially extensive lymphocytic infiltrate can appear monotonous and can be mistaken for malignant lymphoma arising in lymphocytic thyroiditis.[18–21]

Follicular-Patterned Neoplasms

Thyroid (FNA) cannot distinguish between benign and malignant nonpapillary follicular and Hurthle cell lesions; both benign and malignant lesions demonstrate similar cytomorphology.[22]

Follicular/Follicular Neoplasm with Oncocytic Features (Hurthle Cell Neoplasm)

This term is used to describe the FNA features seen in both benign and malignant tumors, including follicular adenoma and carcinoma and oncocytic follicular adenoma and carcinoma. The cytologic diagnosis of "neoplasm" reflects the limitations of thyroid cytology,[23,24] since the diagnosis of follicular carcinoma can only be made with histologic evidence of capsular and/or vascular invasion.[25–27] Several authors have shown that, at most, only 20–30% of cases diagnosed as "follicular neoplasm" are diagnosed as malignant on histological examination, with the remainder representing benign follicular adenomas or cellular adenomatoid nodules.[28,29]

The FNA of a follicular neoplasm is usually hyper-cellular and show a monotonous population of either follicular or Hurthle cells with minimal or absent background colloid. The cells can be seen as three dimensional groups or microfollicles with prominent nuclear overlapping and crowding. Random nuclear atypia is also commonly observed in oncocytic follicular (Hurthle cell) lesions; this can be seen in the form of nuclear enlargement, multi-nucleation, cellular pleomorphism, and prominent nucleoli. Some authors have reported the presence of intra-cytoplasmic lumens and transgressing vessels in FNA specimens of neoplastic oncocytic follicular (Hurthle cell) lesions.[30]

Papillary Thyroid Carcinoma and Its Variants

The cytodiagnosis of papillary thyroid carcinoma (PTC) is based on characteristic nuclear morphology regardless of cytoplasmic features, growth pattern, special stains and immunohistochemical markers. This holds true for a majority of cases of PTC, though some variants of PTC may be difficult to diagnose at the cytologic level.[31,32]

The FNA specimen of PTC is usually cellular and shows tumor cells arranged in papillary groups, three-dimensional clusters or as single cells in a background of watery or thick "ropy" colloid. Additional features that can be seen are nuclear or calcific debris, macrophages, and stromal fragments.

The individual tumor cells are enlarged and elongated, or oval in shape, with eosinophilic cytoplasm. The cytoplasmic eosinophilia is more pronounced in Romanowsky stained preparations, but can be indistinct in alcohol fixed Papanicolaou stained preparations and monolayer preparations.[8] The nuclei show nuclear membrane thickening, chromatin clearing, grooves, and inclusions (Figure 7.2). The nucleoli are usually small and eccentric. Some of these features are not specific for papillary carcinoma. Intranuclear grooves and inclusions can be seen in other benign and malignant conditions of thyroid, including Hashimoto's thyroiditis, nodular goiter, hyalinizing trabecular neoplasm, Hurthle cell tumors, and medullary carcinoma.[33,34]

The cytologic interpretation of Follicular variant of papillary carcinoma (FVPTC) can be challenging due to a paucity of diagnostic nuclear features. The cytologic samples from FVPTC usually show enlarged follicular cells arranged in monolayer sheets and follicular groups in a background of thin and thick colloid. The individual tumor cells show nuclear elongation, chromatin clearing, and thick nuclear membranes, but nuclear grooves and inclusions are usually scarce. Thus, a majority of cytologic samples of FVPTC are diagnosed as "suspicious for papillary carcinoma."[35]

The cytologic samples in tall cell variant of papillary carcinoma demonstrate elongated cells with sharp cytoplasmic borders, granular eosinophilic cytoplasm, and variably sized nuclei with the other typical nuclear features of papillary carcinoma.[36]

Warthin-Like variant of PTC

Warthin-like variant of PTC can show papillary fragments or cellular groups of oncocytic cells with PTC nuclei infiltrated by a lymphocytes and plasma cells. Aspirates from this form of PTC can be mistaken for chronic lymphocytic thyroiditis. The tumor cells from warthin-like variant, however, have distinct PTC nuclei which do not resemble oncocytic follicular (Hurthle) cells.[37]

Medullary Thyroid Carcinoma

Medullary thyroid carcinoma (MTC) arises from the C-cells of the thyroid and constitutes about 10% of all malignant thyroid tumors. This thyroid tumor is unique among thyroid tumors due to its clinical presentation, potential hereditary associations, and variable morphology.[6]

The FNA specimens from MTC can display a spectrum of morphologic pattern similar to surgical pathology specimens. The majority of MTC FNA cases are cellular specimens consisting of round to oval cells arranged loosely cohesive groups or as single cells.

The tumor cells show ample granular cytoplasm with eccentric nuclei imparting a plasmacytoid appearance to tumor cells (Figure 7.3). The nuclear chromatin is similar to that seen in neuroendocrine tumors. Intranuclear inclusions and multinucleated cells can also be seen. The tumor

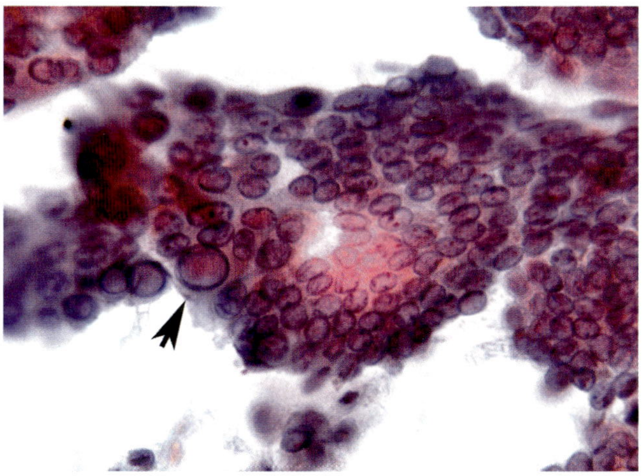

FIG. 7.2. FNA specimen of papillary thyroid carcinoma showing all major diagnostic features. The cells are enlarged with oval nuclei, intranuclear groves, eccentric nucleoli, chromatin clearing and intranuclear inclusions (*arrowhead*) (Papanicolaou stained alcohol fixed smear, 60×).

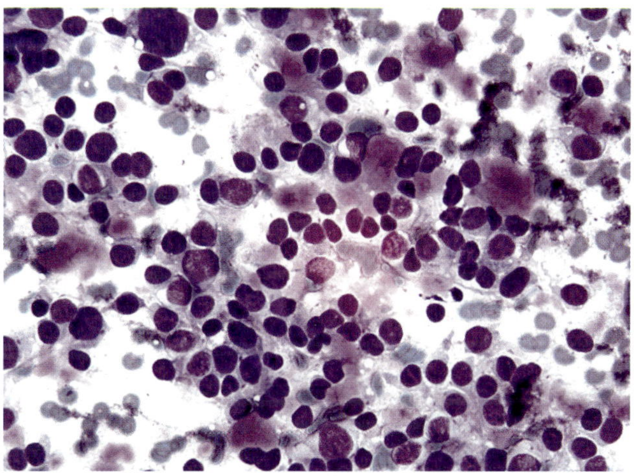

FIG. 7.3. FNA specimen of medullary thyroid carcinoma showing round to oval tumor cells with eccentric nuclei (plasmacytoid appearance) and eosinophilic cytoplasm (Diff-Quik® stained air dried smear, 40×).

cells can assume a "spindle shape" and appear mesenchymal in origin. Acellular amyloid can be seen, and this substance can be distinguished from the thick colloid by performing a Congo-red stain. The diagnosis of MTC can be confirmed by performing immunostains for calcitonin and thyroglobulin.[38]

Anaplastic Carcinoma

Anaplastic carcinoma of the thyroid is one of the most aggressive and fatal human tumors. It usually presents in older individuals and is more common in regions of endemic goiter. The aspirates from anaplastic carcinoma usually do not pose any diagnostic difficulties; they can be readily classified as malignant because of extreme cellular pleomorphism and obvious malignant features.[7]

Role of Special Studies in the Diagnosis of Thyroid Tumors in Cytologic Specimens

Immunohistochemistry

All follicular derived thyroid lesions, whether benign or malignant, commonly express transcription factor (TTF-1) and thyroglobulin. This immunostaining panel is helpful in differentiating primary vs. secondary tumors of the thyroid. The diagnosis of medullary carcinoma can be established in FNA specimens by performing immunostains for calcitonin and calcitonin gene related peptide (CGRP). Medullary carcinoma also stains positive for carcinoembryonic antigen (CEA), chromogranin, and synaptophysin.[38]

Several reports have been published regarding the use of various immunohistochemical markers that can differentiate papillary carcinoma from other follicular derived lesions of the thyroid. From an extensive list of these markers, the ones that have shown some promise include cytokeratin-19, HBME-1, and Galectin-3. However, none of these have proven to be specific since all can be expressed in some benign lesions of thyroid. In addition, spurious staining of benign thyroid epithelium in chronic lymphocytic thyroiditis can lead to false positive diagnosis of malignancy.[39–41] Therefore, it is suggested that if the confirmation of cytologic diagnosis of papillary cancer requires use of immunohistochemistry, then it should be carried out by employing an immunopanel consisting of markers mentioned above in a sample containing enough cells or in cell block preparations.

Molecular Genetics/Diagnosis

In the past decade, the literature on thyroid gland has been focused mainly on the role of various biologic events and genetic determinants in the pathogenesis of various thyroid tumors, and many of these studies have examined the mutations present in FNA specimens.

RET/PTC Oncogenes

Rearrangements of RET gene, known as RET/PTC have been identified in papillary carcinoma of thyroid.[42] RET/PTC 1 and 3 are the most common forms that occur in sporadic papillary carcinoma.[43] The prevalence of RET/PTC in papillary carcinoma varies significantly among various geographic regions[42,44,45]; in US, it ranges from 11 to 43%.[42] Several authors have investigated the expression of RET/PTC rearrangements in thyroid aspirates to establish the diagnosis of papillary thyroid carcinoma. Domingues et al found RET/PTc rearrangements in 25% of FNA specimens of histologically confirmed cases of PTC,[46] whereas Sapio et al found 17% and Pizzolanti et al found 6% F NA samples from histologically confirmed PTC showing RET/PTC rearrangements.[47,48] It has been reported that RET/PTC expression can also occur in some benign lesions. These include hyalinizing trabecular neoplasm,[49] Hahsimoto's thyroiditis[50] and hyperplastic nodules and follicular adenoma.[51,52] Thus, employing only RET/PTC analysis of FNA specimen to establish the diagnosis of PTC does not appear to be a reliable test.

B-RAF

Recently, an activating mutation in BRAF was described in 29–69% of human papillary thyroid cancers. BRAF mutational analysis of FNA samples has been shown to be of value in the diagnosis of papillary thyroid carcinoma. Pizzolanti et al found BRAF mutations in 11/16 (69%) of the FNA samples of the histologically confirmed PTC. Interestingly, in two cases, the cytologic diagnosis was suspicious but not conclusive for PTC. Similar findings have been reported by other investigators.[48] These results appear to justify the role of BRAF mutational analysis to diagnose PTC in inconclusive thyroid FNA specimens. It is well established that BRAF mutations are more common in classic variant of PTC as compared to FVPTC and as mentioned above, the FNA diagnosis of suspicious for papillary carcinoma is most commonly rendered for FVPTC cases because of paucity of diagnostic nuclear features.[48,53–57] Thus, the potential utility of BRAF test in suspicious for PTC FNA cases may be of limited value in clinical practice. Some authors have suggested that since BRAF mutations and RET/PTC rearrangements are independent of each other, it may be helpful to analyze both markers in a given thyroid FNA specimen to establish the diagnosis of PTC.[48]

DNA Microarray Analysis

Recently, DNA microarray analysis of the thyroid FNA samples have been shown to successfully distinguish between majority of the benign and malignant thyroid lesions. Lubitz et al evaluated 22 FNA samples by unsupervised hierarchical cluster analysis using a list of 25 differentially expressed genes. These authors found that their FNA cohort could be separated into three clusters: malignant, benign, and indeterminate.

The benign and malignant groups were in complete concordance with histologic follow-up except one case. Interestingly, in the indeterminate group, two cases were FVPTC on histologic examination.[58]

All above-mentioned studies show a great promise in improving the diagnostic efficacy of thyroid FNA, however, in our view, cytomorphology still remains the gold standard in the clinical management of thyroid nodules.

References

1. Baloch ZW, Cibas ES, Clark DP, et al. The National Cancer Institute Thyroid fine needle aspiration state of the science conference: a summation. *Cytojournal*. 2008;5:6.
2. Cooper DS, Doherty GM, Haugen BR, et al. Management guidelines for patients with thyroid nodules and differentiated thyroid cancer. *Thyroid*. 2006;16:109–142.
3. Baskin HJ, Duick DS. The endocrinologists' view of ultrasound guidelines for fine needle aspiration. *Thyroid*. 2006;16:207–208.
4. Guidelines of the Papanicolaou Society of Cytopathology for the examination of fine-needle aspiration specimens from thyroid nodules. The Papanicolaou Society of Cytopathology Task Force on Standards of Practice. *Diagn Cytopathol*. 1996;15:84–89.
5. American Association of Clinical Endocrinologists and Associazione Medici Endocrinologi medical guidelines for clinical practice for the diagnosis and management of thyroid nodules. *Endocr Pract*. 2006;12:63–102.
6. Murray D. *The Thyroid Gland*. Malden, MA: Blackwell; 1998:295–380.
7. Baloch Z, LiVolsi VA. Pathology of the thyroid gland. In: LiVolsi VA, Asa S, eds. *Endocrine Pathology*. Philadelphia, PA: Churchill Livingston; 2002:61–88.
8. Kini SR. *Guides to Clinical Aspiration Biopsy Thyroid*. 2nd ed. New York, NY: Igaku-Shoin; 1996.
9. Layfield LJ, Wax T, Jones C. Cytologic distinction of goiterous nodules from morphologically normal thyroid: analyses of cytomorphologic features. *Cancer*. 2003;99:217–222.
10. Baloch ZW, Sack MJ, Yu GH, Livolsi VA, Gupta PK. Fine-needle aspiration of thyroid: an institutional experience. *Thyroid*. 1998;8:565–569.
11. Oertel YC, Oertel JE. Thyroid cytology and histology. *Baillieres Best Pract Res Clin Endocrinol Metab*. 2000;14:541–557.
12. Centeno BA, Szyfelbein WM, Daniels GH, Vickery AL Jr. Fine needle aspiration biopsy of the thyroid gland in patients with prior Graves' disease treated with radioactive iodine. Morphologic findings and potential pitfalls. *Acta Cytol*. 1996;40:1189–1197.
13. Anderson SR, Mandel S, LiVolsi VA, Gupta PK, Baloch ZW. Can cytomorphology differentiate between benign nodules and tumors arising in Graves' disease? *Diagn Cytopathol*. 2004;31:64–67.
14. Kim WB, Han SM, Kim TY, et al. Ultrasonographic screening for detection of thyroid cancer in patients with Graves' disease. *Clin Endocrinol (Oxf)*. 2004;60:719–725.
15. Cantalamessa L, Baldini M, Orsatti A, Meroni L, Amodei V, Castagnone D. Thyroid nodules in Graves disease and the risk of thyroid carcinoma. *Arch Intern Med*. 1999;159:1705–1708.
16. Carson HJ, Castelli MJ, Gattuso P. Incidence of neoplasia in Hashimoto's thyroiditis: a fine-needle aspiration study. *Diagn Cytopathol*. 1996;14:38–42.
17. Liu LH, Bakhos R, Wojcik EM. Concomitant papillary thyroid carcinoma and Hashimoto's thyroiditis. *Semin Diagn Pathol*. 2001;18:99–103.
18. Kumar N, Ray C, Jain S. Aspiration cytology of Hashimoto's thyroiditis in an endemic area. *Cytopathology*. 2002;13:31–39.
19. MacDonald L, Yazdi HM. Fine needle aspiration biopsy of Hashimoto's thyroiditis. Sources of diagnostic error. *Acta Cytol*. 1999;43:400–406.
20. Mechler C, Bounacer A, Suarez H, et al. Papillary thyroid carcinoma: 6 cases from 2 families with associated lymphocytic thyroiditis harbouring RET/PTC rearrangements. *Br J Cancer*. 2001;85:1831–1837.
21. Kumarasinghe MP, De Silva S. Pitfalls in cytological diagnosis of autoimmune thyroiditis. *Pathology*. 1999;31:1–8.
22. Baloch ZW, Fleisher S, LiVolsi VA, Gupta PK. Diagnosis of "follicular neoplasm": a gray zone in thyroid fine-needle aspiration cytology. *Diagn Cytopathol*. 2002;26:41–44.
23. Renshaw AA. Follicular lesions of the thyroid. *Am J Clin Pathol*. 2001;115:782–785.
24. Sidawy MK, Del Vecchio DM, Knoll SM. Fine-needle aspiration of thyroid nodules: correlation between cytology and histology and evaluation of discrepant cases. *Cancer*. 1997;81:253–259.
25. Pu RT, Yang J, Wasserman PG, Bhuiya T, Griffith KA, Michael CW. Does Hurthle cell lesion/neoplasm predict malignancy more than follicular lesion/neoplasm on thyroid fine-needle aspiration? *Diagn Cytopathol*. 2006;34:330–334.
26. Deveci MS, Deveci G, LiVolsi VA, Baloch ZW. Fine-needle aspiration of follicular lesions of the thyroid. Diagnosis and follow-up. *Cytojournal*. 2006;3:9.
27. Clary KM, Condel JL, Liu Y, Johnson DR, Grzybicki DM, Raab SS. Interobserver variability in the fine needle aspiration biopsy diagnosis of follicular lesions of the thyroid gland. *Acta Cytol*. 2005;49:378–382.
28. Tuttle RM, Lemar H, Burch HB. Clinical features associated with an increased risk of thyroid malignancy in patients with follicular neoplasia by fine-needle aspiration. *Thyroid*. 1998;8:377–383.
29. Yang J, Schnadig V, Logrono R, Wasserman PG. Fine-needle aspiration of thyroid nodules: a study of 4703 patients with histologic and clinical correlations. *Cancer*. 2007;111:306–315.
30. Elliott DD, Pitman MB, Bloom L, Faquin WC. Fine-needle aspiration biopsy of Hurthle cell lesions of the thyroid gland: a cytomorphologic study of 139 cases with statistical analysis. *Cancer*. 2006;108:102–109.
31. Oertel YC. Fine-needle aspiration in the evaluation of thyroid neoplasms. *Endocr Pathol*. 1997;8:215–224.
32. Das DK, Mallik MK, Sharma P, et al. Papillary thyroid carcinoma and its variants in fine needle aspiration smears. A cytomorphologic study with special reference to tall cell variant. *Acta Cytol*. 2004;48:325–336.
33. Baloch ZW, LiVolsi VA. Cytologic and architectural mimics of papillary thyroid carcinoma. Diagnostic challenges in fine-needle aspiration and surgical pathology specimens. *Am J Clin Pathol*. 2006;125 Suppl:S135–S144.

34. Albores-Saavedra J, Wu J. The many faces and mimics of papillary thyroid carcinoma. *Endocr Pathol.* 2006;17:1–18.
35. Zacks JF, de las Morenas A, Beazley RM, O'Brien MJ. Fine-needle aspiration cytology diagnosis of colloid nodule versus follicular variant of papillary carcinoma of the thyroid. *Diagn Cytopathol.* 1998;18:87–90.
36. Solomon A, Gupta PK, LiVolsi VA, Baloch ZW. Distinguishing tall cell variant of papillary thyroid carcinoma from usual variant of papillary thyroid carcinoma in cytologic specimens. *Diagn Cytopathol.* 2002;27:143–148.
37. Baloch ZW, LiVolsi VA. Warthin-like papillary carcinoma of the thyroid. *Arch Pathol Lab Med.* 2000;124:1192–1195.
38. Collins BT, Cramer HM, Tabatowski K, Hearn S, Raminhos A, Lampe H. Fine needle aspiration of medullary carcinoma of the thyroid. Cytomorphology, immunocytochemistry and electron microscopy. *Acta Cytol.* 1995;39:920–930.
39. Cheung CC, Ezzat S, Freeman JL, Rosen IB, Asa SL. Immunohistochemical diagnosis of papillary thyroid carcinoma. *Mod Pathol.* 2001;14:338–342.
40. Sapio MR, Guerra A, Posca D, et al. Combined analysis of galectin-3 and BRAFV600E improves the accuracy of fine-needle aspiration biopsy with cytological findings suspicious for papillary thyroid carcinoma. *Endocr Relat Cancer.* 2007;14:1089–1097.
41. Barroeta JE, Baloch ZW, Lal P, Pasha TL, Zhang PJ, LiVolsi VA. Diagnostic value of differential expression of CK19, Galectin-3, HBME-1, ERK, RET, and p16 in benign and malignant follicular-derived lesions of the thyroid: an immunohistochemical tissue microarray analysis. *Endocr Pathol.* 2006;17:225–234.
42. Nikiforov YE. RET/PTC rearrangement in thyroid tumors. *Endocr Pathol.* 2002;13:3–16.
43. Fischer AH, Bond JA, Taysavang P, Battles OE, Wynford-Thomas D. Papillary thyroid carcinoma oncogene (RET/PTC) alters the nuclear envelope and chromatin structure. *Am J Pathol.* 1998;153:1443–1450.
44. Zou M, Shi Y, Farid NR. Low rate of ret proto-oncogene activation (PTC/retTPC) in papillary thyroid carcinomas from Saudi Arabia. *Cancer.* 1994;73:176–180.
45. Motomura T, Nikiforov YE, Namba H, et al. Ret rearrangements in Japanese pediatric and adult papillary thyroid cancers. *Thyroid.* 1998;8:485–489.
46. Domingues R, Mendonca E, Sobrinho L, Bugalho MJ. Searching for RET/PTC rearrangements and BRAF V599E mutation in thyroid aspirates might contribute to establish a preoperative diagnosis of papillary thyroid carcinoma. *Cytopathology.* 2005;16:27–31.
47. Sapio MR, Posca D, Raggioli A, et al. Detection of RET/PTC, TRK and BRAF mutations in preoperative diagnosis of thyroid nodules with indeterminate cytological findings. *Clin Endocrinol (Oxf).* 2007;66:678–683.
48. Pizzolanti G, Russo L, Richiusa P, et al. Fine-needle aspiration molecular analysis for the diagnosis of papillary thyroid carcinoma through BRAF V600E mutation and RET/PTC rearrangement. *Thyroid.* 2007;17:1109–1115.
49. Papotti M, Volante M, Giuliano A, et al. RET/PTC activation in hyalinizing trabecular tumors of the thyroid. *Am J Surg Pathol.* 2000;24:1615–1621.
50. Wirtschafter A, Schmidt R, Rosen D, et al. Expression of the RET/PTC fusion gene as a marker for papillary carcinoma in Hashimoto's thyroiditis [see comments]. *Laryngoscope.* 1997;107:95–100.
51. Elisei R, Romei C, Vorontsova T, et al. RET/PTC rearrangements in thyroid nodules: studies in irradiated and not irradiated, malignant and benign thyroid lesions in children and adults. *J Clin Endocrinol Metab.* 2001;86:3211–3216.
52. Inaba M, Umemura S, Satoh H, et al. Expression of RET in follicular cell-derived tumors of the thyroid gland: prevalence and implication of morphological type. *Pathol Int.* 2003;53:146–153.
53. Daum G, Eisenmann-Tappe I, Fries HW, Troppmair J, Rapp UR. The ins and outs of Raf kinases. *Trends Biochem Sci.* 1994;19:474–480.
54. Cohen Y, Xing M, Mambo E, et al. BRAF mutation in papillary thyroid carcinoma. *J Natl Cancer Inst.* 2003;95:625–627.
55. Kimura ET, Nikiforova MN, Zhu Z, Knauf JA, Nikiforov YE, Fagin JA. High prevalence of BRAF mutations in thyroid cancer: genetic evidence for constitutive activation of the RET/PTC-RAS-BRAF signaling pathway in papillary thyroid carcinoma. *Cancer Res.* 2003;63:1454–1457.
56. Fagin JA. How thyroid tumors start and why it matters: kinase mutants as targets for solid cancer pharmacotherapy. *J Endocrinol.* 2004;183:249–256.
57. Soares P, Trovisco V, Rocha AS, et al. BRAF mutations and RET/PTC rearrangements are alternative events in the etiopathogenesis of PTC. *Oncogene.* 2003;22:4578–4580.
58. Lubitz CC, Ugras SK, Kazam JJ, et al. Microarray analysis of thyroid nodule fine-needle aspirates accurately classifies benign and malignant lesions. *J Mol Diagn.* 2006;8:490–498.

8 Well-Differentiated Papillary Thyroid Carcinoma

Lori A. Erickson and Ricardo V. Lloyd

Introduction

Papillary thyroid carcinoma (PTC) is a malignant epithelial tumor showing follicular differentiation and distinctive nuclear features.[1] Papillary thyroid carcinoma is the most common thyroid carcinoma, accounting for 80% of thyroid carcinomas.[2] Numerous variants of PTC have been described, some of which behave more aggressively than conventional PTC. Three distinct molecular alterations are associated with PTC and are mutually exclusive.[3] These include somatic BRAF point mutations, RET/PTC rearrangements, and somatic RAS point mutations. These molecular alterations are also associated with particular clinicopathologic features of PTC as well as particular subtypes of PTC.

Clinical Features

PTC can occur at any age, but most tumors develop in patients between 20 and 50 years of age, and women are affected more commonly than men.[1] PTC accounts for at least 80% of adult and 90% of pediatric thyroid carcinomas.[1] PTC has been identified with Graves, Hashimoto thyroiditis, and hyperplastic nodules and can arise in ectopic thyroid tissue (struma ovarii).

Radiation exposure is a risk factor for the development of PTC.[4] PTC in pediatric patients who were involved in the Chernobyl nuclear accident were associated with a short latency, young age, an almost equal sex ratio, aggressive behavior with intraglandular spread, soft tissue invasion, metastases, and a solid growth pattern.[5–7] Radiation induced tumors frequently show RET/PTC rearrangements, but show a low prevalence of BRAF mutations.[8] Radiographically, PTCs are well demarcated or irregular masses on ultrasound and cold nodules on radioactive iodine scan.

PTC is often treated by near total thyroidectomy with ipsilateral lymph node dissection. Radioactive iodine can also then be administered in attempt to ablate any possible remaining tumor including metastatic sites or suppression of thyroid stimulating hormone secretion without radioactive iodine. The overall prognosis for patients with PTC is excellent, with greater than 90% overall survival.[1] PTC has a propensity to metastasize to ipsilateral cervical lymph nodes and may spread to lung.[2] Unfavorable prognostic features include older age, male gender, large tumor size, multicentricity, vascular invasion, extrathyroidal extension, distant metastases, aneuploidy, high microscopic grade, and progression to poorly differentiated carcinoma.[2] Other poor prognostic features include tumor necrosis, numerous mitoses, and marked nuclear atypia.[9] Recognition of the variants of PTC (Table 8.1) is important as the tall cell variant,[10–12] columnar variant,[13] solid variant, and Hurthle cell variant[14] may be more aggressive tumors.

The increasing incidence of thyroid carcinoma in the United States is mainly due to increasing diagnosis of papillary thyroid carcinomas (PTC), particularly small papillary cancers.[15] Papillary microcarcinoma is defined as a PTC measuring 1 cm or less. These microcarcinomas are often incidental findings in thyroids removed for benign clinical nodules or thyroiditis,[16] and the majority are cured by lobectomy alone. Studies have identified these tumors in 7–35% of autopsies[17,18] and in 7% of surgical cases in patients undergoing surgery for presumably benign disease.[17] The treatment for papillary microcarcinomas has been controversial. Papillary microcarcinomas presenting clinically as a mass or a metastasis are usually treated as a clinical cancer.[16] Up to 5% of these tumors may be associated with capsular invasion or metastases.[19] Incidentally, clinically occult papillary microcarcinomas are less aggressive than those presenting clinically.[20] Clinically overt papillary microcarcinomas are larger and more frequently show multifocality, extrathyroidal extension, vascular invasion, metastases, and recurrence than those discovered incidentally.[20] Familial papillary thyroid microcarcinomas can also behave aggressively.[21]

Follicular variant of PTC (FVPTC) (Lindsay tumor) is the most common variant of PTC and one of the most challenging to diagnose. The histologic features of these tumors were recognized more than 50 years ago.[22,23] These tumors were originally

J.L. Hunt (ed.), *Molecular Pathology of Endocrine Diseases*, Molecular Pathology Library 3,
DOI 10.1007/978-1-4419-1707-2_8, © Springer Science+Business Media, LLC 2010

TABLE 8.1. Variants of papillary thyroid carcinoma.

Papillary microcarcinoma
Follicular variant of papillary thyroid carcinoma
Tall cell variant of papillary thyroid carcinoma
Columnar variant of papillary thyroid carcinoma
Diffuse sclerosing variant of papillary thyroid carcinoma
Solid variant of papillary thyroid carcinoma
Oxyphilic (oncocytic/Hurthle cell) variant of papillary thyroid carcinoma
Warthin-like variant of papillary thyroid carcinoma
Cribriform-morular variant of papillary thyroid carcinoma
Papillary thyroid carcinoma with Nodular Fasciitis-like Stroma
Papillary thyroid carcinoma with Lipomatous Stroma
Clear cell variant of papillary thyroid carcinoma

classified as a type of follicular carcinoma, but were later classified as a type of papillary carcinoma, follicular variant.[24,25] Recent reports have suggested that this tumor may be overdiagnosed by pathologists. A recent study has shown that even experienced thyroid pathologists have low concordance in diagnoses of FVPTC, although increased concordance was noted in tumors associated with metastases.[26] Follicular variant of PTC behaves and is treated similarly to conventional PTC.

Recognition of the variants of PTC is important as some of them including the tall cell variant,[10,11,27] columnar variant,[13] solid variant, and oxyphilic variant[14] may behave more aggressively. The tall cell variant is an uncommon, aggressive variant of PTC, which is more common in elderly males.[10,28] This aggressive tumor is associated with extrathyroidal disease, recurrence, vascular invasion, metastases, decreased survival, and death in 20–25% of patients.[10] The tall cell variant shows increased expression of c-Met, a factor of invasion which correlates with extracapsular spread, and muscle invasion, than classic PTC and FVPTC.[29] The columnar variant of PTC is a rare, aggressive variant of PTC that occurs over a wide age range, can metastasize widely, and usually does not respond to radioactive iodine or chemotherapy.[13,30]

The solid variant of PTC is uncommon, comprising only 2.6% (20 of 756) of papillary thyroid carcinomas at the Mayo Clinic between 1962 and 1989.[31] The solid variant of papillary carcinoma was associated with slightly increased distant metastases and less favorable prognosis than classical PTC.[31] An AMES (Age, Metastasis, Extent and Size) risk classification study of 121 PTC found that among variants of PTC, solid cell variant has the highest proportion of high-risk tumor classified by the AMES criteria (75%), followed by tall cell variant with 33.3% of high risk patients, while only 8.3% of classic PTC were classified as high-risk.[32] The solid cell variant of PTC is more common in children. This variant was the most common subtype of PTC in Belarusian children after the Chernobyl accident, comprising 34% of the PTCs.[33] These tumors were associated with lymph node metastases, extrathyroidal extension, vascular invasion, slightly more distant metastases, and less favorable prognosis than conventional PTC.

The oxyphilic (Hurthle cell) variant of PTC is uncommon. While some have found these tumors to behave similarly to conventional PTC, others have identified more aggressive behavior.[34,35] A study of 1,552 patients with thyroid carcinoma included 42 cases of Hurthle cell variant of PTC with generally favorable 5- and 10-year survival rates of 94 and 87%.[14] Unfavorable prognostic factors included older age, extrathyroidal extension, tumor stage, and metastases. Tumors with features of both oxyphilic PTC and tall cell variant may behave more aggressively.[34]

The Warthin-like variant of PTC resembles Warthin tumor of the salivary gland with its oxyphilic cells and lymphocytic stroma.[36] Overall, these tumors behave like conventional PTC. Similar to conventional PTC, a Warthin-like variant of PTC has been documented in association with an anaplastic thyroid carcinoma.[37]

The diffuse sclerosing variant of PTC was described in 1985.[38] These tumors are more common in women and in younger individuals. The diffuse sclerosing variant of PTC shows aggressive features with increased cervical lymph node involvement and lung metastases.[39–41] The overall outcome has been controversial with some studies showing a worse prognosis with decreased disease-free survival.[39] However, others have found that in spite of aggressive histologic features such as large tumor size and extensive lymph node metastases, overall survival is not significantly different from conventional PTC.[40,42]

Histologic Features

Grossly, PTCs are often ill-defined, infiltrative, firm, single, or multiple masses with a granular whitish appearance.[2] The tumors are usually 2–3 cm in size but can be extremely small and not identifiable grossly. Classically, PTCs are composed of fibrovascular papillae lined by follicular cells with enlarged, irregular nuclei showing nuclear clearing ("Orphan Annie" nuclei), longitudinal nuclear grooves, and intranuclear holes (cytoplasmic invaginations into the nucleus) (Figure 8.1). The colloid in PTC is often darker than that of the surrounding thyroid, and psammoma bodies are seen in approximately 50% of cases. The stroma is usually abundant, fibrous, and sclerotic, although cystic change is not uncommon. Fine needle aspiration biopsies of PTC are cellular and show papillary structures with branching or sheets of cuboidal or columnar cells with enlarged irregular nuclei, nuclear grooves, and nuclear pseudoinclusions. PTC must be differentiated from Graves disease with papillary hyperplasia as well as thyroid neoplasms. Both Graves and PTC can show a papillary architecture, but the cytologic features of PTC are helpful in separating PTC from Graves. In difficult cases of Graves disease with papillary hyperplasia, p27 protein expression is helpful as Graves disease shows higher levels of p27 expression when compared to PTC.[43]

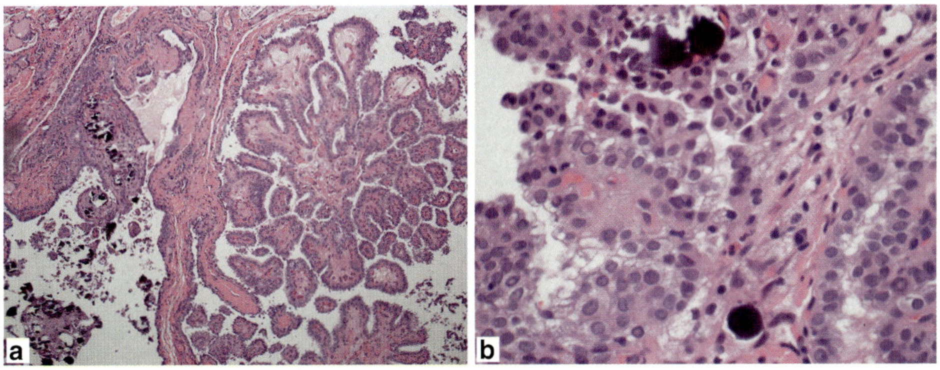

FIG. 8.1. Papillary thyroid carcinoma. (**a**) Classic papillary thyroid carcinoma showing papillae with fibrovascular cores covered by epithelial cells. Psammomatous calcifications are also present. (**b**) High power view of papillary thyroid carcinoma showing enlarged irregular nuclei with nuclear clearing, nuclear grooves and intranuclear holes.

Histologic variants of PTC are important to recognize as the molecular features and biologic behavior may differ from classic PTC, and they can be mistaken for other tumors (Figure 8.2, Table 8.1). FVPTC can have a microfollicular pattern (Figure 8.2a), a macrofollicular pattern, a diffuse pattern, or mixed patterns. These tumors can be particularly difficult to diagnose on fine needle aspiration biopsy. The diffuse pattern of FVPTC is seen in younger patients, is often multicentric, and shows extrathyroidal extension, nodal metastases, and vascular invasion.[44,45] Differentiating FVPTC from a follicular neoplasm can be extremely difficult. Important criteria to diagnose FVPTC are nuclear pseudo-inclusions (cytoplasmic invaginations into the nucleus), abundant nuclear grooves, and ground glass nuclei (Figure 8.2b).[26] Immunohistochemical markers, particularly when used in panels, such as HBME-1, galectin-3, and cytokeratin 19 can also be helpful. The tall cell variant of PTC has prominent papillary structures lined by cells in which height of cell at least twice the width, basally located nuclei, abundant eosinophilic, oxyphilic cytoplasm, (Figure 8.2c) and often a lymphocytic infiltrate. The columnar cell variant shows a prominent papillary architectural pattern with elongated cells with nuclear stratification and scant cytoplasm. Tumors can show both tall cell and columnar features,[46] areas of solid growth, organoid or glandular features,[47] foci of solid spindle-cells,[30] and microfollicular[34] and follicular growth patterns.[48] Encapsulated columnar-cell PTCs have a better prognosis than tumors that are unencapsulated and invasive into adjacent thyroid or extrathyroid tissue.[30,48] The diffuse sclerosing variant of PTC shows diffuse involvement of one or both lobes of the thyroid, extensive squamous metaplasia, numerous psammoma bodies, interstitial fibrosis, a marked lymphocytic infiltrate, and can show widespread intrathyroid lymphatic invasion (Figure 8.2h).[39] The solid cell variant of PTC has a solid architectural pattern of growth and cytologic features classic of PTC (Figure 8.2e). The oxyphilic (Hurthle cell) variant of PTC has a papillary architectural pattern, oxyphilic cytoplasm, and nuclear features are characteristic of PTC. The papillae are lined by a single layer of oxyphilic cells with nuclear features of PTC (Figure 8.2f). Oxyphilic PTC must be differentiated from Hurthle cell neoplasms showing papillary architecture and oxyphilic papillary hyperplasia in Hashimoto thyroiditis and Graves disease. In 1995, the Warthin-like variant of PTC was described as "a peculiar thyroid tumor of follicular epithelial differentiation with distinctly papillary architecture, oxyphilic cytology, and lymphocytic infiltrates in papillary stalks" was described.[36] The Warthin-like variant of PTC resembles Warthin tumor of the salivary gland with its oxyphilic cells and lymphocytic stroma (Figure 8.2g).[36] Warthin-like PTCs can be mistaken for benign lymphoepithelial lesions of the thyroid, Hurthle cell carcinoma, and tall cell variant of PTC in both cytology and histology specimens.[49] A helpful low-power clue to the diagnosis of Warthin-like PTC is a prominent lymphoplasmacytic infiltrate, but cytologic features classic of PTC are most useful in separating the Warthin-like variant of PTC from benign lymphoepithelial lesions of the thyroid and Hurthle cell carcinoma. The cells in the Warthin-like variant can be elongated, but the height of the cells is not at least twice the width as is seen in the tall cell variant of PTC. The nuclear stratification and scant cytoplasm are helpful in differentiating the columnar variant from the tall cell variant of PTC.

A variety of other variants of PTC have been described. PTC with nodular fasciitis-like stroma can be mistaken for a mesenchymal tumor, a carcinosarcoma, or an anaplastic thyroid carcinoma.[50] The tumors show a prominent spindle cell stroma, reminiscent of nodular fasciitis in which small tubules and nests of epithelioid cells with cytologic features characteristic of PTC. Foci of squamous differentiation and/or papillae may be seen.[50] PTC can also show a lipomatous stroma.[27] The clear cell variant of PTC is uncommon, but appears to behave like conventional PTC.[51,52] Metastatic papillary lesions to the thyroid, such as from kidney, nasopharynx, among other sites also need to be differentiated from PTC.

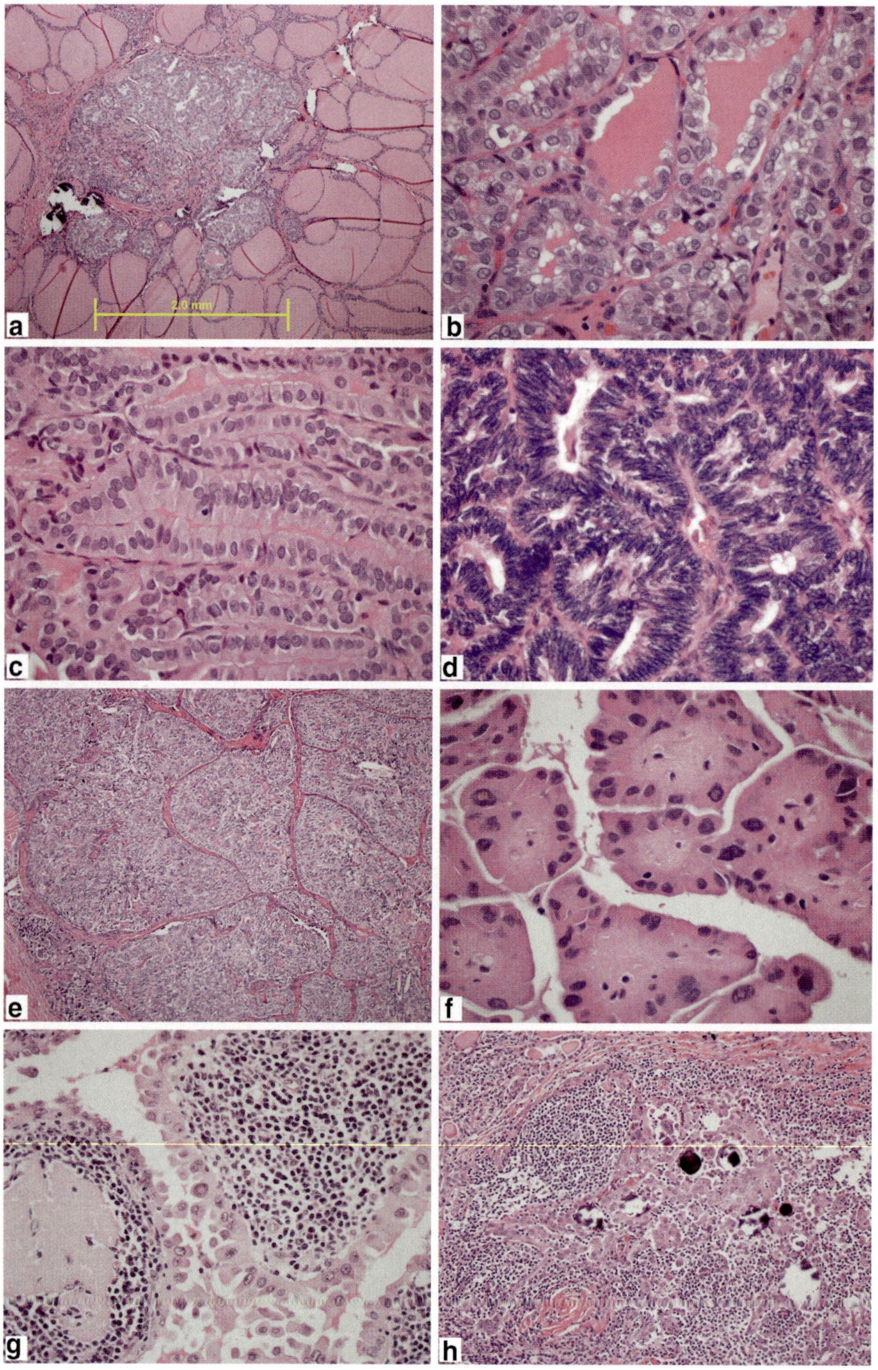

FIG. 8.2. Variants of papillary thyroid carcinoma (PTC). (**a**) Papillary thyroid microcarcinoma measuring less than 1 cm. (**b**) Follicular variant of PTC with follicular growth pattern and cytologic features of PTC. (**c**) The tall cell variant of PTC has prominent papillary structures lined by cells in which height of cell at least twice the width, basally located nuclei, abundant, eosinophilic cytoplasm. (**d**) Columnar variant of PTC a prominent papillary architectural pattern with elongated cells with nuclear stratification. (**e**) Solid variant of PTC showing cytologic features of PTC but a solid architectural pattern. (**f**) Oxyphilic variant of papillary thyroid carcinoma showing cells with nuclear features of PTC, but abundant oxyphilic cytoplasm. (**g**) Warthin-like variant of PTC with oxyphilic cells showing intranuclear holes and a prominent lymphocytic stroma. (**h**) Diffuse sclerosing variant of PTC.

Immunohistochemistry

PTCs are positive for thyroglobulin, thyroid transcription factor-1 (TTF-1), and cytokeratins and are negative for chromogranin, synaptophysin, and calcitonin. Immunohistochemical and molecular markers have been very useful for diagnosing and predicting the behavior of papillary thyroid carcinomas. Although not specific, a number of immunohistochemical markers (Figure 8.3) have been utilized singly and in panels have shown promise in helping to confirm a diagnosis of

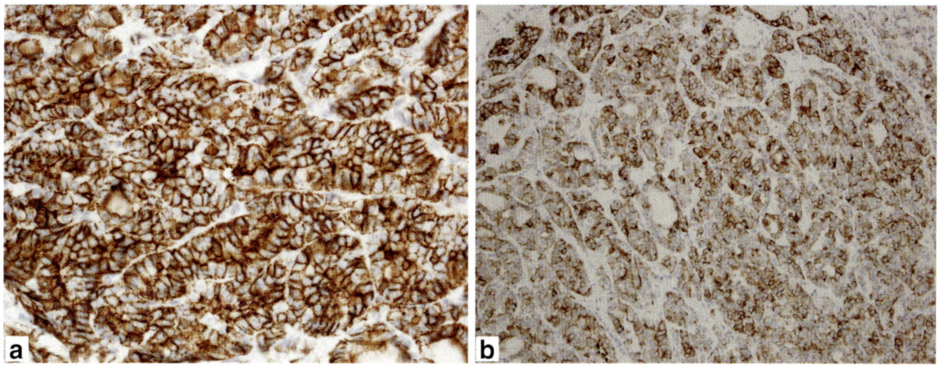

FIG. 8.3. Immunohistochemical studies of PTC. (**a**) HBME1 immunostain showing positive staining in the PTC. (**b**) Cytokeratin 19 immunostain positive in a PTC.

PTC including HMBE-1,[53–59] galectin-3,[53–55,58,60] cytokeratin 19,[53–55,58,59] and CITED-1.[54,55,58,59,61,62]

A study of 67 PTC and a variety of benign thyroid tumors showed expression of galectin-3, fibronectin-1, CITED-1, HBME-1, and cytokeratin 19 were significantly associated with PTC with coexpression of multiple antibodies showing increased specificity for carcinomas, while loss of sets of markers such as galectin-3 or fibronectin-1, and HBME-1 was highly specific for benign lesions.[54] A panel consisting of galectin-3, fibronectin-1, and HBME-1 was most helpful for the diagnosis of PTC.[54] However, galectin-3, cytokeratin 19, and fibronectin as single markers showed focal staining in nonneoplastic thyroid tissue, and the seven neoplasms in the study of undermined malignant potential showed intermediate staining between the benign and malignant tumors.[54] A study from Mayo Clinic also found a panel of markers consisting of HBME-1, galectin-3, and CK19 or a panel consisting of HMBE-1, CITED-1, and galectin-3 to be most effective in distinguishing follicular adenoma from FVPTC.[58] Similarly, single markers were useful, but none was completely specific for FVPTC.[58] Nasr et al found HBME1 to be the most sensitive and specific single marker for PTC, but concluded that a combination of HBME1 and CK19 had the greatest diagnostic utility in differentiating PTC from benign mimics.[59] Another study evaluating multiple immunohistochemical markers also found HBME-1 to be the most specific single marker, but again noted increased specificity when panels of markers such as HMBE-1, galectin-3, and CK19 or HBME-1, CITED-1, and cytokeratin19 were used.[55] They also noted that while these markers are helpful in separating FVPTC from follicular adenoma, particularly when used in panels, an additional group of diagnostically challenging encapsulated follicular lesions with questionable features of PTC showed intermediate staining patterns indicating that these markers may be less useful in borderline lesions.[55] Thus, HMBE-1 appears to be a particularly useful marker in differentiating FVPTC from follicular adenoma, but a panel of immunohistochemical markers including HBME-1, galectin-3, CITED-1, and/or CK19 appears to be most useful.

Genetics of Papillary Thyroid Carcinoma

Three distinct molecular alterations are associated with PTC and are mutually exclusive.[3] These include somatic BRAF point mutations, RET/PTC rearrangements, and somatic RAS point mutations. These molecular alterations are also associated with particular clinicopathologic features of PTC as well as particular subtypes of PTC.

BRAF

In 2002, Davies et al reported somatic BRAF mutations in the majority of melanomas studied and at lower frequency in a wide variety of human cancers, and noted that growth in cancer cell lines with BRAF mutation was independent of RAS function.[63] Numerous studies soon followed regarding somatic BRAF mutation in thyroid tumors.[64–68] BRAF mutation was found to be the most common genetic abnormality in PTC, occurring in 36–69% of cases.[69] The overwhelming majority of mutations are in exon 15, nucleotide 1799 (V600E mutation), but other mutations have been identified in rare cases.[70,71]

The BRAF gene codes for a serine/threonine kinase signaling protein, which along with ARAF and RAF1, are involved in the RAS/RAF/MEK/ERK/MAPK signaling pathway that relays signals from the cell membrane to the nucleus regulating expression of genes involved in cell growth, differentiation and cell death. Tumor suppressor genes and thyroid iodide-metabolizing genes are down-regulated, while cancer promoting molecules including VEGF, matrix metalloproteinases, NF-kappaB, and c-Met are up-regulated.[72] The three RAF genes code for cytoplasmic serine/threonine kinases that are regulated by binding RAS.[63] When RAS becomes activated and it activates BRAF. Mutation of BRAF is an alternative route for activation of the MAP kinase signaling pathway that is independent of RAS.[63] BRAF mutation V600E mimics the phosphorylation of the activation segment of BRAF, thus BRAF becomes activated independent of RAS. RAS function is not required for the growth of cancer cell lines with BRAF point mutations.[63] Recently therapeutic strategies

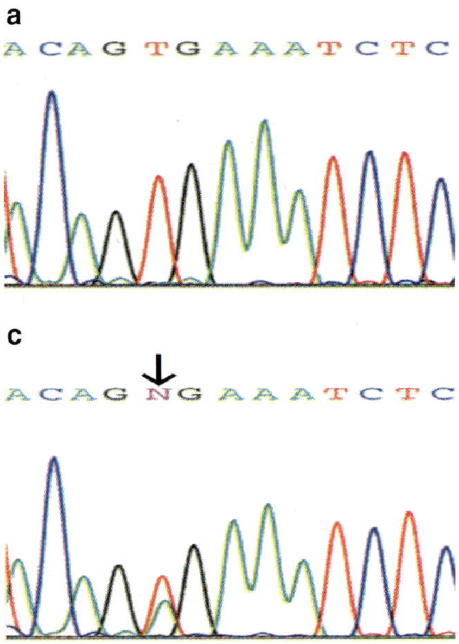

FIG. 8.4. Direct sequencing for BRAF mutation in papillary thyroid carcinomas. A classic papillary thyroid carcinoma showing wild-type BRAF sequence in forward direction (**a**) and reverse direction (**b**). Another classic papillary thyroid carcinoma showing a T to A transversion at nucleotide 1799 in forward direction (**c**) and reverse direction (**d**).

and MEK inhibitors have been proposed to target the MAPK pathway that is aberrantly activated by BRAF mutation.[73,74]

Clinical and pathologic features are associated with BRAF associated PTC (Figure 8.4). BRAF associated PTC most commonly occur in older patients and are uncommon in children.[75–77] Unlike RET/PTC mutation associated PTC, BRAF associated PTC generally are not associated with radiation.[75,78] However, the oncogenic AKAP9-BRAF fusion was recently been identified is associated with radiation induced PTC.[79] This rearrangement of BRAF via paracentric inversion of chromosome 7q results in an in-frame fusion between the AKAP9 gene and BRAF resulting in a fusion protein that lacks the autoinhibitory N-terminal portion of BRAF and has elevated kinase activity is a novel mechanism of MAPK pathway activation.[79]

Somatic BRAF mutation has also been associated with more aggressive tumors in some studies and with particular subtypes of PTC.[69,70,76,77,80–83] BRAF mutation has been associated with clinicopathological features of PTC that are conventionally known to predict tumor progression and recurrence, including, older patient age, extrathyroidal extension, lymph node metastasis, and advanced tumor stages, treatment failure, and tumor recurrence in patients with conventionally low-risk clinicopathological factors.[72] In a study of 96 cases of PTC, BRAF mutations were identified in 42% of cases and associated with older patient age, typical papillary appearance or the tall cell variant, a higher rate of extrathyroidal extension, and more advanced tumor stage at presentation.[77] The diagnostic utility of BRAF mutation was evaluated in 71 thyroid fine needle aspiration (FNA) specimens, and BRAF mutation was detected in 31 of 58 PTC and in none of the 13 non-PTC lesions.[84] The PTC harboring BRAF mutation had higher extrathyroidal invasion and/or lymph node metastasis than PTC with wild-type BRAF.[84] A multicenter study of 219 patients with PTC found a significant association between BRAF mutation and extrathyroidal extension, lymph node metastases, and advanced tumor stage at initial surgery. This association remained significant on multivariate analysis, adjusting for conventional predictors of recurrence, but excluding PTC subtype, but it was lost when tumor subtype was included.[80] However, BRAF mutation remained associated with tumor recurrence on multivariate analysis even with PTC subtype, and BRAF mutation was an independent predictor of recurrence in patients with low stage disease and absence of I131 avidity and treatment failure in recurrent disease.[80] Another study found that BRAF positive tumors correlated with early recurrences and negative radioiodine scans which are associated with worse outcome as treatment with radioactive iodine is not effective.[82] They suggested that this is due to impairment of the sodium iodine symporter targeting the membrane mediated transport of iodine into the thyroid follicular cells.[82] Another study found BRAF mutation associated with recurrence in low-risk patients with conventional PTC, but this association was lost in multivariate analyses when factors of age, gender, tumor size, extrathyroidal extension, multifocality, and lymph node metastasis were included.[81] A recent study of 500 consecutive cases of PTC found BRAF mutation in 219 cases (43.8%), BRAF mutation was associated with extrathyroidal invasion, multicentricity, nodal metastases, absence of tumor capsule in particular in FVPTC, and micropapillary thyroid carcinomas.[85] However not all studies have found BRAF mutation to be associated with aggressive behavior.[86,87] In addition to PTC, BRAF mutations are also present in poorly differentiated and anaplastic carcinomas arising from PTC.[88]

Frequencies of BRAF mutation vary among different variants of PTC. BRAF mutations are frequently identified in the tall cell variant of PTC[77] and PTC with a papillary or mixed follicular/papillary architecture, including conventional PTC, papillary microcarcinoma, Warthin-like PTC, oncocytic/oxyphilic/Hurthle cell variant of PTC,[69,76,89] but are less common in FVPTC.[69,76] BRAF mutation is common in the tall cell variant of PTC.[64,77,88,90] BRAF mutations have been identified in up to 67% of cases of tall cell variant of PTC.[64] BRAF mutations are identified in 75% of Warthin-like variant of PTC.[76] BRAF mutations are commonly seen in the oxyphilic variant of PTC, occurring in 55% of cases.[76] BRAF mutations are also identified in the diffuse sclerosing variant of PTC.[91] A novel BRAF triplet deletion has recently been reported in a PTC with a predominantly solid growth pattern.[70] The deletion leads to the replacement of a valine and a lysine by a glutamate in the BRAF activation segment (BRAF(VK600-1E)).[70] The columnar variant of PTC does not appear to show increased frequency of BRAF mutation (unpublished observations).

BRAF somatic point mutations are identified in 28–42% of papillary thyroid microcarcinomas.[76,91,92] A recent study of tumors from patients with diverse genetic backgrounds showed no differences in BRAF mutation rates in tumors from Russian patients when compared to Japanese patients.[92] BRAF mutation did not significantly correlate with the gender, age at presentation, metastatic indices or with papillary, mixed papillary and follicular, and solid/trabecular features among the papillary microcarcinomas, however papillary microcarcinomas of follicular morphology had fewer BRAF mutations, while those with co-occurrence with less differentiated components showed more frequent BRAF mutation.[92]

BRAF mutations are less frequently associated with FVPTC than with other types.[69,76] Interestingly, a study including 54 cases of FVPTC showed the less common BRAF(K601E) mutation in 7%.[76] Recent studies have compared genetic alterations of FVPTC with those of classic PTC.[64,83] A study from Mayo Clinic found BRAF mutation in 38% of PTC, including 20% of FVPTC.[64] Another study comparing genetic alterations in FVPTC showed BRAF mutation in 1 of 13 (7.6%) cases, RET rearrangement in 5 of 12 cases (41.7%), RAS mutation in 6 of 24 cases (25%), as compared to classic PTC which showed BRAF mutation in 3 of 10 cases (30%), no RAS mutations, and RET rearrangement in 5 of 11 cases (45%). One FVPTC exhibited simultaneous RAS mutation and RET/PTC1 rearrangement.[83] Another study compared the genetic alterations of 30 cases of FVPTC with 46 non-FVPTC.[93] The cases of FVPTC showed one RET/PTC rearrangement (3%) and 13 RAS mutations (43%), while the non-FVPTC cases showed 13 RET/PTC rearrangements (28%) and no RAS mutations confirming the high frequency of RAS point mutations in FVPTC.[93]

A recent study microdissecting different components from 44 PTC found that different structural components within the same tumor had identical BRAF mutation status in 93% (41 of 44) of tumors, while only 7% (3 of 44) of tumors showed BRAF mutation only in the papillary component and not in the follicular component. Similarly, 92% (11 of 12) of lymph node metastases showed BRAF mutation patterns identical to the respective primary tumor.[89] Thus, the cells in PTC appear to be homogeneous in regard to the mutational status, and the results support the reliability of molecular diagnostic testing of PTC in preoperative biopsies as the BRAF status would not depend on which tumor component was sampled.[89] A study evaluating the diagnostic utility of BRAF mutation in thyroid FNA specimens found a high degree of specificity for BRAF mutation by analysis of FNA specimens.[84] BRAF mutation analysis can be useful for the diagnosis of PTC in cases of cytologically indeterminate fine needle aspiration specimens.[84]

RET/PTC

The RET gene is located on 10q11.2.[94] There are many types of RET rearrangements, all of which result in the fusion of the tyrosine kinase domain of RET to the 5′ portion of different genes.[95] There are at least ten different RET/PTC rearrangements. The most common rearrangements are RET/PTC1 and RET/PTC3.[95] RET/PTC1 is the most common overall accounting for two-thirds of RET rearrangements (Figure 8.5). RET/PTC1 is more common in classic PTC with papillary growth, microcarcinomas, and benign behavior.[95] RET/PTC3 correlates with the solid variant of PTC and more aggressive behavior.[95,96] A study from an iodine-rich, nonirradiated area of Japan found the overall frequency of RET/PTC rearrangements in PTC to be 28%, with increased frequency in younger patients (41% in patients less than 20 years of age).[97] The prevalence rate of RET/PTC1 was similar regardless of age, but RET/PTC3 rearrangements were more common among patients less than 20 years-old and in tumors with a solid growth pattern.[97] A study including 17 patients with multifocal PTC found only 2 (12%) patients had identical RET/PTC rearrangements in multiple tumors.[98] Fifteen of the 17 (88%) cases showed diverse rearrangements among the tumors in each patient, indicating that individual tumors arise independently in a background of genetic or environmental susceptibility.[98] An RET/PTC model of thyroid tumor has been reported in transgenic mice.[99] However, not all transgenic mice with overexpression of RET/PTC in their thyroids develop thyroid tumors, other genetic lesions are likely needed for PTC to develop.[99]

RET/PTC is associated with radiation-related PTC, both in patients who have received external radiation for disease[100] and after the Chernobyl diseaster.[101,102] Chernobyl-associated PTC with short latency periods (within 1 year of exposure) are most commonly associated with RET/PTC3, regardless of age.[96,103–105] Late onset PTC (greater than 1 year after exposure) more often show RET/PTC1.[96,103–105]

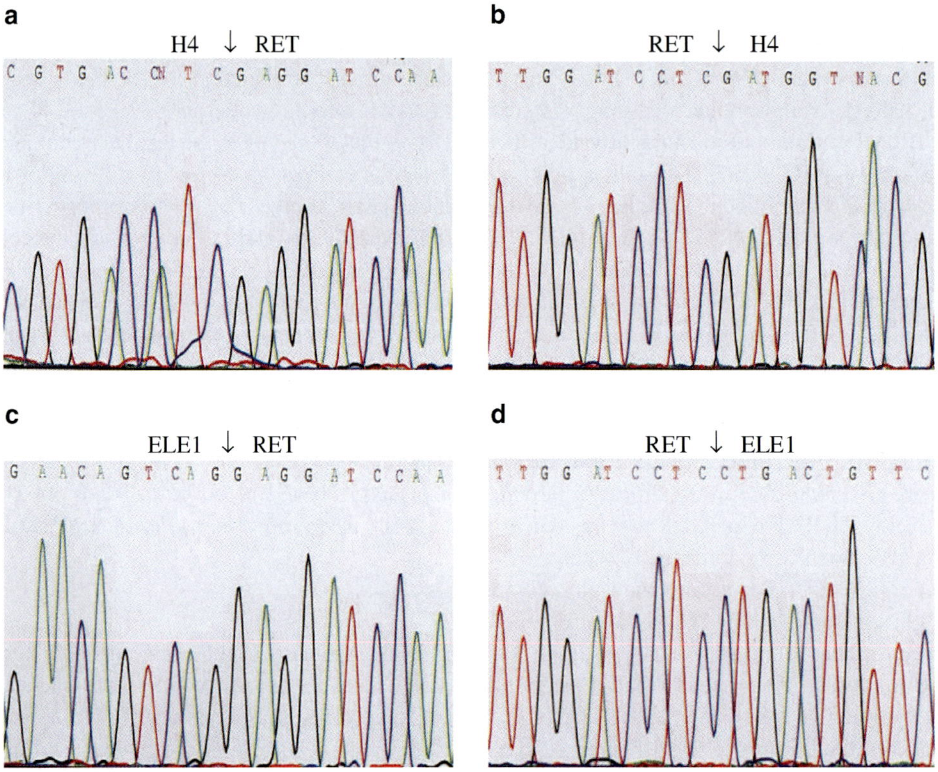

FIG. 8.5. Direct sequencing showed RET/PTC1 rearrangement (H4 and RET fusion) in a papillary thyroid carcinoma ((**a**) forward direction; (**b**) reverse direction). Another papillary thyroid carcinoma showing RET/PTC3 rearrangement (ELE1 and RET fusion). ((**c**) forward direction; (**d**) reverse direction).

RET/PTC rearrangement is a common genetic alteration in PTC with a prevalence that varies among geographical sites and tumor subtypes.[95] Overall, approximately 20–30% of sporadic adult PTC have RET/PTC rearrangement.[1] RET/PTC rearrangements are associated with younger age, papillary histology, psammoma bodies, and lymph node metastases.[77,97] RET/PTC rearrangements are the most common genetic alteration in PTC in children.[77,95,106] RET rearrangements are more commonly detected in incidentally discovered microcarcinomas than in clinically evident PTC, suggesting that RET plays a role in the initiation of thyroid tumorigenesis but is not required for further progression of the tumor.[107] RET rearrangements are not associated with aggressive features such as large tumor size, extrathyroidal extension, metastases, or with poorly differentiated or anaplastic thyroid carcinomas.[108] Generally, RET/PTC rearrangements are associated with well-differentiated PTC, and the subset of RET/PTC positive PTC do not progress to more aggressive, less differentiated tumor phenotypes.[108]

RET/PTC1 tends to be more common in papillary microcarcinomas, tumors with typical papillary growth, and a more benign clinical course, while RET/PTC3 is more common in the solid variant of PTC and more aggressive tumor behavior.[95] In a study of 21 papillary thyroid microcarcinomas by interphase fluorescence in situ hybridization, RET rearrangements were detected in 52% of microcarcinomas, a significantly higher frequency than that found in clinically evident PTC.[107] The authors concluded that the high frequency of RET rearrangements in microcarcinomas suggests that RET plays a role in the initiation of thyroid tumorigenesis but does not seem to be necessary for the further progression of the tumor.[107] In a series of 201 PTC, RET rearrangements were detected in 81 (40.3%) of PTC and correlated with "classic" morphological features of papillary cancer or with the microcarcinoma subtype.[108] A study evaluated the RET/PTC-1, -2, and -3 by PCR analysis in thyroid microcarcinomas and clinically evident PTC to determine its role in early stage versus developed PTC and to examine the diversity of RET/PTC in multifocal disease.[98] Thirty-nine occult papillary thyroid microcarcinomas were analyzed from 21 patients, and 30 microcarcinomas (77%) had RET/PTC rearrangements, 12 of which were RET/PTC1, three RET/ PTC2, six RET/PTC3, and nine had multiple RET/PTC rearrangements.[98] RET/PTC rearrangements were identified in 47% of clinically evident tumors.[98] Of the 17 patients with multifocal disease, identical RET/PTC rearrangements were identified in multiple tumors in two of the patients, while the other 15 patients had diverse rearrangements among their tumors.[98] The authors concluded that RET/PTC rearrangements may have a role in early-stage papillary thyroid carcinogenesis, but they are less important in determining progression to clinically-evident disease, and the diversity of RET/PTC rearrangements among multifocal tumors suggests that individual tumors arise independently in a background of genetic or environmental susceptibility.[98]

A recent study found RET rearrangements in 35.8% (14 of 39 cases) of cases of FVPTC. The prevalence of RET/PTC1 and RET/PTC3 were almost equal in classic PTC and FVPTC, but the tall cell cases showed only RET/PTC3 rearrangements.[109] p53 mutations are usually associated with poorly differentiated and anaplastic thyroid carcinoma, but p53 positivity was found in 61% of tall cell PTC when compared with 11% of common PTC.[110] The diffuse sclerosing variant is seen both in the setting of radiation-induced and in sporadic PTC, with RET/PTC1 being more common than RET/PTC3.[111] RET/PTC3 is more common in the solid/follicular variant, while RET/PTC1 associated with papillary carcinomas of the classic and diffuse sclerosing variants.[111] Another study of PTC in children exposed to radiation identified RET/PTC3 in 79% of solid variant of PTC, whereas only 7% had RET/PTC1 rearrangement.[96]

There are reports of RET/PTC in Hashimoto thyroiditis,[112,113] but others have found no RET/PTC rearrangements in Hashimoto thyroiditis or PTC arising in the background of Hashimoto thyroiditis in contrast to 33% prevalence in PTC not associated with Hashimoto thyroiditis.[114] Expression of wild-type RET was found in more than half of the PTC.[114] If there is an association between Hashimoto thyroiditis and PTC, the molecular basis is thought to be different from the RET/PTC rearrangement.[114] Also, variability in RET/PTC mRNA levels may contribute to inconsistencies in the reported detection rates.[115]

RAS

There are three RAS genes, H-RAS, K-RAS, and N-RAS. Mutational activation of RAS proto-oncogenes results in activation of the MAP kinase pathway. Although RAS point mutations occur relatively frequently in follicular thyroid carcinoma, poorly differentiated thyroid carcinoma, and anaplastic thyroid carcinoma, RAS point mutations occur only in a minority of PTC.[77,93] However, the prevalence of H-RAS, K-RAS, and N-RAS gene mutations in thyroid tumors according to malignancy and histology is controversial.[116] Different studies have identified different frequencies of mutations. A recent study of 96 unselected PTC found 15% had RAS mutations.[77] RAS mutations are more common in the FVPTC,[77,93] occurring in up to 43% of cases.[93] RAS mutations have correlated with less prominent nuclear features of PTC.[77] The prognostic significance of RAS mutations in PTC is controversial. A low rate of lymph node metastases has been reported in patients with PTC with RAS mutation.[77] Others have found RAS mutations to be more common in PTC associated with recurrence or death from disease,[117] while others have found RAS mutations not related to prognosis.[118] RAS mutations have correlated with the histologic differentiation of thyroid carcinomas overall, with higher rates of RAS mutation seen in poorly differentiated carcinomas than in well-differentiated carcinomas.[119] Thus, RAS mutations may be important in the progression from well-differentiated carcinoma to poorly differentiated thyroid carcinoma.[119] However, others have found RAS mutations to be equally prevalent in benign and malignant thyroid neoplasms and have suggested that it may be an early event in thyroid tumorigenesis.[120] Hence, the role of RAS mutations in thyroid carcinoma remains unclear.

Epigenetic Studies

Gene methylation is an important mechanism in regulating gene expression, while aberrant gene methylation can result in the inappropriate silencing of genes particularly tumor suppressor genes. PTEN, RASSF1A,[64] TIMP3 (tissue inhibitor of metalloproteinase-3), SLC5A8, DAPK (death-association protein kinase), and retinoic acid receptor B2 (RARB2) are tumor suppressor genes inappropriately silenced in thyroid carcinomas.,[121] with TIMP3, SCL5A8, and DAPK particularly important in PTC.[122] TIMP3 inhibits metalloproteinase-3 thereby inhibiting the degradation of interstitial matrix.[123] TIMP3 also inhibits angiogenesis by blocking vascular endothelial growth factor (VEGF) binding to VEGF receptor-2.[123] SLC5A8 is a proposed thyroid apical iodide transporter with proapoptotic functions which is down-regulated in classic PTC and methylated in 90% of classic PTC and 20% of other PTCs.[124] Low SLC5A8 expression was also associated with BRAF mutation.[124] DAPK also has proapoptotic functions and is methylated in a variety of cancers including PTC.[122,125] Aberrant methylation of tumor suppressor genes TIMP3, SCL5A8, and DAPK has been associated with features of aggressiveness in PTC, including extrathyroidal extension, lymph node metastases, multifocality, and advanced tumor stages.[122,125] Interestingly, methylation of these genes was also associated with BRAF mutation and classic and tall cell subtypes of PTC.[122] These genes, and others may be epigenetically modified in concert, and silencing of multiple genes increases with tumor progression.[125] These results suggest that aberrant methylation and hence silencing of TIMP3, SLC5A8, DAPK, and RARbeta2, in association with BRAF mutation, may be an important step in PTC tumorigenesis and progression.[122] Another study found a trend toward hypermethylation of multiple markers with hypermethylation of multiple markers detected in 25% of hyperplasias, 38% of adenomas, 48% of thyroid carcinomas, and 100% of thyroid cancer cell lines with a subset of markers appearing to be modified in concert and increasing methylation with cancer progression.[125]

Aberrant methylation of thyroid stimulating hormone receptor (TSHR) expression can silence this gene in PTC.[126] A recent study showed methylation of TSHR gene in 59% of PTC, 47% of follicular thyroid carcinomas, and no methylation in the follicular adenomas and normal thyroid tissues studied.[126] TSHR was normally expressed at the protein and mRNA level in thyroid tumor cell lines, where the TSHR gene was unmethylated, but it was silenced when the TSHR promoter was hypermethylated. They proposed a potential use of demethylating agents in conjunction with TSH-promoted radioiodine therapy for epithelial thyroid cancers.[126]

Gene Expression Profiling

Gene expression profiling has identified over and underexpression of a variety of genes in PTC. In an early study of gene expression array profiling of PTC, Huang et al[62] found that PTC showed concordant expression of many genes and distinct clustered profiles. Genes encoding adhesion and extracellular matrix proteins showed increased expression in PTC.[62] Genes overexpressed in PTC included MET, LGALS3, KRT19, DPP4, MDK, TIMP1, and FN1, as well as genes not previously identified in PTC such as CITED1, CHI3L1, ODZ1, N33, SFTPB, and SCEL.[62] Tumor suppressor genes, thyroid function proteins, and fatty acid binding proteins were underexpressed.[62] The microarrays are useful in identifying markers for further evaluation by other means. The authors demonstrated by immunohistochemical studies that 49 of 52 PTC were positive for CITED1 and 39 of 52 for SFTPB, while follicular thyroid carcinoma and normal thyroid tissues were negative.[62] Genes underexpressed in PTC included tumor suppressor genes, thyroid function-related proteins, and fatty acid binding proteins.[62] Another microarray expression analyses of six PTC showed expression changes in four genes not previously implicated in thyroid carcinogenesis, identified two distinct groups of genes that were either over- or underexpressed when compared with normal thyroid, and identified five genes that could collectively distinguish the PTC from follicular thyroid carcinoma.[127] PTC showed overexpression of CITED1, claudin-10, IGFBP6 but showed no change in the expression of caveolin-1 or -2.[127] However, FTC did not express CLDN10 and had decreased expression of IGFBP6 and/or CAV1 and CAV2.[127] Thus, the distinctive expression profiles indicate PTC and follicular carcinomas are different tumors and suggest markers that may be diagnostically useful.[127] Although DNA array analyses in papillary thyroid carcinoma are helpful in enabling the analysis of gene expression of thousands of genes simultaneously, limitations of DNA array analyses include the use of different platforms, intra-individual versus inter-individual comparisons, different reference tissues, and differences in data analysis methods complicates comparisons between different studies.[128] To date, only a few new molecular markers have been adapted for clinical use from gene expression profiling.

Other Genetic Studies

Other modalities have been utilized to study PTC including microRNA profiling, loss of heterozygosity and cytogenetic analyses. microRNAs are single-stranded, noncoding RNAs, 21–23 nucleotides in length, that negatively regulate gene expression.[129] microRNA expression profiles have been studied in PTC.[130–132] Different microRNA expression profiles have differentiated PTC cell lines with BRAF mutations as well as those with RET/PTC1 from normal thyroid cell lines.[130,131] Recently, a study characterized microRNAs signatures on microRNA obtained formalin-fixed paraffin-embedded PTC and identified 13 upregulated and 26 down regulated microRNAs in PTC compared to multinodular goiter.[132]

Loss of heterozygosity of tumor suppressor genes demonstrate that classic PTC have the lowest frequency of allelic loss (7%), followed by FVPTC (19%), tall cell (20%), and oncocytic (34%).[133] Allelic loss associated with increasing tumor size, but not with age, gender, extrathyroidal extension, or lymph node metastases.[133] Cytogenetic analysis of 94 PTC showed clonal chromosomal changes in 37 cases (40%) with structural cytogenetic abnormalities in 18 cases, including rearrangements of chromosomes 1, 3, 7, and 10 as well as novel breakpoint cluster regions.[134] The most common breakpoint loci 1p32–36, 1p11–13, 1q, 3p25–26, 7q34–36, and 10q11.2.[134] Karyotypic features correlated with some variants of PTC. FVPTC showed some chromosomal aberrations found in thyroid follicular adenomas: a del(11)(q13q13), a t(2;3)(q13;p35), and gains of chromosomes 3, 5, 7, 9, 12, 14, 17, and 20.[134] Of the tall cell PTC, four of the seven tumors had clonal cytogenetic changes, 3 (75%) of which were anomalies of chromosome 2 that lead to overrepresentation of the long arm of this chromosome. Noted also in these series was an association between complex karyotypes and tumors with poorly differentiated histotypes.

Hereditary Papillary Thyroid Carcinoma

Introduction

The overwhelming majority of PTC occurs sporadically, but familial cases have been identified.[21,135–142] PTC has also been reported with ataxia telangiectasia,[143] Gardner syndrome and Cowden syndrome.[135] The cribriform-morular variant of PTC is characteristically occurring in the familial setting.

Clinical

The cribriform-morular variant of PTC can occur as a sporadic tumor,[144] but characteristically occurs in the setting of familial adenomatous polyposis (FAP) and germ line mutations in the *APC* gene on chromosome 5q21–22.[144–148] The cribriform-morular variant of PTC may be solitary or multiple and occurs predominantly in young women. Although the tumors are often well demarcated, total thyroidectomy has been advocated by some because of the frequent multicentricity of the tumor.[146] These tumors behave similarly to conventional PTC.

Histologic Features

The tumor cells have cytologic features of PTC, but are hyperchromatic. The architecture is characterized by cribriform areas with anastomosing bars and arches without intervening

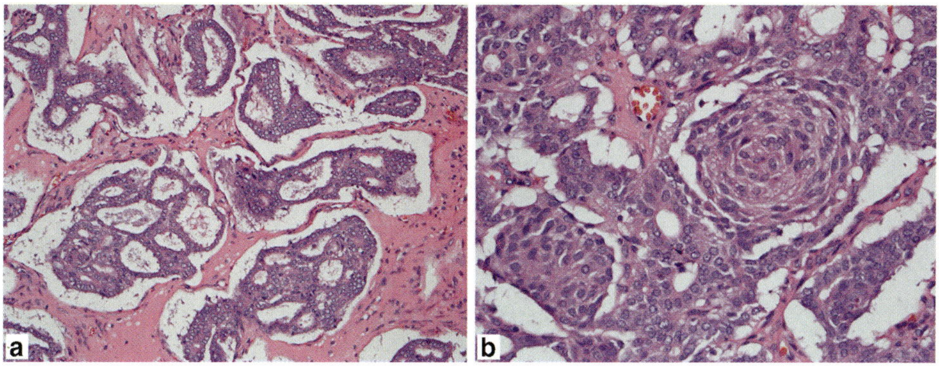

FIG. 8.6. Cribriform-morular variant of papillary thyroid carcinoma (PTC). (**a**) Cribriform-morular variant of PTC with cribriform structures. (**b**) Areas of morular growth in a cribriform-morular variant of PTC.

stroma and areas solid/trabecular and morular growth (Figure 8.6).[147]

Immunohistochemistry

The cribriform-morular variant of PTC shows focal positivity for thyroglobulin.[1] Beta-catenin is also positive in these tumors.

Genetic Findings

Patients with FAP may present with this thyroid tumor before their colon findings are known.[146] Hence, patients diagnosed with the cribriform-morular variant of PTC should be evaluated for the possibility of FAP. A recent study of five young women with the cribriform-morular variant of PTC found two patients with attenuated FAP.[148] The *CTNNB1* gene is located on chromosome 3p21 which encodes beta-catenin. Germline *APC* mutation was identified in only one FAP patient, but somatic mutation analysis of exon 3 of the beta-catenin gene (*CTNNB1*) revealed alterations in seven tumors from all five individuals.[148] Two different tumors from two patients with the multicentric PTC had different somatic mutations of the *CTNNB1* gene suggesting that accumulation of mutant beta-catenin contributes to the development of the cribriform-morular variant of PTC.[148] A report of two FAP kindreds with thyroid cancer with two novel germline *APC* mutations suggested that genetic alterations in FAP-associated thyroid cancer involve loss of function of *APC* along with the gain of function of RET/PTC.[147]

Conclusion

As PTC is the most common endocrine malignancy and is increasing in incidence, molecular genetic discoveries will play an increasingly important role in elucidating the pathogenesis and providing diagnostic and prognostic markers for these neoplasms.

References

1. DeLellis RA, Lloyd RV, Heitz PU, Eng C. *Pathology and Genetics of Tumours of Endocrine Organs. World Health Organization Classification of Tumours*. Lyon: IARC; 2004:320.
2. Rosai J, Carcangiu ML, DeLellis RA. *Tumors of the Thyroid Gland. Atlas of Tumor Pathology*. Vol 5, 3rd Series edition. Washington, DC: Armed Forces Institute of Pathology; 1992:343.
3. Melillo RM, Castellone MD, Guarino V, et al. The RET/PTC-RAS-BRAF linear signaling cascade mediates the motile and mitogenic phenotype of thyroid cancer cells. *J Clin Invest*. 2005;115:1068–1081.
4. Calandra DB, Shah KH, Lawrence AM, Paloyan E. Total thyroidectomy in irradiated patients. A twenty-year experience in 206 patients. *Ann Surg*. 1985;202:356–360.
5. Furmanchuk AW, Averkin JI, Egloff B, et al. Pathomorphological findings in thyroid cancers of children from the Republic of Belarus: a study of 86 cases occurring between 1986 ('post-Chernobyl') and 1991. *Histopathology*. 1992;21:401–408.
6. Unger K, Zurnadzhy L, Walch A, et al. RET rearrangements in post-Chernobyl papillary thyroid carcinomas with a short latency analysed by interphase FISH. *Br J Cancer*. 2006;94:1472–1477.
7. Williams ED, Abrosimov A, Bogdanova T, et al. Thyroid carcinoma after Chernobyl latent period, morphology and aggressiveness. *Br J Cancer*. 2004;90:2219–2224.
8. Nikiforova MN, Ciampi R, Salvatore G, et al. Low prevalence of BRAF mutations in radiation-induced thyroid tumors in contrast to sporadic papillary carcinomas. *Cancer Lett*. 2004;209:1–6.
9. Akslen LA, LiVolsi VA. Prognostic significance of histologic grading compared with subclassification of papillary thyroid carcinoma. *Cancer*. 2000;88:1902–1908.
10. Johnson TL, Lloyd RV, Thompson NW, Beierwaltes WH, Sisson JC. Prognostic implications of the tall cell variant of papillary thyroid carcinoma. *Am J Surg Pathol*. 1988;12:22–27.
11. Michels JJ, Jacques M, Henry-Amar M, Bardet S. Prevalence and prognostic significance of tall cell variant of papillary thyroid carcinoma. *Hum Pathol*. 2007;38:212–219.
12. Moreno Egea A, Rodriguez Gonzalez JM, Sola Perez J, Soria Cogollos T, Parrilla Paricio P. Prognostic value of the tall cell

variety of papillary cancer of the thyroid. *Eur J Surg Oncol.* 1993;19:517–521.
13. Ferreiro JA, Hay ID, Lloyd RV. Columnar cell carcinoma of the thyroid: report of three additional cases. *Hum Pathol.* 1996;27: 1156–1160.
14. Besic N, Hocevar M, Zgajnar J, Petric R, Pilko G. Aggressiveness of therapy and prognosis of patients with Hurthle cell papillary thyroid carcinoma. *Thyroid.* 2006;16:67–72.
15. Davies L, Welch HG. Increasing incidence of thyroid cancer in the United States, 1973–2002. *JAMA.* 2006;295:2164–2167.
16. Baloch ZW, LiVolsi VA. Microcarcinoma of the thyroid. *Adv Anat Pathol.* 2006;13:69–75.
17. de Matos PS, Ferreira AP, Ward LS. Prevalence of papillary microcarcinoma of the thyroid in Brazilian autopsy and surgical series. *Endocr Pathol.* 2006;17:165–173.
18. Harach HR, Franssila KO, Wasenius VM. Occult papillary carcinoma of the thyroid. A "normal" finding in Finland. A systematic autopsy study. *Cancer.* 1985;56:531–538.
19. Haas SN. Management of papillary microcarcinoma of the thyroid. *S D Med.* 2006;59:425–427.
20. Lo CY, Chan WF, Lang BH, Lam KY, Wan KY. Papillary microcarcinoma: is there any difference between clinically overt and occult tumors? *World J Surg.* 2006;30:759–766.
21. Lupoli G, Vitale G, Caraglia M, et al. Familial papillary thyroid microcarcinoma: a new clinical entity. *Lancet.* 1999;353:637–639.
22. Crile G Jr, Hazard JB. Relationship of the age of the patient to the natural history and prognosis of carcinoma of the thyroid. *Ann Surg.* 1953;138:33–38.
23. Hazard JB, Crile G Jr, Dinsmore RS, Hawk WA, Kenyon R. Neoplasms of the thyroid: classification, morphology, and treatment. *AMA Arch Pathol.* 1955;59:502–513.
24. Lindsay S. Natural history of thyroid carcinoma. *Ariz Med.* 1960;17:623–627.
25. Chem KT, Rosai J. Follicular variant of thyroid papillary carcinoma: a clinicopathologic study of six cases. *Am J Surg Pathol.* 1977;1:123–130.
26. Lloyd RV, Erickson LA, Casey MB, et al. Observer variation in the diagnosis of follicular variant of papillary thyroid carcinoma. *Am J Surg Pathol.* 2004;28:1336–1340.
27. Vestfrid MA. Papillary carcinoma of the thyroid gland with lipomatous stroma: report of a peculiar histological type of thyroid tumour. *Histopathology.* 1986;10:97–100.
28. Hawk WA, Hazard JB. The many appearances of papillary carcinoma of the thyroid. *Cleve Clin Q.* 1976;43:207–215.
29. Nardone HC, Ziober AF, LiVolsi VA, et al. c-Met expression in tall cell variant papillary carcinoma of the thyroid. *Cancer.* 2003;98:1386–1393.
30. Evans HL. Columnar-cell carcinoma of the thyroid. A report of two cases of an aggressive variant of thyroid carcinoma. *Am J Clin Pathol.* 1986;85:77–80.
31. Nikiforov YE, Erickson LA, Nikiforova MN, Caudill CM, Lloyd RV. Solid variant of papillary thyroid carcinoma: incidence, clinical-pathologic characteristics, molecular analysis, and biologic behavior. *Am J Surg Pathol.* 2001;25:1478–1484.
32. Keelawat S, Poumsuk U. Association between different variants of papillary thyroid carcinoma and risk-group according to AMES (age, metastasis, extent and size) classification system. *J Med Assoc Thai.* 2006;89:484–489.
33. Nikiforov Y, Gnepp DR. Pediatric thyroid cancer after the Chernobyl disaster. Pathomorphologic study of 84 cases (1991–1992) from the Republic of Belarus. *Cancer.* 1994;74:748–766.
34. Mai KT, Thomas J, Yazdi HM, Commons AS, Lamba M, Stinson AW. Pathologic study and clinical significance of Hurthle cell papillary thyroid carcinoma. *Appl Immunohistochem Mol Morphol.* 2004;12:329–337.
35. Herrera MF, Hay ID, Wu PS, et al. Hurthle cell (oxyphilic) papillary thyroid carcinoma: a variant with more aggressive biologic behavior. *World J Surg.* 1992;16:669–674. discussion 774–775.
36. Apel RL, Asa SL, LiVolsi VA. Papillary Hurthle cell carcinoma with lymphocytic stroma. "Warthin-like tumor" of the thyroid. *Am J Surg Pathol.* 1995;19:810–814.
37. Lam KY, Lo CY, Wei WI. Warthin tumor-like variant of papillary thyroid carcinoma: a case with dedifferentiation (anaplastic changes) and aggressive biological behavior. *Endocr Pathol.* 2005;16:83–89.
38. Vickery AL Jr, Carcangiu ML, Johannessen JV, Sobrinho-Simoes M. Papillary carcinoma. *Semin Diagn Pathol.* 1985;2:90–100.
39. Carcangiu ML, Bianchi S. Diffuse sclerosing variant of papillary thyroid carcinoma. Clinicopathologic study of 15 cases. *Am J Surg Pathol.* 1989;13:1041–1049.
40. Soares J, Limbert E, Sobrinho-Simoes M. Diffuse sclerosing variant of papillary thyroid carcinoma. A clinicopathologic study of 10 cases. *Pathol Res Pract.* 1989;185:200–206.
41. Falvo L, Giacomelli L, D'Andrea V, Marzullo A, Guerriero G, de Antoni E. Prognostic importance of sclerosing variant in papillary thyroid carcinoma. *Am Surg.* 2006;72:438–444.
42. Thompson LD, Wieneke JA, Heffess CS. Diffuse sclerosing variant of papillary thyroid carcinoma: a clinicopathologic and immunophenotypic analysis of 22 cases. *Endocr Pathol.* 2005;16:331–348.
43. Erickson LA, Yousef OM, Jin L, Lohse CM, Pankratz VS, Lloyd RV. p27kip1 expression distinguishes papillary hyperplasia in Graves' disease from papillary thyroid carcinoma. *Mod Pathol.* 2000;13:1014–1019.
44. Ivanova R, Soares P, Castro P, Sobrinho-Simoes M. Diffuse (or multinodular) follicular variant of papillary thyroid carcinoma: a clinicopathologic and immunohistochemical analysis of ten cases of an aggressive form of differentiated thyroid carcinoma. *Virchows Arch.* 2002;440:418–424.
45. Mizukami Y, Nonomura A, Michigishi T, Ohmura K, Noguchi M, Ishizaki T. Diffuse follicular variant of papillary carcinoma of the thyroid. *Histopathology.* 1995;27:575–577.
46. Akslen LA, Varhaug JE. Thyroid carcinoma with mixed tall-cell and columnar-cell features. *Am J Clin Pathol.* 1990;94: 442–445.
47. Gaertner EM, Davidson M, Wenig BM. The columnar cell variant of thyroid papillary carcinoma. Case report and discussion of an unusually aggressive thyroid papillary carcinoma. *Am J Surg Pathol.* 1995;19:940–947.
48. Evans HL. Encapsulated columnar-cell neoplasms of the thyroid. A report of four cases suggesting a favorable prognosis. *Am J Surg Pathol.* 1996;20:1205–1211.
49. Baloch ZW, LiVolsi VA. Warthin-like papillary carcinoma of the thyroid. *Arch Pathol Lab Med.* 2000;124:1192–1195.
50. Chan JK, Carcangiu ML, Rosai J. Papillary carcinoma of thyroid with exuberant nodular fasciitis-like stroma. Report of three cases. *Am J Clin Pathol.* 1991;95:309–314.
51. Carcangiu ML, Sibley RK, Rosai J. Clear cell change in primary thyroid tumors. A study of 38 cases. *Am J Surg Pathol.* 1985;9:705–722.

52. Variakojis D, Getz ML, Paloyan E, Straus FH. Papillary clear cell carcinoma of the thyroid gland. *Hum Pathol.* 1975; 6:384–390.
53. Casey MB, Lohse CM, Lloyd RV. Distinction between papillary thyroid hyperplasia and papillary thyroid carcinoma by immunohistochemical staining for cytokeratin 19, galectin-3, and HBME-1. *Endocr Pathol.* 2003;14:55–60.
54. Prasad ML, Pellegata NS, Huang Y, Nagaraja HN, de la Chapelle A, Kloos RT. Galectin-3, fibronectin-1, CITED-1, HBME1 and cytokeratin-19 immunohistochemistry is useful for the differential diagnosis of thyroid tumors. *Mod Pathol.* 2005;18:48–57.
55. Scognamiglio T, Hyjek E, Kao J, Chen YT. Diagnostic usefulness of HBME1, galectin-3, CK19, and CITED1 and evaluation of their expression in encapsulated lesions with questionable features of papillary thyroid carcinoma. *Am J Clin Pathol.* 2006;126:700–708.
56. de Matos PS, Ferreira AP, de Oliveira Facuri F, Assumpcao LV, Metze K, Ward LS. Usefulness of HBME-1, cytokeratin 19 and galectin-3 immunostaining in the diagnosis of thyroid malignancy. *Histopathology.* 2005;47:391–401.
57. Barroeta JE, Baloch ZW, Lal P, Pasha TL, Zhang PJ, LiVolsi VA. Diagnostic value of differential expression of CK19, Galectin-3, HBME-1, ERK, RET, and p16 in benign and malignant follicular-derived lesions of the thyroid: an immunohistochemical tissue microarray analysis. *Endocr Pathol.* 2006;17:225–234.
58. Nakamura N, Erickson LA, Jin L, et al. Immunohistochemical separation of follicular variant of papillary thyroid carcinoma from follicular adenoma. *Endocr Pathol.* 2006;17:213–223.
59. Nasr MR, Mukhopadhyay S, Zhang S, Katzenstein AL. Immunohistochemical markers in diagnosis of papillary thyroid carcinoma: utility of HBME1 combined with CK19 immunostaining. *Mod Pathol.* 2006;19:1631–1637.
60. Gaffney RL, Carney JA, Sebo TJ, et al. Galectin-3 expression in hyalinizing trabecular tumors of the thyroid gland. *Am J Surg Pathol.* 2003;27:494–498.
61. Prasad ML, Pellegata NS, Kloos RT, Barbacioru C, Huang Y, de la Chapelle A. CITED1 protein expression suggests Papillary Thyroid Carcinoma in high throughput tissue microarray-based study. *Thyroid.* 2004;14:169–175.
62. Huang Y, Prasad M, Lemon WJ, et al. Gene expression in papillary thyroid carcinoma reveals highly consistent profiles. *Proc Natl Acad Sci USA.* 2001;98:15044–15049.
63. Davies H, Bignell GR, Cox C, et al. Mutations of the BRAF gene in human cancer. *Nature.* 2002;417:949–954.
64. Nakamura N, Carney JA, Jin L, et al. RASSF1A and NORE1A methylation and BRAFV600E mutations in thyroid tumors. *Lab Invest.* 2005;85:1065–1075.
65. Cohen Y, Xing M, Mambo E, et al. BRAF mutation in papillary thyroid carcinoma. *J Natl Cancer Inst.* 2003;95:625–627.
66. Fukushima T, Suzuki S, Mashiko M, et al. BRAF mutations in papillary carcinomas of the thyroid. *Oncogene.* 2003;22: 6455–6457.
67. Kimura ET, Nikiforova MN, Zhu Z, Knauf JA, Nikiforov YE, Fagin JA. High prevalence of BRAF mutations in thyroid cancer: genetic evidence for constitutive activation of the RET/PTC-RAS-BRAF signaling pathway in papillary thyroid carcinoma. *Cancer Res.* 2003;63:1454–1457.
68. Soares P, Trovisco V, Rocha AS, et al. BRAF mutations and RET/PTC rearrangements are alternative events in the etiopathogenesis of PTC. *Oncogene.* 2003;22:4578–4580.
69. Trovisco V, Vieira de Castro I, Soares P, et al. BRAF mutations are associated with some histological types of papillary thyroid carcinoma. *J Pathol.* 2004;202:247–251.
70. Trovisco V, Soares P, Soares R, Magalhaes J, Sa-Couto P, Sobrinho-Simoes M. A new BRAF gene mutation detected in a case of a solid variant of papillary thyroid carcinoma. *Hum Pathol.* 2005;36:694–697.
71. Moretti S, Macchiarulo A, De Falco V, et al. Biochemical and molecular characterization of the novel BRAF(V599Ins) mutation detected in a classic papillary thyroid carcinoma. *Oncogene.* 2006;25:4235–4240.
72. Xing M. BRAF mutation in papillary thyroid cancer: pathogenic role, molecular bases, and clinical implications. *Endocr Rev.* 2007;28:742–762.
73. Liu D, Hu S, Hou P, Jiang D, Condouris S, Xing M. Suppression of BRAF/MEK/MAP kinase pathway restores expression of iodide-metabolizing genes in thyroid cells expressing the V600E BRAF mutant. *Clin Cancer Res.* 2007;13:1341–1349.
74. Ball DW, Jin N, Rosen DM, et al. Selective growth inhibition in BRAF mutant thyroid cancer by the mitogen-activated protein kinase kinase 1/2 inhibitor AZD6244. *J Clin Endocrinol Metab.* 2007;92:4712–4718.
75. Powell N, Jeremiah S, Morishita M, et al. Frequency of BRAF T1796A mutation in papillary thyroid carcinoma relates to age of patient at diagnosis and not to radiation exposure. *J Pathol.* 2005;205:558–564.
76. Trovisco V, Soares P, Preto A, et al. Type and prevalence of BRAF mutations are closely associated with papillary thyroid carcinoma histotype and patients' age but not with tumour aggressiveness. *Virchows Arch.* 2005;446:589–595.
77. Adeniran AJ, Zhu Z, Gandhi M, et al. Correlation between genetic alterations and microscopic features, clinical manifestations, and prognostic characteristics of thyroid papillary carcinomas. *Am J Surg Pathol.* 2006;30:216–222.
78. Collins BJ, Schneider AB, Prinz RA, Xu X. Low frequency of BRAF mutations in adult patients with papillary thyroid cancers following childhood radiation exposure. *Thyroid.* 2006; 16:61 66.
79. Ciampi R, Knauf JA, Kerler R, et al. Oncogenic AKAP9-BRAF fusion is a novel mechanism of MAPK pathway activation in thyroid cancer. *J Clin Invest.* 2005;115:94–101.
80. Xing M, Westra WH, Tufano RP, et al. BRAF mutation predicts a poorer clinical prognosis for papillary thyroid cancer. *J Clin Endocrinol Metab.* 2005;90:6373–6379.
81. Kim TY, Kim WB, Rhee YS, et al. The BRAF mutation is useful for prediction of clinical recurrence in low-risk patients with conventional papillary thyroid carcinoma. *Clin Endocrinol (Oxf).* 2006;65:364–368.
82. Riesco-Eizaguirre G, Gutierrez-Martinez P, Garcia-Cabezas MA, Nistal M, Santisteban P. The oncogene BRAF V600E is associated with a high risk of recurrence and less differentiated papillary thyroid carcinoma due to the impairment of Na+/I- targeting to the membrane. *Endocr Relat Cancer.* 2006;13:257–269.
83. Di Cristofaro J, Marcy M, Vasko V, et al. Molecular genetic study comparing follicular variant versus classic papillary thyroid carcinomas: association of N-ras mutation in codon 61 with follicular variant. *Hum Pathol.* 2006;37:824–830.
84. Jin L, Sebo TJ, Nakamura N, et al. BRAF mutation analysis in fine needle aspiration (FNA) cytology of the thyroid. *Diagn Mol Pathol.* 2006;15:136–143.

85. Lupi C, Giannini R, Ugolini C, et al. Association of BRAF V600E mutation with poor clinicopathological outcomes in 500 consecutive cases of papillary thyroid carcinoma. *J Clin Endocrinol Metab*. 2007;92:4085–4090.
86. Kim TY, Kim WB, Song JY, et al. The BRAF mutation is not associated with poor prognostic factors in Korean patients with conventional papillary thyroid microcarcinoma. *Clin Endocrinol (Oxf)*. 2005;63:588–593.
87. Liu RT, Chen YJ, Chou FF, et al. No correlation between BRAFV600E mutation and clinicopathological features of papillary thyroid carcinomas in Taiwan. *Clin Endocrinol (Oxf)*. 2005;63:461–466.
88. Nikiforova MN, Kimura ET, Gandhi M, et al. BRAF mutations in thyroid tumors are restricted to papillary carcinomas and anaplastic or poorly differentiated carcinomas arising from papillary carcinomas. *J Clin Endocrinol Metab*. 2003;88:5399–5404.
89. Abrosimov A, Saenko V, Rogounovitch T, et al. Different structural components of conventional papillary thyroid carcinoma display mostly identical BRAF status. *Int J Cancer*. 2007;120:196–200.
90. Frattini M, Ferrario C, Bressan P, et al. Alternative mutations of BRAF, RET and NTRK1 are associated with similar but distinct gene expression patterns in papillary thyroid cancer. *Oncogene*. 2004;23:7436–7440.
91. Lee JH, Lee ES, Kim YS, Won NH, Chae YS. BRAF mutation and AKAP9 expression in sporadic papillary thyroid carcinomas. *Pathology*. 2006;38:201–204.
92. Sedliarou I, Saenko V, Lantsov D, et al. The BRAFT1796A transversion is a prevalent mutational event in human thyroid microcarcinoma. *Int J Oncol*. 2004;25:1729–1735.
93. Zhu Z, Gandhi M, Nikiforova MN, Fischer AH, Nikiforov YE. Molecular profile and clinical-pathologic features of the follicular variant of papillary thyroid carcinoma. An unusually high prevalence of ras mutations. *Am J Clin Pathol*. 2003;120: 71–77.
94. Pasini B, Hofstra RM, Yin L, et al. The physical map of the human RET proto-oncogene. *Oncogene*. 1995;11: 1737–1743.
95. Nikiforov YE. RET/PTC rearrangement in thyroid tumors. *Endocr Pathol*. 2002;13:3–16.
96. Nikiforov YE, Rowland JM, Bove KE, Monforte-Munoz H, Fagin JA. Distinct pattern of ret oncogene rearrangements in morphological variants of radiation-induced and sporadic thyroid papillary carcinomas in children. *Cancer Res*. 1997;57:1690–1694.
97. Nakazawa T, Kondo T, Kobayashi Y, et al. RET gene rearrangements (RET/PTC1 and RET/PTC3) in papillary thyroid carcinomas from an iodine-rich country (Japan). *Cancer*. 2005;104:943–951.
98. Sugg SL, Ezzat S, Rosen IB, Freeman JL, Asa SL. Distinct multiple RET/PTC gene rearrangements in multifocal papillary thyroid neoplasia. *J Clin Endocrinol Metab*. 1998;83: 4116–4122.
99. de Groot JW, Links TP, Plukker JT, Lips CJ, Hofstra RM. RET as a diagnostic and therapeutic target in sporadic and hereditary endocrine tumors. *Endocr Rev*. 2006;27:535–560.
100. Collins BJ, Chiappetta G, Schneider AB, et al. RET expression in papillary thyroid cancer from patients irradiated in childhood for benign conditions. *J Clin Endocrinol Metab*. 2002;87:3941–3946.
101. Bounacer A, Wicker R, Caillou B, et al. High prevalence of activating ret proto-oncogene rearrangements, in thyroid tumors from patients who had received external radiation. *Oncogene*. 1997;15:1263–1273.
102. Rabes HM, Klugbauer S. Molecular genetics of childhood papillary thyroid carcinomas after irradiation: high prevalence of RET rearrangement. *Recent Results Cancer Res*. 1998;154:248–264.
103. Rabes HM, Demidchik EP, Sidorow JD, et al. Pattern of radiation-induced RET and NTRK1 rearrangements in 191 post-chernobyl papillary thyroid carcinomas: biological, phenotypic, and clinical implications. *Clin Cancer Res*. 2000;6: 1093–1103.
104. Rabes HM. Gene rearrangements in radiation-induced thyroid carcinogenesis. *Med Pediatr Oncol*. 2001;36:574–582.
105. Thomas GA, Bunnell H, Cook HA, et al. High prevalence of RET/PTC rearrangements in Ukrainian and Belarussian post-Chernobyl thyroid papillary carcinomas: a strong correlation between RET/PTC3 and the solid-follicular variant. *J Clin Endocrinol Metab*. 1999;84:4232–4238.
106. Fenton CL, Lukes Y, Nicholson D, Dinauer CA, Francis GL, Tuttle RM. The ret/PTC mutations are common in sporadic papillary thyroid carcinoma of children and young adults. *J Clin Endocrinol Metab*. 2000;85:1170–1175.
107. Corvi R, Martinez-Alfaro M, Harach HR, Zini M, Papotti M, Romeo G. Frequent RET rearrangements in thyroid papillary microcarcinoma detected by interphase fluorescence in situ hybridization. *Lab Invest*. 2001;81:1639–1645.
108. Tallini G, Santoro M, Helie M, et al. RET/PTC oncogene activation defines a subset of papillary thyroid carcinomas lacking evidence of progression to poorly differentiated or undifferentiated tumor phenotypes. *Clin Cancer Res*. 1998;4:287–294.
109. Basolo F, Giannini R, Monaco C, et al. Potent mitogenicity of the RET/PTC3 oncogene correlates with its prevalence in tall-cell variant of papillary thyroid carcinoma. *Am J Pathol*. 2002;160:247–254.
110. Ruter A, Dreifus J, Jones M, Nishiyama R, Lennquist S. Overexpression of p53 in tall cell variants of papillary thyroid carcinoma. *Surgery*. 1996;120:1046–1050.
111. Santoro M, Thomas GA, Vecchio G, et al. Gene rearrangement and Chernobyl related thyroid cancers. *Br J Cancer*. 2000;82:315–322.
112. Wirtschafter A, Schmidt R, Rosen D, et al. Expression of the RET/PTC fusion gene as a marker for papillary carcinoma in Hashimoto's thyroiditis. *Laryngoscope*. 1997;107:95–100.
113. Arif S, Blanes A, Diaz-Cano SJ. Hashimoto's thyroiditis shares features with early papillary thyroid carcinoma. *Histopathology*. 2002;41:357–362.
114. Nikiforova MN, Caudill CM, Biddinger P, Nikiforov YE. Prevalence of RET/PTC rearrangements in Hashimoto's thyroiditis and papillary thyroid carcinomas. *Int J Surg Pathol*. 2002;10:15–22.
115. Rhoden KJ, Johnson C, Brandao G, Howe JG, Smith BR, Tallini G. Real-time quantitative RT-PCR identifies distinct c-RET, RET/PTC1 and RET/PTC3 expression patterns in papillary thyroid carcinoma. *Lab Invest*. 2004;84:1557–1570.
116. Vasko V, Ferrand M, Di Cristofaro J, Carayon P, Henry JF, de Micco C. Specific pattern of RAS oncogene mutations in follicular thyroid tumors. *J Clin Endocrinol Metab*. 2003;88: 2745–2752.

117. Hara H, Fulton N, Yashiro T, Ito K, DeGroot LJ, Kaplan EL. N-ras mutation: an independent prognostic factor for aggressiveness of papillary thyroid carcinoma. *Surgery*. 1994;116: 1010–1016.
118. Capella G, Matias-Guiu X, Ampudia X, de Leiva A, Perucho M, Prat J. Ras oncogene mutations in thyroid tumors: polymerase chain reaction-restriction-fragment-length polymorphism analysis from paraffin-embedded tissues. *Diagn Mol Pathol*. 1996;5:45–52.
119. Motoi N, Sakamoto A, Yamochi T, Horiuchi H, Motoi T, Machinami R. Role of ras mutation in the progression of thyroid carcinoma of follicular epithelial origin. *Pathol Res Pract*. 2000;196:1–7.
120. Namba H, Rubin SA, Fagin JA. Point mutations of ras oncogenes are an early event in thyroid tumorigenesis. *Mol Endocrinol*. 1990;4:1474–1479.
121. Xing M. Gene methylation in thyroid tumorigenesis. *Endocrinology*. 2007;148:948–953.
122. Hu S, Liu D, Tufano RP, et al. Association of aberrant methylation of tumor suppressor genes with tumor aggressiveness and BRAF mutation in papillary thyroid cancer. *Int J Cancer*. 2006;119:2322–2329.
123. Qi JH, Ebrahem Q, Moore N, et al. A novel function for tissue inhibitor of metalloproteinases-3 (TIMP3): inhibition of angiogenesis by blockage of VEGF binding to VEGF receptor-2. *Nat Med*. 2003;9:407–415.
124. Porra V, Ferraro-Peyret C, Durand C, et al. Silencing of the tumor suppressor gene SLC5A8 is associated with BRAF mutations in classical papillary thyroid carcinomas. *J Clin Endocrinol Metab*. 2005;90:3028–3035.
125. Hoque MO, Rosenbaum E, Westra WH, et al. Quantitative assessment of promoter methylation profiles in thyroid neoplasms. *J Clin Endocrinol Metab*. 2005;90:4011–4018.
126. Xing M, Usadel H, Cohen Y, et al. Methylation of the thyroid-stimulating hormone receptor gene in epithelial thyroid tumors: a marker of malignancy and a cause of gene silencing. *Cancer Res*. 2003;63:2316–2321.
127. Aldred MA, Huang Y, Liyanarachchi S, et al. Papillary and follicular thyroid carcinomas show distinctly different microarray expression profiles and can be distinguished by a minimum of five genes. *J Clin Oncol*. 2004;22:3531–3539.
128. Eszlinger M, Krohn K, Kukulska A, Jarzab B, Paschke R. Perspectives and limitations of microarray based gene expression profiling of thyroid tumors. *Endocr Rev*. 2007;28(3):322–338.
129. Ruvkun G. Molecular biology. Glimpses of a tiny RNA world. *Science*. 2001;294:797–799.
130. Cahill S, Smyth P, Denning K, et al. Effect of BRAFV600E mutation on transcription and post-transcriptional regulation in a papillary thyroid carcinoma model. *Mol Cancer*. 2007;6:21.
131. Cahill S, Smyth P, Finn SP, et al. Effect of ret/PTC 1 rearrangement on transcription and post-transcriptional regulation in a papillary thyroid carcinoma model. *Mol Cancer*. 2006;5:70.
132. Tetzlaff MT, Liu A, Xu X, et al. Differential expression of miRNAs in papillary thyroid carcinoma compared to multinodular goiter using formalin fixed paraffin embedded tissues. *Endocr Pathol*. 2007;18:163–173.
133. Hunt JL, Fowler M, Lomago D, et al. Tumor suppressor gene allelic loss profiles of the variants of papillary thyroid carcinoma. *Diagn Mol Pathol*. 2004;13:41–46.
134. Roque L, Nunes VM, Ribeiro C, Martins C, Soares J. Karyotypic characterization of papillary thyroid carcinomas. *Cancer*. 2001;92:2529–2538.
135. Alsanea O, Clark OH. Familial thyroid cancer. *Curr Opin Oncol*. 2001;13:44–51.
136. Corvi R, Lesueur F, Martinez-Alfaro M, et al. RET rearrangements in familial papillary thyroid carcinomas. *Cancer Lett*. 2001;170:191–198.
137. Eng C. Familial papillary thyroid cancer – many syndromes, too many genes? *J Clin Endocrinol Metab*. 2000;85: 1755–1757.
138. Frich L, Glattre E, Akslen LA. Familial occurrence of nonmedullary thyroid cancer: a population-based study of 5673 first-degree relatives of thyroid cancer patients from Norway. *Cancer Epidemiol Biomarkers Prev*. 2001;10:113–117.
139. Gorson D. Familial papillary carcinoma of the thyroid. *Thyroid*. 1992;2:131–132.
140. Malchoff CD, Sarfarazi M, Tendler B, Forouhar F, Whalen G, Malchoff DM. Familial papillary thyroid carcinoma is genetically distinct from familial adenomatous polyposis coli. *Thyroid*. 1999;9:247–252.
141. Malchoff CD, Malchoff DM. Familial papillary thyroid carcinoma. *Cancer Treat Res*. 2004;122:381–387.
142. McKay JD, Williamson J, Lesueur F, et al. At least three genes account for familial papillary thyroid carcinoma: TCO and MNG1 excluded as susceptibility loci from a large Tasmanian family. *Eur J Endocrinol*. 1999;141:122–125.
143. Narita T, Takagi K. Ataxia-telangiectasia with dysgerminoma of right ovary, papillary carcinoma of thyroid, and adenocarcinoma of pancreas. *Cancer*. 1984;54:1113–1116.
144. Cameselle-Teijeiro J, Chan JK. Cribriform-morular variant of papillary carcinoma: a distinctive variant representing the sporadic counterpart of familial adenomatous polyposis-associated thyroid carcinoma? *Mod Pathol*. 1999;12:400–411.
145. Chan JK, Loo KT. Cribriform variant of papillary thyroid carcinoma. *Arch Pathol Lab Med*. 1990;114:622–624.
146. Harach HR, Williams GT, Williams ED. Familial adenomatous polyposis associated thyroid carcinoma: a distinct type of follicular cell neoplasm. *Histopathology*. 1994;25:549–561.
147. Soravia C, Sugg SL, Berk T, et al. Familial adenomatous polyposis-associated thyroid cancer: a clinical, pathological, and molecular genetics study. *Am J Pathol*. 1999;154:127–135.
148. Xu B, Yoshimoto K, Miyauchi A, et al. Cribriform-morular variant of papillary thyroid carcinoma: a pathological and molecular genetic study with evidence of frequent somatic mutations in exon 3 of the beta-catenin gene. *J Pathol*. 2003;199:58–67.

9
Well-Differentiated Thyroid Follicular Carcinoma

Todd G. Kroll

Introduction

Tumors that arise from follicular epithelial cells of the human thyroid gland are common in clinical practice and can be detected in up to 50% of adults by ultrasonography.[1–3] Fortunately, less than 20% of palpable thyroid tumors are carcinomas, and these make up only about 1% of all cancers.[4] Approximately 80% of thyroid cancers are papillary carcinomas that have an excellent prognosis with an overall patient survival of 90–95%.[5] Another 15% of thyroid carcinomas are follicular and Hürthle cell carcinomas that have a good prognosis with an overall patient survival of 75–80%.[4,6–12] Papillary, follicular, and Hürthle cell carcinomas are thought to arise from the same type of precursor thyroid follicular epithelial cell, although each has unique morphologic and clinical features. Well-differentiated thyroid carcinomas have the potential to progress to aggressive clinical disease that may be rapidly lethal, particularly in older patients.

Two overriding clinical problems must be addressed to improve the care of patients with thyroid carcinoma. First, differentiating benign from malignant thyroid tumors must be improved, so that each patient can be treated more specifically and accurately for their particular thyroid disease. Second, identification and treatment of thyroid carcinomas that are resistant to radio-iodine therapy must be improved because no effective therapy for these advanced thyroid cancers is yet available. Recent insights into the molecular pathogenesis of thyroid carcinomas suggest new approaches to these clinical problems. This is important because thyroid carcinoma is the most common cancer of endocrine organs and has been increasing in incidence.[13–15]

The superficial location of the thyroid gland in the anterior neck has facilitated identification, pathologic evaluation, and experimental analyses of thyroid tumors. As such, the thyroid presents an excellent model of epithelial cell-derived cancer. This model has evolved into a histologic-molecular paradigm because different histologic subtypes of thyroid carcinoma contain different somatic mutations that determine biologic features of the cancers. This chapter is focused on the molecular pathology, genetic alterations, clinical-pathologic correlates, and molecular mechanisms of well-differentiated follicular and Hürthle cell carcinomas. Epidemiologic studies suggest a strong inherited predisposition for thyroid carcinoma[16,17] and preliminary data on inherited follicular and Hürthle cell carcinomas are also briefly considered.

Follicular Thyroid Carcinoma

Well-differentiated follicular thyroid carcinoma is a thyroid cancer that has follicular cell differentiation and invasive growth. Follicular carcinomas are most often unilateral, light tan/beige, firm but not hard and variegated in appearance (Figure 9.1a). Pathologic diagnosis of follicular carcinoma is based mainly on morphologic patterns in thyroid tumor sections that have been stained with hematoxylin and eosin.[5] The growth patterns typically seen in follicular carcinomas include microfollicular, trabecular, and/or solid architectures (Figure 9.1b). Identification of invasion into blood vessels, the tumor capsule, and adjacent normal thyroid tissue and/or extra-thyroidal tissues is essential for making the diagnosis of follicular carcinoma (Figure 9.1c). Importantly, the nuclei of follicular carcinomas are small, round, regular, well-dispersed, and lack morphologic features of papillary thyroid carcinoma such as nuclear clearing, elongation, overlap, irregularity, grooves, and pseudo-inclusions.[5] Even so, the differential diagnosis of follicular from papillary carcinomas can be difficult even for experienced endocrine pathologists.[18–20] Well-differentiated follicular carcinomas are often encapsulated (Figure 9.1a) and express differentiation markers such as thyroglobulin (Figure 9.1d). Follicular carcinomas tend to present at slightly older age and lack regional lymph node spread compared to papillary carcinomas.[5,10] Although some geographical variation exists, the incidence of follicular carcinoma has declined over the past 35 years,[7,11,21] most likely because of: (a) earlier clinical detection and removal of small thyroid tumors,[15] (b) evolution of criteria that more broadly define the pathologic diagnosis of papillary carcinoma[13]

J.L. Hunt (ed.), *Molecular Pathology of Endocrine Diseases*, Molecular Pathology Library 3,
DOI 10.1007/978-1-4419-1707-2_9,

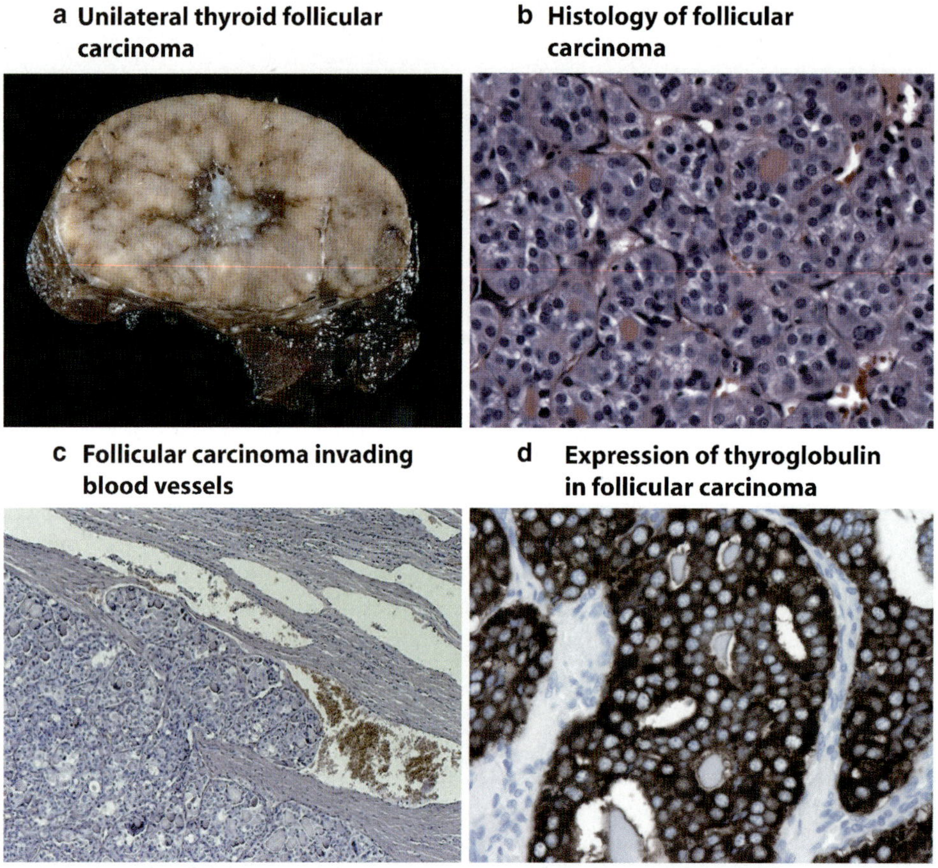

FIG. 9.1. Well-differentiated follicular thyroid carcinoma. (**a**) A well-differentiated follicular carcinoma that is unilateral and encapsulated has replaced most of the normal parenchyma in one thyroid lobe. A central scar is apparent at the fine needle aspiration biopsy site. (**b**) Follicular carcinomas have microfollicular, trabecular and/or solid growth patterns. Small, round, well-dispersed nuclei that lack elongation, overlap or grooves are characteristic. (**c**) Vascular invasion by a thyroid follicular carcinoma. (**d**) Well-differentiated follicular carcinomas immunoreact strongly with antibodies against thyroid antigens such as thyroglobulin, the biosynthetic precursor of thyroid hormones.

and (c) a reduction in endemic goiter from iodine deficiency, a risk factor for follicular carcinoma that has decreased after the introduction of dietary iodine.[22,23]

Hürthle Cell Thyroid Carcinoma

Hürthle cell carcinoma is a thyroid cancer that has follicular cell differentiation, invasive growth, and histologic features similar to, but distinct from follicular carcinoma. The most recent classification of thyroid tumors by the World Health Organization categorizes Hürthle cell carcinoma as a variant of follicular carcinoma,[5] but there is considerable evidence to indicate that Hürthle cell and follicular thyroid carcinomas represent distinct biologic entities. The unique features of Hurthle cell lesions, as compared to follicular lesions, include: (a) distinct morphologic features, (b) more frequent resistance to radio-iodine therapy,[24–26] (c) increased frequency of local recurrence, lymph node metastases and possibly a worse prognosis,[9,27–29] (d) lack of *RAS* mutations,[30] (e) lack of *PPAR*γ rearrangements,[30,31] (f) different patterns and higher levels of loss of hetereozygosity[32–34] and (g) *RET* rearrangements in up to 50% of cases,[35,36] (although the exact nature of these Hurthle cell thyroid tumors with RET rearrangements remains to be clarified).[37]

Well-differentiated Hürthle cell carcinoma presents most often as a unilateral tumor that is encapsulated and soft with a distinctive mahagony brown appearance (Figure 9.2a). The mahagony color results from excessive biogenesis and accumulation of normal and abnormal mitochondria within the tumor cytoplasm (Figure 9.2b). Over production of mitochondria produce a pink, granular (oncocytic) cytoplasm on hematoxylin and eosin staining (Figure 9.2c). It is said that the pink Hürthle "oncocytes" must make up at least 75% of tumor cells to diagnose a Hürthle cell tumor,[5] but this is a somewhat arbitrary designation. Round, well-dispersed nuclei that vary in size and have prominent, central purple-pink (amphophilic) nucleoli are characteristic of Hürthle cell carcinoma (Figure 9.2c). Hürthle cell carcinomas exhibit microfollicular, trabecular, and/or solid architectural patterns

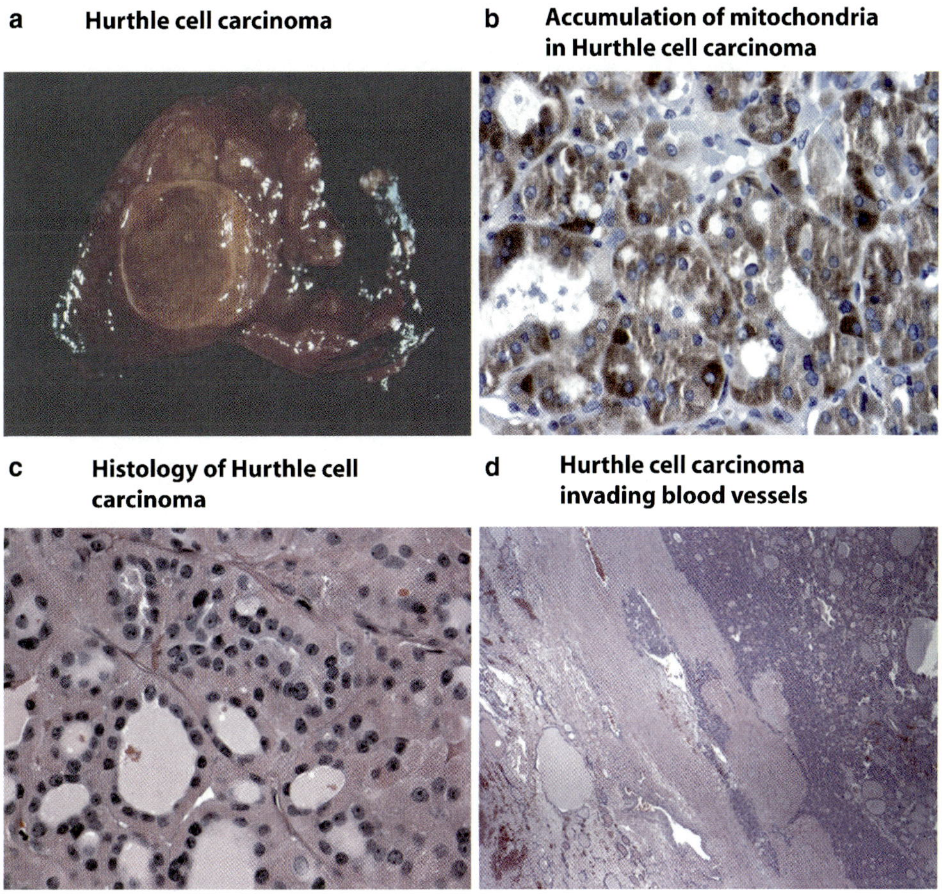

FIG. 9.2. Well-differentiated Hürthle cell thyroid carcinoma. (**a**) A Hürthle cell carcinoma that is unilateral and encapsulated has a characteristic mahogany brown appearance. (**b**) Excessive biogenesis and accumulation of abnormal and normal mitochondria are present in Hürthle carcinoma cells, as illustrated here by immunostaining with an antibody against a mitochondrial antigen. (**c**) Hürthle cell carcinomas have microfollicular, trabecular and/or solid histologic growth patterns. Round, well-dispersed nuclei with prominent central nucleoli are characteristic. (**d**) Vascular and capsular invasion by a Hürthle cell carcinoma.

and invade blood vessels (Figure 9.2d), the tumor capsule (Figure 9.2d), normal thyroid tissue and/or extra-thyroidal tissues, much like follicular carcinomas. Hürthle cell carcinomas are a biologically more heterogeneous group of thyroid cancers than follicular carcinomas.

Immunohistochemistry

Immunohistochemistry can assist in the pathologic diagnoses of well-differentiated thyroid carcinomas. Both follicular and Hürthle cell carcinomas immunoreact strongly with antibodies against thyroid follicular cell antigens such as thyroglobulin (Figure 9.1d), the major protein precursor of thyroid hormones, and TTF-1 (Figure 9.3a), a transcription factor that regulates the expression of genes in thyroid and lung epithelial cells. Immunoreactivity against thyroglobulin is a diagnostic adjunct that is used to differentiate follicular and Hürthle cell carcinomas from medullary thyroid carcinomas, which are thyroglobulin negative and exhibit diverse morphologic patterns. Thyroglobulin and TTF-1 also help distinguish thyroid from nonthyroid carcinomas at metastatic sites. The detection of thyroglobulin in the serum is used routinely to screen for recurrence after the primary treatment of thyroid carcinoma.

Additional immunohistochemical assays are employed by some pathology laboratories[38] to help distinguish follicular carcinomas from benign follicular adenomas and hyperplastic thyroid nodules or from the follicular variant of papillary carcinoma. For example, cytoplasmic staining for galectin 3, a β-galactoside-binding lectin, is observed in 30–80% of follicular carcinomas and higher numbers of papillary carcinomas but is low in normal thyroid tissues and many benign thyroid tumors.[39–53] Galectin-3 immunoreagents tend to cross-react with lymphocytes and therefore may generate background in thyroiditis cases and in papillary carcinomas with lymphocytic infiltration. 30–80% of follicular carcinomas also immunoreact with the HBME-1 antigen in membranous, apical and/or cytoplasmic patterns, whereas HBME-1 immunoreactivity in benign colloid nodules and follicular adenomas is usually weak and focal.[30,39,42,54–60] Lack of HBME-1 immunoreactivity has been reported to correlate with the presence of the

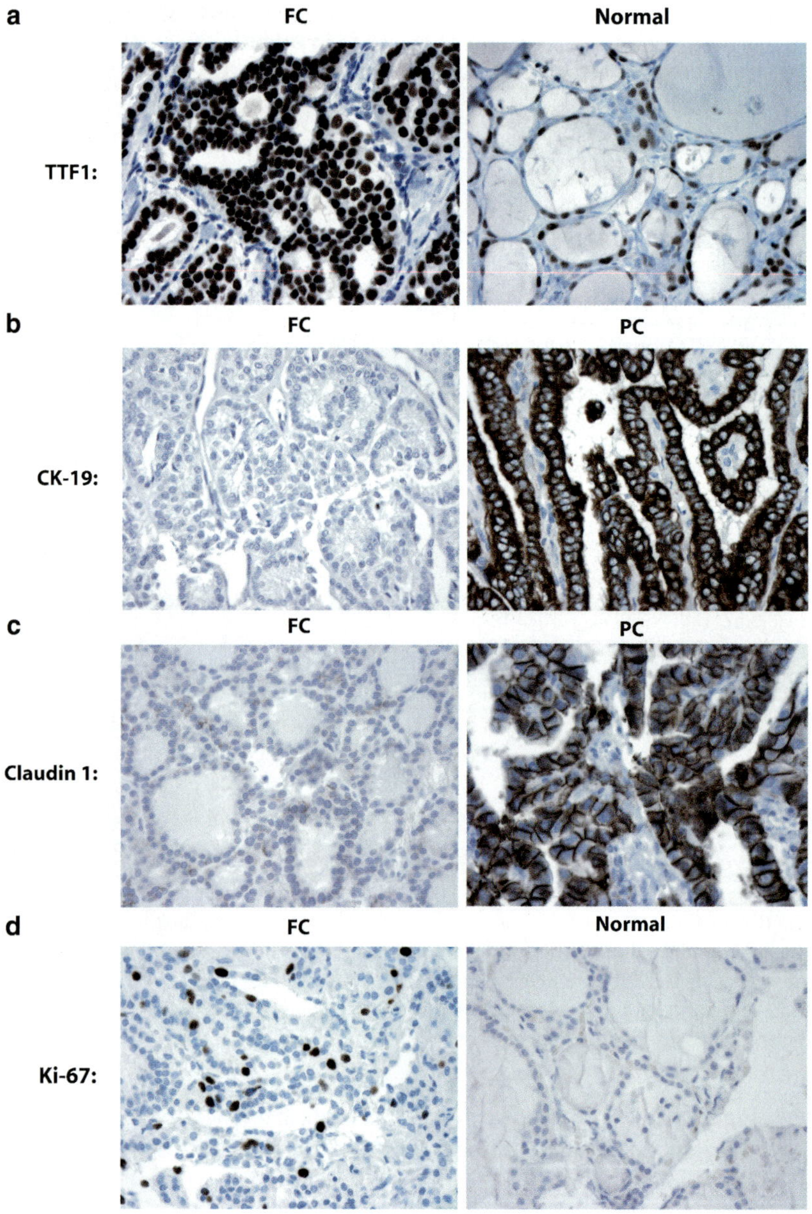

FIG. 9.3. Immunoreactivity of well-differentiated thyroid follicular carcinoma. (**a**) Follicular carcinomas (FC) immunoreact strongly with antibodies against thyroid antigens such as thyroid transcription factor 1 (TTF-1) that is expressed in the nuclei of normal thyroid cells. (**b**) Most follicular carcinomas (FC) immunoreact weakly and focally with antibodies against cytokeratin 19 (CK-19), whereas most papillary carcinomas (PC) immunoreact strongly for CK-19. (**c**) Most follicular carcinomas (FC) immunoreact weakly with antibodies against claudin-1, whereas most papillary carcinomas (PC) immunoreact strongly for claudin-1. (**d**) Follicular carcinomas (FC) often exhibit increased proliferation relative to normal thyroid tissues (NL) or benign thyroid tumors as measured by nuclear immunoreactivity for the Ki-67 antigen. Immunoreactivity is *brown* and the counterstain is *blue*.

PAX8–PPARγ gene fusion in follicular carcinomas.[30] The extent of galectin-3 and HBME-1 immunoreactivity vary considerably in different reports and depends on the antibodies and tissue processing that are used.

Follicular and Hürthle cell carcinomas immunoreact weakly with immunoreagents against the intermediate filament protein CK-19, and this can assist in differential diagnosis from papillary carcinoma in some situations. CK-19 is expressed strongly and diffusely in the cytoplasm of >85% of papillary carcinomas, whereas lighter and focal staining is observed in <15% of follicular and Hürthle cell carcinomas[54,59,61–69] (Figure 9.3b). Membrane staining for claudin-1, a protein of epithelial cell junctions, also may aid in differentiating papillary from follicular and Hürthle cell carcinomas (unpublished data) (Figure 9.3c). Well-differentiated thyroid carcinomas tend to lose expression of these differentiation markers as they progress to poorly differentiated or anaplastic thyroid carcinoma forms.

Follicular and Hürthle cell carcinomas exhibit increased cell proliferation over normal thyroid tissues and benign thyroid tumors, and this can be measured by the nuclear expression of Ki-67, an in situ proliferation marker[70–74] (Figure 9.3d). Hürthle cell carcinomas tend to be more proliferative than follicular carcinomas. However, Ki-67 staining varies widely in thyroid tumors of the same class, including follicular adenomas and Hürthle cell adenomas, and this has limited the diagnostic utility of Ki-67.

The extent and pattern of immunohistochemical staining for the above antigens are important in their interpretation. Thus, each laboratory must validate their immunohistochemical assays with well-defined series of thyroid tumors. In the past, an endogenous biotin-like activity has often generated background in thyroid tissues when performing immunohistochemistry with the classic avidin–biotin complex technique.[75,76] This complication has been circumvented in recent years by use of nonbiotin, polymer-based detection reagents. As a general rule, Hürthle cell carcinomas stain less uniformly and with more cytoplasmic background than follicular carcinomas.[42,57–59,77]

Somatic Mutations

Somatic mutations are fundamental drivers in the pathogenesis of thyroid carcinoma and can be divided into two basic classes: (a) mutations that are present in both thyroid and nonthyroid cancers such as point mutations in *RAS* (G-protein), *BRAF* (serine/threonine kinase), and *PI3KCA* (phosphatidylinositol-3-kinase) and (b) mutations that are specific for thyroid tumors such as rearrangements of *PPAR*γ (nuclear receptor), *RET* (tyrosine kinase), and *NTRK1* (tyrosine kinase) genes (Figure 9.4). *RAS* and *PPAR*γ mutations characterize the majority (70–80%) of well-differentiated follicular carcinomas and appear to be mutually exclusive in individual follicular carcinomas. These mutations are rarely observed in Hürthle cell carcinomas and are thought to arise early in tumorigenesis because they are present in low stage follicular carcinomas and in a subset of follicular adenomas that do not have morphologic signs of invasion. Such follicular adenomas with *RAS* or *PPAR*γ mutations are either true benign thyroid tumors that require additional cellular changes before they progress to invasive carcinoma or are early carcinomas in which invasion has not yet developed or has been missed because of practical limitations of tissue sampling. This distinction may be more academic than practical because both scenarios may portend an increased risk of malignancy relative to thyroid follicular adenomas as a group.

RAS Mutations

RAS point mutations were among the first somatic mutations identified in cancer tissues[78–80] and were the first recurrent mutations identified in sporadic thyroid follicular carcinomas. *RAS* mutations are common in follicular carcinomas (approximately 45%) and follicular adenomas (approximately 20%) but rare in Hürthle cell carcinomas and adenomas,[30,81–89] demonstrating that most follicular and Hürthle cell carcinomas develop through different molecular pathways. *RAS* mutations have also been detected in a small subset (approximately 10%) of thyroid papillary carcinomas[88] that tend to have a follicular growth pattern (follicular variant), tumor encapsulation, vascular invasion, and infrequent lymph node spread,[90] features that are more common in follicular than papillary carcinomas. It will be important to determine whether follicular-patterned papillary carcinomas with *RAS* mutations are "hybrid" thyroid carcinomas that possess mixed morphologic, genetic and clinical characteristics of follicular and papillary carcinoma or are follicular carcinomas that have focal morphologic nuclear alterations that lead to the diagnosis of papillary carcinoma.

In well-differentiated thyroid follicular carcinoma, *N-RAS* mutations seem to predominate over *K-RAS* and *H-RAS* mutations and codon 61 mutations in *N-RAS* may be the most prevalent.[30,87,91–93] In contrast, mutations in *K-RAS* may be more frequent in papillary carcinomas,[82,83,94] radiation-associated thyroid carcinomas,[83] and aggressive thyroid carcinomas.[94] Clinical and pathologic features that appear to correlate with *RAS* mutations in follicular carcinoma patients include older patient age, higher stage at presentation and larger, less differentiated thyroid tumors.[30,85,94–96]

The oncogenic contribution of *RAS* mutations to thyroid carcinoma has been demonstrated experimentally in transgenic mouse models.[97–99] However, mutant *RAS* is insufficient to induce rapid development of follicular carcinoma in vivo or to produce a fully transformed phenotype in thyroid cells in vitro.[100–104] Thus, additional cellular alterations appear to be necessary to manifest a fully invasive follicular carcinoma phenotype. RAS proteins are coupled to growth factor receptors such as receptor tyrosine kinases, bind GTP and propagate signals from the thyroid cell membrane to downstream molecular effectors such as BRAF, the mitogen-activated protein kinases MEK and ERK, Rac1-Rho, Ral-GDS, and PI3K (Figure 9.4). RAS proteins are activated constitutively by mutations in codon 61 that inhibit intrinsic GTPase activity or by mutations in codons 12 or 13 that tend to increase the affinity of RAS for GTP. RAS induces proliferation, survival, de-differentiation, genomic instability, and transformation in thyroid cells. Interestingly, mutations in *RAS* have been observed most often in follicular carcinomas, whereas mutations in *RET*, *NTRK1*, and *BRAF*, molecules also involved in the *RAS* signaling pathway (Figure 9.4), have been observed most often in papillary carcinomas. It will be important to determine how follicular and papillary carcinomas that have different morphologic and clinical tendencies appear to arise from the same *RAS* mutations. Collaborating mutations and/or other cellular alterations may be involved.

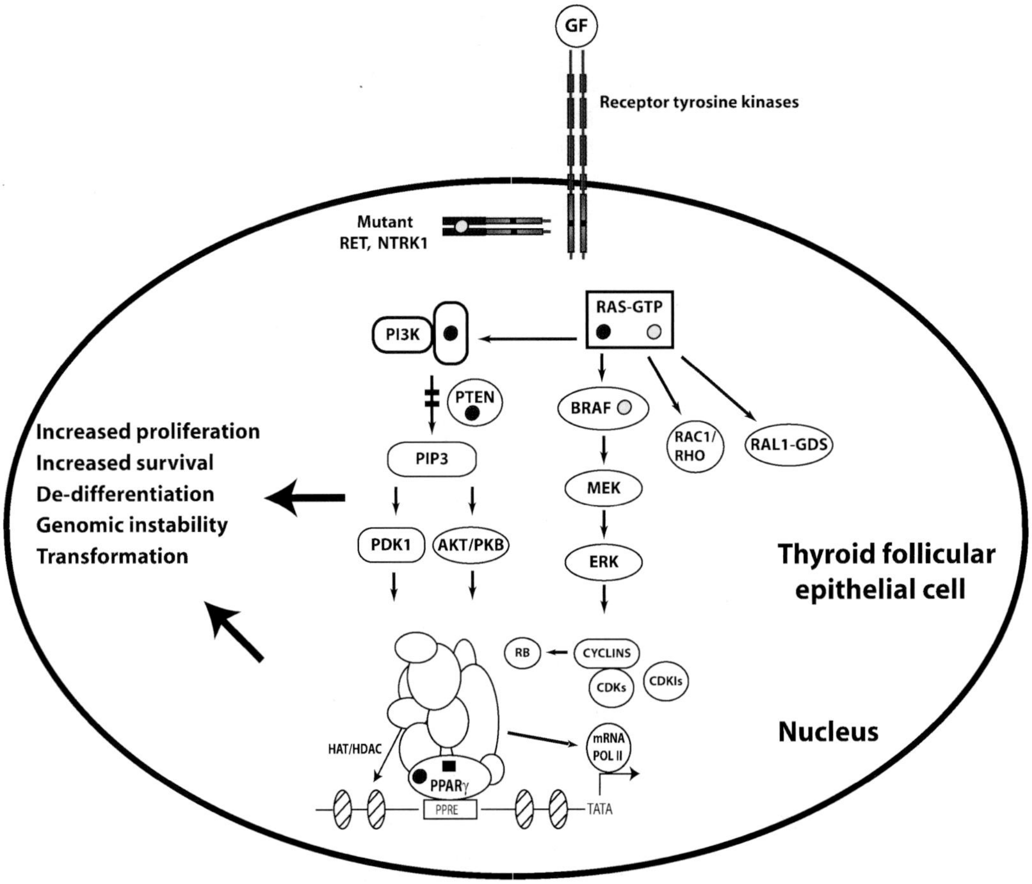

Fig. 9.4. Schematic depiction of molecular pathways in follicular thyroid carcinoma. The RAS/PI3K/AKT/PDK1 pathway is implicated in thyroid follicular carcinoma based on mutations (*red circles*) in *RAS* (~40%), *PI3KCA* (~10%) and *PTEN* (~5%). *PPARγ* mutations (*red circle*) have also been identified in follicular carcinomas (~30%) and may be linked functionally to RAS/PI3K/AKT/PDK1 through PDK1 but additional experiments are required to confirm this connection. On the other hand, the RAS/BRAF/MEK/ERK pathway has been implicated in papillary thyroid carcinoma based on mutations (*light blue circles*) in *RET* (~25%) and *NTRK1* (~10%), *RAS* (~10%) and *BRAF* (~40%) in papillary carcinoma tissues. Both RAS/PI3K/AKT/PDK1 and RAS/BRAF/MEK/ERK regulate multiple cellular processes related to tumorigenesis. Activation of these pathways by mutations increases cell proliferation, survival, de-differentiation, genomic instability and transformation and contributes to biologic and clinical phenotypes in follicular and papillary thyroid carcinoma. *GF* growth factor; *RET* RET receptor tyrosine kinase; *NTRK1* NTRK1 receptor tyrosine kinase; *PTEN* phosphatase and tensin homologue deleted from chromosome 10; *PI3K* phosphatidylinositol 3′-kinase; *PIP3* phosphatidlyinositol-3-4-5-triphosphate; *PDK1* 3-phosphoinositide-dependent protein kinase-1; *AKT/PKB* AKT serine/threonine protein kinase/protein kinase B; *RAS* GTP-activated RAS G protein; *BRAF* BRAF serine/threonine kinase; *MEK* mitogen activated protein kinase ERK kinase; *ERK* extracellular regulated kinase; *RAC1/RHO* RAC1 small GTPase, Rho family; *RAL1-GDS* RAL1 small G protein; *RB* retinoblastoma protein; *CDKs* cyclin-dependent kinases; *CDKIs* cyclin-dependent kinase inhibitors; *HAT* histone acetyltransferase; *HDAC* histone deacetylase; *PPRE* PPARγ response element; *TATA* TATA box; *mRNA pol II* mRNA polymerase II.

PPARγ Mutations

Somatic mutations in *PPARγ* have been identified in 25–55% of follicular thyroid carcinomas[30,31,105–111] in pathologically well-defined series that separate follicular from Hürthle cell carcinomas. *PPARγ* mutations are gene rearrangements that were discovered by cloning[105] of a chromosomal translocation t(2;3)(q13;p25) in follicular thyroid tumors.[105,112–118] t(2;3) juxtaposes the promoter region and 5′ coding sequences of the *PAX8* gene on chromosome 2 with coding and 3′ noncoding sequences of the *PPARγ* gene on chromosome 3 (Figure 9.5a). The *PAX8* promoter is active in thyroid epithelial cells and drives expression of chimeric *PAX8–PPARγ* fusion mRNA and protein (Figure 9.5a). Another *PPARγ* mutation encoded by t(3;7)(p25;q34) has been identified recently in <3% of thyroid follicular carcinomas.[118,119] t(3;7) juxtaposes the promoter region and 5′ coding sequences of the *CREB3L2* gene on chromosome 7 with coding and noncoding 3′ sequences of the *PPARγ* gene on chromosome 3 (Figure 9.5b). The *CREB3L2* promoter is active in thyroid epithelial cells and drives expression of chimeric *CREB3L2–PPARγ* fusion mRNA and

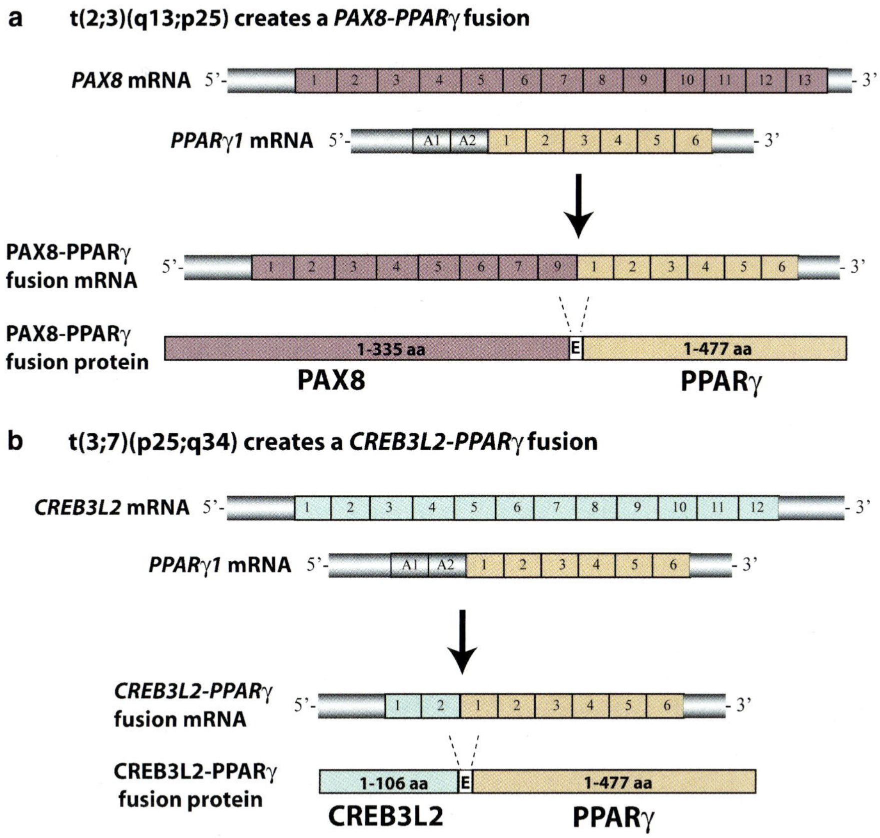

FIG. 9.5. PPARγ fusion mutations in thyroid follicular carcinoma. (**a**) t(2;3)(q13;p25) leads to fusion of the *PAX8* and *PPARγ* genes in 25–35% of thyroid follicular carcinomas. t(2;3)(q13;p25) results in expression of chimeric fusion mRNA that is thyroid-specific and composed of exons 1-7, 1-8, 1-9, or 1-7+9 (shown) of *PAX8* fused to exons 1-6 of *PPARγ*. *PAX8–PPARγ* fusion mRNA encodes a PAX8–PPARγ fusion protein that has been shown to stimulate growth and transformation in thyroid epithelial cells. The paired (DNA binding) domain of PAX8 and all functional domains (AF1, DNA binding, RXR dimerization, ligand binding and transactivation) of PPARγ are present in the PAX8–PPARγ fusion protein. (**b**) t(3;7)(p25;q34) leads to fusion of the *CREB3L2* and *PPARγ* genes in <3% of thyroid follicular carcinomas. t(3;7)(p25;q34) results in expression of chimeric fusion mRNA that is thyroid-specific and composed of exons 1-2 of *CREB3L2* fused to exons 1-6 of *PPARγ*. *CREB3L2–PPARγ* mRNA encodes a CREB3L2–PPARγ fusion protein that has been shown to stimulate the growth of thyroid epithelial cells. Identical functional domains of wild-type PPARγ1 are present in the PAX8–PPARγ and CREB3L2–PPARγ fusion proteins.

protein[119] (Figure 9.5b). These discoveries of *PAX8–PPARγ* and *CREB3L2–PPARγ* demonstrate that a family of related *PPARγ* mutations exists in follicular carcinoma.

PPARγ rearrangements are rare in Hürthle cell carcinomas,[30,31,106,109,111] arguing that follicular and Hürthle cell carcinomas develop through different molecular pathways. Most studies have also shown that *PPARγ* rearrangements occur at relatively low frequency in follicular adenomas[30,31,106–108,110,120] and the follicular variant of papillary carcinoma,[31,105–108] with a couple exceptions.[111,121] The biologic relationships of follicular adenomas and papillary carcinomas with *PPARγ* rearrangements to follicular carcinomas with *PPARγ* rearrangements are not yet clear in part because the histologic diagnoses of follicular-patterned tumors is imprecise and approached somewhat differently by different pathologists.[18,19] mRNA expression profiles argue that follicular carcinomas with *PPARγ* rearrangements are a distinct biologic entity[109,120,122] and that follicular adenomas and follicular carcinomas with *PPARγ* rearrangements are closely related, if not identical, thyroid tumors,[120] although the latter data requires verification. The possibility that *PPARγ* rearrangements mark a subset of follicular carcinomas, some even before histologic evidence of invasion is present, supports the idea that the molecular diagnosis of *PPARγ* rearrangements may be useful in fine needle aspiration biopsies to detect a subset of thyroid carcinomas prior to surgery.[123]

PPARγ rearrangements can be detected in thyroid follicular carcinomas by reverse transcription-polymerase chain reaction (RT-PCR), immunohistochemistry (Figure 9.6a) or fluorescence in situ hybridization (FISH) (Figure 9.6b). Dual color FISH using a probe set that flanks the *PPARγ* gene is particularly informative because it can identify *PPARγ* rearrangements, deletions, amplifications, and clonality in a single assay in clinical or research specimens.[31,123] For example, FISH on paraffin sections of follicular carcinomas, demonstrates two alleles in each nucleus for a normal diploid

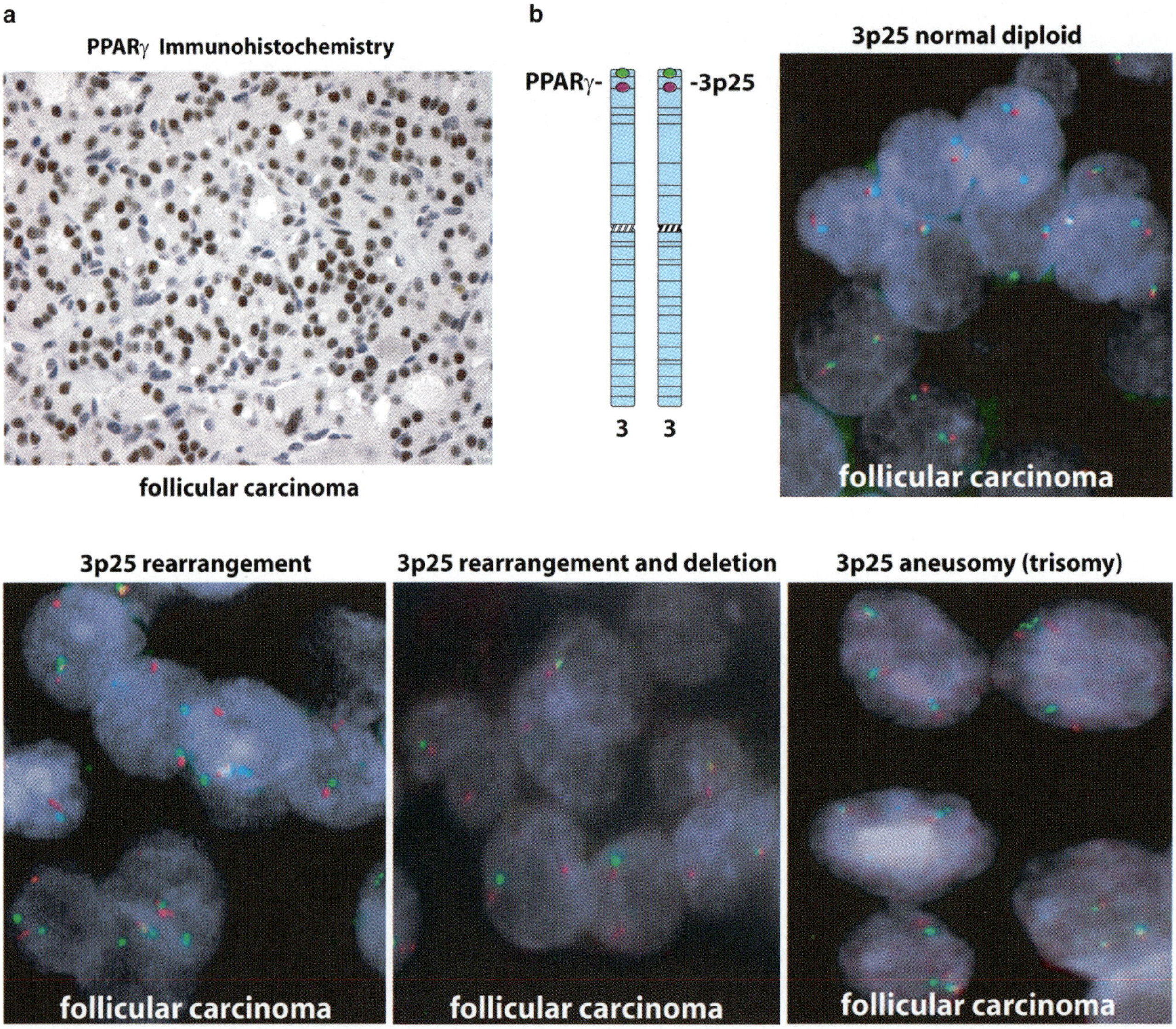

FIG. 9.6. PPARγ fusion mutations are present in a subset of thyroid follicular carcinomas. (**a**) High nuclear PPARγ immunoreactivity can detect PPARγ fusion proteins in a subset of thyroid follicular carcinomas using a PPARγ monoclonal antibody. Low levels of PPARγ protein are expressed in normal thyroid cells. PPARγ immunoreactivity in follicular carcinoma cells is *brown* and the counterstain is *blue*. (**b**) FISH with probes flanking the *PPARγ* gene can detect *PPARγ* fusion mutations in paraffin sections of thyroid follicular carcinomas. FISH demonstrates two alleles per nucleus at the normal diploid *PPARγ* locus, one split allele in each nucleus for a balanced *PPARγ* fusion rearrangement, and one split allele and a signal loss for concomitant *PPARγ* fusion rearrangement and 3p25 deletion. 3p25 aneusomy such as trisomy at the *PPARγ* locus can be detected with the same FISH assay.

PPARγ locus, one split allele in each nucleus for a balanced *PPARγ* rearrangement, and one split allele plus a signal loss for concomitant *PPARγ* rearrangement and 3p25 deletion (Figure 9.6b). In addition, aneusomy at the *PPARγ* locus can be detected by increased 3p25 copy number (Figure 9.6b).

Clinical-pathologic correlates of *PPARγ* rearrangements have been investigated in patients with thyroid follicular carcinoma. Follicular carcinomas with *PPARγ* rearrangements tend to have well-defined vascular invasion,[30,31,110,121] no lymph node metastases,[30,31] presentation at younger patient age,[30,31,110,121] solid/nested tumor histology[31] and little 3p25 aneusomy[31] when compared to follicular carcinomas without *PPARγ* rearrangements. Follicular carcinomas with *PPARγ* rearrangements metastasize in some cases.[110,113]

Experimental work has shown that fusion mutations underlie the pathogenesis of cancer and *PPARγ* rearrangements are no exception. PPARγ is a ligand-activated transcription factor that binds in a protein complex to PPARγ response elements and regulates the transcription of target genes (Figure 9.4). All functional domains of wild-type PPARγ1 are present in PAX8–PPARγ and CREB3L2–PPARγ (Figure 9.5), suggesting that PPARγ-related activities are critical in the oncogenic function of PPARγ fusion proteins. The paired domain of PAX8 and the transactivation domain of CREB3L2 are retained in PAX8–PPARγ and CREB3L2–PPARγ, respectively, suggesting that PAX8- and CREB3L2-related functions are also important. Consistent with this possibility, wild-type PAX8 is required for the development of thyroid follicular cell lineage[124] and exhibits transforming activity in vitro.[125] In addition, PAX5 is a frequent target of mutations and rearrangements in B cell lymphoblastic leukemia[126–128] and the paired domains of PAX3 and PAX7 are rearranged as fusion proteins in alveolar rhabdomyosarcoma.[129–131] Moreover, the BZIP domain of CREB3L2 is rearranged as a fusion protein in fibromyxoid sarcoma.[132]

Potent growth activities for the PAX8–PPARγ and CREB3L2–PPARγ fusion proteins have been demonstrated. Primary human thyroid follicles and follicular epithelial cell monolayers can be isolated from normal thyroid tissues removed by surgery for thyroid tumors[133] (Figure 9.7a). PAX8–PPARγ and CREB3L2–PPARγ have been shown to stimulate proliferation of primary human thyroid cells by 20–30% on day 3 after electroporation[119] (Figure 9.7b). PAX8–PPARγ also induces proliferation, anchorage-independent growth, and transformation and inhibits apoptosis in immortalized human thyroid cell lines.[134,135] Initial functional studies indicated that PAX8–PPARγ has little transcriptional activity at PPARγ response elements and inhibits transcription by wild-type PPARγ in a dominant negative manner,[105] suggesting a model in which PAX8–PPARγ acts in part by blocking transcriptional activities of PPARγ. This model is consistent with: (a) the growth inhibitory effects of PPARγ ligands on thyroid[134–144] and nonthyroid cancer cell lines, (b) the low levels of wild-type PPARγ in thyroid tumor tissues that lack *PPARγ* mutations,[31,110,145] (c) rare inactivating point mutations in wild-type *PPARγ* in colon carcinoma tissues,[146] and (d) inhibition of PPARγ expression and transcriptional activity in a mouse model of aggressive thyroid follicular carcinoma that arises after overexpression of a mutant thyroid hormone receptor β.[140,147,148] Even so, dominant negative activity is probably not the most important functional aspect of PPARγ fusion proteins because: (a) the CREB3L2–PPARγ fusion protein, which contains the same PPARγ domains as PAX8–PPARγ (Figure 9.5), exhibits robust transcriptional activity at PPARγ response elements (unpublished data), (b) transcriptional activity of PPARγ fusion proteins may depend on cell context and type of PPARγ response element examined,[149] (c) expression profiling indicates that some PPARγ-responsive genes are up regulated in follicular carcinomas with PAX8–PPARγ[109,120,122] and (d) some inhibitory effects of PPARγ ligands on cell growth result from PPRE-independent effects.[150,151] Furthermore, PPARδ not PPARγ is the predominate PPAR that is expressed in thyroid cells and tissues.[74] PPARδ regulates thyroid cell proliferation by a cyclin E1-dependent mechanism[74] and controls PPARγ transcriptional responses.[152] Thus, fundamental mechanisms of *PPARγ* mutations in follicular carcinoma remain to be elucidated. Expression profiling suggests that NORE1A, FGD1, ANGPTL4, CCND1, CTBP2, EGFR, or other molecular pathways may be involved.[109,120,122,153]

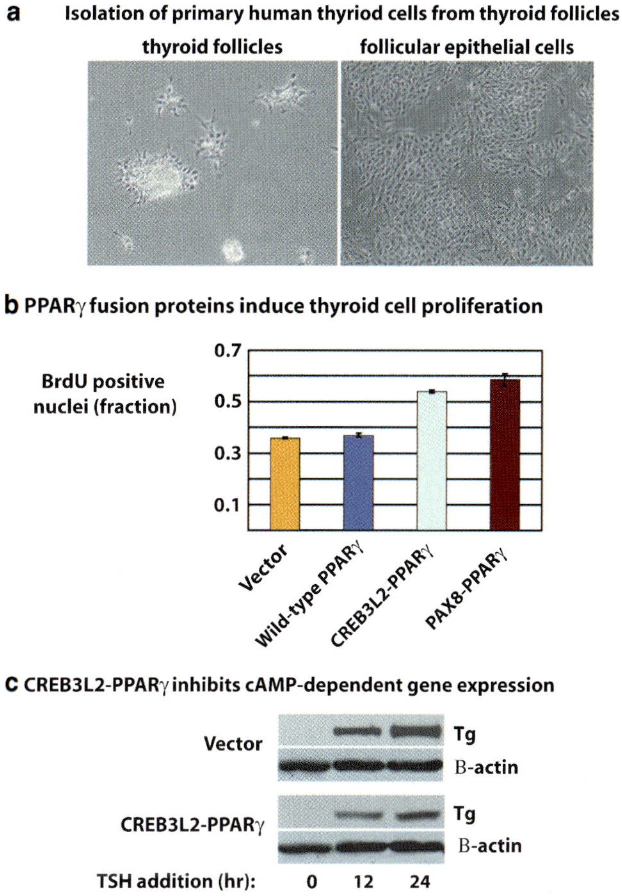

FIG. 9.7. PPARγ fusion proteins regulate the growth of primary human thyroid epithelial cells. (**a**) Intact thyroid follicles and monolayers of thyroid follicular epithelial cells can be isolated from normal human thyroid tissues that are removed by surgery for thyroid tumors. (**b**) Electroporation of primary human thyroid cells demonstrates that the PAX8–PPARγ and CREB3L2–PPARγ fusion proteins induce proliferation by 25–30% over vector and wild-type PPARγ controls. Overexpression of wild-type and PPARγ fusion proteins was confirmed by immunoblots. (**c**) The CREB3L2–PPARγ fusion protein inhibits by fourfold the expression of native thyroglobulin in primary human thyroid cells that have been treated with thyroid stimulating hormone (TSH). TSH is the major regulator of thyroid cell proliferation and differentiation in vivo and induces thyroglobulin by a cAMP-dependent mechanism.

An important aspect of fusion mutations in cancer is that they often identify novel growth pathways and a new thyroid signaling system has been detected by investigation of CREB3L2–PPARγ. Wild-type CREB3L2 is a BZIP transcription factor with a transmembrane domain that is cleaved by intra-membrane proteolysis, thereby releasing CREB3L2 to the nucleus to regulate gene expression.[119] Wild-type CREB3L2 is localized in the cell membrane, cytoplasm, and nucleus of normal thyroid cells based on antisera that are specific to CREB3L2 domains (unpublished data). The CREB3L2–PPARγ fusion protein lacks the DNA binding domain of CREB3L2 and has little ability to stimulate transcription from cAMP response elements, in marked contrast to wild-type CREB3L2.[119] CREB3L2–PPARγ also inhibits the native expression of thyroglobulin in primary thyroid cells that have been treated with thyroid stimulating hormone[119] (Figure 9.7c). Thus, CREB3L2–PPARγ likely acts in follicular carcinoma in part by inhibiting cAMP-dependent thyroid genes and disrupts the CREB3L2 pathway. In contrast, the PAX8–PPARγ fusion protein may have less effects on thyroid cell differentiation.[120,122]

PI3KCA and *PTEN* Mutations

Somatic mutations in the PI3K/PIP3/AKT/PDK1 pathway have been implicated in well-differentiated follicular thyroid carcinoma. The PI3K/PIP3/AKT/PDK1 pathway is activated by growth factors and receptor tyrosine kinases and regulates multiple cell processes related to tumorigenesis. PI3K (phosphatidylinositol 3′-kinase) generates PIP3 (phosphatidlyinositol-3-4-5-triphosphate) at thyroid cell membranes and PIP3 activates AKT, PDK1, and other downstream signaling molecules (Figure 9.4. Somatic mutations in *PI3KCA*, which encodes the p110α catalytic subunit of PI3K, have been identified in 7–13% of thyroid follicular carcinomas[154–156] and *PI3KCA* copy number changes have been detected in 24–29% of follicular carcinomas.[155–157] *PI3KCA* mutations in follicular carcinomas may correlate with metastatic disease,[154] but additional patients are needed to verify this association. *PI3KCA* mutations are more frequent in anaplastic thyroid carcinoma than in follicular carcinoma,[154,156,158] consistent with an association with clinical aggressiveness. Mutations in exons 9 (helical region) and 20 (kinase region) of *PI3KCA* are common in breast, ovarian, colorectal, and brain cancers[159–162] and contribute functionally to these malignancies.[163,164]

PTEN (phosphatase and tensin homologue deleted from chromosome 10) encodes a dual-specificity phosphatase that inhibits the PI3K/PIP3/AKT/PDK1 pathway.[165] Germ-line mutations[166] or deletions in *PTEN* cause Cowden Syndrome, which is associated with the development of benign and malignant tumors including breast and thyroid follicular carcinomas. Mice engineered to be heterozygous for *PTEN* (+/–) develop thyroid and other tumors.[167,168] Deletions of *PTEN* have been noted in up to 27% of sporadic follicular thyroid carcinomas[169–172] and *PTEN* mutations have been identified in sporadic follicular carcinomas as well.[170] PTEN protein is reduced in a significant fraction of thyroid follicular tumors.[173,174]

RET Mutations

RET rearrangements have been identified in approximately 50% of Hürthle cell carcinomas and adenomas,[35,36] a somewhat surprising finding because *RET* rearrangements were long considered to be specific for papillary thyroid carcinoma.[175–178] Although the exact nature of Hürthle cell tumors with *RET* rearrangements is not yet certain, they may be variants of papillary carcinoma.[179] Papillary carcinomas with oncocytic cytoplasm are recognizable,[5,180–182] and Hürthle cell tumors can have nuclear hyperchromasia that may obscure nuclear alterations used for pathologic diagnosis of papillary carcinoma.[37] Interestingly, Hürthle cell tumors with *RET* rearrangements exhibit frequent lymph node metastases,[35,37] a feature common to papillary carcinomas.

Other Chromosomal Rearrangements and Deletions

Moderate numbers of chromosomal alterations have been described in well-differentiated follicular and Hürthle cell carcinomas.[183] Balanced and unbalanced t(7;8)(p15;q24) has been noted in some follicular carcinomas, but the rearrangement breakpoints have not yet been cloned.[184] Loss of heterozygosity and comparative genomic hybridization studies indicate that genetic losses predominate over genetic gains in follicular and Hürthle cell carcinomas. Consistent chromosome losses in follicular carcinomas occur at the chromosome 2p,[32,185–187] 2q,[32,185,186] 3p,[183,185–190] 7q,[186,191,192] 9,[185,186,188,193,194] 10q,[171,195,196] 11q,[185,187,194,196–198] 13q,[185,186,195,196] 17q,[199] 18q,[185,188,196] and 22q[185,186,194,200,201] loci. Hürthle cell carcinomas harbor frequent losses at 1q, 8q, 9q, 14q, and 17p[188,193,199] in addition to those above.

DNA regions that exhibit consistent loss of heterozygosity are thought to encode tumor suppressor genes and Hunt et al[189,202,203] have undertaken a genotyping analyses of polymorphic short tandem repeats in follicular carcinomas to determine whether loss of heterozygosity correlates with useful clinical parameters. The biologic rationale for this approach is supported by high numbers of mutations and deletions identified recently in carcinoma tissues by direct sequencing of long regions of DNA.[204–208] DNA losses are more prevalent in widely invasive Hürthle cell carcinomas than in follicular carcinomas or follicular adenomas and correlate statistically with the degree of tumor invasiveness[202] and with genetic heterogeneity. Patients with recurrent and lethal follicular carcinomas have the highest number of DNA losses.[203] Interestingly, specific DNA losses do not correlate consistently with specific thyroid tumor types, suggesting that this approach provides a general measure of genetic instability that may be useful for prognostication of thyroid carcinoma in patients.

Expression Profiling

Expression profiling has been employed with thyroid tumor tissues to identify genes and pathways that are important in

TABLE 9.1. Selected expression profiling studies on well-differentiated follicular and Hurthle cell thyroid carcinoma.

Study	Separation	Classifier set	Validation	Selected genes
Huang et al[215] Oligonucleotide array	FC vs. PC	83–143 genes	RTPCR, IHC	CITED1, SFTPB
Barden et al[209] Oligonucleotide array	FC vs. FA	105 genes	RTPCR, IB	DDIT3
Aldred et al[214] Oligonucleotide array	FC vs. PC	5 genes	qRTPCR	CAV1, CAV2 CITED1, CLDN10, IGFBP6
Chevillard et al[210] cDNA array	FC vs. FA vs. PC	23–80 genes	qRTPCR	T, MCM7, RAP2A ID4, SELENBP1
Finley et al[211] Oligonucleotide array	FC vs. FA vs. PC	627 genes	NA	TROP2, MSG1 TNC, TTF3, FABP4, EDM3
Takano et al[216] SAGE	FC and HC vs. FA	1 gene	qRTPCR	TTF3
Cerutti et al[217] SAGE	FC vs. FA	17–73 genes	qRTPCR, IHC	DDIT3, ARG2, ITM1 C1LORF24
Weber et al[213] Oligonucleotide array	FC vs. FA	3 genes	qRTPCR, IHC	CCND2, PCSK2, GDF-15
Fryknas et al[212] cDNA array	FC vs. FA	10 gene	qRTPCR	FHL1, IFITM3, C4.4A, PLA2R1, HBB, FBXW2
Baris et al[219] cDNA array	HC vs. PC, oncocytic	83 genes	qRTPCR, IHC	ADA, IEF2S2, TIMP1, COL8A1, CCND1
Netea-Maier et al[218] Mass spectroscopy	FC vs. FA	37 proteins	IHC	HSPGP96, PDIA3

SAGE serial analyses of gene expression; *FC* follicular carcinoma; *PC* papillary carcinoma; *FA* follicular adenoma; *HC* Hurthle cell carcinoma; *RTPCR* reverse transcription polymerase chain reaction; *qRTPCR* quantitative reverse transcription polymerase chain reaction; *IHC* immunohistochemistry; *IB* immunoblot.

cancer pathogenesis, provide molecular-based classification of thyroid cancer subtypes and correlate gene expression patterns with important clinical variables. A major finding from mRNA expression profiling studies (Table 9.1) is that follicular carcinomas cluster separately from follicular adenomas[209–213] and papillary carcinomas based on gene expression signatures.[210,211,214,215] This observation is supported by other techniques such as serial analysis of gene expression[216,217] and mass spectroscopy of proteins that are expressed in thyroid tumors.[218] mRNA Expression profiles also distinguish Hürthle cell carcinomas from follicular carcinomas, follicular adenomas, and oncocytic papillary carcinomas.[216,219] These data provide proof-of-principle that gene expression patterns underlie thyroid carcinogenesis and may be useful in diagnosis or treatment of patients with thyroid tumors. In fact, expression profiling has been applied to fine needle aspiration biopsies from thyroid tumors ex vivo to separate papillary carcinomas from benign thyroid tumors.[272] Interestingly, there is little overlap in the gene classifiers identified in profiling studies from different laboratories, most likely because of different patient materials,[215] tissue processing,[214] RNA quality, sample sizes, expression platforms, and statistical methodologies employed. Thus, validation with techniques such as quantitative RTPCR and immunohistochemistry and robust correlation with prospective patient parameters and long term outcomes will be required if profiling is to be applied for routine clinical use.

A second major finding from profiling experiments is that mRNA expression signatures in thyroid carcinomas correlate with specific somatic mutations. For example, well-differentiated follicular carcinomas that harbor the *PAX8–PPARγ* fusion cluster away from follicular carcinomas without *PAX8–PPARγ*,[109,122,220] follicular adenomas, papillary carcinomas and normal thyroid tissues.[109] These data argue that follicular carcinomas with *PAX8–PPARγ* are a distinct biologic entity[31,122] and suggest that metabolic, proliferation, signal transduction and growth factor pathways are altered by PAX8–PPARγ. Follicular carcinomas with and without *PAX8–PPARγ* were said to be morphologically indistinguishable in these studies,[109,220] although histologic tendencies in follicular carcinomas with *PAX8–PPARγ* have been noted previously.[30,31] mRNA expression profiling has also identified subgroups of papillary carcinomas that exhibit separate *BRAF*, *RET*, or *RAS* mutations,[221] indicating that mutation status is a primary determinant of gene expression and may correlate more strongly with gene expression than with classic tumor morphology.[221]

MicroRNAs

Investigations of microRNAs in thyroid carcinoma tissues suggest both a functional role and diagnostic potential. MicroRNAs are small noncoding oligonucleotides that are believed to regulate the expression of multiple target genes. Alterations in the expression of microRNAs in cancer[222–226] have created great interest because many microRNAs function by binding the 3′ untranslated region of mRNA to control its degradation and translation.[227,228] Several studies have focused on microRNAs in thyroid papillary carcinoma[229–234] and shown that engineered overexpression of selected microRNAs can stimulate the growth of follicular[235] or papillary[229,231,232] thyroid carcinoma cell lines. Fewer studies have investigated microRNAs in well-differentiated follicular and Hürthle cell carcinomas, but

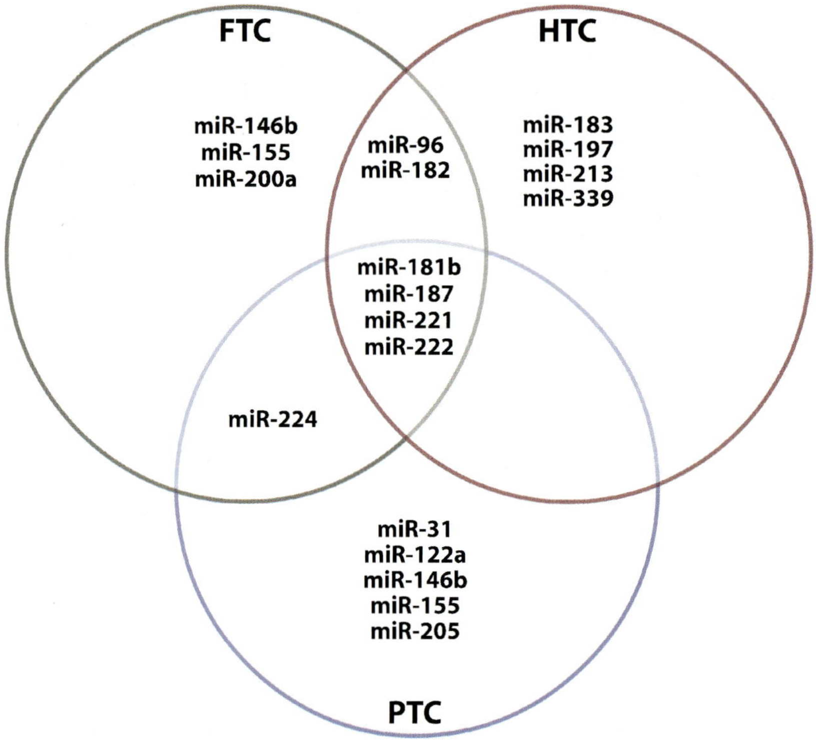

Fig. 9.8. A subset of MicroRNAs are overexpressed in follicular carcinoma, Hürthle cell carcinoma and papillary carcinoma tissues. MicroRNAs have been found to be over and under expressed in thyroid carcinomas and their expression can divide thyroid carcinomas into histologic subtypes. *Circles* show selected microRNAs that are overexpressed highly in thyroid carcinomas and thought to downregulate the expression of genes that encode proteins. MicroRNAs such as MiR-188b, MiR-187, MiR-221 and MiR222 are expressed in all three thyroid carcinoma types, MiR-146b, MiR-155 and MiR-200a are overexpressed selectively in follicular carcinomas, and MiR-183, MiR-197, MiR-213 and MiR-339 are overexpressed selectively in Hürthle cell carcinomas. Altered expression of microRNAs may contribute to the formation and phenotype of well-differentiated thyroid cancer.

both upregulation (Figure 9.8) and downregulation of microRNA expression have been observed.[229,235] In these studies, the expression microRNAs in follicular tumors, Hürthle cell tumors, and papillary carcinomas appears to be more similar to each other than in medullary thyroid carcinomas, as would be expected from their common origin from thyroid follicular cells. Unsupervised hierarchical clustering based on microRNA expression also segregated thyroid tumors into the classic histologic categories of follicular tumor, Hürthle cell tumor, papillary carcinoma, and medullary carcinoma,[229] supporting the idea that microRNAs contribute to thyroid cancer phenotype. Separation of follicular from Hürthle cell carcinomas by microRNA expression provides additional evidence that these are distinct thyroid cancer groups. Clustering of follicular adenomas with follicular carcinomas and Hürthle cell adenomas with Hürthle cell carcinomas is consistent with the progression of some adenomas to carcinoma, a possibility that requires further investigation. Interestingly, deregulation of miR-200A may be particularly important in follicular carcinomas with the *PAX8–PPAR*γ fusion[109] and distinct microRNA expression patterns correlate with specific *BRAF*, *RET*, or *PAX8–PPAR*γ[229] mutations, although there is considerable variability in the expression of microRNAs in thyroid tumors of the same histologic type.

Inherited Well-Differentiated Thyroid Carcinoma

Epidemiologic studies indicate that thyroid carcinoma arising from follicular epithelial cells occurs in families more often than expected by chance.[17,236,237] Most studies have suggested a predisposition to familial papillary carcinoma,[236] but follicular carcinoma is an inherited component of Cowden Disease that results from germ-line mutations in the *PTEN* tumor suppressor gene.[166] In addition, families with Hürthle cell carcinomas and other oncocytic tumors have been linked to the 19p13.2 chromosomal locus,[238,239] although the mutation responsible for this linkage is not yet identified.[240]

Summary

Recent advances in the molecular pathology of thyroid tumors, including well-differentiated follicular and Hürthle cell carcinomas, have identified mechanisms of thyroid carcinogenesis and suggested new approaches to help improve the diagnoses, prognostication, and treatment of thyroid cancer in patients. Somatic mutations are driving molecular events in well-differentiated thyroid carcinoma, and similarities in the mutations in thyroid carcinoma and myeloid leukemia are remarkable – common *N-RAS* mutations,[241–244] *PPARγ* compared to *RARα* rearrangements[245,246] in the same nuclear receptor family and *RET* compared to *FTL3*[247,248] receptor tyrosine kinases. Mutations in both myeloid leukemia and thyroid carcinoma are primary determinates of gene expression, morphology, and clinical phenotype and speak to a shared molecular pathogenesis of cancers arising in very different tissues. Approaches that have been successful in diagnosis and treatment of leukemia may be worthy of consideration in thyroid carcinoma. For example, molecular diagnosis and disease monitoring of mutations are now standard-of-care in many leukemia patients.[249–251] In thyroid carcinoma, molecular diagnostic assays that reflect mutation status, whether based on RTPCR, FISH, DNA sequencing, expression signatures, or other techniques, will be implemented and validated to diagnose thyroid carcinomas more precisely and accurately prior surgery.[123,217,229,231,252–262] Some of the most effective chemotherapies yet initiated for any cancer type are based on mutations and their molecular pathways identified by gene rearrangements.[263–267] Preclinical and clinical studies are underway based on mutations and their molecular pathways in thyroid carcinoma and provide promise for thyroid cancer patients.[268–270] The most valuable agents will be efficacious against advanced stage, poorly differentiated and/or Hürthle cell thyroid carcinomas that are frequently resistant to radio-iodine therapy and lack alternate treatment options. In well-differentiated thyroid follicular carcinoma, the PI3K/PIP3/AKT/PDK1 axis may be particularly important because mutations in *RAS*, *PPARγ*,[271] *PI3KCA*, and *PTEN* are all connected functionally to PI3K/PIP3/AKT/PDK1 signaling. Further investigations into the pathogenesis of thyroid carcinomas will continue to expand our understanding of thyroid cancer mechanisms and provide new opportunities to advance clinical interventions.

References

1. Tan GH, Gharib H. Thyroid incidentalomas: management approaches to nonpalpable nodules discovered incidentally on thyroid imaging. *Ann Intern Med.* 1997;126:226–231.
2. Ezzat S. Sarti DA, Cain DR. *Braunstein GD Thyroid incidentalomas Prevalence by palpation and ultrasonography Arch Intern Med.* 1994;154:1838–1840.
3. Bruneton JN, Balu-Maestro C, Marcy PY, Melia P, Mourou MY. Very high frequency (13 MHz) ultrasonographic examination of the normal neck: detection of normal lymph nodes and thyroid nodules. *J Ultrasound Med.* 1994;13:87–90.
4. Hundahl SA, Fleming ID, Fremgen AM, Menck HR. A National Cancer Data Base report on 53, 856 cases of thyroid carcinoma treated in the U.S., 1985–1995 [see comments]. *Cancer.* 1998;83:2638–2648.
5. DeLellis R, Lloyd R, Heitz P, Eng C, eds. *Pathology and Genetics of Tumours of Endocrine Organs.* Lyon: IARC; 2004.
6. D'Avanzo A, Ituarte P, Treseler P, et al. Prognostic scoring systems in patients with follicular thyroid cancer: a comparison of different staging systems in predicting the patient outcome. *Thyroid.* 2004;14:453–458.
7. Harness JK, Thompson NW, McLeod MK, Eckhauser FE, Lloyd RV. Follicular carcinoma of the thyroid gland: trends and treatment. *Surgery.* 1984;96:972–980.
8. Lang W, Choritz H, Hundeshagen H. Risk factors in follicular thyroid carcinomas. A retrospective follow-up study covering a 14-year period with emphasis on morphological findings. *Am J Surg Pathol.* 1986;10:246–255.
9. DeGroot LJ, Kaplan EL, Shukla MS, Salti G, Straus FH. Morbidity and mortality in follicular thyroid cancer. *J Clin Endocrinol Metab.* 1995;80:2946–2953.
10. Brennan MD, Bergstralh EJ, van Heerden JA, McConahey WM. Follicular thyroid cancer treated at the Mayo Clinic, 1946 through 1970: initial manifestations, pathologic findings, therapy, and outcome. *Mayo Clin Proc.* 1991;66:11–22.
11. Grebe SK, Hay ID. Follicular thyroid cancer. *Endocrinol Metab Clin North Am.* 1995;24:761–801.
12. Evans HL. Follicular neoplasms of the thyroid. A study of 44 cases followed for a minimum of 10 years, with emphasis on differential diagnosis. *Cancer.* 1984;54:535–540.
13. Albores-Saavedra J, Henson DE, Glazer E, Schwartz AM. Changing patterns in the incidence and survival of thyroid cancer with follicular phenotype – papillary, follicular, and anaplastic: a morphological and epidemiological study. *Endocr Pathol.* 2007;18:1–7.
14. Hodgson NC, Button J, Solorzano CC. Thyroid cancer: is the incidence still increasing? *Ann Surg Oncol.* 2004;11:1093–1097.
15. Davies L, Welch HG. Increasing incidence of thyroid cancer in the United States, 1973–2002. *JAMA.* 2006;295:2164–2167.
16. Czene K, Lichtenstein P, Hemminki K. Environmental and heritable causes of cancer among 9.6 million individuals in the Swedish Family-Cancer Database. *Int J Cancer.* 2002;99:260–266.
17. Goldgar DE, Easton DF, Cannon-Albright LA, Skolnick MH. Systematic population-based assessment of cancer risk in first-degree relatives of cancer probands. *J Natl Cancer Inst.* 1994;86:1600–1608.
18. Lloyd RV, Erickson LA, Casey MB, et al. Observer variation in the diagnosis of follicular variant of papillary thyroid carcinoma. *Am J Surg Pathol.* 2004;28:1336–1340.
19. Hirokawa M, Carney JA, Goellner JR, et al. Observer variation of encapsulated follicular lesions of the thyroid gland. *Am J Surg Pathol.* 2002;26:1508–1514.
20. Baloch ZW, Livolsi VA. Follicular-patterned lesions of the thyroid: the bane of the pathologist. *Am J Clin Pathol.* 2002;117:143–150.
21. LiVolsi VA, Asa SL. The demise of follicular carcinoma of the thyroid gland. *Thyroid.* 1994;4:233–236.

22. Farahati J, Geling M, Mader U, et al. Changing trends of incidence and prognosis of thyroid carcinoma in lower Franconia, Germany, from 1981–1995. *Thyroid*. 2004;14:141–147.
23. Williams ED, Doniach I, Bjarnason O, Michie W. Thyroid cancer in an iodide rich area: a histopathological study. *Cancer*. 1977;39:215–222.
24. Stojadinovic A, Hoos A, Ghossein RA, et al. Hürthle cell carcinoma: a 60-year experience. *Ann Surg Oncol*. 2002;9:197–203.
25. Har-El G, Hadar T, Segal K, Levy R, Sidi J. Hürthle cell carcinoma of the thyroid gland. A tumor of moderate malignancy. *Cancer*. 1986;57:1613–1617.
26. Grossman RF, Clark OH. Hürthle cell carcinoma. *Cancer Control*. 1997;4:13–17.
27. Kushchayeva Y, Duh QY, Kebebew E, D'Avanzo A, Clark OH. Comparison of clinical characteristics at diagnosis and during follow-up in 118 patients with Hürthle cell or follicular thyroid cancer. *Am J Surg*. 2008;195:457–462.
28. Shaha AR, Loree TR, Shah JP. Prognostic factors and risk group analysis in follicular carcinoma of the thyroid. *Surgery*. 1995;118:1131–1136. discussion 1136–1138.
29. Evans HL, Vassilopoulou-Sellin R. Follicular and Hürthle cell carcinomas of the thyroid: a comparative study. *Am J Surg Pathol*. 1998;22:1512–1520.
30. Nikiforova MN, Lynch RA, Biddinger PW, et al. RAS point mutations and PAX8-PPAR gamma rearrangement in thyroid tumors: evidence for distinct molecular pathways in thyroid follicular carcinoma. *J Clin Endocrinol Metab*. 2003;88:2318–2326.
31. French CA, Alexander EK, Cibas ES, et al. Genetic and biological subgroups of low-stage follicular thyroid cancer. *Am J Pathol*. 2003;162:1053–1060.
32. Tung WS, Shevlin DW, Kaleem Z, Tribune DJ, Wells SA Jr, Goodfellow PJ. Allelotype of follicular thyroid carcinomas reveals genetic instability consistent with frequent nondisjunctional chromosomal loss. *Genes Chromosomes Cancer*. 1997;19:43–51.
33. Semple RK, Meirhaeghe A, Vidal-Puig AJ, et al. A dominant negative human peroxisome proliferator-activated receptor (PPAR){alpha} is a constitutive transcriptional corepressor and inhibits signaling through all PPAR isoforms. *Endocrinology*. 2005;146:1871–1882.
34. Farrand K, Delahunt B, Wang XL, et al. High resolution loss of heterozygosity mapping of 17p13 in thyroid cancer: Hürthle cell carcinomas exhibit a small 411-kilobase common region of allelic imbalance, probably containing a novel tumor suppressor gene. *J Clin Endocrinol Metab*. 2002;87:4715–4721.
35. Cheung CC, Ezzat S, Ramyar L, Freeman JL, Asa SL. Molecular basis off Hürthle cell papillary thyroid carcinoma. *J Clin Endocrinol Metab*. 2000;85:878–882.
36. Chiappetta G, Toti P, Cetta F, et al. The RET/PTC oncogene is frequently activated in oncocytic thyroid tumors (Hürthle cell adenomas and carcinomas), but not in oncocytic hyperplastic lesions. *J Clin Endocrinol Metab*. 2002;87:364–369.
37. Belchetz G, Cheung CC, Freeman J, Rosen IB, Witterick IJ, Asa SL. Hürthle cell tumors: using molecular techniques to define a novel classification system. *Arch Otolaryngol Head Neck Surg*. 2002;128:237–240.
38. Fischer S, Asa SL. Application of immunohistochemistry to thyroid neoplasms. *Arch Pathol Lab Med*. 2008;132:359–372.
39. Papotti M, Rodriguez J, De Pompa R, Bartolazzi A, Rosai J. Galectin-3 and HBME-1 expression in well-differentiated thyroid tumors with follicular architecture of uncertain malignant potential. *Mod Pathol*. 2005;18:541–546.
40. Weber KB, Shroyer KR, Heinz DE, Nawaz S, Said MS, Haugen BR. The use of a combination of galectin-3 and thyroid peroxidase for the diagnosis and prognosis of thyroid cancer. *Am J Clin Pathol*. 2004;122:524–531.
41. Oestreicher-Kedem Y, Halpern M, Roizman P, et al. Diagnostic value of galectin-3 as a marker for malignancy in follicular patterned thyroid lesions. *Head Neck*. 2004;26:960–966.
42. Prasad ML, Pellegata NS, Huang Y, Nagaraja HN, de la Chapelle A, Kloos RT. Galectin-3, fibronectin-1, CITED-1, HBME1 and cytokeratin-19 immunohistochemistry is useful for the differential diagnosis of thyroid tumors. *Mod Pathol*. 2005;18:48–57.
43. Saggiorato E, Aversa S, Deandreis D, et al. Galectin-3: presurgical marker of thyroid follicular epithelial cell-derived carcinomas. *J Endocrinol Invest*. 2004;27:311–317.
44. Bartolazzi A, Orlandi F, Saggiorato E, et al. Galectin-3-expression analysis in the surgical selection of follicular thyroid nodules with indeterminate fine-needle aspiration cytology: a prospective multicentre study. *Lancet Oncol*. 2008; 9:543–549.
45. Cvejic DS, Savin SB, Petrovic IM, Paunovic IR, Tatic SB, Havelka MJ. Galectin-3 expression in papillary thyroid carcinoma: relation to histomorphologic growth pattern, lymph node metastasis, extrathyroid invasion, and tumor size. *Head Neck*. 2005;27:1049–1055.
46. Fernandez PL, Merino MJ, Gomez M, et al. Galectin-3 and laminin expression in neoplastic and non-neoplastic thyroid tissue. *J Pathol*. 1997;181:80–86.
47. Herrmann ME, LiVolsi VA, Pasha TL, Roberts SA, Wojcik EM, Baloch ZW. Immunohistochemical expression of galectin-3 in benign and malignant thyroid lesions. *Arch Pathol Lab Med*. 2002;126:710–713.
48. Kovacs RB, Foldes J, Winkler G, Bodo M, Sapi Z. The investigation of galectin-3 in diseases of the thyroid gland. *Eur J Endocrinol*. 2003;149:449–453.
49. Gasbarri A, Martegani MP, Del Prete F, Lucante T, Natali PG, Bartolazzi A. Galectin-3 and CD44v6 isoforms in the preoperative evaluation of thyroid nodules. *J Clin Oncol*. 1999;17:3494–3502.
50. Chiariotti L, Berlingieri MT, Battaglia C, et al. Expression of galectin-1 in normal human thyroid gland and in differentiated and poorly differentiated thyroid tumors. *Int J Cancer*. 1995; 64:171–175.
51. Inohara H, Honjo Y, Yoshii T, et al. Expression of galectin-3 in fine-needle aspirates as a diagnostic marker differentiating benign from malignant thyroid neoplasms. *Cancer*. 1999;85:2475–2484.
52. Orlandi F, Saggiorato E, Pivano G, et al. Galectin-3 is a presurgical marker of human thyroid carcinoma. *Cancer Res*. 1998;58: 3015–3020.
53. Xu XC. el-Naggar AK, Lotan R. Differential expression of galectin-1 and galectin-3 in thyroid tumors. Potential diagnostic implications. *Am J Pathol*. 1995;147:815–822.
54. de Matos PS, Ferreira AP, de Oliveira Facuri F, Assumpcao LV, Metze K, Ward LS. Usefulness of HBME-1, cytokeratin 19 and galectin-3 immunostaining in the diagnosis of thyroid malignancy. *Histopathology*. 2005;47:391–401.
55. Miettinen M, Karkkainen P. Differential reactivity of HBME-1 and CD15 antibodies in benign and malignant thyroid tumours. Preferential reactivity with malignant tumours. *Virchows Arch*. 1996;429:213–219.
56. Rezk S, Khan A. Role of immunohistochemistry in the diagnosis and progression of follicular epithelium-derived thyroid

carcinoma. *Appl Immunohistochem Mol Morphol*. 2005; 13:256–264.
57. Saggiorato E, De Pompa R, Volante M, et al. Characterization of thyroid 'follicular neoplasms' in fine-needle aspiration cytological specimens using a panel of immunohistochemical markers: a proposal for clinical application. *Endocr Relat Cancer*. 2005;12:305–317.
58. Choi YL, Kim MK, Suh JW, et al. Immunoexpression of HBME-1, high molecular weight cytokeratin, cytokeratin 19, thyroid transcription factor-1, and E-cadherin in thyroid carcinomas. *J Korean Med Sci*. 2005;20:853–859.
59. Cheung CC, Ezzat S, Freeman JL, Rosen IB, Asa SL. Immunohistochemical diagnosis of papillary thyroid carcinoma. *Mod Pathol*. 2001;14:338–342.
60. Mase T, Funahashi H, Koshikawa T, et al. HBME-1 immunostaining in thyroid tumors especially in follicular neoplasm. *Endocr J*. 2003;50:173–177.
61. Cerilli LA, Mills SE, Rumpel CA, Dudley TH, Moskaluk CA. Interpretation of RET immunostaining in follicular lesions of the thyroid. *Am J Clin Pathol*. 2002;118:186–193.
62. Nasser SM, Pitman MB, Pilch BZ, Faquin WC. Fine-needle aspiration biopsy of papillary thyroid carcinoma: diagnostic utility of cytokeratin 19 immunostaining. *Cancer*. 2000;90:307–311.
63. Lam KY, Lui MC, Lo CY. Cytokeratin expression profiles in thyroid carcinomas. *Eur J Surg Oncol*. 2001;27:631–635.
64. Khurana KK, Truong LD, LiVolsi VA, Baloch ZW. Cytokeratin 19 immunolocalization in cell block preparation of thyroid aspirates. An adjunct to fine-needle aspiration diagnosis of papillary thyroid carcinoma. *Arch Pathol Lab Med*. 2003;127:579–583.
65. Baloch ZW, Abraham S, Roberts S, LiVolsi VA. Differential expression of cytokeratins in follicular variant of papillary carcinoma: an immunohistochemical study and its diagnostic utility. *Hum Pathol*. 1999;30:1166–1171.
66. Sahoo S, Hoda SA, Rosai J, DeLellis RA. Cytokeratin 19 immunoreactivity in the diagnosis of papillary thyroid carinoma: a note of caution. *Am J Clin Pathol*. 2001;116:696–702.
67. Beesley MF, McLaren KM. Cytokeratin 19 and galectin-3 immunohistochemistry in the differential diagnosis of solitary thyroid nodules. *Histopathology*. 2002;41:236–243.
68. Raphael SJ, McKeown-Eyssen G, Asa SL. High-molecular-weight cytokeratin and cytokeratin-19 in the diagnosis of thyroid tumors. *Mod Pathol*. 1994;7:295–300.
69. Fonseca E, Nesland JM, Hoie J, Sobrinho-Simoes M. Pattern of expression of intermediate cytokeratin filaments in the thyroid gland: an immunohistochemical study of simple and stratified epithelial-type cytokeratins. *Virchows Arch*. 1997;430:239–245.
70. Kjellman P, Wallin G, Hoog A, Auer G, Larsson C, Zedenius J. MIB-1 index in thyroid tumors: a predictor of the clinical course in papillary thyroid carcinoma. *Thyroid*. 2003;13:371–380.
71. Rickert D, Mittermayer C, Lindenfelser R, Biesterfeld S. MIB-1 immunohistometry of follicular adenoma and follicular carcinoma of the thyroid gland. *Anal Quant Cytol Histol*. 2000;22:229–234.
72. Erickson LA, Jin L, Wollan PC, Thompson GB, van Heerden J, Lloyd RV. Expression of p27kip1 and Ki-67 in benign and malignant thyroid tumors. *Mod Pathol*. 1998;11:169–174.
73. Erickson LA, Jin L, Goellner JR, et al. Pathologic features, proliferative activity, and cyclin D1 expression in Hürthle cell neoplasms of the thyroid. *Mod Pathol*. 2000;13:186–192.
74. Zeng L, Geng Y, Tretiakova M, Yu X, Sicinski P, Kroll T. Peroxisome proliferator-activated receptor-delta induces cell proliferation by a novel cyclin E1-dependent mechanism and is upregulated in thyroid tumors. *Cancer Res*. 2008;68(16):6578–6586.
75. Kashima K, Yokoyama S, Daa T, Nakayama I, Nickerson PA, Noguchi S. Cytoplasmic biotin-like activity interferes with immunohistochemical analysis of thyroid lesions: a comparison of antigen retrieval methods. *Mod Pathol*. 1997; 10:515–519.
76. Srivastava A, Tischler AS, Delellis RA. Endogenous biotin staining as an artifact of antigen retrieval with automated immunostaining. *Endocr Pathol*. 2004;15:175–178.
77. Volante M, Bozzalla-Cassione F, DePompa R, et al. Galectin-3 and HBME-1 expression in oncocytic cell tumors of the thyroid. *Virchows Arch*. 2004;445:183–188.
78. Murray MJ, Cunningham JM, Parada LF, Dautry F, Lebowitz P, Weinberg RA. The HL-60 transforming sequence: a ras oncogene coexisting with altered myc genes in hematopoietic tumors. *Cell*. 1983;33:749–757.
79. Karnoub AE, Weinberg RA. Ras oncogenes: split personalities. *Nat Rev Mol Cell Biol*. 2008;9:517–531.
80. Bos JL. ras oncogenes in human cancer: a review. *Cancer Res*. 1989;49:4682–4689.
81. Shi YF, Zou MJ, Schmidt H, et al. High rates of ras codon 61 mutation in thyroid tumors in an iodide-deficient area. *Cancer Res*. 1991;51:2690–2693.
82. Wright PA, Lemoine NR, Mayall ES, et al. Papillary and follicular thyroid carcinomas show a different pattern of ras oncogene mutation. *Br J Cancer*. 1989;60:576–577.
83. Wright PA, Williams ED, Lemoine NR, Wynford-Thomas D. Radiation-associated and 'spontaneous' human thyroid carcinomas show a different pattern of ras oncogene mutation. *Oncogene*. 1991;6:471–473.
84. Lemoine NR, Mayall ES, Wyllie FS, et al. Activated ras oncogenes in human thyroid cancers. *Cancer Res*. 1988;48:4459–4463.
85. Manenti G, Pilotti S, Re FC, Della Porta G, Pierotti MA. Selective activation of ras oncogenes in follicular and undifferentiated thyroid carcinomas. *Eur J Cancer*. 1994;30A:987–993.
86. Lemoine NR, Mayall ES, Wyllie FS, et al. High frequency of ras oncogene activation in all stages of human thyroid tumorigenesis. *Oncogene*. 1989;4:159–164.
87. Fukushima T, Suzuki S, Mashiko M, et al. BRAF mutations in papillary carcinomas of the thyroid. *Oncogene*. 2003;22:6455–6457.
88. Namba H, Rubin SA, Fagin JA. Point mutations of ras oncogenes are an early event in thyroid tumorigenesis. *Mol Endocrinol*. 1990;4:1474–1479.
89. Soares P, Trovisco V, Rocha AS, et al. BRAF mutations and RET/PTC rearrangements are alternative events in the etiopathogenesis of PTC. *Oncogene*. 2003;22:4578–4580.
90. Zhu Z, Gandhi M, Nikiforova MN, Fischer AH, Nikiforov YE. Molecular profile and clinical-pathologic features of the follicular variant of papillary thyroid carcinoma. An unusually high prevalence of ras mutations. *Am J Clin Pathol*. 2003;120:71–77.
91. Banito A, Pinto AE, Espadinha C, Marques AR, Leite V. Aneuploidy and RAS mutations are mutually exclusive events in the development of well-differentiated thyroid follicular tumours. *Clin Endocrinol (Oxf)*. 2007;67:706–711.
92. Oyama T, Suzuki T, Hara F, et al. N-ras mutation of thyroid tumor with special reference to the follicular type. *Pathol Int*. 1995;45:45–50.

93. Vasko V, Ferrand M, Di Cristofaro J, Carayon P, Henry JF, de Micco C. Specific pattern of RAS oncogene mutations in follicular thyroid tumors. *J Clin Endocrinol Metab.* 2003;88:2745–2752.
94. Garcia-Rostan G, Zhao H, Camp RL, et al. ras mutations are associated with aggressive tumor phenotypes and poor prognosis in thyroid cancer. *J Clin Oncol.* 2003;21:3226–3235.
95. Hara H, Fulton N, Yashiro T, Ito K, DeGroot LJ, Kaplan EL. N-ras mutation: an independent prognostic factor for aggressiveness of papillary thyroid carcinoma. *Surgery.* 1994;116:1010–1016.
96. Basolo F, Pisaturo F, Pollina LE, et al. N-ras mutation in poorly differentiated thyroid carcinomas: correlation with bone metastases and inverse correlation to thyroglobulin expression. *Thyroid.* 2000;10:19–23.
97. Santelli G, de Franciscis V, Chiappetta G, et al. Thyroid specific expression of the Ki-ras oncogene in transgenic mice. *Adv Exp Med Biol.* 1993;348:59–62.
98. Aguirre AJ, Bardeesy N, Sinha M, et al. Activated Kras and Ink4a/Arf deficiency cooperate to produce metastatic pancreatic ductal adenocarcinoma. *Genes Dev.* 2003;17:3112–3126.
99. Rochefort P, Caillou B, Michiels FM, et al. Thyroid pathologies in transgenic mice expressing a human activated Ras gene driven by a thyroglobulin promoter. *Oncogene.* 1996;12:111–118.
100. Santoro M, Melillo RM, Grieco M, Berlingieri MT, Vecchio G, Fusco A. The TRK and RET tyrosine kinase oncogenes cooperate with ras in the neoplastic transformation of a rat thyroid epithelial cell line. *Cell Growth Differ.* 1993;4:77–84.
101. Fusco A, Berlingieri MT, Di Fiore PP, Portella G, Grieco M, Vecchio G. One- and two-step transformations of rat thyroid epithelial cells by retroviral oncogenes. *Mol Cell Biol.* 1987;7:3365–3370.
102. Gire V, Marshall CJ, Wynford-Thomas D. Activation of mitogen-activated protein kinase is necessary but not sufficient for proliferation of human thyroid epithelial cells induced by mutant Ras. *Oncogene.* 1999;18:4819–4832.
103. Gire V, Wynford-Thomas D. RAS oncogene activation induces proliferation in normal human thyroid epithelial cells without loss of differentiation. *Oncogene.* 2000;19:737–744.
104. Fagin JA. Minireview: branded from the start-distinct oncogenic initiating events may determine tumor fate in the thyroid. *Mol Endocrinol.* 2002;16:903–911.
105. Kroll TG, Sarraf P, Pecciarini L, et al. *PAX8-PPARg*1 fusion oncogene in human thyroid carcinoma. *Science.* 2000;289:1357–1360.
106. Nikiforova MN, Biddinger PW, Caudill CM, Kroll TG, Nikiforov YE. PAX8-PPARgamma rearrangement in thyroid tumors: RT-PCR and immunohistochemical analyses. *Am J Surg Pathol.* 2002;26:1016–1023.
107. Marques AR, Espadinha C, Catarino AL, et al. Expression of PAX8-PPARgamma1 rearrangements in both follicular thyroid carcinomas and adenomas. *J Clin Endocrinol Metab.* 2002;87:3947–3952.
108. Lacroix L, Mian C, Barrier T, et al. PAX8 and peroxisome proliferator-activated receptor gamma 1 gene expression status in benign and malignant thyroid tissues. *Eur J Endocrinol.* 2004;151:367–374.
109. Giordano TJ, Au AY, Kuick R, et al. Delineation, functional validation, and bioinformatic evaluation of gene expression in thyroid follicular carcinomas with the PAX8-PPARG translocation. *Clin Cancer Res.* 2006;12:1983–1993.
110. Dwight T, Thoppe SR, Foukakis T, et al. Involvement of the PAX8/peroxisome proliferator-activated receptor gamma rearrangement in follicular thyroid tumors. *J Clin Endocrinol Metab.* 2003;88:4440–4445.
111. Cheung L, Messina M, Gill A, et al. Detection of the PAX8-PPAR gamma fusion oncogene in both follicular thyroid carcinomas and adenomas. *J Clin Endocrinol Metab.* 2003;88:354–357.
112. Jenkins RB, Hay ID, Herath JF, et al. Frequent occurrence of cytogenetic abnormalities in sporadic nonmedullary thyroid carcinoma. *Cancer.* 1990;66:1213–1220.
113. Roque L, Castedo S, Clode A, Soares J. Deletion of 3p25→pter in a primary follicular thyroid carcinoma and its metastasis. *Genes Chromosomes Cancer.* 1993;8:199–203.
114. Bondeson L, Bengtsson A, Bondeson AG, et al. Chromosome studies in thyroid neoplasia. *Cancer.* 1989;64:680–685.
115. Roque L, Castedo S, Gomes P, Soares P, Clode A, Soares J. Cytogenetic findings in 18 follicular thyroid adenomas. *Cancer Genet Cytogenet.* 1993;67:1–6.
116. Teyssier JR, Liautaud-Roger F, Ferre D, Patey M, Dufer J. Chromosomal changes in thyroid tumors. Relation with DNA content, karyotypic features, and clinical data. *Cancer Genet Cytogenet.* 1990;50:249–263.
117. Sozzi G, Miozzo M, Cariani TC, et al. A t(2;3)(q12-13;p24-25) in follicular thyroid adenomas. *Cancer Genet Cytogenet.* 1992;64:38–41.
118. Lui WO, Kytola S, Anfalk L, Larsson C, Farnebo LO. Balanced translocation (3;7)(p25;q34): another mechanism of tumorigenesis in follicular thyroid carcinoma? *Cancer Genet Cytogenet.* 2000;119:109–112.
119. Lui W, Zeng L, Rehrmann V, et al. *CREB3L2-PPARg* fusion mutation identifies a thyroid signaling pathway regulated by intra-membrane proteolysis. *Cancer Res.* 2008;68(17):7156–7164.
120. Lacroix L, Lazar V, Michiels S, et al. Follicular thyroid tumors with the PAX8-PPARgamma1 rearrangement display characteristic genetic alterations. *Am J Pathol.* 2005;167:223–231.
121. Castro P, Rebocho AP, Soares RJ, et al. PAX8-PPARgamma rearrangement is frequently detected in the follicular variant of papillary thyroid carcinoma. *J Clin Endocrinol Metab.* 2006;91:213–220.
122. Lui WO, Foukakis T, Liden J, et al. Expression profiling reveals a distinct transcription signature in follicular thyroid carcinomas with a PAX8-PPAR(gamma) fusion oncogene. *Oncogene.* 2005;24:1467–1476.
123. French C, Fletcher J, Cibas E, Caulfield C, Allard P, Kroll T. Molecular detection of *PPARg* rearrangements and thyroid carcinoma in pre-operative fine needle aspiration biopsies. *Endocr Pathol.* 2008;19(3):166–174.
124. Mansouri A, Chowdhury K, Gruss P. Follicular cells of the thyroid gland require Pax8 gene function. *Nat Genet.* 1998;19:87–90.
125. Maulbecker CC, Gruss P. The oncogenic potential of Pax genes. *EMBO J.* 1993;12:2361–2367.
126. Cazzaniga G, Daniotti M, Tosi S, et al. The paired box domain gene PAX5 is fused to ETV6/TEL in an acute lymphoblastic leukemia case. *Cancer Res.* 2001;61:4666–4670.

127. Iida S, Rao PH, Nallasivam P, et al. The t(9;14)(p13;q32) chromosomal translocation associated with lymphoplasmacytoid lymphoma involves the PAX-5 gene. *Blood.* 1996;88:4110–4117.
128. Mullighan CG, Goorha S, Radtke I, et al. Genome-wide analysis of genetic alterations in acute lymphoblastic leukaemia. *Nature.* 2007;446:758–764.
129. Galili N, Davis RJ, Fredericks WJ, et al. Fusion of a fork head domain gene to PAX3 in the solid tumour alveolar rhabdomyosarcoma. *Nat Genet.* 1993;5:230–235.
130. Barr FG, Galili N, Holick J, Biegel JA, Rovera G, Emanuel BS. Rearrangement of the PAX3 paired box gene in the paediatric solid tumour alveolar rhabdomyosarcoma. *Nat Genet.* 1993;3:113–117.
131. Shapiro DN, Sublett JE, Li B, Downing JR, Naeve CW. Fusion of PAX3 to a member of the forkhead family of transcription factors in human alveolar rhabdomyosarcoma. *Cancer Res.* 1993;53:5108–5112.
132. Storlazzi CT, Mertens F, Nascimento A, et al. Fusion of the FUS and BBF2H7 genes in low grade fibromyxoid sarcoma. *Hum Mol Genet.* 2003;12:2349–2358.
133. Williams DW, Wynford-Thomas D. Human thyroid epithelial cells. *Methods Mol Biol.* 1997;75:163–172.
134. Martelli ML, Iuliano R, Le Pera I, et al. Inhibitory effects of peroxisome proliferator-activated receptor gamma on thyroid carcinoma cell growth. *J Clin Endocrinol Metab.* 2002;87:4728–4735.
135. Powell J, Wang X, Allard B, et al. The PAX8/PPARg fusion oncoprotein transforms immortalized human thyrocytes through a mechanism probably involving wild-type PPARg inhibition. *Oncogene.* 2004;23:3634–3641.
136. Klopper JP, Hays WR, Sharma V, Baumbusch MA, Hershman JM, Haugen BR. Retinoid X receptor-gamma and peroxisome proliferator-activated receptor-gamma expression predicts thyroid carcinoma cell response to retinoid and thiazolidinedione treatment. *Mol Cancer Ther.* 2004;3:1011–1020.
137. Park JW, Zarnegar R, Kanauchi H, et al. Troglitazone, the peroxisome proliferator-activated receptor-gamma agonist, induces antiproliferation and redifferentiation in human thyroid cancer cell lines. *Thyroid.* 2005;15:222–231.
138. Aiello A, Pandini G, Frasca F, et al. Peroxisomal proliferator-activated receptor-gamma agonists induce partial reversion of epithelial-mesenchymal transition in anaplastic thyroid cancer cells. *Endocrinology.* 2006;147:4463–4475.
139. Hayashi N, Nakamori S, Hiraoka N, et al. Antitumor effects of peroxisome proliferator activate receptor gamma ligands on anaplastic thyroid carcinoma. *Int J Oncol.* 2004;24:89–95.
140. Kato Y, Ying H, Zhao L, et al. PPARgamma insufficiency promotes follicular thyroid carcinogenesis via activation of the nuclear factor-kappaB signaling pathway. *Oncogene.* 2006;25:2736–2747.
141. Ohta K, Endo T, Haraguchi K, Hershman JM, Onaya T. Ligands for peroxisome proliferator-activated receptor gamma inhibit growth and induce apoptosis of human papillary thyroid carcinoma cells. *J Clin Endocrinol Metab.* 2001;86:2170–2177.
142. Copland JA, Marlow LA, Kurakata S, et al. Novel high-affinity PPARgamma agonist alone and in combination with paclitaxel inhibits human anaplastic thyroid carcinoma tumor growth via p21WAF1/CIP1. *Oncogene.* 2006;25:2304–2317.
143. Chen Y, Wang SM, Wu JC, Huang SH. Effects of PPARgamma agonists on cell survival and focal adhesions in a Chinese thyroid carcinoma cell line. *J Cell Biochem.* 2006;98: 1021–1035.
144. Frohlich E, Machicao F, Wahl R. Action of thiazolidinediones on differentiation, proliferation and apoptosis of normal and transformed thyrocytes in culture. *Endocr Relat Cancer.* 2005;12:291–303.
145. Aldred MA, Morrison C, Gimm O, et al. Peroxisome proliferator-activated receptor gamma is frequently downregulated in a diversity of sporadic nonmedullary thyroid carcinomas. *Oncogene.* 2003;22:3412–3416.
146. Sarraf P, Mueller E, Smith WM, et al. Loss-of-function mutations in PPAR gamma associated with human colon cancer. *Mol Cell.* 1999;3:799–804.
147. Ying H, Suzuki H, Furumoto H, et al. Alterations in genomic profiles during tumor progression in a mouse model of follicular thyroid carcinoma. *Carcinogenesis.* 2003;24:1467–1479.
148. Ying H, Suzuki H, Zhao L, Willingham MC, Meltzer P, Cheng SY. Mutant thyroid hormone receptor beta represses the expression and transcriptional activity of peroxisome proliferator-activated receptor gamma during thyroid carcinogenesis. *Cancer Res.* 2003;63:5274–5280.
149. Au AY, McBride C, Wilhelm KG Jr, et al. PAX8-peroxisome proliferator-activated receptor gamma (PPARgamma) disrupts normal PAX8 or PPARgamma transcriptional function and stimulates follicular thyroid cell growth. *Endocrinology.* 2006;147:367–376.
150. Baek SJ, Wilson LC, Hsi LC, Eling TE. Troglitazone, a peroxisome proliferator-activated receptor gamma (PPAR gamma) ligand, selectively induces the early growth response-1 gene independently of PPAR gamma. A novel mechanism for its anti-tumorigenic activity. *J Biol Chem.* 2003;278: 5845–5853.
151. Palakurthi SS, Aktas H, Grubissich LM, Mortensen RM, Halperin JA. Anticancer effects of thiazolidinediones are independent of peroxisome proliferator-activated receptor gamma and mediated by inhibition of translation initiation. *Cancer Res.* 2001;61:6213–6218.
152. Shi Y, Hon M, Evans RM. The peroxisome proliferator-activated receptor delta, an integrator of transcriptional repression and nuclear receptor signaling. *Proc Natl Acad Sci USA.* 2002;99:2613–2618.
153. Foukakis T, Au AY, Wallin G, et al. The Ras effector NORE1A is suppressed in follicular thyroid carcinomas with a PAX8-PPARgamma fusion. *J Clin Endocrinol Metab.* 2006;91: 1143–1149.
154. Garcia-Rostan G, Costa AM, Pereira-Castro I, et al. Mutation of the PIK3CA gene in anaplastic thyroid cancer. *Cancer Res.* 2005;65:10199–10207.
155. Wang Y, Hou P, Yu H, et al. High prevalence and mutual exclusivity of genetic alterations in the phosphatidylinositol-3-kinase/akt pathway in thyroid tumors. *J Clin Endocrinol Metab.* 2007;92:2387–2390.
156. Hou P, Liu D, Shan Y, et al. Genetic alterations and their relationship in the phosphatidylinositol 3-kinase/Akt pathway in thyroid cancer. *Clin Cancer Res.* 2007;13:1161–1170.
157. Wu G, Mambo E, Guo Z, et al. Uncommon mutation, but common amplifications, of the PIK3CA gene in thyroid tumors. *J Clin Endocrinol Metab.* 2005;90:4688–4693.
158. Santarpia L, El-Naggar AK, Cote GJ, Myers JN, Sherman SI. Phosphatidylinositol 3-kinase/akt and ras/raf-mitogen-activated

protein kinase pathway mutations in anaplastic thyroid cancer. *J Clin Endocrinol Metab*. 2008;93:278–284.
159. Broderick DK, Di C, Parrett TJ, et al. Mutations of PIK3CA in anaplastic oligodendrogliomas, high-grade astrocytomas, and medulloblastomas. *Cancer Res*. 2004;64:5048–5050.
160. Campbell IG, Russell SE, Choong DY, et al. Mutation of the PIK3CA gene in ovarian and breast cancer. *Cancer Res*. 2004;64:7678–7681.
161. Saal LH, Holm K, Maurer M, et al. PIK3CA mutations correlate with hormone receptors, node metastasis, and ERBB2, and are mutually exclusive with PTEN loss in human breast carcinoma. *Cancer Res*. 2005;65:2554–2559.
162. Samuels Y, Wang Z, Bardelli A, et al. High frequency of mutations of the PIK3CA gene in human cancers. *Science*. 2004;304:554.
163. Kang S, Bader AG, Vogt PK. Phosphatidylinositol 3-kinase mutations identified in human cancer are oncogenic. *Proc Natl Acad Sci USA*. 2005;102:802–807.
164. Bader AG, Kang S, Vogt PK. Cancer-specific mutations in PIK3CA are oncogenic in vivo. *Proc Natl Acad Sci USA*. 2006;103:1475–1479.
165. Eng C. Role of PTEN, a lipid phosphatase upstream effector of protein kinase B, in epithelial thyroid carcinogenesis. *Ann N Y Acad Sci*. 2002;968:213–221.
166. Liaw D, Marsh DJ, Li J, et al. Germline mutations of the PTEN gene in Cowden disease, an inherited breast and thyroid cancer syndrome. *Nat Genet*. 1997;16:64–67.
167. Di Cristofano A, Pesce B, Cordon-Cardo C, Pandolfi PP. Pten is essential for embryonic development and tumour suppression. *Nat Genet*. 1998;19:348–355.
168. Podsypanina K, Ellenson LH, Nemes A, et al. Mutation of Pten/Mmac1 in mice causes neoplasia in multiple organ systems. *Proc Natl Acad Sci USA*. 1999;96:1563–1568.
169. Dahia PL, Marsh DJ, Zheng Z, et al. Somatic deletions and mutations in the Cowden disease gene, PTEN, in sporadic thyroid tumors. *Cancer Res*. 1997;57:4710–4713.
170. Halachmi N, Halachmi S, Evron E, et al. Somatic mutations of the PTEN tumor suppressor gene in sporadic follicular thyroid tumors. *Genes Chromosomes Cancer*. 1998;23:239–243.
171. Yeh JJ, Marsh DJ, Zedenius J, et al. Fine-structure deletion mapping of 10q22-24 identifies regions of loss of heterozygosity and suggests that sporadic follicular thyroid adenomas and follicular thyroid carcinomas develop along distinct neoplastic pathways. *Genes Chromosomes Cancer*. 1999;26: 322–328.
172. Frisk T, Foukakis T, Dwight T, et al. Silencing of the PTEN tumor-suppressor gene in anaplastic thyroid cancer. *Genes Chromosomes Cancer*. 2002;35:74–80.
173. Gimm O, Perren A, Weng LP, et al. Differential nuclear and cytoplasmic expression of PTEN in normal thyroid tissue, and benign and malignant epithelial thyroid tumors. *Am J Pathol*. 2000;156:1693–1700.
174. Bruni P, Boccia A, Baldassarre G, et al. PTEN expression is reduced in a subset of sporadic thyroid carcinomas: evidence that PTEN-growth suppressing activity in thyroid cancer cells mediated by p27kip1. *Oncogene*. 2000;19:3146–3155.
175. Kimura ET, Nikiforova MN, Zhu Z, Knauf JA, Nikiforov YE, Fagin JA. High prevalence of BRAF mutations in thyroid cancer: genetic evidence for constitutive activation of the RET/PTC-RAS-BRAF signaling pathway in papillary thyroid carcinoma. *Cancer Res*. 2003;63:1454–1457.
176. Santoro M, Carlomagno F, Hay ID, et al. Ret oncogene activation in human thyroid neoplasms is restricted to the papillary cancer subtype. *J Clin Invest*. 1992;89:1517–1522.
177. Fusco A, Grieco M, Santoro M, et al. A new oncogene in human thyroid papillary carcinomas and their lymph- nodal metastases. *Nature*. 1987;328:170–172.
178. Grieco M, Santoro M, Berlingieri MT, et al. PTC is a novel rearranged form of the ret proto-oncogene and is frequently detected in vivo in human thyroid papillary carcinomas. *Cell*. 1990;60:557–563.
179. Maxwell EL, Palme CE, Freeman J. Hürthle cell tumors: applying molecular markers to define a new management algorithm. *Arch Otolaryngol Head Neck Surg*. 2006;132:54–58.
180. Carcangiu ML, Bianchi S, Savino D, Voynick IM, Rosai J. Follicular Hürthle cell tumors of the thyroid gland. *Cancer*. 1991;68:1944–1953.
181. Berho M, Suster S. The oncocytic variant of papillary carcinoma of the thyroid: a clinicopathologic study of 15 cases. *Hum Pathol*. 1997;28:47–53.
182. Herrera MF, Hay ID, Wu PS, et al. Hürthle cell (oxyphilic) papillary thyroid carcinoma: a variant with more aggressive biologic behavior. *World J Surg*. 1992;16:669–674. discussion 774–775.
183. Rodrigues-Serpa A, Catarino A, Soares J. Loss of heterozygosity in follicular and papillary thyroid carcinomas. *Cancer Genet Cytogenet*. 2003;141:26–31.
184. Roque L, Clode A, Belge G, et al. Follicular thyroid carcinoma: chromosome analysis of 19 cases. *Genes Chromosomes Cancer*. 1998;21:250–255.
185. Roque L, Rodrigues R, Pinto A, Moura-Nunes V, Soares J. Chromosome imbalances in thyroid follicular neoplasms: a comparison between follicular adenomas and carcinomas. *Genes Chromosomes Cancer*. 2003;36:292–302.
186. Kitamura Y, Shimizu K, Ito K, Tanaka S, Emi M. Allelotyping of follicular thyroid carcinoma: frequent allelic losses in chromosome arms 7q, 11p, and 22q. *J Clin Endocrinol Metab*. 2001;86:4268–4272.
187. Ward LS, Brenta G, Medvedovic M, Fagin JA. Studies of allelic loss in thyroid tumors reveal major differences in chromosomal instability between papillary and follicular carcinomas. *J Clin Endocrinol Metab*. 1998;83:525–530.
188. Segev DL, Saji M, Phillips GS, et al. Polymerase chain reaction-based microsatellite polymorphism analysis of follicular and Hürthle cell neoplasms of the thyroid. *J Clin Endocrinol Metab*. 1998;83:2036–2042.
189. Hunt JL, Yim JH, Tometsko M, Finkelstein SD, Swalsky P, Carty SE. Loss of heterozygosity of the VHL gene identifies malignancy and predicts death in follicular thyroid tumors. *Surgery*. 2003;134:1043–1047. discussion 1047–1048.
190. Herrmann MA, Hay ID, Bartelt DH Jr, et al. Cytogenetic and molecular genetic studies of follicular and papillary thyroid cancers. *J Clin Invest*. 1991;88:1596–1604.
191. Zhang JS, Nelson M, McIver B, et al. Differential loss of heterozygosity at 7q31.2 in follicular and papillary thyroid tumors. *Oncogene*. 1998;17:789–793.
192. Trovato M, Fraggetta F, Villari D, et al. Loss of heterozygosity of the long arm of chromosome 7 in follicular and anaplastic thyroid cancer, but not in papillary thyroid cancer. *J Clin Endocrinol Metab*. 1999;84:3235–3240.
193. Frisk T, Kytola S, Wallin G, Zedenius J, Larsson C. Low frequency of numerical chromosomal aberrations in follicular

thyroid tumors detected by comparative genomic hybridization. *Genes Chromosomes Cancer*. 1999;25:349–353.
194. Kitamura Y, Shimizu K, Tanaka S, Ito K, Emi M. Allelotyping of anaplastic thyroid carcinoma: frequent allelic losses on 1q, 9p, 11, 17, 19p, and 22q. *Genes Chromosomes Cancer*. 2000;27:244–251.
195. Zedenius J, Wallin G, Svensson A, et al. Deletions of the long arm of chromosome 10 in progression of follicular thyroid tumors. *Hum Genet*. 1996;97:299–303.
196. Zedenius J, Wallin G, Svensson A, et al. Allelotyping of follicular thyroid tumors. *Hum Genet*. 1995;96:27–32.
197. Nord B, Larsson C, Wong FK, Wallin G, Teh BT, Zedenius J. Sporadic follicular thyroid tumors show loss of a 200-kb region in 11q13 without evidence for mutations in the MEN1 gene. *Genes Chromosomes Cancer*. 1999;26:35–39.
198. Matsuo K, Tang SH, Fagin JA. Allelotype of human thyroid tumors: loss of chromosome 11q13 sequences in follicular neoplasms. *Mol Endocrinol*. 1991;5:1873–1879.
199. Grebe SK, McIver B, Hay ID, et al. Frequent loss of heterozygosity on chromosomes 3p and 17p without VHL or p53 mutations suggests involvement of unidentified tumor suppressor genes in follicular thyroid carcinoma. *J Clin Endocrinol Metab*. 1997;82:3684–3691.
200. Hemmer S, Wasenius VM, Knuutila S, Franssila K, Joensuu H. DNA copy number changes in thyroid carcinoma. *Am J Pathol*. 1999;154:1539–1547.
201. Hemmer S, Wasenius VM, Knuutila S, Joensuu H, Franssila K. Comparison of benign and malignant follicular thyroid tumours by comparative genomic hybridization. *Br J Cancer*. 1998;78:1012–1017.
202. Hunt JL, Livolsi VA, Baloch ZW, et al. A novel microdissection and genotyping of follicular-derived thyroid tumors to predict aggressiveness. *Hum Pathol*. 2003;34:375–380.
203. Hunt JL, Yim JH, Carty SE. Fractional allelic loss of tumor suppressor genes identifies malignancy and predicts clinical outcome in follicular thyroid tumors. *Thyroid*. 2006;16:643–649.
204. Ruan Y, Ooi HS, Choo SW, et al. Fusion transcripts and transcribed retrotransposed loci discovered through comprehensive transcriptome analysis using Paired-End diTags (PETs). *Genome Res*. 2007;17:828–838.
205. Greenman C, Stephens P, Smith R, et al. Patterns of somatic mutation in human cancer genomes. *Nature*. 2007;446:153–158.
206. Davies H, Hunter C, Smith R, et al. Somatic mutations of the protein kinase gene family in human lung cancer. *Cancer Res*. 2005;65:7591–7595.
207. Sjoblom T, Jones S, Wood LD, et al. The consensus coding sequences of human breast and colorectal cancers. *Science*. 2006;314:268–274.
208. Wood LD, Parsons DW, Jones S, et al. The genomic landscapes of human breast and colorectal cancers. *Science*. 2007;318:1108–1113.
209. Barden CB, Shister KW, Zhu B, et al. Classification of follicular thyroid tumors by molecular signature: results of gene profiling. *Clin Cancer Res*. 2003;9:1792–1800.
210. Chevillard S, Ugolin N, Vielh P, et al. Gene expression profiling of differentiated thyroid neoplasms: diagnostic and clinical implications. *Clin Cancer Res*. 2004;10:6586–6597.
211. Finley DJ, Zhu B, Barden CB, Fahey TJ 3rd. Discrimination of benign and malignant thyroid nodules by molecular profiling. *Ann Surg*. 2004;240:425–436. discussion 436–437.
212. Fryknas M, Wickenberg-Bolin U, Goransson H, et al. Molecular markers for discrimination of benign and malignant follicular thyroid tumors. *Tumour Biol*. 2006;27:211–220.
213. Weber F, Shen L, Aldred MA, et al. Genetic classification of benign and malignant thyroid follicular neoplasia based on a three-gene combination. *J Clin Endocrinol Metab*. 2005; 90:2512–2521.
214. Aldred MA, Huang Y, Liyanarachchi S, et al. Papillary and follicular thyroid carcinomas show distinctly different microarray expression profiles and can be distinguished by a minimum of five genes. *J Clin Oncol*. 2004;22:3531–3539.
215. Huang Y, Prasad M, Lemon WJ, et al. Gene expression in papillary thyroid carcinoma reveals highly consistent profiles. *Proc Natl Acad Sci USA*. 2001;98:15044–15049.
216. Takano T, Miyauchi A, Yoshida H, Kuma K, Amino N. High-throughput differential screening of mRNAs by serial analysis of gene expression: decreased expression of trefoil factor 3 mRNA in thyroid follicular carcinomas. *Br J Cancer*. 2004;90:1600–1605.
217. Cerutti JM, Delcelo R, Amadei MJ, et al. A preoperative diagnostic test that distinguishes benign from malignant thyroid carcinoma based on gene expression. *J Clin Invest*. 2004;113:1234–1242.
218. Netea-Maier RT, Hunsucker SW, Hoevenaars BM, et al. Discovery and validation of protein abundance differences between follicular thyroid neoplasms. *Cancer Res*. 2008;68:1572–1580.
219. Baris O, Mirebeau-Prunier D, Savagner F, et al. Gene profiling reveals specific oncogenic mechanisms and signaling pathways in oncocytic and papillary thyroid carcinoma. *Oncogene*. 2005;24:4155–4161.
220. Lacroix L, Ripoche H, Lazar V, et al. Molecular signatures of thyroid follicular tumors presenting the PAX8-PPARG1 rearrangement. *Thyroid*. 2003;13:699.
221. Giordano TJ, Kuick R, Thomas DG, et al. Molecular classification of papillary thyroid carcinoma: distinct BRAF, RAS, and RET/PTC mutation-specific gene expression profiles discovered by DNA microarray analysis. *Oncogene*. 2005;24:6646–6656.
222. Schetter AJ, Leung SY, Sohn JJ, et al. MicroRNA expression profiles associated with prognosis and therapeutic outcome in colon adenocarcinoma. *JAMA*. 2008;299:425–436.
223. Esquela-Kerscher A, Slack FJ. Oncomirs – microRNAs with a role in cancer. *Nat Rev Cancer*. 2006;6:259–269.
224. Calin GA, Croce CM. MicroRNA signatures in human cancers. *Nat Rev Cancer*. 2006;6:857–866.
225. Lu J, Getz G, Miska EA, et al. MicroRNA expression profiles classify human cancers. *Nature*. 2005;435:834–838.
226. Volinia S, Calin GA, Liu CG, et al. A microRNA expression signature of human solid tumors defines cancer gene targets. *Proc Natl Acad Sci USA*. 2006;103:2257–2261.
227. Ambros V. The functions of animal microRNAs. *Nature*. 2004;431:350–355.
228. Bartel DP. MicroRNAs: genomics, biogenesis, mechanism, and function. *Cell*. 2004;116:281–297.
229. Nikiforova MN, Tseng GC, Steward D, Diorio D, Nikiforov YE. MicroRNA expression profiling of thyroid tumors: biological significance and diagnostic utility. *J Clin Endocrinol Metab*. 2008;93:1600–1608.
230. He H, Jazdzewski K, Li W, et al. The role of microRNA genes in papillary thyroid carcinoma. *Proc Natl Acad Sci USA*. 2005;102:19075–19080.

231. Pallante P, Visone R, Ferracin M, et al. MicroRNA deregulation in human thyroid papillary carcinomas. *Endocr Relat Cancer*. 2006;13:497–508.
232. Visone R, Russo L, Pallante P, et al. MicroRNAs (miR)-221 and miR-222, both overexpressed in human thyroid papillary carcinomas, regulate p27Kip1 protein levels and cell cycle. *Endocr Relat Cancer*. 2007;14:791–798.
233. Cahill S, Smyth P, Denning K, et al. Effect of BRAFV600E mutation on transcription and post-transcriptional regulation in a papillary thyroid carcinoma model. *Mol Cancer*. 2007;6:21.
234. Cahill S, Smyth P, Finn SP, et al. Effect of ret/PTC 1 rearrangement on transcription and post-transcriptional regulation in a papillary thyroid carcinoma model. *Mol Cancer*. 2006;5:70.
235. Weber F, Teresi RE, Broelsch CE, Frilling A, Eng C. A limited set of human MicroRNA is deregulated in follicular thyroid carcinoma. *J Clin Endocrinol Metab*. 2006;91:3584–3591.
236. Malchoff CD, Malchoff DM. The genetics of hereditary nonmedullary thyroid carcinoma. *J Clin Endocrinol Metab*. 2002;87:2455–2459.
237. Hemminki K, Eng C, Chen B. Familial risks for nonmedullary thyroid cancer. *J Clin Endocrinol Metab*. 2005;90:5747–5753.
238. Canzian F, Amati P, Harach HR, et al. A gene predisposing to familial thyroid tumors with cell oxyphilia maps to chromosome 19p13.2. *Am J Hum Genet*. 1998;63:1743–1748.
239. Harach HR, Lesueur F, Amati P, et al. Histology of familial thyroid tumours linked to a gene mapping to chromosome 19p13.2. *J Pathol*. 1999;189:387–393.
240. Maximo V, Botelho T, Capela J, et al. Somatic and germline mutation in GRIM-19, a dual function gene involved in mitochondrial metabolism and cell death, is linked to mitochondrion-rich (Hürthle cell) tumours of the thyroid. *Br J Cancer*. 2005;92:1892–1898.
241. Coghlan DW, Morley AA, Matthews JP, Bishop JF. The incidence and prognostic significance of mutations in codon 13 of the N-ras gene in acute myeloid leukemia. *Leukemia*. 1994;8:1682–1687.
242. Neubauer A, Dodge RK, George SL, et al. Prognostic importance of mutations in the ras proto-oncogenes in de novo acute myeloid leukemia. *Blood*. 1994;83:1603–1611.
243. Radich JP, Kopecky KJ, Willman CL, et al. N-ras mutations in adult de novo acute myelogenous leukemia: prevalence and clinical significance. *Blood*. 1990;76:801–807.
244. Stirewalt DL, Kopecky KJ, Meshinchi S, et al. FLT3, RAS, and TP53 mutations in elderly patients with acute myeloid leukemia. *Blood*. 2001;97:3589–3595.
245. Jansen JH, Mahfoudi A, Rambaud S, Lavau C, Wahli W, Dejean A. Multimeric complexes of the PML-retinoic acid receptor alpha fusion protein in acute promyelocytic leukemia cells and interference with retinoid and peroxisome-proliferator signaling pathways. *Proc Natl Acad Sci USA*. 1995;92:7401–7405.
246. Okuda T, Cai Z, Yang S, et al. Expression of a knocked-in AML1-ETO leukemia gene inhibits the establishment of normal definitive hematopoiesis and directly generates dysplastic hematopoietic progenitors. *Blood*. 1998;91:3134–3143.
247. Nakao M, Yokota S, Iwai T, et al. Internal tandem duplication of the flt3 gene found in acute myeloid leukemia. *Leukemia*. 1996;10:1911–1918.
248. Gilliland DG, Griffin JD. Role of FLT3 in leukemia. *Curr Opin Hematol*. 2002;9:274–281.
249. Ross DM, Hughes TP. Current and emerging tests for the laboratory monitoring of chronic myeloid leukaemia and related disorders. *Pathology*. 2008;40:231–246.
250. Gilliland DG, Tallman MS. Focus on acute leukemias. *Cancer Cell*. 2002;1:417–420.
251. Mrozek K, Bloomfield CD. Clinical significance of the most common chromosome translocations in adult acute myeloid leukemia. *J Natl Cancer Inst Monogr*. 2008;(39):52–57.
252. Cheung CC, Carydis B, Ezzat S, Bedard YC, Asa SL. Analysis of ret/PTC gene rearrangements refines the fine needle aspiration diagnosis of thyroid cancer. *J Clin Endocrinol Metab*. 2001;86:2187–2190.
253. Chung KW, Yang SK, Lee GK, et al. Detection of BRAFV600E mutation on fine needle aspiration specimens of thyroid nodule refines cyto-pathology diagnosis, especially in BRAF600E mutation-prevalent area. *Clin Endocrinol (Oxf)*. 2006;65:660–666.
254. Cohen Y, Rosenbaum E, Clark DP, et al. Mutational analysis of BRAF in fine needle aspiration biopsies of the thyroid: a potential application for the preoperative assessment of thyroid nodules. *Clin Cancer Res*. 2004;10:2761–2765.
255. Jin L, Sebo TJ, Nakamura N, et al. BRAF mutation analysis in fine needle aspiration (FNA) cytology of the thyroid. *Diagn Mol Pathol*. 2006;15:136–143.
256. Pizzolanti G, Russo L, Richiusa P, et al. Fine-needle aspiration molecular analysis for the diagnosis of papillary thyroid carcinoma through BRAF V600E mutation and RET/PTC rearrangement. *Thyroid*. 2007;17:1109–1115.
257. Rowe LR, Bentz BG, Bentz JS. Utility of BRAF V600E mutation detection in cytologically indeterminate thyroid nodules. *Cytojournal*. 2006;3:10.
258. Salvatore G, Giannini R, Faviana P, et al. Analysis of BRAF point mutation and RET/PTC rearrangement refines the fine-needle aspiration diagnosis of papillary thyroid carcinoma. *J Clin Endocrinol Metab*. 2004;89:5175–5180.
259. Sapio MR, Posca D, Raggioli A, et al. Detection of RET/PTC, TRK and BRAF mutations in preoperative diagnosis of thyroid nodules with indeterminate cytological findings. *Clin Endocrinol (Oxf)*. 2007;66:678–683.
260. Xing M, Tufano RP, Tufaro AP, et al. Detection of BRAF mutation on fine needle aspiration biopsy specimens: a new diagnostic tool for papillary thyroid cancer. *J Clin Endocrinol Metab*. 2004;89:2867–2872.
261. Foukakis T, Gusnanto A, Au AY, et al. A PCR-based expression signature of malignancy in follicular thyroid tumors. *Endocr Relat Cancer*. 2007;14:381–391.
262. Denning KM, Smyth PC, Cahill SF, et al. A molecular expression signature distinguishing follicular lesions in thyroid carcinoma using preamplification RT-PCR in archival samples. *Mod Pathol*. 2007;20:1095–1102.
263. Tallman MS, Andersen JW, Schiffer CA, et al. All-trans retinoic acid in acute promyelocytic leukemia: long-term outcome and prognostic factor analysis from the North American Intergroup protocol. *Blood*. 2002;100:4298–4302.
264. Weisberg E, Boulton C, Kelly LM, et al. Inhibition of mutant FLT3 receptors in leukemia cells by the small molecule tyrosine kinase inhibitor PKC412. *Cancer Cell*. 2002;1:433–443.

265. Kelly LM, Yu JC, Boulton CL, et al. CT53518, a novel selective FLT3 antagonist for the treatment of acute myelogenous leukemia (AML). *Cancer Cell*. 2002;1:421–432.
266. Druker BJ, Sawyers CL, Kantarjian H, et al. Activity of a specific inhibitor of the BCR-ABL tyrosine kinase in the blast crisis of chronic myeloid leukemia and acute lymphoblastic leukemia with the Philadelphia chromosome. *N Engl J Med*. 2001;344:1038–1042.
267. Druker BJ, Talpaz M, Resta DJ, et al. Efficacy and safety of a specific inhibitor of the BCR-ABL tyrosine kinase in chronic myeloid leukemia. *N Engl J Med*. 2001;344:1031–1037.
268. Carlomagno F, Vitagliano D, Guida T, et al. ZD6474, an orally available inhibitor of KDR tyrosine kinase activity, efficiently blocks oncogenic RET kinases. *Cancer Res*. 2002;62:7284–7290.
269. Carlomagno F, Vitagliano D, Guida T, et al. The kinase inhibitor PP1 blocks tumorigenesis induced by RET oncogenes. *Cancer Res*. 2002;62:1077–1082.
270. Carlomagno F, Vitagliano D, Guida T, et al. Efficient inhibition of RET/papillary thyroid carcinoma oncogenic kinases by 4-amino-5-(4-chloro-phenyl)-7-(t-butyl)pyrazolo[3, 4-d]pyrimidine (PP2). *J Clin Endocrinol Metab*. 2003;88:1897–1902.
271. Yin Y, Yuan H, Wang C, et al. 3-phosphoinositide-dependent protein kinase-1 activates the peroxisome proliferator-activated receptor-gamma and promotes adipocyte differentiation. *Mol Endocrinol*. 2006;20:268–278.
272. Lubitz CC, Ugras SK, Kazam JJ, et al. Microarray analysis of thyroid nodule fine-needle aspirates accurately classifies benign and malignant lesions. *J Mol Diagn*. 2006;8:490–498.

10 Poorly Differentiated and Undifferentiated Thyroid Carcinomas

Jennifer L. Hunt and Virginia A. LiVolsi

Introduction

The definition of poorly differentiated thyroid carcinoma has been the source of great controversy in the pathology literature.[1] Many definitions and schemes have been proposed, but little consensus exists about what defines a poorly differentiated thyroid carcinoma (PDTCA). Because of this, the clinical behavior is not well defined and the clinicopathologic features affecting prognosis remain largely unknown.

In contrast, anaplastic thyroid carcinoma (ATC, also called "undifferentiated thyroid carcinoma") is pathologically fairly well characterized; clinically it affects a unique group of patients, which further enables a straight-forward diagnosis.

This chapter will discuss the clinical and histologic features, immunohistochemical staining patterns, and the molecular genetics of each of these two thyroid tumor categories.

Poorly Differentiated Thyroid Carcinoma

No standardized definitions exist for the grading of the differentiation of thyroid carcinoma, other than the dogma that follicular carcinoma and papillary carcinomas are considered to be well-differentiated tumors and anaplastic carcinoma is considered to be undifferentiated. Grading of tumors that exist in the spectrum between these two extremes is surrounded by some degree of controversy both in the literature and in practice. Grading is further complicated by the fact that PDTCAs may be derived from well-differentiated tumors and varying amounts of these well-differentiated elements can be represented in the histologic sections of any particular tumor.

As with other organ systems, tumor differentiation does play a key role in prognostication for thyroid tumors. But, in thyroid carcinoma, the independent prognostic value or independent impact of differentiation on prognosis is less clear. In fact, the influence of standard variables, such as age, gender, tumor size, extrathyroidal extension of tumor, and metastasis is so strong that prognosis is heavily influenced by these factors.[2] The strongest argument for assessing differentiation can be found in the many papers that have demonstrated survival disadvantage when higher grade histologic features are identified.[3–5] Even when poorly differentiated areas are entirely well contained within otherwise well-differentiated tumors, the presence of this more aggressive morphology likely impacts survival.[3] Unfortunately, in treatment protocols for thyroid carcinoma, there are no additional therapies that have proven to be of great value when poorly differentiated components are identified.[6–8] Although chemotherapy and external beam radiation therapy have been used in some series, dramatic improvement in survival has not been shown and these treatments are usually reserved for the palliative setting.[9,10]

When tumors are well-differentiated, tumor histologic grading is probably not essential. Patients with these well-differentiated tumors tend to have an excellent survival and differences based on traditional nuclear and histologic grading will not impact greatly on prognosis.[3] When tumors transition into less well-differentiated lesions, however, it is more important to note the presence of histologically aggressive features.[11,12] The pathologist should therefore be familiar with the features of poorly differentiated tumors.

Histology

The growth pattern of a thyroid tumor provides one of the most important diagnostic features for differentiation in thyroid carcinomas.[1] However, some classification schemes include specific subtypes of thyroid cancer as PDTCA, i.e., tall cell papillary carcinoma or Hurthle cell carcinoma.[13,14] These latter entities have been fairly well described both morphologically and be clinicopathologic features and hence should not be added to the mix of PDTCA. Growth patterns that are considered to be less well-differentiated include insular, trabecular, and solid growth.[6] Various studies have demonstrated that these growth patterns are associated with a worse prognosis.[13] Unfortunately, the studies are

J.L. Hunt (ed.), *Molecular Pathology of Endocrine Diseases*, Molecular Pathology Library 3,
DOI 10.1007/978-1-4419-1707-2_10, © Springer Science+Business Media, LLC 2010

highly variable about what is considered the minimal amount needed to classify a tumor as "poorly differentiated".[14] Various proposed cut-offs have included >10%, >40%, and >70%.[14,15] Because of these inconsistencies, it is difficult to compare the different studies and to arrive at a conclusion about the true impact of these growth patterns on prognosis.

In 1984, Carcangiu and Rosai described 25 cases of a new form of PDTCA that had a poor prognosis and a unique histologic appearance; they designated this tumor as "insular carcinoma".[16] The insular growth pattern shows large nests of cells with small round nuclei. The nests are surrounded by a rich vascular network. This tumor designation has now been used for several decades, but it is now controversial whether this is a distinct tumor type or simply a pattern of poor differentiation.[17–21] In fact, insular growth patterns can be seen focally or even diffusely in all types of well-differentiated carcinomas.[6,14] Pure insular growth in tumors is relatively uncommon and is most certainly associated with a poor prognosis.[21]

Some studies have shown that even a minor insular growth pattern component is significant for prognosis in an otherwise well-differentiated tumor but others have argued that it is not significant.[22] Trabecular and solid growth are the other two growth patterns that have been described as indicative of a less well-differentiated tumor.[6,21] These are less reliable features, however, since trabecular and solid growth can be seen as a minor component of benign follicular lesion as well.[8]

There are a host of other histologic features that are relied upon to supplement the growth pattern in making a diagnosis of poorly differentiated carcinoma. These include extensive vascular invasion, nuclear atypia, increased mitotic activity, and tumor necrosis.[1,23] A recent proposal from a group of endocrine pathologists suggests that the minimal features that should be used for a diagnosis of PDTCA should be (a) solid, trabecular, or insular growth, (b) absence of conventional papillary carcinoma nuclear features, and (c) presence of at least one of the following features: convoluted nuclei, mitotic activity >3 per 10 high power fields, or coagulative necrosis.[1]

Immunohistochemistry and Genetics

The immunohistochemical staining patterns and the molecular mutational profiles of poorly differentiated tumors have studied. At the very basic level, most of these tumors will express thyroid transcription factor (TTF) and thyroglobulin at least focally.

In terms of tumor markers, the results for PDTCAs are sparse. The best studied genetic alteration is in the p53 gene. The results for expression of p53 in insular carcinoma in particular have been mixed, with some studies showing significant expression and others showing no expression.[24,25] These discrepancies may be related to the original classification of the tumors, or to the methods used for detection, or they may just reflect the fact that PDTCA remains a very heterogeneous group of tumors. Another tumor marker that has been studied is the KIT gene, which is a receptor tyrosine kinase. The KIT gene has been best studied at the molecular level in gastrointestinal stromal tumors, which harbor both over-expression and somatic mutations. In these tumors, remarkable results have been achieved when patients are treated with targeted therapies against receptor tyrosine kinase.[26,27] Expression of KIT is seen in some PDTCAs, but is highly variable. Importantly, the KIT expression is not associated with mutations in the commonly mutated exons for the KIT gene. Therefore, it is unlikely that agents targeting receptor tyrosine kinases will be of value in treating PDTCA.[28] Very few other immunohistochemical markers have shown any prognostic significance in PDTCA.[29]

Another immunomarker that may be helpful is Ki67 since PDTCA often have significant mitotic activity and this stain may allow numerical assessment of this activity.

Very little work has been done with PDTCA and the other oncogene mutations that are associated with thyroid carcinoma, such as *BRAF*, *RAS*, and the tumor translocations. There do appear to be different expression profiles between well-differentiated tumors and PDTCAs.[30] Specifically, PDTCA appears to have alterations of key activators and negative regulators in the MAP-kinase pathways.[30,31] There is also evidence that cyclin D1 and e-cadherin are over-expressed in PDTCA, and low p27KIP1 expression and high proliferative rates have been associated with a poorer prognosis.[32,33] Finally, CTNNB1, which is the gene that encodes beta-catenin, has been shown to harbor mutations and altered expression by immunohistochemistry in PDTCA.[34,35]

Anaplastic Thyroid Carcinoma

The terminology for ATC has changed over the years. In the 1930s, ATCs were designated as sarcomas,[36] but in the 1950s to 1960s, it was recognized that these tumors were actually carcinomas with spindle and giant cells (sarcomatoid carcinoma).[37,38] Some ATCs have an epithelioid pattern (at least in part) and usually these resemble large cell lung carcinoma or even frank squamous differentiation may be noted. The association with a well-differentiated carcinoma in many cases also lends support to the notion that they are carcinomas. A particular example is the entity of spindle cell squamous cell carcinoma arising in association with tall cell variant papillary carcinoma.[39]

Many tumors that had been designated as "small cell anaplastic thyroid carcinoma" before the use of immunohistochemistry were reclassified as medullary carcinomas and lymphomas when markers for these tumors came into use.[40,41] What was uniformly recognized throughout the decades was the aggressive behavior of ATC.[42]

ATCs represent an extremely aggressive tumor that is at the extreme end of the differentiation spectrum; they have also been designated as "undifferentiated thyroid carcinoma".

These tumors usually present in patients older than 60 years of age, often with a rapidly enlarging neck mass.[43] Patients may come to medical attention because of respiratory distress, which may even necessitate an emergent tracheostomy. The major differential from the clinical perspective is lymphoma (markedly different therapy and prognosis).

Undifferentiated carcinomas frequently develop in patients who have a history of thyroid disease. This can include multinodular goiter or possibly even a history of a well-differentiated carcinoma.[44] Some patients will have a component of a well-differentiated thyroid carcinoma in their tumor specimens, when there is adequate material for representative sampling. The well-differentiated tumors most commonly reported in combination with ATC are papillary carcinoma, Hurthle cell carcinoma or follicular carcinoma. Concordant well-differentiated components are present in up to 50% of well sampled ATCs.[45]

The prognosis for ATC is dismal. Survival for ATC is usually measured in months, with mean survival in larger series ranging from 3 to 6 months.[46,47] However, there are rare cases that have a better prognosis. These are usually restricted to otherwise well-differentiated tumors with early incidental anaplastic transformation or rare cases that can be completely removed with negative margins.[48]

Histology

ATCs can exhibit various morphologies from very bland to the highly pleomorphic tumors. They can be composed of a wide variety of cell types, as well, including spindle cells, giant cells, squamoid cells or even more rare variant morphologies like the rhabdoid subtype.[49–51] These variant morphologies do not have significant differences in prognosis. An unusual morphologic feature of ATC is its propensity to invade into vessels. The invasion can have a unique appearance that resembles colonization or replacement, but not destruction of the vessel wall by anaplastic tumor cells.[52]

The major differential diagnoses for ATC will include both benign and malignant tumors. The benign lesions that are in the differential diagnosis are spindle cell metaplasia, post-FNA spindle cell nodules, nodular fasciitis like areas, and Riedel's thyroiditis.[53–59] All of these entities can have spindle cell areas of varying cellularity. However, they should not harbor the pleomorphic cells and mitotic activity of ATC. The malignant tumors in the differential diagnosis for ATC include sarcomas, carcinoma with thymus like differentiation (CASTLE), spindle epithelial tumor of thymus origin (SETTLE), which are both discussed in chapter 12 and squamous cell carcinoma of the head and neck secondarily involving the thyroid.[60–65] Other entities in the differential diagnosis include solitary fibrous tumor, neural and smooth muscle tumors, and metastases from sarcomas.[66,67] Some of these may be resolved with an immunohistochemical staining panel (Table 10.1).

Immunohistochemistry

Immunohistochemical stains are often necessary in the work-up of ATC because this tumor is frequently essentially undifferentiated by light microscopy. But, there are some significant disadvantages of immunohistochemistry, again related to the undifferentiated nature of these tumors. Up to 30%

TABLE 10.1. Differential diagnosis for anaplastic thyroid carcinoma with morphologic, immunohistochemical and molecular profiles.

Tumor type	Morphology	Immunohistochemistry	Molecular
Spindle cell metaplasia	Bland spindle cells arranged in fascicles	(+) TTF-1 (+) Thyroglobulin	Unknown
Spindle cell nodules, post-FNA	Plump spindle cells in intersecting bundles with admixed inflammation and vessels	(+) SMA (+) Factor VIII and CD31	Unknown
Riedel's thyroiditis	Dense collagen with lymphocytes	None	Unknown
Angiosarcoma	Highly atypical vascular endothelial cells with slit like spaces	(+) Factor VIII (+) CD31 (+/−) Cytokeratins	Unknown
CASTLE	Lymphoepithelioma or squamous cell like tumor.	(+) CD5 (+) CD 20 (−) Thyroglobulin	Unknown
SETTLE	Compact spindle cells with glandular component	(+) Cytokeratins (−) Thyroglobulin (−) CD5 (−) CD20	KRAS mutation (codon 12 and 15 in one case)
Squamous cell carcinoma	Squamous differentiation	(+) Cytokeratins (+) p63 (+/−) TTF and thyroglobulin (30–60%)	BRAF negative
Anaplastic thyroid carcinoma	Spindle cell, giant cell, squamoid, paucicellular, rhabdoid	(+) Cytokeratin (30–50%) (−) TTF-1 (+/−) Thyroglobulin (+) Vimentin (+/−) p63 (+) p53 (50–60%)	BRAF positive (40–60%) p53 mutations (40%)

of ATC will not stain for any epithelial markers, and most will not stain for markers of thyroid origin, such as TTF-1 or thyroglobulin.[52,68] It may be necessary to utilize a number of anticytokeratin antibodies to demonstrate epithelial differentiation. High molecular weight cytokeratins are somewhat more frequently found in ATCs than the low or intermediate molecular weight moieties (P. J. Zhang MD, personal communication). Recently, it has been shown that Pax8 expression may also be helpful in resolving difficult cases of ATC, since up to 79% of these tumors will be positive for this marker.[69] ATCs, no matter what the morphological appearance, should be considered to be carcinomas, since older studies of ultrastructure of these lesions showed epithelial characteristics.[52] The morphology and the clinical history may be necessary to resolve these difficult differential diagnoses.

Immunohistochemistry targets for potential prognostic and therapeutic value have also been investigated. One study of ATC suggested that these tumors express targets that are associated with potential targeted therapies, including beta-catenin (in 41%), aurora A (in 41%), cyclin E (in 67%), cyclin D1 (in 77%), and EGFR (in 84%).[32] Over-expression of platelet derived growth factor and Her2/neu have also been seen in a subset of ATC.[70]

Molecular Genetics

Much of the early work in the molecular mutational analysis of ATC was done in an attempt to prove its origin from well-differentiated carcinomas. Several different studies have demonstrated that ATC and well-differentiated carcinoma that occur concurrently have similar mutational profiles in terms of both tumor suppressor gene mutational profiles and somatic oncogene mutations.[71–73]

The presence of specific mutations in ATC may have diagnostic applications. As can be seen from the above discussion of the variable and non-specific immunohistochemical staining pattern of these tumors, some cases remain very difficult to classify. Mutational assessment has also been suggested as potentially promising for the incorporation of targeted therapies into the fairly unsuccessful treatment regimens for this aggressive disease. Early studies in cell lines do suggest that some of the targeted therapies can control cell growth of ATC,[74–76] but initial human trials have not been promising for showing objective responses.[77,78]

Oncogenes

The oncogene mutations that are seen in both papillary carcinoma and follicular derived carcinomas are also seen in ATC. This includes the BRAF point mutation, which is found in a highly variable number of ATCs, ranging from 10 to 50%.[72,79–82] Up to 30% of ATCs have been found to harbor RAS point mutations.[82–84] The finding of these mutations in ATCs probably reflects the fact that many of these high-grade tumors derive from well-differentiated precursor lesions, even when the well-differentiated component is no longer histologically apparent.[80,81]

Other mutations, including both copy number changes and somatic point mutations have also been seen in ATC.[85,86] For example, CyclinD1 copy number alterations have been noted, as have losses of 7q and 13q, using a comparative genomic hybridization (CGH) approach.[85,87]

Activation of the PI3K/Akt pathway by various copy number alterations and mutations are seen in up to 81% of ATCs.[88] Another gene that appears to be involved in progression of ATC is the CTNNB1 gene, encoding for beta-catenin. Both altered expression and somatic mutations have been identified in CTNNB1 in ATCs.[34,35]

Tumor Suppressor Genes

ATC has been show to have a much higher burden of somatic mutations than any of the other thyroid carcinomas, particularly in terms of tumor suppressor genes. These can be evidenced by CGH studies demonstrating consistent loss mutations at specific tumor suppressor gene locations, and by loss of heterozygosity alterations where targeted analysis can be done for specific tumor suppressor genes.[86,89] The most commonly studied tumor suppressor gene in ATC is the p53 gene. Between 50 and 100% of ATCs will harbor point mutations in the p53 gene, and many will have loss of heterozygosity of the p53 gene as well.[24,71,82,90,91] These tumors also frequently have over-expression of p53 at the immunohistochemical level, though there is not always correlation between expression and mutation.[80,92] This contrasts with well-differentiated thyroid carcinomas, which have low rates of p53 alterations.[93,94]

Epigenetics

ATC has not been extensively studied for changes or alterations in promoter methylation. The one gene that has been identified as having promoter methylation in ATC is the RASSF1A gene, which is tumor suppressor gene located on chromosome 3p21.3.[95] Approximately one-third of ATCs have promoter methylation of the RASSF1A gene, which parallels the rate seen for PTC; follicular carcinoma appears to have a much higher rate of RASSF1A promoter methylation.[95,96]

References

1. Volante M, Collini P, Nikiforov Y, et al. Poorly differentiated thyroid carcinoma: the Turin proposal for the use of uniform diagnostic criteria and an algorithmic diagnostic approach. *Am J Surg Pathol.* 2007;31(8):1256–1264.
2. Cady B. Hayes Martin Lecture. Our AMES is true: how an old concept still hits the mark: or, risk group assignment points the arrow to rational therapy selection in differentiated thyroid cancer. *Am J Surg.* 1997;174(5):462–468.
3. Akslen LA, LiVolsi VA. Poorly differentiated thyroid carcinoma – it is important. *Am J Surg Pathol.* 2000;24(2): 310–313.

4. Patel KN, Shaha AR. Locally advanced thyroid cancer. *Curr Opin Otolaryngol Head Neck Surg*. 2005;13(2):112–116.
5. Haq M, Harmer C. Differentiated thyroid carcinoma with distant metastases at presentation: prognostic factors and outcome. *Clin Endocrinol*. 2005;63(1):87–93.
6. Volante M, Landolfi S, Chiusa P, et al. Poorly differentiated carcinomas of the thyroid with trabecular, insular, and solid patterns: a clinicopathologic study of 183 patients. *Cancer*. 2004;100(5):950–957.
7. Nishiyama RH. Another dissertation on poorly differentiated carcinomas: is it really necessary? *Adv Anat Pathol*. 1999;6(5): 281–286.
8. Albores-Saavedra J, Carrick K. Where to set the threshold between well differentiated and poorly differentiated follicular carcinomas of the thyroid. *Endocr Pathol*. 2004;15(4): 297–305.
9. Kebebew E, Greenspan FS, Clark OH, et al. Anaplastic thyroid carcinoma. Treatment outcome and prognostic factors. *Cancer*. 2005;103(7):1330–1335.
10. Sanders Jr EM, Jr LiVolsi V, Brierly J, et al. An evidence-based review of poorly differentiated thyroid cancer. *World J Surg*. 2007;31(5):934–945.
11. Pilotti S, Collini P, Mariani L, et al. Poorly differentiated forms of papillary thyroid carcinoma: distinctive entities or morphological patterns? *Semin Diagn Pathol*. 1995;12(3):249–255.
12. Sywak M, Pasieka JL, Ogilvie T. A review of thyroid cancer with intermediate differentiation. *J Surg Oncol*. 2004;86(1): 44–54.
13. Sakamoto A, Kasai N, Sugano H. Poorly differentiated carcinoma of the thyroid. A clinicopathologic entity for a high-risk group of papillary and follicular carcinomas. *Cancer*. 1983;52(10):1849–1855.
14. Yamashita H, Noguchi Y, Noguchi S, et al. Significance of an insular component in follicular thyroid carcinoma with distant metastasis at initial presentation. *Endocr Pathol*. 2005; 16(1):41–48.
15. Volante M, Cavallo GP, Papotti M. Prognostic factors of clinical interest in poorly differentiated carcinomas of the thyroid. *Endocr Pathol*. 2004;15(4):313–317.
16. Carcangiu ML, Zampi G, Rosai J. Poorly differentiated ("insular") thyroid carcinoma. A reinterpretation of Langhans' "wuchernde Struma". *Am J Surg Pathol*. 1984;8(9):655–668.
17. Chao TC, Lin JD, Chen MF. Insular carcinoma: infrequent subtype of thyroid cancer with aggressive clinical course. *World J Surg*. 2004;28(4):393–396.
18. Pilotti S, Collini P, Mariani L, et al. Insular carcinoma: a distinct de novo entity among follicular carcinomas of the thyroid gland. *Am J Surg Pathol*. 1997;21(12):1466–1473.
19. Falvo L, Catania A, Diandrea V, et al. Prognostic factors of insular versus papillary/follicular thyroid carcinoma. *Am Surg*. 2004;70(5):461–466.
20. Collini P, Sampietro G, Rosai J, et al. Minimally invasive (encapsulated) follicular carcinoma of the thyroid gland is the low-risk counterpart of widely invasive follicular carcinoma but not of insular carcinoma. *Virchows Arch*. 2003;442(1):71–76.
21. Sobrinho-Simoes M, Sambade C, Fonseca E, et al. Poorly differentiated carcinomas of the thyroid gland: a review of the clinicopathologic features of a series of 28 cases of a heterogeneous, clinically aggressive group of thyroid tumors. *Int J Surg Pathol*. 2002;10(2):123–131.
22. Sasaki A, Daa T, Kashima K, et al. Insular component as a risk factor of thyroid carcinoma. *Pathol Int*. 1996;46(12):939–946.
23. Hiltzik DD, Carlson DL, Tuttle RM, et al. Poorly differentiated thyroid carcinomas defined on the basis of mitosis and necrosis: a clinicopathologic study of 58 patients. *Cancer*. 2006;106(6): 1286–1295.
24. Lam KY, Lo CY, Chan KW, et al. Insular and anaplastic carcinoma of the thyroid: a 45-year comparative study at a single institution and a review of the significance of p53 and p21. *Ann Surg*. 2000;231(3):329–338.
25. Takeuchi Y, Das T, Kashima K, et al. Mutations of p53 in thyroid carcinoma with an insular component. *Thyroid*. 1999;9(4):377–381.
26. Rubin BP, Heinrich MC, Corless CL. Gastrointestinal stromal tumour. *Lancet*. 2007;369(9574):1731–1741.
27. Fletcher JA, Rubin BP. KIT mutations in GIST. *Curr Opin Genet Dev*. 2007;17(1):3–7.
28. Broecker-Preuss M, Sheiu SY, Worm K, et al. Expression and mutation analysis of the tyrosine kinase c-kit in poorly differentiated and anaplastic thyroid carcinoma. *Horm Metab Res*. 2008;40(10):685–691.
29. Pulcrano M, Boukheris H, Talbot M, et al. Poorly differentiated follicular thyroid carcinoma: prognostic factors and relevance of histological classification. *Thyroid*. 2007;17(7):639–646.
30. Montero-Conde C, Martin-Campos JM, Lerma E, et al. Molecular profiling related to poor prognosis in thyroid carcinoma. Combining gene expression data and biological information. *Oncogene*. 2008;27(11):1554–1561.
31. Rodrigues RF, Roque L, King T, et al. Poorly differentiated and anaplastic thyroid carcinomas: chromosomal and oligo-array profile of five new cell lines. *Br J Cancer*. 2007;96(8): 1237–1245.
32. Wiseman SM, Masoudi H, Niblock P, et al. Anaplastic thyroid carcinoma: expression profile of targets for therapy offers new insights for disease treatment. *Ann Surg Oncol*. 2007;14(2):719–729.
33. Tallini G, Garcia-Rostan G, Herreo A, et al. Downregulation of p27KIP1 and Ki67/Mib1 labeling index support the classification of thyroid carcinoma into prognostically relevant categories. *Am J Surg Pathol*. 1999;23(6):678–685.
34. Garcia-Rostan G, Camp RL, Herrero A, et al. Beta-catenin dysregulation in thyroid neoplasms: down-regulation, aberrant nuclear expression, and CTNNB1 exon 3 mutations are markers for aggressive tumor phenotypes and poor prognosis. *Am J Pathol*. 2001;158(3):987–996.
35. Garcia-Rostan G, Tallini G, Herrero A, et al. Frequent mutation and nuclear localization of beta-catenin in anaplastic thyroid carcinoma. *Cancer Res*. 1999;59(8):1811–1815.
36. Smith LW. Certain so-called sarcomas of the thyroid. *Arch Pathol*. 1930;10:524–530.
37. Hutter RV, Tollefson HR, DeCosse J, et al. Spindle and giant cell metaplasia in papillary carcinoma of the thyroid. *Am J Surg*. 1965;110(4):660–668.
38. Maddox WA, Knott HW, Dowling EA. Carcinoma of the thyroid: review of fifteen years' experience. 1. Origin of spindle and giant cell carcinoma. 2. Occurrence of thyroid cancer in ectopic thyroid tissue. *Am Surg*. 1971;37(11):653–660.
39. Bronner MP, LiVolsi VA. Spindle cell squamous carcinoma of the thyroid: an unusual anaplastic tumor associated with tall cell papillary cancer. *Mod Pathol*. 1991;4(5):637–643.

40. Wolf BC, Sheahan K, DeCosste D, et al. Immunohistochemical analysis of small cell tumors of the thyroid gland: an Eastern Cooperative Oncology Group study. *Hum Pathol.* 1992;23(11):1252–1261.
41. Mendelsohn G, Baylin SB, Bigner SH, et al. Anaplastic variants of medullary thyroid carcinoma: a light-microscopic and immunohistochemical study. *Am J Surg Pathol.* 1980;4(4): 333–341.
42. O'Neill JP, O'Neill B, Conaron C, et al. Anaplastic (undifferentiated) thyroid cancer: improved insight and therapeutic strategy into a highly aggressive disease. *J Laryngol Otol.* 2005;119(8):585–591.
43. Jiang JY, Tseng FY. Prognostic factors of anaplastic thyroid carcinoma. *J Endocrinol Invest.* 2006;29(1):11–17.
44. Aratake Y, Nomura H, Katami T, et al. Coexistent anaplastic and differentiated thyroid carcinoma. *Am J Clin Pathol.* 2006; 125(3):399–406.
45. Hunt JL. Unusual thyroid tumors: a review of pathologic and molecular diagnosis. *Expert Rev Mol Diagn.* 2005;5(5): 725–734.
46. Besic N, Hocevar M, Zogjnar J, et al. Prognostic factors in anaplastic carcinoma of the thyroid – a multivariate survival analysis of 188 patients. *Langenbecks Arch Surg.* 2005;390(3): 203–208.
47. Goutsouliak V, Hay JH. Anaplastic thyroid cancer in British Columbia 1985–1999: a population-based study. *Clin Oncol (R Coll Radiol).* 2005;17(2):75–78.
48. Yau T, Lo CY, Epstein RJ, et al. Treatment outcomes in anaplastic thyroid carcinoma: survival improvement in young patients with localized disease treated by combination of surgery and radiotherapy. *Ann Surg Oncol.* 2008;15(9):2500–2505.
49. Lai ML, Faa G, Senes C, et al. Rhabdoid tumor of the thyroid gland: a variant of anaplastic carcinoma. *Arch Pathol Lab Med.* 2005;129(3):e55–e57.
50. Carda C, Ferrer J, Vilanova M, et al. Anaplastic carcinoma of the thyroid with rhabdomyosarcomatous differentiation: a report of two cases. *Virchows Arch.* 2005;446(1):46–51.
51. Sato K, Waseda R, Tatsuzawa Y, et al. Papillary thyroid carcinoma with anaplastic transformation showing a rhabdoid phenotype solely in the cervical lymph node metastasis. *Pathol Res Pract.* 2006;202(1):55–59.
52. Carcangiu ML, Steeper T, Zampi G, et al. Anaplastic thyroid carcinoma. A study of 70 cases. *Am J Clin Pathol.* 1985;83(2): 135–158.
53. Shikama Y, Mizukami H, Yagihashi N, et al. Spindle cell metaplasia arising in thyroid adenoma: characterization of its pathology and differential diagnosis. *J Endocrinol Invest.* 2006;29(2):168–171.
54. Aker FV, Bas Y, Ozkara S, et al. Spindle cell metaplasia in follicular adenoma of the thyroid gland: case report and review of the literature. *Endocr J.* 2004;51(5):457–461.
55. Vergilio J, Baloch ZW, LiVolsi VA. Spindle cell metaplasia of the thyroid arising in association with papillary carcinoma and follicular adenoma. *Am J Clin Pathol.* 2002;117(2):199–204.
56. Baloch ZW, Wu H, LiVolsi VA. Post-fine-needle aspiration spindle cell nodules of the thyroid (PSCNT). *Am J Clin Pathol.* 1999;111(1):70–74.
57. Chan JK, Carcangiu ML, Rosai J. Papillary carcinoma of thyroid with exuberant nodular fasciitis-like stroma: report of three cases. *Am J Clin Pathol.* 1991;95(3):309–314.
58. Naganuma H, Iwama N, Nakamura Y, et al. Papillary carcinoma of the thyroid gland forming a myofibroblastic nodular tumor: report of two cases and review of the literature. *Pathol Int.* 2002;52(1):54–58.
59. Wan SK, Chan JK, Tang SK. Paucicellular variant of anaplastic thyroid carcinoma. A mimic of Reidel's thyroiditis. *Am J Clin Pathol.* 1996;105(4):388–393.
60. Roka S, Kojnek G, Schuller J, et al. Carcinoma showing thymic-like elements – a rare malignancy of the thyroid gland. *Br J Surg.* 2004;91(2):142–145.
61. Dorfman DM, Shahsafaei A, Miyauchi A. Intrathyroidal epithelial thymoma (ITET)/carcinoma showing thymus-like differentiation (CASTLE) exhibits CD5 immunoreactivity: new evidence for thymic differentiation. *Histopathology.* 1998;32(2):104–109.
62. Berezowski K, Grimes M, Gal AA, et al. CD5 immunoreactivity of epithelial cells in thymic carcinoma and CASTLE using paraffin-embedded tissue. *Am J Clin Pathol.* 1996; 106(4):483–486.
63. Chan JK, Rosai J. Tumors of the neck showing thymic or related branchial pouch differentiation: a unifying concept. *Hum Pathol.* 1991;22(4):349–367.
64. Erickson ML, Tapia E, Moreno ER, et al. Early metastasizing spindle epithelial tumor with thymus-like differentiation (SETTLE) of the thyroid. *Pediatr Dev Pathol.* 2005;8(5): 599–606.
65. Booya F, Sebo TJ, Kasperbauer JL, et al. Primary squamous cell carcinoma of the thyroid: report of ten cases. *Thyroid.* 2006;16(1):89–93.
66. Rodriguez I, Ayala E, Caballero C, et al. Solitary fibrous tumor of the thyroid gland: report of seven cases. *Am J Surg Pathol.* 2001;25(11):1424–1428.
67. Papi G, Corrado S, LiVolsi VA. Primary spindle cell lesions of the thyroid gland: an overview. *Am J Clin Pathol.* 2006;125(suppl):S95–S123.
68. Miettinen M, Franssila KO. Variable expression of keratins and nearly uniform lack of thyroid transcription factor 1 in thyroid anaplastic carcinoma. *Hum Pathol.* 2000;31(9):1139–1145.
69. Nonaka D, Dhiriboga L, Soslow R, et al. Diagnostic utility of thyroid transcription factors Pax8 and TTF-2 (FoxE1) in thyroid epithelial neoplasms. *Mod Pathol.* 2008;21(2):192–200.
70. Elliott DD, Sherman SL, Bussaldy NL, et al. Growth factor receptors expression in anaplastic thyroid carcinoma: potential markers for therapeutic stratification. *Hum Pathol.* 2008;39(1):15–20.
71. Nikiforov YE. Genetic alterations involved in the transition from well-differentiated to poorly differentiated and anaplastic thyroid carcinomas. *Endocr Pathol.* 2004;15(4):319–327.
72. Begum S, Rosenbaum E, Henrique R, et al. BRAF mutations in anaplastic thyroid carcinoma: implications for tumor origin, diagnosis and treatment. *Mod Pathol.* 2004;17(11): 1359–1363.
73. Hunt JL, Tometsko M, LiVolsi V, et al. Molecular evidence of anaplastic transformation in coexisting well-differentiated and anaplastic carcinomas of the thyroid. *Am J Surg Pathol.* 2003;27(12):1559–1564.
74. Sala E, Mologni L, Truffa S, et al. BRAF silencing by short hairpin RNA or chemical blockade by PLX4032 leads to different responses in melanoma and thyroid carcinoma cells. *Mol Cancer Res.* 2008;6(5):751–759.

75. Leboeuf R, Baumgartner JE, Benezra M, et al. BRAFV600E mutation is associated with preferential sensitivity to mitogen-activated protein kinase kinase inhibition in thyroid cancer cell lines. *J Clin Endocrinol Metab*. 2008;93(6):2194–2201.
76. Hoffmann S, Burchert A, Weinderlich A, et al. Differential effects of cetuximab and AEE 788 on epidermal growth factor receptor (EGF-R) and vascular endothelial growth factor receptor (VEGF-R) in thyroid cancer cell lines. *Endocrine*. 2007;31(2):105–113.
77. Pennell NA, Daniels GH, Haddad Ri, et al. A phase II study of gefitinib in patients with advanced thyroid cancer. *Thyroid*. 2008;18(3):317–323.
78. Stenner F, Liewen H, Zweller M, et al. Targeted therapeutic approach for an anaplastic thyroid cancer in vitro and in vivo. *Cancer Sci*. 2008;99(9):1847–1852.
79. Salvatore G, DeFalco V, Salerno P, et al. BRAF is a therapeutic target in aggressive thyroid carcinoma. *Clin Cancer Res*. 2006;12(5):1623–1629.
80. Quiros RM, Ding H, Gattuso P, et al. Evidence that one subset of anaplastic thyroid carcinomas are derived from papillary carcinomas due to BRAF and p53 mutations. *Cancer*. 2005;103(11):2261–2268.
81. Nikiforova MN, Kimura EJ, Gandhi M, et al. BRAF mutations in thyroid tumors are restricted to papillary carcinomas and anaplastic or poorly differentiated carcinomas arising from papillary carcinomas. *J Clin Endocrinol Metab*. 2003;88(11):5399–5404.
82. Wang HM, Huang YU, Huang JS, et al. Anaplastic carcinoma of the thyroid arising more often from follicular carcinoma than papillary carcinoma. *Ann Surg Oncol*. 2007;14(10):3011–3018.
83. Santarpia L, El Naggar AK, Cote G, et al. PI3K/Akt and Ras/Raf-MAPK pathway mutations in anaplastic thyroid cancer. *J Clin Endocrinol Metab*. 2008;93(1):278–284.
84. Costa AM, Herrerro A, Fresno MF, et al. BRAF mutation associated with other genetic events identifies a subset of aggressive papillary thyroid carcinoma. *Clin Endocrinol (Oxf)*. 2008;68(4):618–634.
85. Rodrigues RF, Roque L, Rosa-Santos J, et al. Chromosomal imbalances associated with anaplastic transformation of follicular thyroid carcinomas. *Br J Cancer*. 2004;90(2):492–496.
86. Miura D, Wada N, Chin K, et al. Anaplastic thyroid cancer: cytogenetic patterns by comparative genomic hybridization. *Thyroid*. 2003;13(3):283–290.
87. Lee JJ, Au AY, Foukakis J, et al. Array-CGH identifies cyclin D1 and UBCH10 amplicons in anaplastic thyroid carcinoma. *Endocr Relat Cancer*. 2008;15(3):801–815.
88. Liu Z, Hou P, Ji M, et al. Highly prevalent genetic alterations in receptor tyrosine kinases and phosphatidylinositol 3-kinase/akt and mitogen-activated protein kinase pathways in anaplastic and follicular thyroid cancers. *J Clin Endocrinol Metab*. 2008;93(8):3106–3116.
89. Kitamura Y, Ahimiu K, Ito K, et al. Allelotyping of anaplastic thyroid carcinoma: frequent allelic losses on 1q, 9p, 11, 17, 19p, and 22q. *Genes Chromosomes Cancer*. 2000;27(3):244–251.
90. Fagin JA, Matsuo L, Karmakar A, et al. High prevalence of mutations of the p53 gene in poorly differentiated human thyroid carcinomas. *J Clin Invest*. 1993;91(1):179–184.
91. Sera N, Ashizawa K, Ando T, et al. Anaplastic changes associated with p53 gene mutation in differentiated thyroid carcinoma after insufficient radioactive iodine (131I) therapy. *Thyroid*. 2000;10(11):975–979.
92. Hosal SA, Apel R, Freeman JL, et al. Immunohistochemical localization of p53 in human thyroid neoplasms: correlation with biological behavior. *Endocr Pathol*. 1997;8(1):21–28.
93. Salvatore D, Celletti A, Fabien N, et al. Low frequency of p53 mutations in human thyroid tumours; p53 and Ras mutation in two out of fifty-six thyroid tumours. *Eur J Endocrinol*. 1996;134(2):177–183.
94. Zafon C, Obois G, Castelivi J, et al. Clinical significance of RET/PTC and p53 protein expression in sporadic papillary thyroid carcinoma. *Histopathology*. 2007;50(2):225–231.
95. Nakamura N, Carney Ja, Jin L, et al. RASSF1A and NORE1A methylation and BRAFV600E mutations in thyroid tumors. *Lab Invest*. 2005;85(9):1065–1075.
96. Xing M, Cohen Y, Mambo E, et al. Early occurrence of RASSF1A hypermethylation and its mutual exclusion with BRAF mutation in thyroid tumorigenesis. *Cancer Res*. 2004;64(5):1664–1668.

11 Medullary Thyroid Carcinoma

Ronald A. DeLellis

Introduction

Medullary thyroid carcinoma (MTC) is currently defined as a malignant thyroid tumor with evidence of C-cell differentiation.[1,2] While earlier reports had alluded to the existence of this tumor type, Robert Horn in 1951 reported a series of 7 cases of a thyroid cancer characterized by sharply defined rounded or ovoid compact cell groups of moderate size in a background of hyalinized connective tissue.[3] He noted that "while not pursuing the rapid course characteristic of the giant cell, spindle cell and small cell thyroid carcinoma, these tumors have by no means the favorable prognosis of malignant adenoma and papillary tumors". The major histopathologic features of this tumor, including the presence of stromal amyloid deposits, were defined in 1959 by Hazard and coworkers who suggested the term, medullary thyroid carcinoma (MTC).[4]

In 1966, Williams proposed that MTCs were derived from the thyroid parafollicular cells based on comparative studies in dogs and other animals.[5] Bussolati and Pearse[6] in the following year demonstrated the parafollicular cell origin of calcitonin, and subsequent studies confirmed the presence of calcitonin in tumor extracts and in the serum of affected patients.[7,8]

Medullary carcinomas comprise up to 10% of all thyroid malignancies in most large clinical series.[1,2,9] In patients with nodular thyroid disease subjected to serum basal and pentagastrin stimulated calcitonin studies, the prevalence of MTC ranges from 0.24 to 2.85% (mean 0.61%) based on nine reported series, primarily from Europe.[10] The studies of Pacini et al have further underscored the high prevalence of MTC in more than 1,300 patients with nodular thyroid disease. In their study, MTC represented 0.57% all thyroid nodules and 15.7% of all incidentally discovered thyroid carcinomas.[10] Cheung et al have shown that the cost effectiveness of routine calcitonin screening in patients with nodular thyroid disease is comparable to measurement of thyroid stimulating hormone, colonoscopy, and mammographic screening.[11]

The incidence of MTC is not increased in humans treated by irradiation to the head and neck. However, data in experimental animals suggest that rats treated with low doses of ^{131}I have an increased incidence of these tumors[12,13] and that high levels of calcium in the drinking water do not appear to potentiate tumor development.

Clinical Features

Medullary thyroid carcinomas may occur sporadically or in association with the multiple endocrine neoplasia (MEN)2 syndromes which are inherited as autosomal document traits (Table 11.1).[14–16] Sporadic tumors account for 75% of cases, while MEN2 associated cases account for the remainder.[2]

Sporadic MTC is primarily a tumor of middle aged adults with a female to male ratio of 1.3:1. Generally, most patients present with a painless tumor nodule that is typically cold on scintigraphic scan. In the series reported by Kebebew et al, nearly 75% of patients presented with a thyroid mass, while 15% had symptoms of dysphagia, dyspnea, or hoarseness.[17] Cervical lymph node metastases may be present, and in some cases, distant metastases may also be evident. Affected patients may present with a variety of signs and symptoms in addition to the thyroid mass. Patients with metastatic disease, for example, may have severe diarrhea or flushing, and these symptoms may be related to the high circulating levels of calcitonin. In Kebebew's series, approximately 10% of patients presented with systemic symptoms.[17] The tumors may produce a wide array of peptides, amines, and prostaglandins that have been implicated in the development of diarrhea, flushing, and other systemic symptoms. They may also produce ACTH and proopiomelanocortins, which have been implicated in the development of Cushing's syndrome. This syndrome occurs in approximately 0.6% of patients with medullary thyroid carcinoma and survival following the recognition of the syndrome is poor.[18] Although very high levels of calcitonin may be present in patients with these tumors, hypocalcemia is virtually nonexistent.

J.L. Hunt (ed.), *Molecular Pathology of Endocrine Diseases*, Molecular Pathology Library 3,
DOI 10.1007/978-1-4419-1707-2_11, © Springer Science+Business Media, LLC 2010

TABLE 11.1. Heritable medullary thyroid carcinoma syndromes.

Syndrome	MIM #[a]	Age at diagnosis[b]	Components
Multiple endocrine neoplasia type 2A (MEN2A)[c]	171400	25–35 year	Medullary thyroid carcinoma (90–100%), pheochromocytoma (40–60%), parathyroid hyperplasia/adenoma (10–30%)
Multiple endocrine neoplasia type 2B (MEN2B)[d]	162300	10–20 year	Medullary thyroid carcinoma (100%), pheochromocytoma (40–60%), neuromas of the tongue and/or ganglioneuromatosis of the intestine, marfanoid habitus and/or medullated corneal nerve fibers
Familial medullary thyroid carcinoma (FMTC)	155240	45–55 year	Medullary thyroid carcinoma (90–100%)

[a]Mendelian inheritance in man number.
[b]The mean age at diagnosis has become substantially younger with the development of biochemical and genetic screening studies.
[c]MEN2A is also known as Sipple syndrome.
[d]MEN2B has been referred to as Wagenmann-Froboese syndrome.

Medullary carcinomas are highly penetrant in the MEN2 syndromes, and it has been estimated that more than 90% of carriers will develop thyroid tumors.[16] MEN2A accounts for more than 75% of all heritable MTC cases. Affected patients also have pheochromocytomas in approximately 40–60% of cases and parathyroid abnormalities, (predominantly chief cell hyperplasia) in 10–30%. Some kindreds with MEN2A or familial MTC (FMTC) may also have cutaneous lichen amyloidosis which typically appears as pruritic plaques over the upper back.[19] The studies of Verga and coworkers have suggested that pruritis has a pivotal role in the development of cutaneous lichen amyloidosis with the amyloidosis developing as a consequence of repeated scratching.[20] Hirschsprung's disease has been associated with MEN2A in a few families.[21]

Patients with MEN2A generally present with thyroid tumors between the ages of 25 and 35. It should be noted, however, that the age of presentation has become progressively younger with the development of calcitonin screening studies in the 1970s and molecular diagnostic testing for mutations of the RET oncogene in the past decade.[16,19] In approximately 10% of patients, pheochromocytomas may become evident before the appearance of the thyroid tumors. Pheochromocytomas in this syndrome are commonly bilateral and multicentric and are preceded in their development by phases of adrenal medullary hyperplasia.[22,23] Malignant pheochromocytomas have been observed in less than 4% of patients with MEN2A. The frequency of malignancy in MEN2A associated pheochromocytomas does not differ significantly from that observed in patients with nonsyndromic tumors. Rare examples of composite pheochromocytomas have been reported in association with MEN2A. Hyperparathyroidism occurs in up to 30% of affected patients, and the resected parathyroid glands typically show evidence of chief cell hyperplasia, which is indistinguishable from that observed in patients with other forms of familial or sporadic hyperplasia.

MEN2B is the most phenotypically distinctive type of the MEN2 syndromes[16,24] and accounts for approximately 5% of the familial forms of MTC. A significant proportion of these cases represent de novo RET mutations. Affected patients have pheochromocytomas in 40–60% of cases, but parathyroid abnormalities, in contrast to MEN2A, are absent. Additionally, patients with MEN2B have neuromas of the tongue and/ or ganglioneuromatosis of the gastrointestinal tract with or without a marfanoid habitus. The MTCs in this syndrome typically have an early onset and an aggressive clinical course. The studies of Leboulleux and coworkers indicate that the stage at diagnosis of MTC is the major prognostic factor in these patients.[25]

Occasional kindreds with familial MTC syndromes may manifest thyroid tumors exclusively, and these patients are classified as familial MTC (FMTC).[26] These patients typically present at the same age as those with nonfamilial MTCs. In fact, a significant proportion of patients presenting with apparent sporadic MTCs will prove to have FMTC on the basis of molecular analysis.[27]

Pathological Features

Medullary carcinomas vary in size from those that are barely visible to those that replace the entire lobe of the thyroid.[1,2] The term "medullary microcarcinoma" has been used to describe those tumors measuring less than 1 cm in diameter (Figure 11.1).[28] The tumors are generally sharply circumscribed but nonencapsulated. Occasionally, however, they may be surrounded by a fibrous capsule. On cross-section,

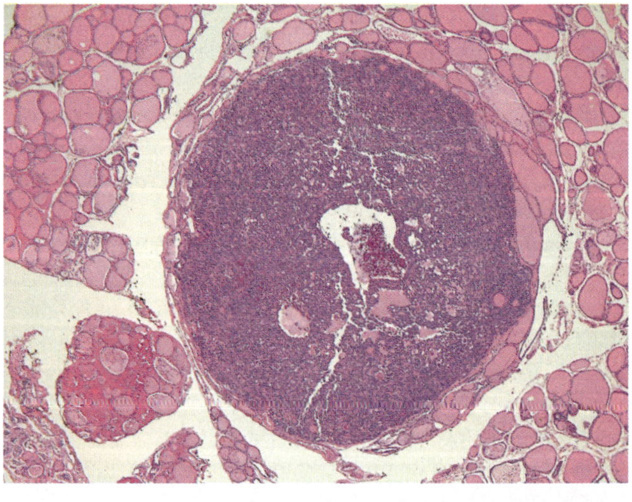

FIG. 11.1. Medullary microcarcinoma. This 0.2 cm tumor was an incidental finding in a patient with multinodular goiter (Hematoxylin and eosin).

many of the tumors are tan to pink with a generally soft consistency. Others are quite firm and fibrotic with areas of granular yellow discoloration that represent focal calcifications. The smaller tumors generally occur at the junction of the upper and middle thirds of the lobes in which C-cells normally predominate. When the tumors become very large, they may replace the entire lobe and extend into the perithyroidal soft tissues and trachea. While sporadic tumors most commonly present as unilateral lesions, the heritable tumors characteristically involve both lobes of the gland and are typically multicentric.

Sporadic and familial medullary carcinomas typically exhibit a wide spectrum of histological patterns that may mimic other primary thyroid tumors, including follicular, papillary, and undifferentiated carcinomas. The prototypic medullary carcinoma has a lobular, trabecular, insular, or sheet-like growth pattern with evidence of focal extension of tumor into the adjacent normal thyroid (Figures 11.2 and 11.3). Individual tumor cells may be round, polygonal, or spindle shaped with frequent admixtures of these cell types (Figure 11.4). In the round and polygonal cells, the nuclei have coarsely clumped or speckled (salt and pepper) chromatin and generally inconspicuous nucleoli. Occasional nuclear pseudoinclusions similar to those seen in papillary carcinomas may be present. Binucleate cells are common and multinucleate giant cells may be evident. Spindle cells have elongated nuclei with chromatin distribution similar to that seen in the polygonal and round cells. Most MTCs exhibit moderate degrees of pleomorphism but mitotic activity is generally low.

The cytoplasm varies from eosinophilic to basophilic and appears finely granular. In some cases, however, the cytoplasm is clear. Occasional mucin positive cytoplasmic vacuoles may be present in some cases. Zaatari et al have found mucicarmine positive deposits in up to 40% of cases.[29] In 17% of cases, mucicarmine positivity was present extracellularly, while in 8% the deposits were intracellular. Both intra- and extra-cellular mucin deposits were present in 17% of cases. Ultrastructurally, the tumors contain dense core secretory granules, in which calcitonin and other peptides are stored.[9]

Foci of necrosis and hemorrhage are uncommon in small tumors, while larger tumors exhibit these features more commonly. Lymphatic and vascular invasion may be seen at the advancing front of the tumor. In advanced cases, foci of lymphatic invasion may be present in the contralateral lobe. Occasionally, nodal and distant metastases may be present in association with tumors measuring less than 1 cm (Figures 11.5 and 11.6).

Some medullary thyroid carcinomas contain prominent areas of fibrosis (Figure 11.7). Stromal amyloid deposits are present in up to 80% of cases. The amyloid deposits are Congo red positive and show typical green birefringence in

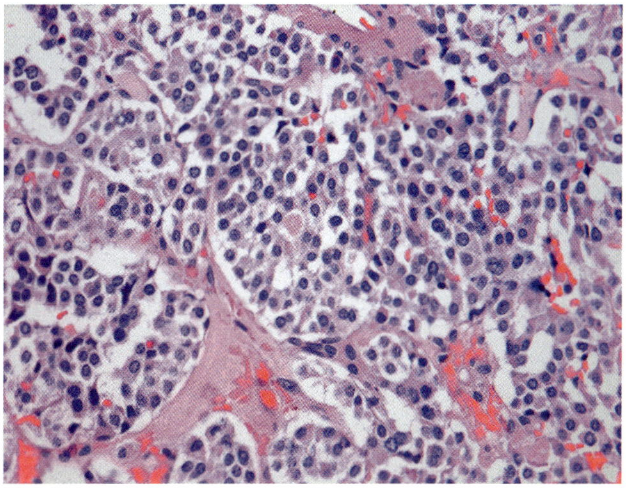

FIG. 11.3. Medullary thyroid carcinoma. This tumor has a nesting growth pattern. While many of the nuclei are central, others are eccentric (Hematoxylin and eosin).

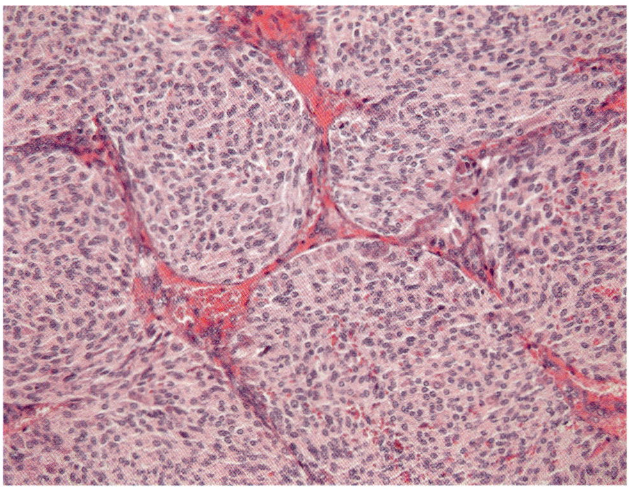

FIG. 11.2. Medullary thyroid carcinoma. This tumor has a lobular growth pattern (Hematoxylin and eosin).

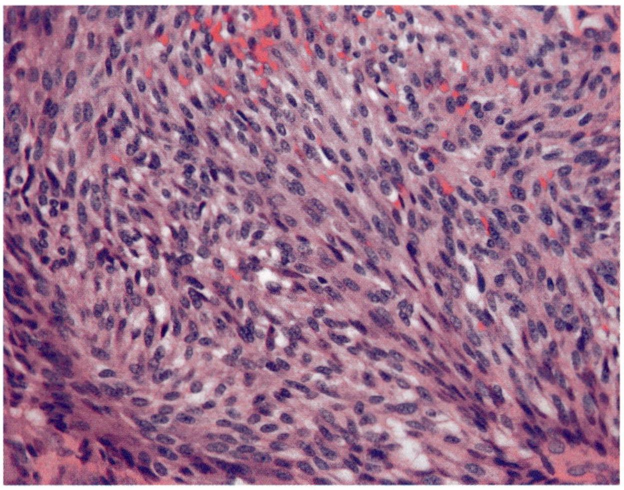

FIG. 11.4. Medullary thyroid carcinoma. This tumor is composed of spindle cells (Hematoxylin and eosin).

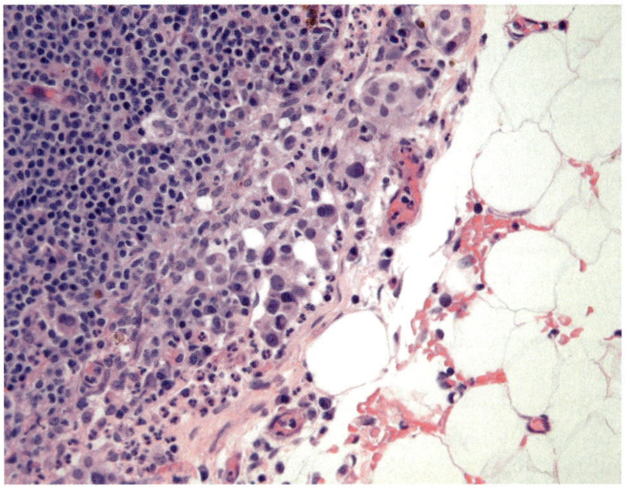

FIG. 11.5. Metastatic medullary thyroid carcinoma in the peripheral sinus of a cervical lymph node. The primary tumor measured 0.9 cm. (Hematoxylin and eosin).

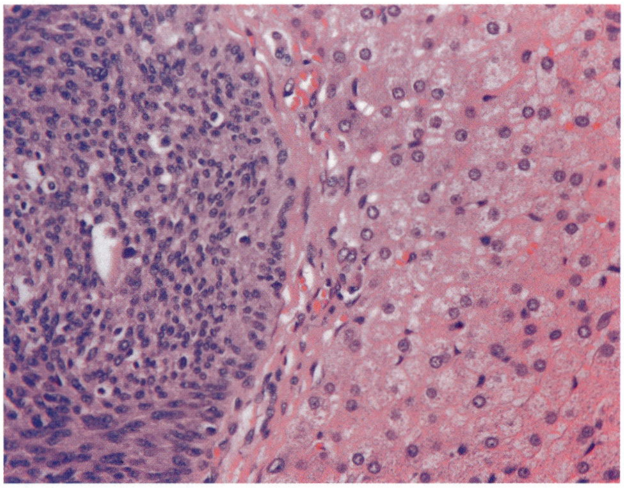

FIG. 11.6. Metastatic medullary thyroid carcinoma in liver. The primary tumor measured 1 cm (Hematoxylin and eosin).

polarized light, while crystal violet stained sections demonstrate metachromasia in the amyloid deposits. Ultrastructurally, the amyloid deposits have a fibrillar ultrastructure that is identical to that seen in other forms of amyloidosis. Antibodies to calcitonin demonstrate positive staining within the amyloid. Although earlier studies had suggested that the amyloid in these tumors was derived from the calcitonin precursor,[30] more recent studies utilizing mass spectrometric analysis indicate that full length calcitonin is the sole constituent of amyloid in medullary carcinoma.[31] In some instances, the amyloid may elicit a foreign body giant cell reaction. Calcification of the amyloid may occur and occasional tumors may contain psammoma bodies. A few medullary carcinomas may consist almost exclusively of amyloid and such cases may be difficult to distinguish from amyloid goiters (Figure 11.8).

Medullary carcinomas are typically argyrophilic with the Grimelius method with the most intensely positive cells having a dendritic morphology. The Masson Fontana stain is usually negative although occasional cases may contain scattered argentaffin positive cells.

In fine needle aspirates, medullary carcinomas are variably cellular depending on the amount of stromal fibrosis or amyloid deposition.[2,32] Cells are usually present singly or in loosely cohesive groups with poorly defined cell margins (Figure 11.9). Aspirates typically appear pleomorphic and while some cells are small and round, others may be cuboidal, polyhedral, or spindle shaped. Occasional tumors may be dominated by one cell type. The nuclei tend to be located eccentrically within the cytoplasm, and this feature imparts a plasmacytoid appearance to the tumor cells. The chromatin is coarsely granular and nucleoli are usually small and inconspicuous. Occasional nuclear pseudoinclusions may be present.

The cytoplasm is generally pale and fibrillary in Papanicolaou stained preparations with occasional areas of process formation.[2,32] In Wright–Giemsa stained slides, cytoplasmic granularity may be evident, and in some instances, the granules

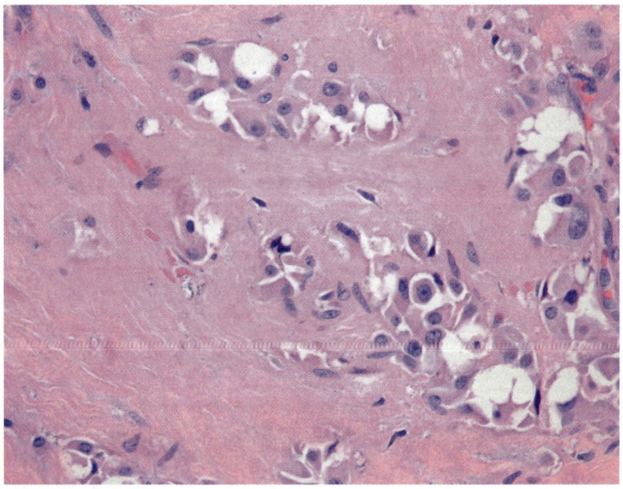

FIG. 11.7. Medullary thyroid carcinoma. This tumor contains abundant fibrous tissue (Hematoxylin and eosin).

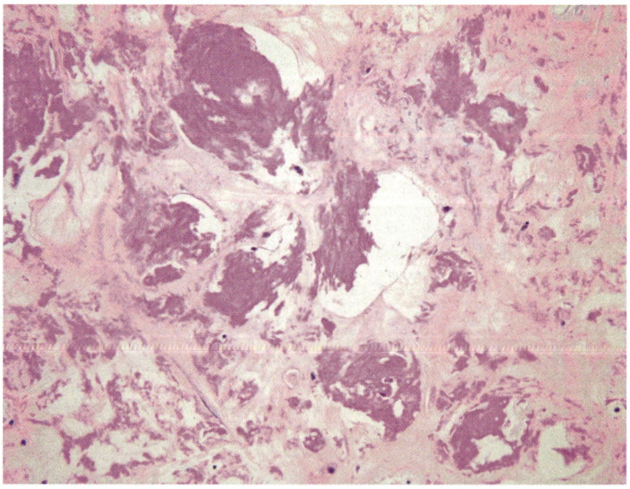

FIG. 11.8. Medullary thyroid carcinoma. This tumor is completely replaced by amyloid deposits (Hematoxylin and eosin).

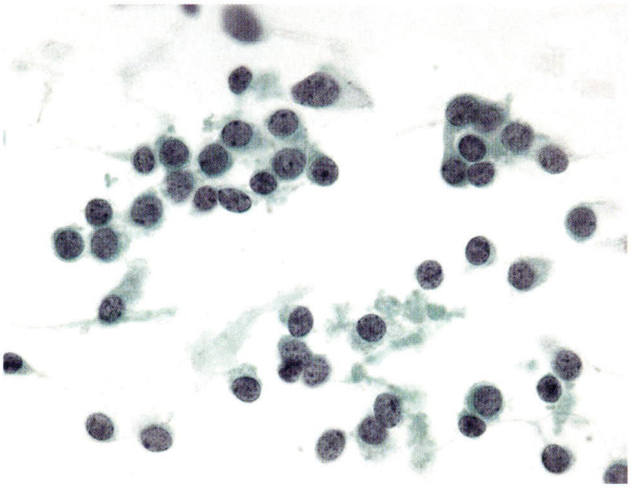

Fig. 11.9. Medullary thyroid carcinoma. This fine needle aspiration contains small cell groups and single cells with eccentric nuclei (Papanicolaou stain).

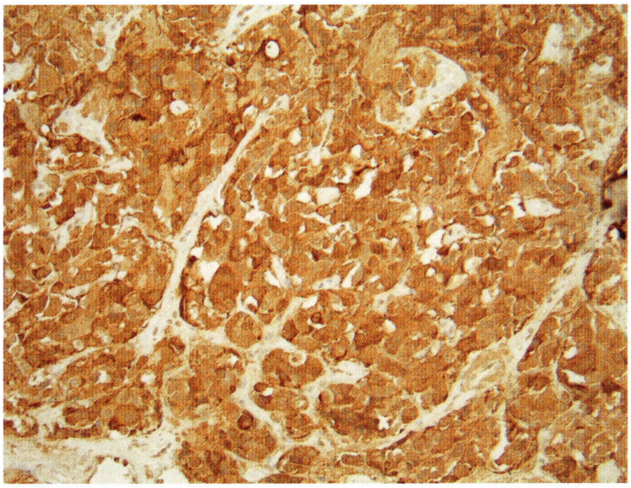

Fig. 11.10. Medullary thyroid carcinoma. This tumor is stained for calcitonin and demonstrates intense reactivity in virtually all of the cells (Immunoperoxidase stain).

appear metachromatic. Amyloid may be indistinguishable from colloid in Papanicolaou stains, but a Congo red stain can be performed to confirm the presence of amyloid. The diagnosis of medullary carcinoma should be confirmed with immunostains for calcitonin or chromogranin.

Medullary thyroid carcinomas demonstrate positivity for thyroid transcription factor-1 (TTF-1), a property that they share with tumors of follicular cell origin.[33] Stains for thyroglobulin are typically negative, although entrapped normal thyroid follicles may stain positively. Medullary carcinomas are typically positive for low molecular weight cytokeratins and typically exhibit a cytokeratin 7 positive/cytokeratin 20 negative phenotype.[34] Vimentin is variably present within the tumor cells, and some tumors contain subpopulations of neurofilament positive cells.[35]

The tumors are typically positive for calcitonin (Figure 11.10) and a wide spectrum of generic neuroendocrine markers including chromogranin and synaptophysin.[36–38] Chromogranin is a sensitive marker for medullary carcinoma and, in fact, may be more sensitive than calcitonin for the identification of this tumor type.[39] Other products found in these tumors include calbindin-D28K and polysialic acid of NCAM.[40,41]

Calcitonin is present in 80–90% of medullary carcinomas (Figure 11.10). Although many cases show extensive calcitonin staining throughout the tumor, others may show only focal and weak reactivity.[42,43] The calcitonin gene related peptide is also commonly present.[44] Some tumors which are negative for calcitonin peptide and the calcitonin gene related peptide usually give positive signals for calcitonin messenger RNA using in situ hybridization.[45]

A variety of other peptides have been localized within these tumors, and their presence has been confirmed by radioimmunoassays of tumor extracts. Both somatostatin and gastrin releasing peptide are present in subpopulations of normal C-cells, and both of these peptides are commonly expressed in medullary carcinomas.[46,47] Generally, somatostatin immunoreactivity is present in single cells or in small cell groups, which most often comprise less than 5% of the tumor cell population. The somatostatin positive cells often have a dendritic morphology with branching cell processes extending between the adjacent tumor cells. Somatostatin receptors are also commonly present within these tumors.

Other peptides that are commonly present include ACTH, leuenkephalin, neurotensin, substance P, vasoactive intestinal peptide, and chorionic gonadotropin.[48–50] In rare instances, the tumors may contain subpopulations of cells immunoreactive for glucagon, gastrin, and insulin.[50] Both catecholamines and serotonin may also be present.[51]

Galectin-3 has been reported in 92% of heritable medullary thyroid carcinomas.[52] The staining is focal in 26% of the carcinomas and diffuse in the remainder. Interestingly, galectin-3 is reduced or absent in nodal metastases, while foci of C-cell hyperplasia are negative for galectin-3.

CEA levels are typically increased in the plasma of patients with MTC,[53,54] and correlative immunohistochemical studies have demonstrated that nearly 100% of the tumors exhibit CEA positivity. Several groups have demonstrated that a subset of MTCs may lose the ability to synthesize and secrete calcitonin while maintaining their capacity for CEA synthesis. In fact, calcitonin negative areas in medullary carcinoma are frequently positive for CEA. The finding of decreasing levels of calcitonin in the face of increasing levels of CEA generally predicts an aggressive clinical course.[55]

Numerous variants of medullary carcinoma have been described. Rarely, medullary carcinomas may exhibit a true *papillary* pattern in which the component tumor cells are aligned along fibrovascular stalks. In the cases described by Kakudo et al,[56] the tumors also exhibited solid foci characteristic of typical medullary carcinoma. The presence of thyroglobulin serves to distinguish these tumors from papillary carcinomas of follicular origin. A pseudopapillary pattern is considerably more common and results from artifactual separation of groups of tumor cells with groups of tumor cells

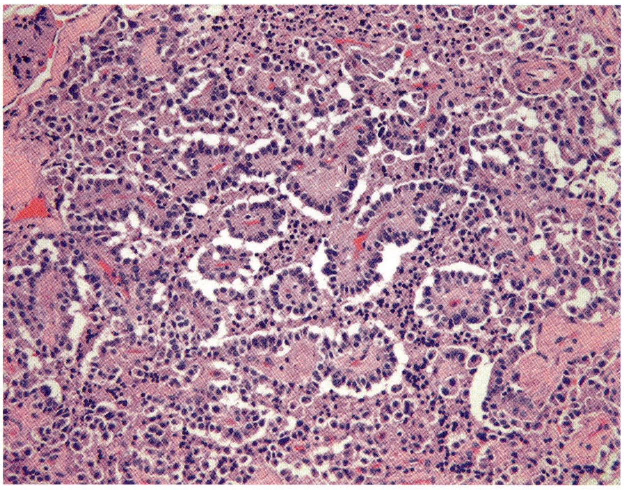

FIG. 11.11. Medullary thyroid carcinoma. This tumor has a pseudopapillary growth pattern (Hematoxylin and eosin).

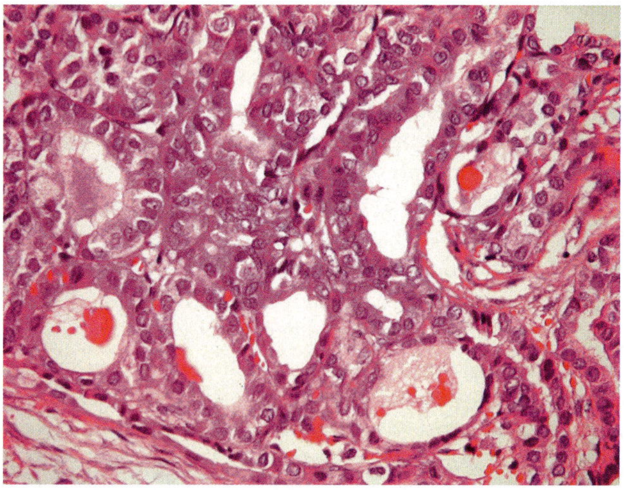

FIG. 11.12. Medullary thyroid carcinoma. This tumor has a follicular growth pattern (Hematoxylin and eosin).

appearing to be attached to stromal elements of the tumor with intervening "empty" spaces (Figure 11.11).

The *follicular variant* is composed wholly or in part of follicular structures and may resemble follicular cell neoplasms.[57] The tumor cells form follicles lined by cells that resemble those seen in the more solid areas of the tumor (Figure 11.12). The lumina of the follicles may appear empty or may contain an eosinophilic material resembling colloid. Although the origin of the colloid-like material is unknown, it most likely represents calcitonin and other secreted proteins. Immunostains for calcitonin have revealed variable degrees of reactivity within the colloid areas while stains for thyroglobulin are negative.

The *small cell* variant is characterized by the presence of cells with round to ovoid hyperchromatic nuclei and scant cytoplasm (Figure 11.13). Some of the tumors may resemble

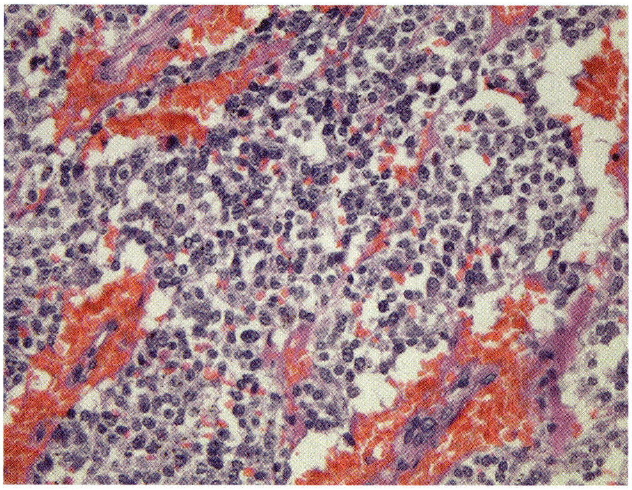

FIG. 11.13. Medullary thyroid carcinoma. This tumor has a small cell pattern (Hematoxylin and eosin).

neuroblastoma.[58] The presence of calcitonin, calcitonin gene related peptide, or other peptides (somatostatin, gastrin releasing peptide) is characteristic of C-cell differentiation in these cases. The small cell variant may exhibit a compact, trabecular or diffuse growth pattern. Mitotic activity may be high and foci of necrosis may be present. This variant may occur in a pure form or may be admixed with more typical foci of tumor. Of note, amyloid may be absent from the small cell variant. The tumor cells may be negative for calcitonin but stains for CEA are usually strongly positive.

Eusebi and coworkers[59] have reported two cases of small cell thyroid carcinoma that were classified as apparent primary oat cell carcinomas. Both tumors were positive for chromogranin and synaptophysin but were negative for thyroglobulin and calcitonin by immunohistochemistry and for calcitonin messenger RNA by in situ hybridization. On the basis of these studies, Eusebi and coworkers concluded that such cases should be separated from small cell medullary carcinomas and should be classified as primary small (oat) cell carcinomas of the thyroid.

The *giant cell* variant is characterized by a predominance of multinucleate giant cells.[60] Typically, the giant cell areas are admixed with foci of more typical medullary carcinoma. The tumor giant cells are typically positive for calcitonin.

The *clear* cell variant is characterized by cells with optically clear cytoplasm. Landon and Ordonez[61] described a medullary carcinoma composed predominantly of large polygonal cells with clear cytoplasm (Figure 11.14). In other areas, the tumor was composed of spindle shaped cells with eosinophilic cytoplasm. The clear cells were negative for mucins and did not contain appreciable amounts of glycogen. The tumor stained positively for calcitonin and contained dense core secretory granules ultrastructurally.

The *melanotic* variant is composed of cells with varying amounts of melanin pigment (Figure 11.15). Marcus and coworkers[62] described a case of nonfamilial medullary thyroid

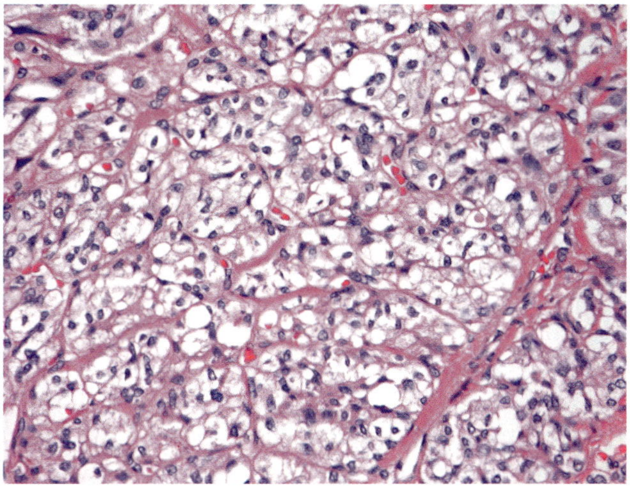

Fig. 11.14. Medullary thyroid carcinoma. This tumor is composed of clear cells (Hematoxylin and eosin).

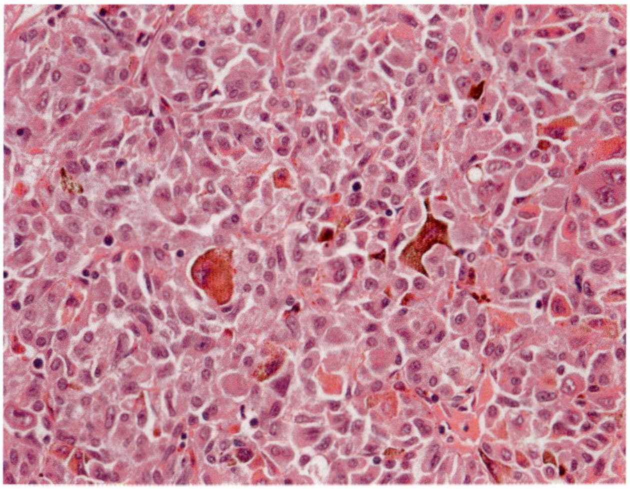

Fig. 11.15. Medullary thyroid carcinoma. This tumor is pigmented and contains melanin deposits in many of the cells (Hematoxylin and eosin).

carcinoma that contained collections of dendritic argentaffin positive cells. The dendritic cells were negative for calcitonin by immunohistochemistry while the remaining cells within the tumor were positive. Ultrastructurally, the argentaffin positive cells contained typical melanosomes. Beerman and coworkers[63] demonstrated both melanosomes and calcitonin containing secretory granules within the same tumor cells.

The *oncocytic variant* is composed of cells with mitochondria rich cytoplasm. In the case reported by Dominguez–Malagon and coworkers, 60–70% of the tumor cells were of the oncocytic type, while the remainder of the tumor had features of conventional medullary carcinoma.[64] The tumor cells had a trabecular arrangement and were separated by an amyloid free fibrous stroma. At the ultrastructural level, the tumor cells contained numerous mitochondria and few membrane bound secretory granules. Tumor cells showed strong positivity for calcitonin, chromogranin, and CEA but were negative for thyroglobulin.

The *squamous variant* is characterized by the presence of cells with varying degrees of squamous metaplasia. The case reported by Dominguez-Malagon[64] was calcitonin negative but showed diffuse positivity for neuron specific enolase and chromogranin and focal positivity for CEA. Focal deposits of stromal amyloid were present in this case. Schröder and coworkers noted foci of squamous metaplasia in metastatic medullary carcinoma.

The *amphicrine variant* is characterized by the presence of cells with varying degrees of mucinous change.[65] Combined alcian blue and Grimelius stains revealed that approximately 5% of the tumor cells were both alcianophilic and argyrophilic. Ultrastructurally, the tumor cells contained both mucin deposits and membrane bound secretory granules.

Occasional medullary carcinomas may be encapsulated and may be arranged in a broad trabecular pattern with an amyloid negative hyalinized stroma (*paraganglioma-like variant*). Huss and Mendelsohn[66] reported two such cases that presented as encapsulated neoplasms resembling hyalinizing trabecular adenoma. In contrast to the latter tumors,[66] however, both cases were calcitonin positive. Rare examples of true paragangliomas have been reported within the thyroid.

Occasional medullary carcinomas may have pseudosarcomatous features and may be reminiscent of angiosarcomas. This variant has been described as the *angiosarcoma-like* or pseudoangiomatous variant.[67]

Virtually all neoplasms of C-cells have been considered to represent carcinomas although occasional examples of C-cell adenomas have been reported.[68] In 1988, Kodama and coworkers[69] reported 2 cases of C-cell adenoma, each of which measured 4 cm in diameter. Both tumors were composed of cells that were fusiform to cuboidal with small elliptical nuclei. Neither tumor contained amyloid or foci of calcification. In contrast to most medullary carcinomas, stains for CEA were negative, and there was no evidence of increased CEA levels in the serum. Calcitonin levels were markedly elevated, and the tumor cells stained strongly for this peptide. The term "C-cell adenoma" has been suggested for completely encapsulated C-cell tumors[70]; however, until more is known about the biology of these tumors, it is best to regard them as encapsulated medullary carcinomas.

The term *medullary microcarcinoma* has been used to describe those tumors measuring less than 1 cm in diameter (Figure 11.1).[28] These tumors may exhibit nesting, trabecular, or diffuse growth patterns. Occasional microcarcinomas may have a microfollicular growth pattern resembling small follicular adenomas or adenomatous foci. Most of the reported cases have been incidental findings in thyroids removed for other reasons or in patients with nodular thyroid disease who have been screened for calcitonin abnormalities. However, occasional microcarcinomas may give rise to nodal and distant metastases. Microcarcinomas may occur sporadically or in association with the MEN2 syndromes.

Differential Diagnosis

Medullary carcinomas may mimic the entire spectrum of benign and malignant thyroid tumors. Papillary/pseudopapillary and other variants may have nuclear pseudoinclusions and psammoma bodies; however, they lack the nuclear clearing that is typically seen in papillary carcinomas. Additionally, medullary carcinomas are positive for chromogranin, calcitonin, and synaptophysin, while papillary carcinomas are negative for these markers. Since medullary carcinomas may contain follicles, they must be distinguished from follicular neoplasms, which are typically positive for thyroglobulin and negative for calcitonin, chromogranin, and synaptophysin. Poorly differentiated carcinomas of insular type are composed of nests and insulae of follicular cells and may contain microfollicles. These tumors are also positive for thyroglobulin and negative for calcitonin, chromogranin, and synaptophysin. Medullary carcinomas of spindle and giant cell types must be distinguished from undifferentiated carcinomas of follicular origin. The latter tumors are negative for neuroendocrine markers, calcitonin, thyroglobulin, and TTF-1.

The distinction of small cell medullary carcinoma from malignant lymphomas may be difficult, particularly in small biopsy or cytological samples. The demonstration of CD45 and other markers of T- and B-cells establishes the diagnosis of lymphoma. Small cell carcinoma of the lungs and other sites may metastasize to the thyroid and may mimic medullary carcinoma of small cell type.[71] Since TTF-1 is expressed both in lung and thyroid tumors, the presence of this marker is not a useful discriminant. Moreover, calcitonin and generic neuroendocrine markers may be present in both tumor types. In these instances, careful clinical and radiological examination may be helpful in identifying a pulmonary primary. Since mucin may be present in medullary carcinomas, these tumors must also be distinguished from mucinous carcinomas that have metastasized to the thyroid. The demonstration of calcitonin in a mucinous tumor within the thyroid establishes its C-cell origin.

Oncocytic medullary carcinomas must be distinguished from oncocytic tumors of follicular cell origin and oncocytic parathyroid neoplasms. The former will be positive for thyroglobulin, while the latter will be positive for parathyroid hormone. The hyalinizing trabecular tumor is typically encapsulated, as are some variants of medullary carcinoma. A trabecular pattern is present in both tumor types and both may exhibit areas of hyalinization resembling amyloid. However, the stroma of medullary carcinoma is positive for amyloid, whereas the stroma of hyalinizing trabecular tumors stains only for collagen. While medullary carcinomas stain positively for calcitonin and CEA, these markers are negative in hyalinizing trabecular tumors. It should be noted that occasional hyalinizing trabecular tumors may be positive for generic neuroendocrine markers.[72]

Medullary carcinomas may be difficult to distinguish from paragangliomas. The latter tumors are positive for chromogranin and synaptophysin but are negative for calcitonin. A population of S-100 positive sustentacular cells is typically present in paragangliomas. Occasional intrathyroidal parathyroid adenomas also may be difficult to distinguish from medullary carcinomas. Parathyroid tumors are also positive for parathyroid hormone and chromogranin, but stains for calcitonin are negative and should serve to distinguish these tumor types.

Heritable Forms of Medullary Thyroid Carcinoma and C-cell Hyperplasia

The histopathological features of the tumors in patients with heritable medullary carcinoma are virtually indistinguishable from those occurring sporadically, except for their bilaterality and multifocality. Studies based on enhanced calcitonin secretory responses to calcium and pentagastrin in patients at risk for the development of heritable forms of these tumors established that the tumors were preceded in their development by C-cell hyperplasia (Figures 11.16 and 11.17).[24,73,74] Detailed clinical and pathological studies have shown that C-cell hyperplasia is characterized by increased numbers of C-cells within follicular spaces.[75] With further progression, C-cells fill and expand the follicles to produce foci of nodular hyperplasia. Transition of this phase of C-cell growth to medullary carcinoma is heralded at the light microscopic level by fine areas of fibrosis between the proliferating C-cells (Figures 11.16b and 11.17c). With further progression, there are increasing degrees of fibrosis between the groups of neoplastic C-cells (Figures 11.16c and 11.17d). At the ultrastructural level, the earliest feature of malignancy is characterized by the extension of intrafollicular C-cells through the follicular basement membranes into the interstitium of the gland. McDermott and coworkers confirmed these observations using an immunoperoxidase technique for the demonstration of type IV collagen in the follicular basement membranes.[76]

The distinction of normal C-cell distribution from the earliest phases of C-cell hyperplasia is both difficult and controversial. Although initial studies suggested that the presence of 10 C-cells per low power field constituted sufficient evidence for C-cell hyperplasia, more recent studies indicate that this diagnosis should be made when there are at least 50 C-cells per low power field.[77] In some regions of the lobes, particularly in the vicinity of solid cell nests, the numbers of C-cells may exceed 50 per low power field in occasional normal individuals (Figure 11.18). In a quantitative image analysis study, Guyetant and colleagues demonstrated that C-cells were more numerous in male patients than in females, correlating with the known higher plasma calcitonin levels in men than in women.[78] Moreover, this study demonstrated the 33% of the adult population, including 15% of women and 41% of men, had evidence of CCH as defined by having at least three microscopic fields (100×) with greater than 50 C-cells.

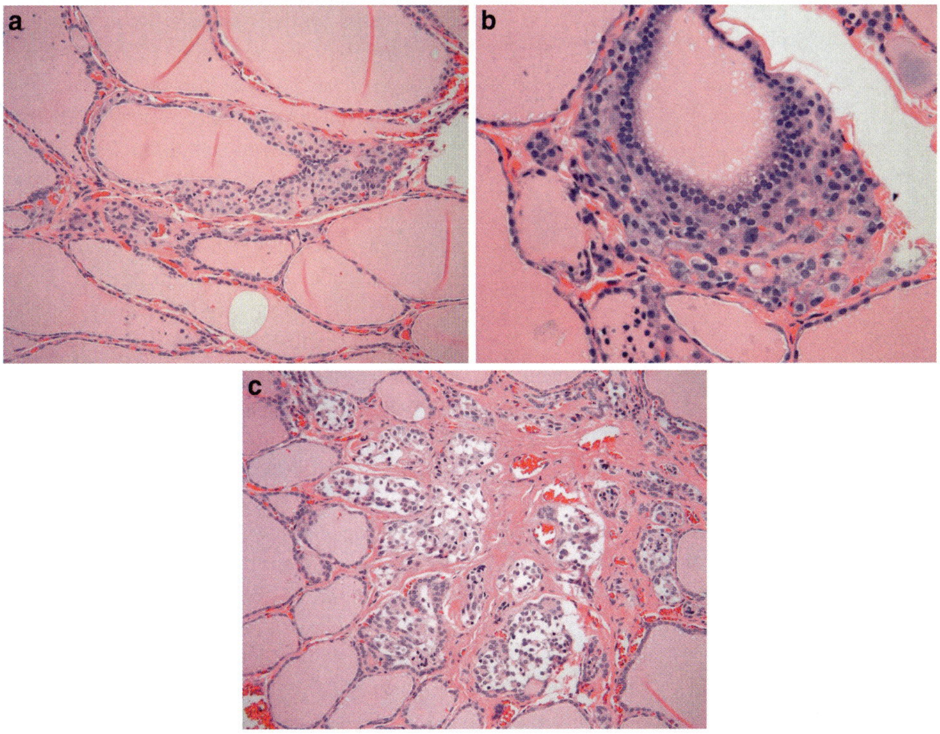

FIG. 11.16. C-cell hyperplasia and medullary thyroid carcinoma in a patient with MEN2A. (**a**) C-cell hyperplasia. The central follicle is surrounded by a collar of C-cells. (**b**) Early medullary thyroid carcinoma arising in association with C-cell hyperplasia. The C-cells in the left portion of the field are surrounded by collagen which is indicative of early stromal invasion. (**c**) Microscopic focus of medullary thyroid carcinoma. The tumor cell nests are surrounded by a dense fibrous stroma (Hematoxylin and eosin).

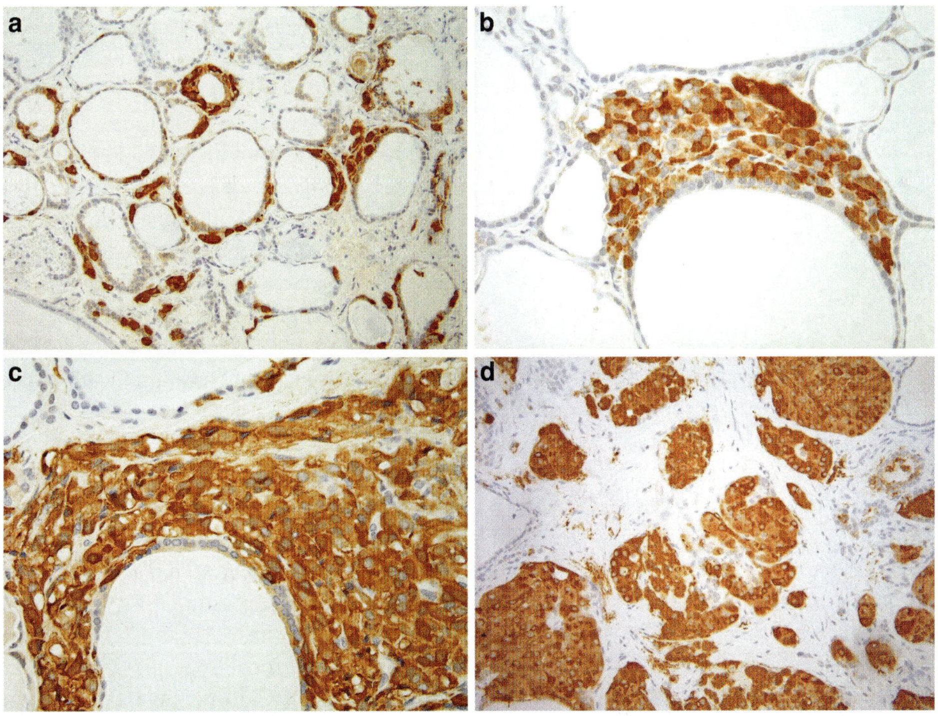

FIG. 11.17. C-cell hyperplasia and medullary thyroid carcinoma in a patient with MEN2A. (**a**) Diffuse C-cell hyperplasia is characterized by an increased number of C-cells. (**b**) C-cell hyperplasia. The proliferation of C-cells around this follicle is eccentric. (**c**) Microscopic medullary thyroid carcinoma. The proliferating C-cells have elicited a mild stromal reaction. (**d**) Small medullary thyroid carcinoma. The tumor cell groups are separated by a prominent fibrous stroma (Immunoperoxidase stain for calcitonin).

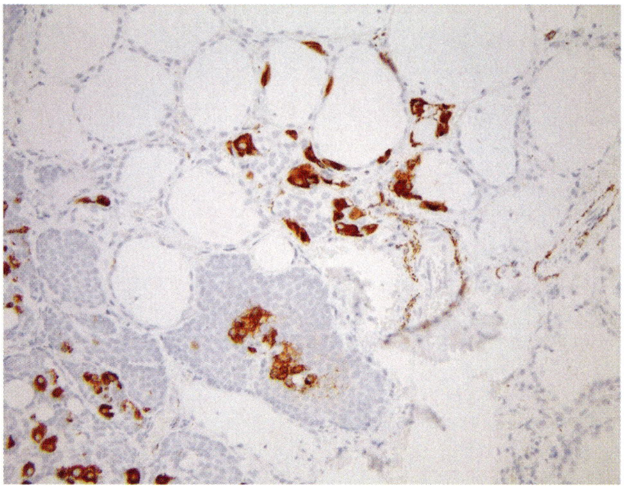

FIG. 11.18. Prominent C-cell populations adjacent to a solid cell nest in an eucalcemic normal adult male (Immunoperoxidase stain for calcitonin).

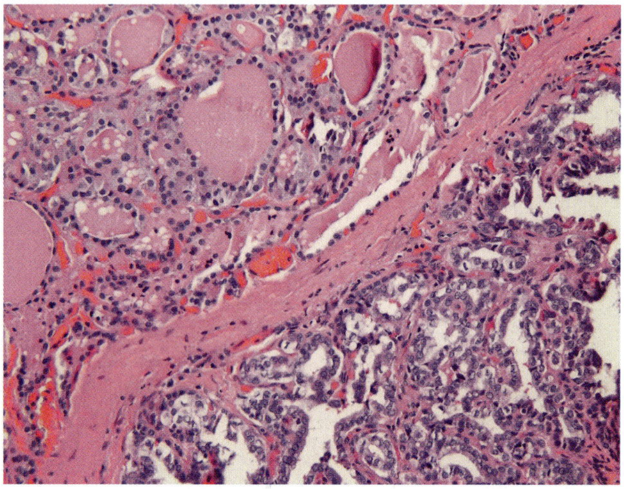

FIG. 11.19. C-cell hyperplasia (*top right*) adjacent to a small papillary carcinoma (*bottom left*) (Hematoxylin and eosin).

These findings suggest that either a substantial portion of the population has CCH or that the criteria for the definition of this entity are inaccurate. Interestingly, abnormal pentagastrin tests are found in only approximately 5% of the normal population as compared to the 30% frequency of CCH, as defined histologically. These observations suggest that there may be considerable variation in C-cell distribution among normal individuals and that these variations may not be accompanied by hypercalcitoninemia.

In addition to its presence in MEN2 syndromes, CCH has been reported in a number of other conditions including hypercalcemia, hypergastrinemia, Hashimoto's thyroiditis, and adjacent to a variety of follicular cell tumors, including follicular adenomas and carcinomas and papillary carcinomas (peritumoral C-cell hyperplasia) (Figure 11.19). This type of hyperplasia has been referred to as physiologic or secondary C-cell hyperplasia, in contrast to MEN2-associated CCH, which has been referred to as primary or "neoplastic" hyperplasia. Perry and coworkers have reported that physiologic CCH is primarily a diffuse process characterized by increased numbers of normal C-cells which can be diagnosed with confidence only on the basis of calcitonin immunostains.[79] "Neoplastic" CCH, on the other hand, involves the proliferation of dysplastic C-cells and can be diagnosed frequently on the basis of H&E stains alone. While "neoplastic"/MEN2-associated CCH is generally regarded as a precursor of MTC, the neoplastic potential of physiologic CCH remains unknown, notwithstanding the rare cases of MTC reported in patients with chronic hypercalcemia.

Carney and coworkers in 1978 proposed that CCH associated with MEN2 syndromes represents a preinvasive carcinoma or carcinoma in situ.[80] Further evidence for the neoplastic nature of CCH has come from Diaz-Cano's molecular studies of microdissected foci of thyroid glands from patients with MEN2A.[81] These studies have shown that foci of CCH are monoclonal with inactivation of the same allele in both thyroid lobes. Moreover, the foci have different secondary alterations involving the tumor suppressor genes p53, RB1, WT1, and NF1. These findings, together with the downregulation of apoptosis, are consistent with an intraepithelial neoplastic process and suggest that early clonal expansions precede migration of C-cell precursors into each thyroid lobe.

Although CCH has been regarded as a precursor and marker of MEN2 associated medullary carcinoma, this view has been challenged by several recent reports. In a series of 30 patients with nodular thyroid disease and abnormal pentagastrin stimulated calcitonin levels, Kaserer et al reported 19 patients (F:M;14:5) with MTC and 11 males but no females with CCH only, as defined by greater than 50 C-cells per low power field.[82] Six of 16 patients with sporadic MTC had concomitant CCH, and three of these patients proved to be new MEN2 index cases, as proven by genetic studies. On the basis of these studies, Kaserer et al concluded that CCH was an unreliable marker for heritable MTC and that CCH had a preneoplastic potential in the absence of RET germline mutations.

In a second study of 16 familial and 34 sporadic MTCs, Kaserer et al noted CCH in 16/16 (100%) of familial cases and in 24/34 (71%) of sporadic cases.[83] Among familial cases, CCH was of neoplastic type in 85% (14/16), nodular type in 6% (1/14), and focal type in 6% (1/14). In sporadic cases, on the other hand, neoplastic CCH was present in 18% (6/34), nodular hyperplasia in 21% (7/34), diffuse hyperplasia in 18% (6/34), and focal hyperplasia in 14% (5/34). There was no evidence of CCH in 29% (10/34) of the sporadic cases. On the basis of this study, Kaserer et al concluded that many sporadic MTCs develop on a background of CCH.[83]

Since there is such a wide variation in C-cell counts in normal thyroid glands, two possible interpretations of these studies are that the observed "CCH" in sporadic tumor cases represents the upper limit of normal C-cell distribution or that it is analogous to the secondary CCH found adjacent to follicular and papillary tumors. Indeed, Mears and Diaz-Cano have reanalyzed the data in the Kaserer study.[84] They concluded that multifocal and bilateral invasive MTCs associated with expansile intraepithelial neoplasia (nodular and neoplastic hyperplasia) represent familial disease in 98% of cases. The probability of sporadic disease associated with nodular and neoplastic C-cell hyperplasia was calculated as 1.87%.[84]

In summary, C-cell distribution has a remarkably wide variation in normal individuals. The current criterion of 50 C-cells per 100× microscopic field is, in all likelihood, an underestimate since up to 40% of normal males would have CCH according to this definition. MEN2-associated CCH has characteristic topographic, cytological, and molecular features, which permit its distinction from secondary C-cell hyperplasia in most cases, and this can be confirmed by the presence of germline RET mutations. Whether physiologic/secondary CCH has a significant preneoplastic potential remains an unanswered question.

Molecular Pathology

A major breakthrough in the study of the molecular origins of familial MTC syndromes was the observation that the putative MEN2A gene mapped to the pericentromeric region of chromosome 10.[85,86] The availability of a number of DNA markers to this region permitted the use of restriction length polymorphisms to identify carriers of this disorder.[87,88] Subsequent studies were successful in mapping the MEN2A and 2B gene to the specific region of chromosome 10 (10q11.2) that contained the RET proto-oncogene and in demonstrating germline missense RET mutations in affected individuals.[89–100]

The RET (*re*arranged during *t*ransfection) proto-oncogene was discovered in 1985 by its ability to transform NIH 3T3 cells.[101,102] The PTC oncogene, a naturally occurring RET rearrangement was subsequently discovered in 1990 in a papillary thyroid carcinoma (PTC).[103] The PTC oncogene develops as a result of translocation involving the 3' area of RET, which contains the tyrosine kinase domain and the 5' area of several genes that are normally expressed in thyroid follicular cells. More than 10 different RET/PTC arrangements have been identified to date.[104–106] These rearrangements induce transformation in vitro and result in constitutive tyrosine kinase activation. There is a considerable variation in the frequency of RET rearrangements in papillary thyroid carcinomas in different geographic areas and in different age groups, ranging from 3 to 67%.[106,107] At least, some of this variability may be related to different pathogenetic mechanisms for the development of these tumors. Studies of transgenic mice have demonstrated that thyroid targeted expression of the RET/PTC oncogene leads to the development of thyroid carcinoma with features of papillary carcinoma, while tissue culture studies have shown that RET/PTC has a direct role in the development of the nuclear features of these tumors.[108,109] In addition to its role in the development of papillary thyroid carcinoma, RET is overexpressed in neuroblastomas, MTC, and pheochromocytomas.[110,111]

The RET proto-oncogene contains 21 exons and encodes a cell surface tyrosine kinase receptor with a cadherin ligand binding site and a cysteine-rich extracellular domain, a transmembrane region and two cytoplasmic tyrosine kinase domains.[102,112] The cadherin binding site plays an important role in cell signaling, while the cysteine rich extracellular domain is important for receptor dimerization. RET is expressed in a variety of neural crest derivatives (C-cells, adrenal medulla, extra-adrenal paraganglia, sympathetic and enteric ganglia), parathyroid gland and urogenital tract.[100,113] Mice homozygous for a targeted RET mutation develop to term but demonstrate both renal agenesis or dysgenesis and absence of enteric neurons, but do not have evidence of neoplastic disorders.[114]

The ligands for RET are members of the glial cell line derived neurotrophic factor family and include glial cell line derived neurotrophic factor (GDNF) and neurturin (NTN).[115–121] GDNF is a crucial survival factor for central and peripheral neurons and is required for the development of the kidney and enteric neurons.[100] The receptors for GDNF family are membrane bound adaptor molecules and RET which form a trimeric receptor system. Glial derived neurotrophic factor binds GDNF Family Receptor alpha-1 (GDNFR-alpha), a glycosyl-phosphatidylinositol-linked protein, that is now known as GFR alpha-1, with high affinity while NTN binds GFR alpha-2. Additional members of the GFR alpha family include GFR-alpha 3 and -alpha 4.[120] Persephin and artemin are additional GDNF-like neurotrophic factors. Upon activation of RET receptors, phosphorylation of intracellular tyrosines leads to the stimulation of downstream signaling pathways including the RAS/ERK, ERK5, p38MAPK, PLCγ, PI3-kinase, JNK, STAT, and SRC cascades.[122]

Activating germline mutations in the RET proto-oncogene resulting in aberrant activation of RET receptors have been characterized in MEN2A, MEN2B, and FMTC (Table 11.2).[16,92–100] The mutations are of the missense type and affect primarily exons 10 and 11 with less frequent mutations affecting exons 13, 14, 15, and 16. Most of the mutations affect the cysteine rich extracellular domain of RET (MEN2A, FMTC). Codon 634 mutations account for approximately 80% of MEN2A patients while codon 609, 618, and 620 mutations account for more than 60% of FMTC cases and those patients with the Hirschsprung's phenotype. In patients with MEN2A, the codon 634 mutations show a strong genotype–phenotype correlation with the development of pheochromocytoma and hyperparathyroidism.[98] Substitution of cysteine with several other amino acids increases the formation of active RET dimers resulting

TABLE 11.2. RET mutations in MEN2 syndromes.

Site	Codon	Syndrome	Frequency (%)
Cysteine-rich domain	609	MEN2A, FMTC	0–1
	611	MEN2A, FMTC	2–3
	618	MEN2A, FMTC	3–5
	620	MEN2A, FMTC	6–8
	630	MEN2A, FMTC	0–1
	634	MEN2A, FMTC	80–90
Transmembrane domain	768	FTMC	Rare
	790	MEN2A	Rare
	791	FMTC	Rare
	804	MEN2A/FMTC	0–1
	844	FMTC	Rare
Tyrosine kinase domain	883	MEN2B	Rare
	891	FMTC	Rare
	918	MEN2B	3–5
	922	MEN2B	Rare

in their transforming potential.[123,124] Mutations affecting codons 768 or 804 (tyrosine kinase domain) may also occur (Table 11.2).

Mutations affecting the tyrosine kinase domain (codon 918) are found in patients with MEN2B and in a subset of sporadic medullary carcinomas.[95–97] This mutation results in the replacement of methionine with threonine. Codon 883 mutations resulting in the substitution of phenylalanine for alanine have also been demonstrated in a small subset of patients with MEN2B.[125,126] The MEN2B mutations result in RET activation in its monomeric form.[123,124] These mutations are present in the catalytic core region of the tyrosine kinase domain, and it has been suggested that they induce a conformational change in this region leading to an increased tyrosine kinase activity or alteration in its substrate specificity.[123] Mutations commonly detected in MEN2A and 2B have high transforming activities for NIH 3T3 cells, suggesting that the underlying tumorigenic mechanism of RET mutations results from dominant oncogenic conversion rather than from a loss of tumor suppressor function.[123,124] Moreover, targeting of MEN2A mutant RET forms to C-cells in transgenic mice results in the development of CCH or MTC in 100% of the animals in addition to mammary and parotid gland carcinomas in approximately 50%.[127] Mutations in the GDNF gene, on the other hand, have not been implicated in the development of the MEN2 syndromes.[128]

The use of molecular genetic testing has had a profound impact on the management of patients with these syndromes.[100,129,130] The decision to perform a prophylactic thyroidectomy is now based exclusively on the use of this type of testing rather than the cumbersome calcium and pentagastrin provocative tests used in the past. Secondly, based on a negative test result family members at risk for the development of the syndrome need not be subjected to additional testing with repeated calcium and pentagastrin provocative tests.

Several studies have assessed the value of genetic analyses as the basis of thyroidectomies in patients with MEN2.[131–133] In a survey of prophylactic thyroidectomies in 75 children and adolescents with proven RET mutations, MTC was found in 61% and C-cell hyperplasia alone was found in 39%. Three patients had nodal metastases. Testing for RET mutations is now the standard of care for patients with MEN2.[134] For patients with MEN2A, a prophylactic thyroidectomy is recommended between the ages of 5 and 10 years. For patients with MEN2B, thyroidectomy before the age of 3 or earlier is recommended. The therapeutic strategy for those patients with mutations associated with FMTC remains to be determined.

The frequency of RET germline mutations in cases of apparent sporadic MTC has been assessed in several studies.[99] In one study, 6 of 101 individuals harbored mutations involving codons 609, 611, 618, or 634.[135] Four of the affected patients were the probands of previously unrecognized kindreds, while the remaining two patients were examples of de novo mutations. Combining the results of several studies, it has been estimated that approximately 7% of patients with apparent sporadic tumors have germline mutations.[99] These findings indicate that analysis of RET should be performed in all patients presenting with apparent sporadic medullary carcinoma.

Somatic mutations in codon 918 have been observed in up to 70% of sporadic MTCs.[96,99] This mutation, which is identical to the 918 germ line mutation in MEN2B, results in the substitution of threonine for methionine. Although Zedenius et al[136] and Eng et al[137] have suggested that sporadic tumors with this mutation pursue a more aggressive course, this point has been controversial.[138] The studies of Eng et al have further suggested that the codon 918 mutation can arise as an event in tumor progression within a single tumor or in a metastatic clone.[137] Somatic mutations in codons 630, 634, 766, 768, 804, and 833 have been observed considerably less commonly than codon 918 mutations in sporadic medullary carcinomas.[99]

The relationship of physiological/secondary CCH to the development of nonfamilial MTC is controversial. Recent studies based on laser capture microdissection studies of 24 cases of CCH either isolated or associated with nonfamilial MTC failed to show RET mutations in foci of CCH, despite the presence of codon 918 mutations in 3 concomitant MTCs.[139]

RET mutations involving codons 620, 630, 634, and 918 have been found in 10–20% of sporadic pheochromocytomas.[140–142] In contrast, RET mutations have not been detected in parathyroid hyperplasias or adenomas, pituitary adenomas, pancreatic endocrine tumors, carcinoids, or neuroblastomas.[143,144]

RET mutations are also responsible for up to 40% of the autosomal dominant forms of Hirschsprung's disease and a subset of patients with sporadic disease.[99,145] Mutations are scattered throughout the gene and result in the loss of function of the RET protein. Rarely, FMTC or MEN2A may be present in association with Hirschsprung's disease, and in 5 kindreds with this association, mutations in codons 618 and 620 were found.[96] In addition to RET, a variety of other genes including GDNF, NTN, endothelin-B and endothelin-B receptor have been implicated in the pathogenesis of Hirschsprung's disease.

Treatment and Prognosis

Surgical treatment of patients with medullary thyroid carcinoma is guided by the pattern of spread of these tumors, which includes central compartment lymph nodes followed by ipsilateral and then contralateral cervical lymph nodes.[146,147] Approximately 50% of patients with palpable primary tumors, in fact, will have evidence of cervical nodal metastases. Both sporadic and heritable MTCs, therefore, are generally treated by total thyroidectomy with central lymph node dissection. In those patients with palpable primary tumors, some surgeons advocate the use of ipsilateral and even contralateral cervical lymph node dissections to optimize the chances for complete local control. Postoperative reduction of basal and stimulated calcitonin levels as well as other biomarkers is highly effective in providing information on biochemical care.

Radioactive iodine, external beam radiation therapy, and conventional chemotherapy generally have not been effective in the treatment of patients with recurrent or metastatic disease. Newer approaches include the use of tyrosine kinase inhibitors that target RET in addition to vascular endothelial growth factor receptors and additional kinase inhibitors in patients with advanced tumors.[148] The challenge for investigators is in analyzing the effect to which RET is being inhibited and correlating these findings with a variety of biomarkers indicative of disease status and outcome data.[148] Approaches for RET negative tumors include the use of angiogenesis inhibitors, proteasome inhibitors, and cytotoxic chemotherapy in combination with tyrosine kinase or angiogenesis inhibitors.

The survival of patients with these tumors is strongly correlated with stage.[149] In general, surgery provides cure in nearly all patients whose tumors measure less than a few millimeters in diameter, in 90% when tumors are less than 1 cm and in 50% with tumors measuring more than 1 cm.[150] Overall, 10-year survival rates range from 75 to 85%. In Kebebew's series of 104 patients with sporadic and heritable MTC, 49.4% of the patients were cured, 12.3% had recurrent tumor, and 38.3% had persistent tumor.[17] The mean follow-up time was 8.6 years with 10.7% and 13.5% cause specific mortalities at 5 and 10 years, respectively. In this series, 32% of the patients with heritable tumors were diagnosed by genetic or biochemical screening studies. These patients had a lower incidence of cervical node metastases than patients with sporadic tumors, and 94.7% were cured at last follow-up. Patients presenting with systemic symptoms of diarrhea, bone pain, and flushing had widespread metastatic disease, and one third of these patients died within 5 years.

As with other thyroid tumors, patient age (greater than 50 years) and stage are the most important prognostic factors. In the study reported by Kebebew et al, age and stage were the only two independent prognostic factors.[17] Male sex approached statistical significance in univariate analyses and most likely represents a minor risk factor. While patients with cervical lymph node metastases were more likely to have recurrent or persistent disease, this parameter was not associated with a significantly higher mortality.

The type of MTC (sporadic MTC, FMTC, MEN2A, MEN2B) has been reported to be an important prognostic factor in some studies. However, when controlling for stage or in multivariate analyses, the subtype of MTC does not appear to be an important prognostic factor.[25]

Numerous histological and immunohistochemical parameters, including cellular composition (spindle cell vs. round cell), pleomorphism, extent of amyloid deposition, immunohistochemical features, and extent of calcitonin staining, have been examined as potential prognostic parameters, and none has proven to be significant in multivariate analyses.[151] Koperek et al have demonstrated that desmoplasia is a reliable and reproducible parameter to predict nodal metastatic potential.[152] However, additional studies will be required to confirm this hypothesis.

Both calcitonin and CEA serum doubling times have been used as prognostic indices in patients with MTC.[153] When calcitonin doubling time was less than 6 months, 5 and 10-year survivals were 25% and 8%, respectively, while doubling times between 6 months and 2 years were associated with 5 and 10-year survivals of 92% and 37%, respectively. In contrast, patients with calcitonin doubling times of greater than 2 years were all alive at the end of the study.

The presence of somatic RET mutation, particularly involving codon 918, has been linked to poor prognosis.[136,137] Elisei and coworkers have shown that somatic RET mutations involving codon 918 were more frequent in large tumors and in those tumors with nodal and distant metastases.[154] Among all prognostic factors found to be correlated with a worse outcome, only advanced stage at diagnosis and the presence of RET mutations showed an independent correlation ($p<0.0001$ and $p=0.01$, respectively). Survival curves of MTC patients showed a significantly lower percentage of surviving patients in the group with RET mutations ($p=0.006$)

Mixed Medullary and Follicular Carcinomas

Tumors with evidence of follicular cell and neuroendocrine differentiation span a spectrum that includes mixed medullary and follicular/papillary carcinomas, medullary carcinoma with thyroglobulin immunoreactivity, and thyroglobulin positive tumors that coexpress neuroendocrine markers.[155–170] Among the latter group are occasional poorly differentiated (insular) carcinomas, mucoepidermoid tumors, and hyalinizing trabecular tumors.[171–173] For example, poorly differentiated carcinomas of the insular type may coexpress thyroglobulin and somatostatin while hyalinizing trabecular tumors may stain positively for neuron specific enolase, chromogranin A, neurotensin, or somatostatin and may contain electron dense neuroendocrine type granules.[171,172]

Mixed medullary and follicular (or papillary) carcinomas represent a rare and controversial entity. They account for 0.13–0.15% of all thyroid tumors and most cases have been sporadic; however, rare examples of familial mixed tumors have also been reported.[170] The median age is 48 years and the mean size of reported tumors is 3.7 cm. Nodal metastases have been reported in nearly 75% of cases. According to the of *WHO Classification of Endocrine Tumours*, mixed tumors are defined as "showing the morphological features of both medullary carcinoma together with immunoreactive calcitonin and the morphological features of follicular (or papillary) carcinomas with immunoreactive thyroglobulin".[174] Although this definition may seem relatively straightforward, the distinction of true thyroglobulin immunoreactivity from passively absorbed or phagocytosed thyroglobulin by tumor cells is often difficult. For example, positive staining for thyroglobulin was observed in 65% primary MTCs, particularly at the junctions of tumor with normal thyroid, but in none of 8 lymph node metastases in one case series.[53]

The first documented case of a true mixed medullary and follicular carcinoma was reported in 1982.[155] Both thyroglobulin and calcitonin were present both in the primary tumor and in its nodal metastases. Ljungberg and coworkers described a group of differentiated thyroid carcinomas with morphological and immunohistochemical evidence of follicular cell (positivity for thyroglobulin) and C-cell differentiation (positivity for calcitonin, neurotensin or somatostatin).[157,158] These workers concluded that differentiated thyroid carcinomas could be regarded as a spectrum of tumor types with pure follicular carcinomas and pure medullary carcinomas representing the two ends of the spectrum, while tumors with biphasic features represented a broad intermediate group.

In a series of 14 cases of thyroglobulin and calcitonin positive MTCs, thyroglobulin and calcitonin were colocalized in the same neoplastic cells in 8 cases using a double immunolabeling procedure.[159] Three of the 8 cases also contained the calcitonin gene related peptide. On the basis of these observations, Holm and coworkers concluded that a common stem cell was the most likely origin of these tumors.[159] Alternative explanations have suggested that mixed follicular and medullary carcinomas represent collision tumors.[160] Using in situ hybridization and immunohistochemistry, Papotti et al demonstrated that most mixed tumors had separate patterns of calcitonin and thyroglobulin gene expression although rare cells with concurrent calcitonin and thyroglobulin expression were found in 2 of 11 cases of their series.[170]

Tumors with mixed papillary and medullary components have also been described. The phenotypic features of the medullary and papillary component are distinct.[161] The papillary components are thyroglobulin positive but are negative for calcitonin and CEA. The medullary components, on the other hand, are calcitonin and CEA positive but negative for thyroglobulin. Both components have been recognized in the primary tumors and in metastatic sites. The existence of such tumors has raised the same histogenetic issues as those of the mixed follicular and medullary carcinomas.

Volante and coworkers have utilized molecular approaches to study a series of 12 mixed medullary and follicular/papillary carcinomas.[169] Following laser capture microdissection, cases were analyzed for mutations in the RET proto-oncogene and allelic losses of nine loci of six chromosomes together with studies of clonality based on the analysis of the androgen receptor gene. These studies supported the view that the two components were derived from different cells since the components of 7 cases consistently showed differences in patterns of RET mutations, allelic losses, and clonal composition. According to their "hostage" hypothesis, Volante et al postulated that entrapped nonneoplastic follicles were stimulated by medullary carcinoma derived trophic factors leading to hyperplastic follicular foci. The nature of the trophic factors, however, remains to be determined. Subsequently, acquired genetic defects in the follicular cells lead to their neoplastic transformation and the development of papillary or follicular carcinoma components that have the capacity to metastasize. These studies have also demonstrated that a subset of "mixed tumors" is composed of a medullary carcinoma containing hyperplastic follicles, based on the fact that such follicles are often polyclonal or oligoclonal.

Rarely, families with RET point mutations develop both MTC and papillary thyroid carcinoma (PTC). These observations suggest that under certain circumstances RET point mutations rather than rearrangements can drive the development of papillary thyroid carcinoma. The mutant RET found in such families scored constitutive kinase activity and mitogenic effects for cultured thyroid follicular cells (PCC13) although at a significantly lower level than RET/PTC1.[175] These findings indicate that RET point mutants can behave as dominant oncogenes for thyroid follicular cells under some circumstances.

It is likely that mixed medullary and follicular/papillary carcinomas represent a heterogeneous group.[168] In addition to those tumors explained by the "hostage" hypothesis, some mixed tumors may represent collision tumors, while a subset may represent medullary carcinomas with thyroglobulin-expressing cells that might be derived from a common stem cell.[168,170]

References

1. Rosai J, Carcangiu MI, DeLellis RA. *Tumors of the Thyroid Gland Atlas of Tumor Pathology*. Armed Forces Institute of Pathology: Washington, DC; 1992:207–258.
2. Matias-Guiu X, DeLellis RA, Moley JF, et al. Medullary thyroid carcinoma. In: DeLellis RA, Lloyd RV, Heitz PU, Eng C, eds. *Pathology and Genetics of Tumours of Endocrine Organs.*

WHO Classification of Tumours. Lyon: IARC Press; 2004:86–91.
3. Horn RC. Carcinoma of the thyroid. Description of a distinctive morphological variant and report of seven cases. *Cancer*. 1951;4:697–707.
4. Hazard JB, Hawke WA, Crile G. Medullary (solid) carcinoma of the thyroid: a clinicopathological entity. *J Clin Endocrinol Metab*. 1959;19:152–161.
5. Williams ED. Histogenesis of medullary carcinoma of the thyroid. *J Clin Pathol*. 1966;19:114–118.
6. Bussolati G, Pearse AGE. Immunofluorescent localization of calcitonin in the 'C'-cells of the dog and pig thyroid. *J Endocrinol*. 1967;37:205–209.
7. Tashjian AH, Melvin EW. Medullary carcinoma of the thyroid gland. Studies of thyrocalcitonin in plasma and tumor extracts. *N Engl J Med*. 1968;279:279–283.
8. Melvin KE, Miller HH, Tashjian AH Jr. Early diagnosis of medullary carcinoma of the thyroid means of calcitonin assay. *N Engl J Med*. 1971;285:1115–1120.
9. DeLellis RA, Wolfe HJ. The pathology of human calcitonin (C)-cell. *Annu Rev Pathol*. 1981;16:25–52.
10. Pacini F, Fontanelli M, Fugazzola L, et al. Routine measurement of serum calcitonin in nodular thyroid disease allows the preoperative diagnosis of unsuspected sporadic medullary thyroid carcinoma. *J Clin Endocrinol Metab*. 1994; 78:826–829.
11. Cheung K, Roman SA, Wang TS, et al. Calcitonin measurement in the evaluation of thyroid nodules in the United States: a cost effectiveness and discussion analysis. *J Clin Endocrinol Metab*. 2008;93:2173–2218.
12. Thurston V, Williams ED. Experimental induction of C-cell tumours in thyroid by increased dietary content of vitamin D3. *Acta Endocrinol*. 1982;100:41–45.
13. Triggs SM, Williams ED. Experimental carcinogenesis in the rat thyroid follicular and C-cells. A comparison of the effect of variation in dietary calcium and of radiation. *Acta Endocrinol*. 1977;858:4–92.
14. DeLellis RA. Multiple endocrine neoplasia syndromes revisited. Clinical, morphological and molecular features. *Lab Invest*. 1995;72:494–505.
15. Lips CMJ, Vasen HFA, Lamers CBHW. Multiple endocrine neoplasia syndromes. *CRC Crit Rev Oncol Hematol*. 1988;2:117–184.
16. Gimm O, Morrison CD, Suster S, et al. Multiple endocrine neoplasia type 2. In: DeLellis RA, Lloyd RV, Heitz PU, Eng C, eds. *Pathology and Genetics of Tumours of Endocrine Organs. WHO Classification of Tumours*. Lyon: IARC Press; 2004:211–217.
17. Kebebew E, Ituarte PHG, Siperstein AE, et al. Medullary thyroid carcinoma. Clinical characteristics; treatment, prognostic factors and a comparison of staging systems. *Cancer*. 2000;88: 1139–1148.
18. Barbosa SL-S, Rodien P, Leboulleux S, et al. Ectopic adrenocorticotropic hormone-syndrome in medullary carcinoma of the thyroid: a retrospective analysis and review of the literature. *Thyroid*. 2005;15:618–623.
19. Gagel RF, Tashjian AH Jr, Cummings T, et al. The clinical outcome of prospective screening for multiple endocrine neoplasia type 2a: an 18 year experience. *N Engl J Med*. 1988;318:478–484.
20. Verga U, Fugazzola L, Cambiaghi S, et al. Frequent association between MEN2A and cutaneous lichen amyloidosis. *Clin Endocrinol (Oxf)*. 2005;59:156–161.
21. Verdy M, Weber AM, Roy CC, et al. Hirschsprung's disease in a family with multiple endocrine neoplasia type 2. *J Pediatr Gastroenterol Nutr*. 1982;1:603–607.
22. DeLellis RA, Wolfe HJ, Gagel RF, et al. Adrenal medullary hyperplasia a morphometric analysis in patients with familial medullary thyroid carcinoma. *Am J Pathol*. 1976;183:177–196.
23. Carney JA, Sizemore GW, Tyce GM. Bilateral adrenal medullary hyperplasia in multiple endocrine neoplasia type 2: the precursor of bilateral pheochromocytoma. *Mayo Clin Proc*. 1975;50:3–10.
24. Carney JA, Sizemore GW, Hayles AB. Multiple endocrine neoplasia type 2B. *Pathobiol Annu*. 1978;8:105–153.
25. Leboulleux S, Travagli JP, Caillou B, et al. Medullary thyroid carcinoma as part of a multiple endocrine neoplasia type 2B syndrome. Influence of the stage on the clinical course. *Cancer*. 2002;94:44–50.
26. Farndon JR, Leight GS, Dilley WG, et al. Familial medullary thyroid carcinoma without associated endocrinopathies: a distinct clinical entity. *Br J Surg*. 1986;73(4):278–281.
27. Elisei R, Romei C, Cosci B, et al. RET genetic screening in patients with medullary thyroid cancer and their relatives: experience with 807 individuals at one center. *J Clin Endocrinol Metab*. 2007;92:4725–4729.
28. Mizukami Y, Kurumaya H, Nonomura A, et al. Sporadic medullary microcarcinoma of the thyroid. *Histopathology*. 1992;21: 373–377.
29. Zaatari GS, Saigo PC, Huvos AG. Mucin production in medullary carcinoma of the thyroid. *Arch Pathol Lab Med*. 1983;107:70–74.
30. Sletton K, Westermark P, Natwig JB. Characterization of amyloid fibril proteins from medullary carcinoma of the thyroid. *J Exp Med*. 1976;143:993–998.
31. Khurana R, Agarwal A, Bajpai VK, et al. Unraveling the amyloid associated with human medullary carcinoma. *Endocrinology*. 2004;154:5465–5470.
32. Kini S. *Thyroid Cytopathology: An Atlas and Text*. Philadelphia: Lippencott Williams and Wilkins; 2008.
33. Kaufmann O, Dietel M. Expression of thyroid transcription factor-1 in pulmonary and extrapulmonary small cell carcinomas and other neuroendocrine carcinomas of various primary sites. *Histopathology*. 2000;36:415–420.
34. Bejarano PA, Nikiforov YE, Swenson ES, Biddinger PW. Thyroid transcription factor-1, thyroglobulin, cytokeratin 7 and cytokeratin 20 in thyroid neoplasms. *Appl Immunohistochem Mol Morphol*. 2000;8:189–194.
35. Kimura N, Nakazato Y, Nagura H, Sasano N. Expression of intermediate filaments in neuroendocrine tumors. *Arch Pathol Lab Med*. 1990;114:506–510.
36. DeLellis RA. The pathology of medullary thyroid carcinoma and its precursors. In: LiVolsi VA, DeLellis RA, eds. *Pathology of the Parathyroid and Thyroid Glands*. Baltimore: Williams and Wilkins; 1993:77–102.
37. Holm R, Sobrinho-Simoes M, Fould NJM, VE JJV. Medullary carcinoma of the thyroid gland: and immunocytochemical study. *Ultrastruct Pathol*. 1985;8:25–41.
38. Portela-Gomes GM, Luckinius GM, Grimeluis L. synaptic vesicle protein 2, a new neuroendocrine cell marker. *Am J Pathol*. 2000;157:1299–1309.
39. Schmid KW, Fisher-Colbrie R, Hagn C, Jasani B, Williams E, Winkler H. Chromogranin A and B and secretogranin II in

medullary carcinomas of the thyroid. *Am J Surg Pathol.* 1987;11:551–556.
40. Katsetos CD, Jami MM, Krishna L, Jackson R, Patchefsky AS, Cooper HS. Novel immunohistochemical localization of 28, 000 molecular weight (Mr) calcium binding protein (Calbindin-D28k) in enterochromaffin cells of the human appendix and neuroendocrine tumors (carcinoids and small cell carcinomas) of the midgut and foregut. *Arch Pathol Lab Med.* 1994;11:633–639.
41. Komminoth P, Roth J, Saremaslani P, Matias-Guiu T, Wolfe HF, Heitz PU. Polysialic acid of the neural cell adhesion molecule in the human thyroid: a marker for medullary thyroid carcinoma and primary C-cell hyperplasia. An immumohistochemical study of 70 thyroid lesions. *Am J Surg Pathol.* 1994;18:399–411.
42. Saad MF, Ordonez NG, Guido JJ, Samaan N. The prognostic value of calcitonin immunostaining in medullary carcinoma of the thyroid. *J Clin Endocrinol Metab.* 1984;59:850–856.
43. Sikri KL, Varndell IM, Hamid QA, et al. Medullary carcinoma of the thyroid. An immunocytochemical and histochemical study of 25 cases using 8 separate markers. *Cancer.* 1985;56:2481–2491.
44. Steenbergh PH, Heppner JW, Zandberg J, et al. Calcitonin gene related peptide coding sequence is conserved in the human genome and is expressed in medullary thyroid carcinoma. *J Clin Endocrinol Metab.* 1984;5:358–360.
45. Zajac JD, Penschow J, Mason T, et al. Identification of calcitonin and calcitonin gene-related peptide messenger RNA in medullary thyroid carcinoma by hybridization histochemistry. *J Clin Endocrinol Metab.* 1986;62:1037–1043.
46. Scopsi L, Ferrari C, Pilotti S, et al. Immunocytochemical localization and identification of prosomatostatin gene products in medullary carcinoma of human thyroid gland. *Hum Pathol.* 1990;21:820–830.
47. Sunday ME, Wolfe HJ, Roos BA, Chin WW, Spindel ER. Gastrin releasing peptide gene expression in developing, hyperplastic and neoplastic thyroid C-cell. *Endocrinology.* 1988;122:1551–1558.
48. Williams ED, Morales AM, Horn RC. Thyroid carcinoma and Cushing's syndrome. A report of two cases with review of the common features of the non-endocrine tumours associated with Cushing's syndrome. *J Clin Pathol.* 1968;21:129–135.
49. Roth KA, Bensch KG, Hoffman AR. Characterization of opioid peptides in human thyroid medullary carcinoma. *Cancer.* 1987;59:850–856.
50. Birkenhäger JC, Upton GV, Seldenrath HJ, Krieger DT, Tashjian AH Jr. Medullary thyroid carcinoma: ectoic production of peptides with ACTH-like, corticotropin-releasing factor-like and prolactin production – stimulating activities. *Acta Endocrinol (Copenh).* 1976;83:280–292.
51. Uribe M, Fenoglio-Preiser CN, Grimes M, Feind C. Medullary carcinoma of the thyroid gland. Clinical, pathological, and immunohistochemical features with review of the literature. *Am J Surg Pathol.* 1985;9:577–594.
52. Faggiano A, Talbot M, Lacroix L, et al. Differential expression of galectin-3 in medullary thyroid carcinoma and C-cell hyperplasia. *Clin Endocrinol.* 2002;57:813–819.
53. DeLellis RA, Rule AH, Spiler I, Nathanson L, Tashjian AH Jr, Wolfe HJ. Calcitonin and carcinoembryonic antigen as tumor markers in medullary thyroid carcinoma. *Am J Clin Pathol.* 1978;70:587–594.
54. Schroder S, Klöppel G. Carcinoembryonic antigen and nonspecific cross-reacting antigen in thyroid cancer. An immunocytochemical study using polyclonal and monoclonal antibodies. *Am J Surg Pathol.* 1987;11:100–108.
55. Mendelsohn G, Wells SA, Baylin SB. Relationship of tissue carcinoembryonic antigen and calcitonin to tumor virulence in medullary thyroid carcinoma. An immunohistochemical study in early, localized and virulent disseminated stages of disease. *Cancer.* 1984;54:657–662.
56. Kakudo K, Miyauchi A, Yakai SI, et al. C-cell carcinoma of the thyroid, papillary type. *Acta Pathol Jpn.* 1979;29:653–659.
57. Harach HR, Williams ED. Glandular (tubular and follicular) variants of medullary carcinoma of the thyroid. *Histopathology.* 1983;7:83–97.
58. Harach HR, Bergholm U. Small cell variant of medullary carcinoma of the thyroid with neuroblastoma-like features. *Histopathology.* 1992;21:378–380.
59. Eusebi V, Damiani S, Riva C, Lloyd RV, Capella C. Calcitonin free oat cell carcinoma of the thyroid gland. *Virchows Arch A Pathol Anat Histopathol.* 1990;417:267–271.
60. Mendelsohn G, Baylin SB, Bigner SH, et al. Anaplastic variants of medullary thyroid carcinoma: a light microscopic and immunohistochemical study. *Am J Surg Pathol.* 1980;4: 333–341.
61. Landon G, Ordóñex NG. Clear cell variant of medullary carcinoma of the thyroid. *Hum Pathol.* 1985;16:844–847.
62. Marcus JN, Dise CA, LiVolsi VA. Melanin production in a medullary thyroid carcinoma. *Cancer.* 1982;49:2518–2526.
63. Beerman H, Rigaud C, Bogomeletz WV, Hollander H, Veldhuizen H. Melanin production in black medullary thyroid cancer (MTC). *Histopathology.* 1990;16:227–234.
64. Dominguez-Malagon H, Delgardo-Chavez R, Torres-Najera M, Gould E, Albores-Saavedra J. Oxyphil and squamous variants of medullary thyroid carcinoma. *Cancer.* 1989;63:1183–1188.
65. Golough R, Us-Krasovec M, Auersperg M, Jancar J, Bondi A, Eusebi V. Amphicrine-composite calcitonin and mucin producing carcinoma of the thyroid. *Ultrastruct Pathol.* 1985; 8:197–206.
66. Huss LJ, Mendlesohn G. Medullary carcinoma of the thyroid gland: an encapsulated variant resembling the hyalinizing trabecular (paraganglioma-like) adenoma of thyroid. *Mod Pathol.* 1990;3:581–585.
67. Laforga JB, Aranda FI. Pseudoangiosarcomatous features in medullary thyroid carcinoma spindle cell variant. Report of a case studied by FNA and immunohistochemistry. *Diagn Cytopathol.* 2007;34:424–428.
68. Beskid M, Lorenc R, Rôsciszewska A. C-cell thyroid adenoma in man. *J Pathol.* 1971;103:3343–3346.
69. Kodama T, Okamoto T, Fujjimoto Y, et al. C-cell adenoma in the thyroid: a rare but distinct clinical entity. *Surgery.* 1988;104:997–1003.
70. Mendelsohn G, Oertel JE. Encapsulated medullary thyroid carcinoma [Abstract]. *Lab Invest.* 1981;44:43A.
71. Matias-Guiu X, LaGuette J, Puras-Gil AM, Rosai J. Metastatic neuroendocrine tumors to the thyroid mimicking medullary carcinoma: a pathological and immunohistochemical study of six cases. *Am J Surg Pathol.* 1997;21:754–762.
72. Shikama Y, Osawa T, Yagihashis N, et al. Neuroendocrine differentiation in hyalinizing trabecular tumors of the thyroid. *Virchows Arch.* 2003;443:792–796.

73. Wolfe HJ, Melvin KE, Cervi-Skinner SJ, et al. C-cell hyperplasia preceding medullary thyroid carcinoma. *N Engl J Med.* 1973;289:437–441.
74. Wells SA, Ontjes DA, Cooper CW, et al. The early diagnosis of medullary carcinoma of the thyroid gland in patients with multiple endocrine neoplasia type II. *Ann Surg.* 1975;182:362–370.
75. DeLellis RA, Nunnemacher G, Wolfe HJ. C-cell hyperplasia: an ultrastructural analysis. *Lab Invest.* 1977;36:237–248.
76. McDermott MB, Swanson PE, Wick MR. Immunostains for collagen type IV discriminate between C-cell hyperplasia and microscopic medullary carcinoma in multiple endocrine neoplasia, type 2A. *Hum Pathol.* 1995;26:1308–1312.
77. Albores-Saavedra J, Monforte H, Nadji M, Morales AR. C-cell hyperplasia in thyroid tissue adjacent to follicular cell tumors. *Hum Pathol.* 1988;19:795–799.
78. Guyetant S, Rousselet MC, Durigon M, et al. Sex related C-cell hyperplasia in the normal human thyroid: a quantitative autopsy study. *J Clin Endocrinol Metab.* 1997;82:42–47.
79. Perry A, Molberg K, Albores-Saavedra J. Physiologic versus neoplastic C-cell hyperplasia of the thyroid: separation of distinct histologic and biologic entities. *Cancer.* 1996;77:750–756.
80. Carney JA, Sizemore GW, Hales AB. Multiple endocrine neoplasia, type 2B. *Pathobiol Annu.* 1978;8:105–153.
81. Diaz-Cano S, DeMiguel M, Blanes A, et al. Germline RET634 mutation positive MEN2A related C-cell hyperplasias have genetic features consistent with intraepithelial neoplasias. *J Clin Endocrinol Metab.* 2001;86:3948–3951.
82. Kaserer K, Scheuba C, Neuhold N, et al. C-cell hyperplasia and medullary thyroid carcinoma in patients routinely screened for serum calcitonin. *Am J Surg Pathol.* 1998;22:722–728.
83. Kaserer K, Scheuba C, Neuhold N, et al. sporadic versus familial medullary thyroid microcarcinoma: a histopathologic study of 50 consecutive patients. *Am J Surg Pathol.* 2001;25:1245–1251.
84. Mears L, Diaz-Cano S. Difference between familial and sporadic medullary thyroid carcinomas (Letter). *Am J Surg Pathol.* 2003;27:266–267.
85. Mathew CG, Chin KS, Easton DF, et al. A linked genetic marker for multiple endocrine neoplasia type 2A on chromosome 10. *Nature.* 1987;328:527–528.
86. Simpson NE, Kidd KK, Goodfellow PJ, et al. Assignment of multiple endocrine neoplasia type 2A to chromosome 10 by linkage. *Nature.* 1987;328:528–530.
87. Ponder BA, Coffe R, Gagel RF, et al. Risk estimation and screening of families of patients with medullary thyroid carcinoma. *Lancet.* 1988;1:397–401.
88. Sobol H, Narod SA, Nakamura Y, et al. Screening for multiple endocrine neoplasia type 2A with DNA polymorphism analysis. *N Engl J Med.* 1989;321:996–1001.
89. Gardner E, Papi L, Easton DF, et al. Genetic linkage studies map the multiple endocrine neoplasia type 2 loci to a small interval of chromosome 10q 11.2. *Hum Mol Genet.* 1993;2:241–246.
90. Lairmore TC, Dou S, Howe JR, et al. A1.5 megabase yeast artificial chromosome contig from human chromosome 10q 11.2 connecting 3 genetic loci (RET, D10S94, and D10S102) closely linked to the MEN2A locus. *Proc Natl Acad Sci USA.* 1993;90:492–496.
91. Mole SE, Mulligan LM, Healey CS, et al. Localization of the gene for localization of the gene for multiple endocrine neoplasia type 2A to a 480 kb region in chromosome band 10q 11.2. *Hum Mol Genet.* 1993;2:247–252.
92. Mulligan LM, Kwok JBJ, Healey CS, et al. Germline mutations of the RET proto-oncogene in multiple endocrine neoplasia type 2A. *Nature.* 1993;363:458–460.
93. Donis-Keller H, Dou S, Chi D, et al. Mutations in the RET proto-oncogene are associated with MEN2A and FMTC. *Hum Mol Genet.* 1993;2:851–856.
94. Mulligan LM, Eng C, Healey CS, et al. Specific mutations of the RET proto-oncogene are related to disease phenotype in MEN2A and FMTC. *Nat Genet.* 1994;6:70–74.
95. Hofstra RM, Landsvater RM, Ceccherini I, et al. A mutation in the RET proto-oncogene associated with multiple endocrine neoplasia type 2B and sporadic medullary thyroid carcinoma. *Nature.* 1994;367:375–376.
96. Eng C, Smith DP, Mulligan LM, et al. Point mutations within the tyrosine kinase domain of the RET proto-oncogene in multiple endocrine neoplasia type 2B and related sporadic tumors. *Hum Mol Genet.* 1994;3:237–241.
97. Carlson KM, Dou S, Chi D, et al. single missense mutation in the tyrosine kinase catalytic domain of the RET proto-oncogene is associated with multiple endocrine neoplasia type 2B. *Proc Natl Acad Sci USA.* 1994;91:1579–1583.
98. Eng C, Clayton D, Schuffenecker I, et al. The relationship between specific RET proto-oncogene mutations and disease phenotype in multiple endocrine neoplasia type 2. International RET mutation consortium analysis. *JAMA.* 1996;276: 1575–1579.
99. Eng C. RET proto-oncogene in the development of human cancer. *J Clin Oncol.* 1999;17:380–393.
100. Hoff AO, Cote GJ, Gagel RF. Multiple endocrine neoplasias. *Annu Rev Physiol.* 2000;62:377–411.
101. Takahashi M, Ritz J, Cooper GM. Activation of a novel human transforming gener, ret by DNA rearrangement. *Cell.* 1985;42: 581–588.
102. Takahashi M, Buma Y, Iwamoto T. Cloning and expression of the ret proto-oncogene encoding a tyrosine kinase with two potential transmembrane domains. *Oncogene.* 1988;3: 571–578.
103. Grieco M, Santoro M, Berlingiere MT, et al. PTC is a novel rearranged form of the ret proto-oncogene and is frequently detected *in vivo* in human papillary carcinomas. *Cell.* 1990;60:557–563.
104. Santoro M, Dathan NA, Berlingieri MT, et al. Molecular characterization of RET/PTC3, a novel rearranged version of the RET proto-oncogene n a human papillary thyroid carcinoma. *Oncogene.* 1990;9:509–516.
105. Klugbauer S, Demidchik EP, Lengfelder E, Rabes HM. Detection of a novel type of RET rearrangement (PTC5) in thyroid carcinomas after Chernobyl and analysis of the involved RET-fused gene RFG5. *Cancer Res.* 1998;58:198–203.
106. LiVolsi VA, Albores-Saavedra J, Asa SL, et al. Papillary carcinoma. In: DeLellis RA, Lloyd RV, Heitz PU, Eng C, eds. *WHO Classification of Tumours.* Lyon: IARC Press; 2004:57–66.
107. Lam AKY, Montore KT, Nolan KA, LiVolsi VA. RET oncogene activation in papillary thyroid carcinoma: Prevalence and implication of the histological parameters. *Hum Pathol.* 1998;19:565–568.

108. Jhiang SM, Sagartz JE, Tong Q, et al. Targeted expression of the ret/PTC1 oncogene induces papillary thyroid carcinomas. *Endocrinology*. 1996;137:375–378.
109. Fischer AH, Bond JA, Taysavang P, Battles OE, Wynford-Thomas D. Papillary thyroid carcinoma oncogene (RET/PTC) alters the nuclear envelope and chromatin structure. *Am J Pathol*. 1998;153:1443–1450.
110. Nagao M, Ishizaka Y, Nakagawora A, et al. expression of ret proto-oncogene in human in neuroblastomas. *Jpn J Cancer Res*. 1990;81:309–312.
111. Santoro M, Rosati R, Grieco M, et al. The ret- proto-oncogene is consistently expressed in human pheochromocytomas and thyroid medullary carcinomas. *Oncogene*. 1990;5:1595–1598.
112. Pasini B, Hofstra RM, Yin L, et al. The physical map of the RET proto-oncogene. *Oncogene*. 1995;11:1737–1743.
113. Pachnis V, Mankoo B, Costantiri F. Expression of the C-ret proto-oncogene during mouse embryogenesis. *Development*. 1993;119:1005–1017.
114. Schuchardt A, D'Agati V, Larsson-Bloomberg L, Costantini F, Pachnis V. Defects in the kidney and enteric nervous system of mice lacking the tyrosine kinase receptor ret. *Nature*. 1994;367:380–383.
115. Durbee P, Marcos-Guiterrez CV, Kilkenny C, et al. Glial cell line derived neurotrophic factor signaling through the RET receptor tyrosine kinase. *Nature*. 1996;381:789–793.
116. Jing S, Wen D, Yu Y, et al. GDNF-induced activation of the ret protein tyrosine kinase is mediated by GDNFR-δ, a novel receptor for GDNF. *Cell*. 1996;85:1113–11124.
117. Treanor JJ, Goodman L, deSauvage F, et al. Characterization of a multicomponent receptor. *Nature*. 1996;381:80–83.
118. Sanicola M, Hession C, Worlely D, et al. GDNF-dependent RET activation can be mediated by two different cell surface accessory proteins. *Proc Natl Acad Sci USA*. 1997;94:6238–6243.
119. Kotzbauer PT, Lampe PA, Heuckeroth RO, et al. Neurtusin, a relative of glial cell line derived neurotropic factor. *Nature*. 1996;384:467–470.
120. Jing S, Yu Y, Fang M, et al. GFR-alpha-2 and GFR-alpha 3 are two new receptors for ligands of the GDNF family. *J Biol Chem*. 1997;272:33111–33117.
121. Baloh RH, Tansey MG, Lampe PA, et al. Artemin, a novel member of GDNF ligand family, supports peripheral and central neurons and signals through the GFR alpha 3-RET receptor complex. *Neuron*. 1998;21:1291–1302.
122. Lai AZ, Gujral TS, Mulligan LM. RET signalling in endocrine tumors: delving deeper into molecular mechanisms. *Endocr Pathol*. 2007;18:57–67.
123. Santoro M, Carlomagno F, Romano A, et al. Activation of RET as a dominant transforming by germline mutations of MEN2A and MEN2B. *Science*. 1995;267:381–383.
124. Iwashita T, Asai N, Murakami H, et al. Identification of tyrosine residues that are essential for transforming activity of the ret proto-oncogene with MEN2A or MEN2B mutations. *Oncogene*. 1976;12:481–487.
125. Gimm O, Marsh DJ, Andrew SD, et al. Germline dinucleotide mutation in codon 883 of the RET proto-oncogene in multiple endocrine neoplasia type 2B without codon 918 mutation. *J Clin Endocrinol Metab*. 1997;81:3902–3904.
126. Smith DP, Houghton C, Ponder BA. Germline mutation of RET codon 883 in two cases of de novo MEN2B. *Oncogene*. 1997;15:1213–1217.
127. Kawai K, Iwashita T, Murakami H, et al. Tissue specific carcinogenesis in neoplasia type 2A mutation. *Cancer Res*. 2000;60:5254–5260.
128. Marsh DJ, Zheng Z, Arnold A, et al. Mutation analysis of glial cell line derived neurotropic factor, a ligand for the RET/co-receptor complex in MEN2 and sporadic neuroendocrine tumors. *J Clin Endocrinol Metab*. 1997;81:3025–3028.
129. Peacock ML, Borst MJ, Sweet JD, Decker RA. Detection of RET mutations in multiple endocrine neoplasia type 2A and familial medullary thyroid carcinoma by denaturing gel electrophoresis. *Hum Mutat*. 1996;7:100–104.
130. Wohllk N, Cote GJ, Evans DB, et al. Application of genetic screening information to the management of medullary thyroid carcinoma and multiple endocrine neoplasia type 2. *Endocrinol Metab Clinics North Am*. 1996;25:1–25.
131. Wells SA, Chi DD, Toshima K, et al. Predictive DNA testing and prophylactic thyroidectomy in patients at risk for multiple endocrine neoplasia type 2A. *Ann Surg*. 1994;220:237–250.
132. Lips CJ, Landsvater RM, Hoppener JW, et al. Clinical screening as compared with DNA analysis in families with multiple endocrine neoplasia type 2A. *N Engl J Med*. 1994; 331:828–835.
133. Dralle H, Gimm O, Simon D, et al. Prophylactic thyroidectomy in 75 children and adolescents with hereditary mudullary thyroid carcinoma: German and Austrian experience. *World J Surg*. 1998;22(7):744–751.
134. Offit K, Biesecker BB, Burt RW, et al. Statement of the American Society of Oncology: genetic testing for cancer susceptibility. *J Clin Oncol*. 1996;14:1730–1736.
135. Wohllk N, Cote GJ, Bugalho MM, et al. Relevance of RET proto-oncogene mutations in sporadic medullary thyroid carcinoma. *J Clin Endocrinol Metab*. 1996;81:3740–3745.
136. Zedenius J, Wallin G, Hamberger B, et al. Somatic and MEN2A de novo mutations identified in the RET proto-oncogene by screening of sporadic MTCs. *Hum Mol Genet*. 1994;3:1259–1262.
137. Eng C, Mulligan LM, Healey CS, et al. Heterogeneous mutation of the RET proto-oncogene in subpopulations of medullary thyroid carcinoma. *Cancer Res*. 1996;56:2167–2170.
138. Marsh DJ, Learoyd DL, Andrew SD, et al. Somatic mutations in the RET proto-oncogene in sporadic medullary thyroid carcinoma. *Clin Endocrinol*. 1996;44:249–257.
139. Saggiorato E, Rapa I, Garino F, et al. Absence of RET gene point mutation in sporadic C-cell hyperplasia. *J Mol Diagn*. 2007;9:214–219.
140. Eng C, Crossey PA, Mulligan LM, et al. Mutations of the RET proto-oncogene and von Hippel Lindau disease tumour suppressor gene in sporadic and syndromic pheochromocytoma. *J Med Genet*. 1995;32:934–937.
141. Lindor LM, Honchel R, Khosla S, et al. Mutations in the RET proto-oncogene in sporadic pheochromocytomas. *J Clin Endocrinol Metab*. 1995;80:627–629.
142. Beldjord B, Desclaux-Arranond F, Raffin-Samson M, et al. The RET proto-oncogene in sporadic pheochromocytomas. Frequent MEN2-like mutations and new molecular defects. *J Clin Endocrinol Metab*. 1995;80:2063–2068.
143. Padberg BC, Schroder S, Jochum W, et al. Absence of RET proto-oncogene point mutations in sporadic hyperplastic and neoplastic lesions of the parathyroid gland. *Am J Pathol*. 1995;147:1600–1607.

144. Komminoth P, Roth J, Mulletta-Feurer S, et al. RET proto-oncogene point mutations in sporadic neuroendocrine tumors. *J Clin Endocrinol Metab*. 1996;81:2041–2046.
145. Eng C, Mulligan LM. Mutations of the RET proto-oncogene in the multiple endocrine neoplasia type 2 syndrome, related sporadic tumours and Hirschsprung disease. *Hum Mut*. 1997;9:97–109.
146. Fialkowski EA, Moley JF. Current approaches to medullary thyroid carcinoma, sporadic and familial. *J Surg Oncol*. 2006;94:737–747.
147. Moley JF, Fialkowski EA. Evidence based approach to the managementof sporadic medullary thyroid carcinoma. *World J Surg*. 2007;31:946–956.
148. Ball DW. Medullary thyroid carcinoma: therapeutic targets and molecular markers. *Curr Opin Oncol*. 2007;19:18–23.
149. Modigliani E, Cohen R, Campos JM, et al. Prognostic factors for survival and for biochemical cure in medullary thyroid carcinoma: results in 819 patients. The GETC Study Group. Groupe d'etude des tumeurs a calcitonine. *Clin Endocrinol (Oxf)*. 1998;48:265–273.
150. Vezzosi D, Bennet A, Caron P. Recent advances in treatment of medullary thyroid carcinoma. *Ann Endocrinol (Paris)*. 2007;68:147–153.
151. Schröder S, Böcker W, Baisch H, et al. Prognostic factors in medullary thyroid carcinoma. Survival in relation to age, sex, stage, histology, immunohistochemistry and DNA content. *Cancer*. 1998;61:806–816.
152. Koporek O, Scheuba C, Cherenko M, et al. Desmoplasia in medullary thyroid carcinoma: a reliable indicator of metastatic potential. *Histopathology*. 2008;52:623–630.
153. Barbet J, Campion L, Kraeber-Bodere F, Chatal JF. Prognostic impact of serum calcitonin and carcinoembryonic antigen doubling times in patients with medullary thyroid carcinoma. *J Clin Endocrinol Metab*. 2005;90:6077–6084.
154. Elisei R, Cosci B, Romei C, et al. Prognostic significance of somatic RET oncogene mutations in sporadic medullary thyroid carcinoma: a 10-year follow-up study. *J Clin Endocrinol Metab*. 2008;93:682 687.
155. Hales M, Rosenau W, Okerlund MD, Galante M. Carcinoma of the thyroid with a mixed medullary and follicular pattern: morphological, immunohistochemical and clinical laboratory studies. *Cancer*. 1982;50:1352–1359.
156. Pfaltz M, Hedinger CE, Muhlethales JP. Mixed medullary and follicular carcinoma of the thyroid. *Virchows Arch [Pathol Anat]*. 1983;400:53–59.
157. Ljungberg O, Ericsson U-B, Bondeson L, Thorell J. A compound follicular-parafollicular cell carcinoma of the thyroid: a new tumor entity? *Cancer*. 1984;52:1053–1061.
158. Ljungberg OB, Bondeson L, Bondeson AG. Differentiated thyroid carcinoma, intermediate type: a new tumor entity with features of follicular and parafollicular cell carcinoma. *Hum Pathol*. 1984;15:218–228.
159. Holm R, Sobrinho-Simoes M, Nesland JM, Sambade C, Johannessen JV. Medullary thyroid carcinoma with thyroglobulin immunoreactivity. A special entity? *Lab Invest*. 1987;57:258–268.
160. LiVolsi VA. Mixed thyroid carcinoma: a real entity? *Lab Invest*. 1987;57:237–239.
161. Albores-Saavedra J, de la Mora TG, de la Torra-Rendon F, Gould E. Mixed medullary-papillary carcinoma of the thyroid: a previously unrecognized variant of thyroid carcinoma. *Hum Pathol*. 1990;21:1151–1155.
162. Mizukami Y, Michigishi T, Nonomura A, et al. Mixed medullary-follicular carcinoma of the thyroid occurring in familial form. *Histopathology*. 1993;22:284–287.
163. Matias-Guiu X, Caixas A, Costa I, Cabezas R, Prat J. Compound medullary-papillary carcinoma of the thyroid: true mixed versus collision tumour. *Histopathology*. 1994;25:183–185.
164. Lax SF, Beham A, Kronberger-Schönecker D, Langsteger W, Denk H. Coexistence of papillary and medullary carcinoma of the thyroid gland-mixed or collision tumors? Clinicopathological analysis of three cases. *Virchows Arch*. 1994;424:441–447.
165. Kobayashi K, Teramoto S, Maeta H, Ishiguro S, Mori T, Horie Y. Simultaneous occurrence of medullary carcinoma and papillary carcinoma of the thyroid. *J Surg Oncol*. 1995;59:276–279.
166. Mizukami Y, Nonomura A, Michigishi T, Noguchi M, Ishizaki T. Mixed medullary-follicular carcinoma of the thyroid gland: a clinicopathologic variant of medullary thyroid carcinoma. *Mod Pathol*. 1996;9:631–635.
167. Papotti M, Negro F, Carney JA, Bussolati G, Lloyd RV. Mixed medullary-follicular carcinoma of the thyroid. A morphological, immunohistochemical and in situ hybridization analysis of 11 cases. *Virchows Arch*. 1997;430:397–405.
168. Matias-Guiu X. Mixed medullary and follicular carcinoma of the thyroid. On the search for its histogenesis. *Am J Pathol*. 1999;155:1413–1418.
169. Volante M, Papotti M, Roth J, et al. Mixed medullary-follicular thyroid carcinoma. Molecular evidence for a dual origin of tumor components. *Am J Pathol*. 1999;155:1499–1509.
170. Pappoti M, Volante M, Komminoth P, Sobrinho-Simoes M, Bussolati G. Thyroid carcinomas with mixed follicular and C-cell differentiation patterns. *Semin Diagn Pathol*. 2000;17:109–119.
171. Katoh R, Jasani B, Williams ED. Hyalinizing trabecular adenomas of the thyroid: a report of three cases with immunohistochemical and ultrastructural studies. *Histopathology*. 1989;15:211–224.
172. Carcangiu ML, Zampi G, Rosai J. Poorly differentiated ("insular") thyroid carcinoma. A reinterpretation of Langhans "wuchernde struma". *Am J Surg Pathol*. 1984;8:655–668.
173. Sobrinho-Simoes M. Poorly differentiated carcinomas of the thyroid. *Endocr Pathol*. 1996;7:99–102.
174. Papotti M, Bussolati G, Kommoth P, et al. Mixed medullary and follicular cell carcinoma. In: DeLellis RA, Lloyd RV, Heitz PU, Eng C, eds. *Pathology and Genetics of Tumours of Endocrine Organs. WHO Classification of Tumours*. Lyon: IARC Press; 2004:92–92.
175. Mellilo RM, Cirafici AM, DeFalco V, et al. The oncogenic activity of RET point mutants for follicular thyroid cells may account for the occurrence of papillary thyroid carcinoma in patients affected by familial medullary thyroid carcinoma. *Am J Pathol*. 2004;165:511–521.

12 Unusual Thyroid Tumors

Jennifer L. Hunt

Introduction

There are a number of tumors of the thyroid gland that do not fit into the conventional categories of follicular and C-cell derived lesions. These tumors tend to be very rare, and the literature regarding molecular alterations in these lesions is sparse. However, as the pathologist may encounter these tumors rarely in practice, they will be reviewed in this chapter.

Mucoepidermoid Carcinoma

Mucoepidermoid carcinoma (MEC) of the thyroid gland is a rare tumor that represents less than 0.5% of all thyroid gland malignancies.[1] The patients affected by this tumor have a broad age range, but they are more common in women than in men.[2] There are no clinical features which will distinguish this tumor from other more typical thyroid gland lesions.

Histologically, MEC has a unique appearance, but with features similar to salivary gland derived MEC.[2] The cellular components include both epidermoid type cells and mucin containing cells.[3] The tumor cells grow in compact nests and clusters that may be surrounded by dense fibrosis.[2] The glandular spaces are lined by mucinous cells that can be either cuboidal or can have goblet cell features.[2] One case has been described that demonstrated ciliated cells as well.[4]

Thyroid MECs usually stain positive for TTF-1 and thyroglobulin, at least focally.[5,6] They will also often stain positive for CEA, and they are negative for calcitonin.[7]

At the molecular level, thyroid MEC has only been rarely studied for molecular mutations. One study of salivary gland MECs also included three cases of thyroid MEC in analyzing the *CRTC1/MAML2* (also known as *MECT1/MAML2*) translocation.[8] This translocation has been identified in approximately 50–60% of salivary gland derived MECs, with higher rates seen in lower grade lesions.[9–11] Interestingly, one of the three thyroid MECs was reportedly positive for the translocation.[8]

Sclerosing Mucoepidermoid Carcinoma with Eosinophia

Sclerosing mucoepidermoid carcinoma with eosinophia (SMECE) is another very rare tumor of the thyroid gland that remains incompletely understood. Patients with these tumors tend to present with a mass lesion.[6] The average age at presentation is around 52 years of age, and there is a strong female predominance. Approximately half of the patients with SMECE will develop recurrent disease or distant metastases.[12]

Most cases of SMECE occur in a background of chronic lymphocytic thyroiditis, particularly those cases with fibrosis (so-called fibrosing Hashimoto's thyroiditis).[6] At low power, the tumor cells grow in small nests and islands, anastomosing cords, and narrow strands.[7] There are four populations of cells that can be identified.[6,13] There is a squamoid component that demonstrates typical intracellular bridges and can have squamous pearl formation.[14] The glandular component has mucous cells that occur either individually or as part of mucinous cysts. There can also be a population of clear cells that are usually found to be rich in glycogen. Finally, there are abundant inflammatory cells in the background of these tumors, including eosinophils, lymphocytes, and plasma cells. SMECE can occasionally be associated with a conventional papillary carcinoma.[6,15]

Immunohistochemical staining for SMECE demonstrates uniform positivity for cytokeratin and variable positivity for TTF-1.[13] p63 has been shown to be positive in these tumors.[4,16] Thyroglobulin is usually negative and calcitonin is always negative.[13] SMECE has not been studied at the molecular level.

Hyalinizing Trabecular Tumor

Hyalinizing trabecular tumor (HTT) is an unusual lesion in the thyroid that has been the subject of some controversy over the past decade and has had several different names.[17]

J.L. Hunt (ed.), *Molecular Pathology of Endocrine Diseases*, Molecular Pathology Library 3,
DOI 10.1007/978-1-4419-1707-2_12, © Springer Science+Business Media, LLC 2010

The tumor was initially described as a paraganglioma-like adenoma of the thyroid because of the unique histologic appearance,[18] but then assumed the more commonly used name of hyalinizing trabecular adenoma.[19] Because of controversy regarding whether these lesions are variants of papillary carcinoma, many pathologists have adopted the terminology of "hyalinizing trabecular tumor" or "hyalinizing trabecular neoplasm".[20] Despite this cautiousness, a recent study of 119 lesions demonstrated that 118 were typical hyalinizing trabecular lesions and no cases had recurrence, metastasis or poor outcome with good long-term follow-up.[21]

HTTs have a characteristic morphology. The growth pattern is strictly trabecular and should not include any follicular growth. There is usually deposition of an eosinophilic extracellular material that stains with collagen type IV and laminin; this can be located central to radiating trabecullae or can be deposited in the stromal compartment of the tumors.[22,23] Because of the growth pattern and the eosinophilic hyaline material, medullary carcinoma should be ruled out with negative calcitonin and positive thyroglobulin stains before making the diagnosis of HTT.[24] They nuclei can have a resemblance to those seen in papillary carcinoma, with intranuclear inclusions, enlargement, clearing, and grooves.[25,26] In fact, this lesion can represent a major pitfall in cytology.[26] Inclusions in the cytoplasm have been described ("yellow bodies") that have a refractile nature and represent giant lysosomes on ultrastructural studies; these have also been seen in papillary carcinomas.[27,28] HTT has the immunohistochemical profile of a follicular derived process, with positive staining with TTF-1 and thyroglobulin stains and negative staining with calcitonin; chromogranin, and NSE can also be positive.[23] One study demonstrated negative cytokeratin-19 staining in HTT and while all papillary carcinoma were positive, though another study found the lesions to be positive for CK19.[29,30] Another study demonstrated galectin-3 staining in 40% of HTTs, while 83% of papillary carcinomas were positive.[31] True paragangliomas of the thyroid gland are quite rare; they can be distinguished from HTT by negative thyroglobulin staining and by the presence of sustentacular cells on S100 stains.[32]

HTT has most commonly been reported to have a benign clinical course and most cases are entirely well encapsulated.[19] Few reports have described a malignant histologic appearance, and one case has been reported to have metastasized.[20] These rare apparently malignant cases have been designated as "hyalinizing trabecular carcinoma" with capsular and vascular invasion.[33–35] Interestingly, many HTTs are reported to coexist with a papillary carcinoma.[30,36]

Because of histologic overlap with and coexistence of HTT and papillary carcinoma, some investigators have studied the mutational profiles of HTT to investigate genetic similarities with papillary carcinoma. In several series, between 30% and 66% of HTTs have proven to have the RET–PTC translocation that is characteristic of papillary carcinoma.[37–40] The presence of this mutation in HTTs has been used as evidence that HTT is directly related to papillary carcinoma. Interestingly, recent studies of BRAF mutations in HTT has shown that these tumors do not harbor the characteristic point mutations that is seen in papillary carcinomas.[38] Additionally, RAS mutations have not been identified in HTTs.[21]

Tumors with Thymus-Like Differentiation

Two types of tumors of the thyroid gland have been reported to have thymus-like differentiation: carcinoma with thymus-like elements (CASTLE) and spindle epithelial tumor with thymus-like differentiation (SETTLE). Both of these tumors are extremely rare, with very few cases having been reported in the literature. Therefore, experience with these lesions is quite limited and represents the result of examination of only case reports. SETTLE usually is reported to have a reasonably good prognosis, though there are several case reports of patients who have metastases. It has been postulated that these tumors are derived from remnants of thymus within the thyroid gland, or possibly from remnants of the ultimobranchial body.

Carcinoma with Thymus-Like Elements

This very rare tumor has only been reported in about 30 cases in the literature.[41] CASTLE tends to occur in adults, particularly in the fifth decade. Many of these tumors are slow growing and indolent, but occasional aggressive tumors have also been reported.[42]

Grossly, these tumors have a lobular appearance, with multiple lobules of tumor surrounded by fibrous bands. Histologically, the tumor has a unique appearance that can include squamous-like differentiation or features that resemble lymphoepithelial carcinoma or basaloid squamous cell carcinoma. In the lymphoepithelial type of pattern, there are vesicular nuclei growing in a syncytial pattern with variable lymphoplasmacytic infiltrates.[43,44] The tumor cells are negative for thyroglobulin and calcitonin, and may be positive with markers for thymic differentiation, such as CD5.[45–47] CASTLE has not been studied at the molecular level.

Spindle Epithelial Tumor with Thymus-Like Differentiation

SETTLE tumors usually arise in young patients, often in children, with the average age of cases reported in the literature is 18 years.[43] Most of these tumors are reported to have a relatively benign clinical course, but up to 17% of cases are reported with metastases,[48–50] and 13% of patients are reported to die from disease. The tumors are usually biphasic in nature, with the two components including a cellular spindle cell component that is composed of elongated cells with some deposition of fibrous tissue. The second component, which can merge indistinguishably with the spindle cell component, is a glandular or epithelial component. These glandular cells can even be mucinous in nature, though more commonly they consist of nondescript tubules and cystic spaces. Sometimes respiratory type epithelium can be seen. In other cases, well developed epithelial cells are not seen and these are termed "monophasic", but collections of intracellular fluid and cystic mucinous areas may be seen even in these predominantly spindle cell tumors.[51] There is usually low mitotic activity.

At the IHC level, SETTLE is usually negative for thyroglobulin and TTF-1, and should always be negative for calcitonin and CEA.[52] Similar to thymomas, these tumors are positive for cytokeratins and bcl-2. SMA and vimentin have also been reported to be positive. Electron microscopy demonstrates that the tumor has prominent desmosomes and tonofilament bundles, which are seen in thymomas as well. Although this tumor has been postulated to also arise from thymus inclusions or other thymic derivatives, this origin has been disputed since CD5 and CD20, both of which can be expressed in some thymic lesions, are negative in SETTLE.

The molecular mutational profile of these tumors has been largely unexplored. One case has been investigated at the molecular level and was positive for a KRAS mutation and negative for p53 mutations.[53] The differential diagnosis for SETTLE includes other spindle cell neoplasms, including most importantly medullary carcinoma, synovial sarcoma, and anaplastic carcinoma. One recent study used fluorescent in situ hybridization to study a series of 11 cases of SETTLE and 2 unresolved cases for the SS18/SSX1 and SS18/SSX2 translocations that is seen in synovial sarcoma. All 11 of the SETTLE cases were negative for the translocation and the 2 other cases were positive, suggesting that they were true synovial sarcomas of thyroid origin.[54]

References

1. Cameselle-Teijeiro J. Mucoepidermoid carcinoma and solid cell nests of the thyroid. *Hum Pathol.* 1996;27(8):861-863.
2. Wenig BM, Adair CF, Heffess CS. Primary mucoepidermoid carcinoma of the thyroid gland: a report of six cases and a review of the literature of a follicular epithelial-derived tumor. [see comment]. *Hum Pathol.* 1995;26(10):1099–1108.
3. Katoh R, Sugai T, Ono S, et al. Mucoepidermoid carcinoma of the thyroid gland. *Cancer* 1990;65(7):2020–2027.
4. Ando M, Nakanishi Y, Asai M, et al. Mucoepidermoid carcinoma of the thyroid gland showing marked ciliation suggestive of its pathogenesis. *Pathol Int.* 2008;58(11):741–744.
5. Rocha AS, Soares P, Machado JC, et al. Mucoepidermoid carcinoma of the thyroid: a tumour histotype characterised by P-cadherin neoexpression and marked abnormalities of E-cadherin/catenins complex. *Virchows Arch.* 2002;440(5):498–504.
6. Baloch ZW, Solomon AC, LiVolsi VA. Primary mucoepidermoid carcinoma and sclerosing mucoepidermoid carcinoma with eosinophilia of the thyroid gland: a report of nine cases. *Mod Pathol.* 2000;13(7):802–807.
7. Hunt JL: Unusual thyroid tumors: a review of pathologic and molecular diagnosis. *Expert Rev Mol Diagn.* 2005;5(5):725–734.
8. Tirado Y, Williams MD, Hanna EY, et al. CRTC1/MAML2 fusion transcript in high grade mucoepidermoid carcinomas of salivary and thyroid glands and Warthin's tumors: implications for histogenesis and biologic behavior. *Genes Chromosomes Cancer.* 2007;46(7):708–715.
9. Okabe M, Miyabe S, Nagatsuka H, et al. MECT1-MAML2 fusion transcript defines a favorable subset of mucoepidermoid carcinoma. *Clin Cancer Res.* 2006;12(13):3902–3907.
10. Behboudi A, Enlund F, Winnes M, et al. Molecular classification of mucoepidermoid carcinomas-prognostic significance of the MECT1-MAML2 fusion oncogene. *Genes Chromosomes Cancer.* 2006;45(5):470–481.
11. Coxon A, Rozenblum E, Park YS, et al. Mect1---Maml2 fusion oncogene linked to the aberrant activation of cyclic AMP/CREB regulated genes. *Cancer Res.* 2005;65(16):7137–7144.
12. Shehadeh NJ, Vernick J, Lonardo F, et al. Sclerosing mucoepidermoid carcinoma with eosinophilia of the thyroid: a case report and review of the literature. *Am J Otolaryngol.* 2004;25(1):48–53.
13. Albores-Saavedra J, Gu X, Luna MA. Clear cells and thyroid transcription factor I reactivity in sclerosing mucoepidermoid carcinoma of the thyroid gland. *Ann Diagn Pathol.* 2003;7(6):348–353.
14. Geisinger KR, Steffee CH, McGee RS, et al. The cytomorphologic features of sclerosing mucoepidermoid carcinoma of the thyroid gland with eosinophilia. *Am J Clin Pathol.* 1998;109(3):294–301.
15. Arezzo A, Patetta R, Ceppa P, et al. Mucoepidermoid carcinoma of the thyroid gland arising from a papillary epithelial neoplasm. *Am Surg.* 1998;64(4):307–311.
16. Hunt JL, LiVolsi VA, Barnes EL. p63 expression in sclerosing mucoepidermoid carcinomas with eosinophilia arising in the thyroid. *Mod Pathol.* 2004;17(5):526–529.
17. LiVolsi VA. Hyalinizing trabecular tumor of the thyroid: adenoma, carcinoma, or neoplasm of uncertain malignant potential? *Am J Surg Pathol.* 2000;24(12):1683–1684.
18. Chetty R, Beydoun R, LiVolsi VA. Paraganglioma-like (hyalinizing trabecular) adenoma of the thyroid revisited. *Pathology.* 1994;26(4):429–431.
19. Carney JA, Ryan J, Goellner JR. Hyalinizing trabecular adenoma of the thyroid gland. *Am J Surg Pathol.* 1987;11(8):583–591.
20. Sambade C, Franssila K, Cameselle-Teijeiro J, et al. Hyalinizing trabecular adenoma: a misnomer for a peculiar tumor of the thyroid gland. *Endocr Pathol.* 1991;2:83–91.
21. Carney JA, Hirokawa M, Lloyd RV, et al. Hyalinizing trabecular tumors of the thyroid gland are almost all benign. *Am J Surg Pathol.* 2008;32(1):1877–1889.
22. Katoh R, Muramatsu A, Kawaoi A, et al. Alteration of the basement membrane in human thyroid diseases: an immunohistochemical study of type IV collagen, laminin and heparan sulphate proteoglycan. *Virchows Archiv A, Pathol Anat Histopathol.* 1993;423(6):417–424.
23. Katoh R, Jasani B, Williams ED. Hyalinizing trabecular adenoma of the thyroid. A report of three cases with immunohistochemical and ultrastructural studies. *Histopathol.* 1989;15(3):211–224.
24. Huss LJ, Mendelsohn G. Medullary carcinoma of the thyroid gland: an encapsulated variant resembling the hyalinizing trabecular (paraganglioma-like) adenoma of thyroid. *Mod Pathol.* 1990;3(5):581–585.

25. Goellner JR, Carney JA. Cytologic features of fine-needle aspirates of hyalinizing trabecular adenoma of the thyroid. *Am J Clin Pathol.* 1989;91(2):115–119.
26. Casey MB, Sebo TJ, Carney JA. Hyalinizing trabecular adenoma of the thyroid gland: cytologic features in 29 cases. *Am J Surg Pathol.* 2004;28(7):859–867.
27. Rothenberg HJ, Goellner JR, Carney JA. Prevalence and incidence of cytoplasmic yellow bodies in thyroid neoplasms. *Arch Pathol Lab Med.* 2003;127(6):715–717.
28. Rothenberg HJ, Goellner JR, Carney JA. Hyalinizing trabecular adenoma of the thyroid gland: recognition and characterization of its cytoplasmic yellow body. *Am J Surg Pathol.* 1999;23(1): 118–125.
29. Hirokawa M, Carney JA, Ohtsuki Y. Hyalinizing trabecular adenoma and papillary carcinoma of the thyroid gland express different cytokeratin patterns. *Am J Surg Pathol.* 2000;24(6): 877–881.
30. Fonseca E, Nesland JM, Sobrinho-Simoes M. Expression of stratified epithelial-type cytokeratins in hyalinizing trabecular adenomas supports their relationship with papillary carcinomas of the thyroid. *Histopathology.* 1997;31(4):330–335.
31. Gaffney RL, Carney JA, Sebo TJ, et al. Galectin-3 expression in hyalinizing trabecular tumors of the thyroid gland. *Am J Surg Pathol.* 2003;27(4):494–498.
32. LaGuette J, Matias-Guiu X, Rosai J. Thyroid paraganglioma: a clinicopathologic and immunohistochemical study of three cases. *Am J Surg Pathol.* 1997;21(7):748–753.
33. Gonzalez-Campora R, Fuentes-Vaamonde E, Hevia-Vazquez A, et al. Hyalinizing trabecular carcinoma of the thyroid gland: report of two cases of follicular cell thyroid carcinoma with hyalinizing trabecular pattern. *Ultrastruct Pathol.* 1998;22(1):39–46.
34. Molberg K, Albores-Saavedra J. Hyalinizing trabecular carcinoma of the thyroid gland. *Hum Pathol.* 1994;25(2):192–197.
35. McCluggage WG, Sloan JM. Hyalinizing trabecular carcinoma of thyroid gland. *Histopathology*. 1996;28(4):357–362.
36. Papotti M, Riella P, Montemurro F, et al. Immunophenotypic heterogeneity of hyalinizing trabecular tumours of the thyroid. *Histopathology.* 1997;31(6):525–533.
37. Cheung CC, Boerner SL, MacMillan CM, et al. Hyalinizing trabecular tumor of the thyroid: a variant of papillary carcinoma proved by molecular genetics. *Am J Surg Pathol.* 2000;24(12):1622–626.
38. Salvatore G, Chiappetta G, Nikiforov YE, et al. Molecular profile of hyalinizing trabecular tumours of the thyrod: high prevalence of RET/PTC rearrangements and absence of B-raf and N-ras piont mutations. *Eur J Cancer.* 2005;41:816–821.
39. Lloyd RV. Hyalinizing trabecular tumors of the thyroid: a variant of papillary carcinoma? *Adv Anat Pathol.* 2002;9(1):7–11.
40. Papotti M, Volante M, Giuliano A, et al. RET/PTC activation in hyalinizing trabecular tumors of the thyroid. *Am J Surg Pathol.* 2000;24(12):1615–1621.
41. Roka S, Kornek G, Schuller J, et al. Carcinoma showing thymic-like elements--a rare malignancy of the thyroid gland. *Br J Surg.* 2004;91(2):142–145.
42. Cappelli C, Tironi A, Marchetti GP, et al. Aggressive thyroid carcinoma showing thymic-like differentiation (CASTLE): case report and review of the literature. *Endocr J* 2008;55(4):685–690.
43. Chan JK, Rosai J. Tumors of the neck showing thymic or related branchial pouch differentiation: a unifying concept. *Hum Pathol.* 1991;22(4):349–367.
44. Ahuja AT, Chan ES, Allen PW, et al. Carcinoma showing thymiclike differentiation (CASTLE tumor). *AJNR: Am J Neuroradiol.* 1998;19(7):1225–1228.
45. Ito Y, Miyauchi A, Nakamura Y, et al. Clinicopathologic significance of intrathyroidal epithelial thymoma/carcinoma showing thymus-like differentiation: a collaborative study with Member Institutes of The Japanese Society of Thyroid Surgery. *Am J Clin Pathol.* 2007;127(2):230–236.
46. Dorfman DM, Shahsafaei A, Miyauchi A. Intrathyroidal epithelial thymoma (ITET)/carcinoma showing thymus-like differentiation (CASTLE) exhibits CD5 immunoreactivity: new evidence for thymic differentiation. *Histopathology.* 1998;32(2):104–109.
47. Yamazaki M, Fujii S, Daiko H, et al. Carcinoma showing thymus-like differentiation (CASTLE) with neuroendocrine differentiation. *Pathol Int.* 2008;58(12):775–779.
48. Cheuk W, Jacobson AA, Chan JK: Spindle epithelial tumor with thymus-like differentiation (SETTLE): a distinctive malignant thyroid neoplasm with significant metastatic potential. *Mod Pathol.* 2000;13(10):1150–1155.
49. Erickson ML, Tapia B, Moreno ER, et al. Early metastasizing spindle epithelial tumor with thymus-like differentiation (SETTLE) of the thyroid. *Pediatr Dev Pathol.* 2005;8(5):599–606.
50. Raffel A, Cupisti K, Rees M, et al. Spindle epithelial tumour with thymus-like differentiation (SETTLE) of the thyroid gland with widespread metastases in a 13-year-old girl. *Clin Oncol (R Coll Radiol)* 2003;15(8):490–495.
51. Chetty R, Goetsch S, Nayler S, et al. Spindle epithelial tumour with thymus-like element (SETTLE): the predominantly monophasic variant. Histopathology. 1998;33(1):71–74.
52. Su L, Beals T, Bernacki EG, et al. Spindle epithelial tumor with thymus-like differentiation: a case report with cytologic, histologic, immunohistologic, and ultrastructural findings. *Mod Pathol.* 1997;10(5):510–514.
53. Xu B, Hirokawa M, Yoshimoto K, et al. Spindle epithelial tumor with thymus-like differentiation of the thyroid: a case report with pathological and molecular genetics study. *Hum Pathol* 2003;34(2):190–193.
54. Folpe AL, Lloyd RV, Bacchi CE, et al. Spindle Epithelial Tumor with Thymus-Like Differentiation (SETTLE): A Morphological, Immunohistochemical and Molecular Genetic Study of 11 Cases. *Am J Surg Pathol.* 2009;33(8):1179–1186.

13
Hematopoietic Tumors of the Thyroid

Lawrence Tsao and Eric Hsi

Introduction

Primary lymphoma of the thyroid gland is a relatively uncommon disease. The term "primary thyroid lymphoma" (PTL) is a nonspecific, broad term referring to any lymphoma restricted to the thyroid gland. Further classification of PTL is clinically necessary and should be based on histologic, phenotypic, and molecular features using the current World Health Organization (WHO) classification system. Both Hodgkin and many types of non-Hodgkin lymphomas can occur as a PTL. However, the most common types of PTL are extranodal marginal zone B-cell lymphoma of mucosa-associated lymphoid tissue (MALT lymphomas) and diffuse large B-cell lymphomas, NOS (DLBCL).

The molecular genetic changes of PTL vary with the type of lymphoma. In many cases, it is unclear whether PTL are truly distinct entities from their systemic counterparts. For example, follicular lymphomas of the thyroid are identical to systemic follicular lymphomas histologically and phenotypically, and even show identical molecular abnormalities (i.e., IGH/BCL2 translocations). Therefore, in many instances, the molecular genetics of the PTL are simply that of the systemic counterpart of the particular subtype.

MALT lymphomas and DLBCL of the thyroid, although histologically and phenotypically indistinguishable from their counterparts, at other sites show distinct molecular pathogenesis from MALT lymphomas and DLBCL of other sites. The association with chronic lymphocytic thyroiditis has long been established by epidemiologic studies. Recent studies have implicated numerous molecular lesions and pathways, including proliferation and antiapoptotic targets, in the pathogenesis and progression of chronic lymphocytic thyroiditis to MALT lymphoma in the thyroid. However, the data is currently still limited. In this chapter, we review, specifically, MALT lymphomas and DLBCL of the thyroid.

Background

PTL is an uncommon disease accounting for approximately 1–5% of all primary thyroid neoplasms[1,2] and 2–7% of extranodal lymphomas.[1,3] Characteristically, PTL presents in older females (M:F 2.5–30, median age 59.5–66.3 years) most commonly as a thyroid mass.[4–6] Thyroid dysfunction can be present especially with concurrent chronic lymphocytic thyroiditis, which has been observed in a third to >90% of the cases.[4,5] At presentation, PTL are most commonly low stage (IE or IIE) and demonstrate a relatively good response to combined modality therapy (CMT) including surgical, radiation, and/or chemotherapy.[7–9] Localized PTL treated with CMT has overall good 5-year survival ranging from 70 to 90%.[7–9] DLBCL and high grade histologic subtypes show a relatively worse prognosis when compared to MALT lymphomas and low grade histologic subtypes.[4–6,10] In PTL with mixed histologic types, especially DLBCL and MALT lymphomas, the prognosis is dictated by high grade histology.[4,6] Of the prognostic factors, the histologic type, stage, and patient performance status are consistently significant.

Although almost all histologic types of lymphomas, including Burkitt lymphoma,[5] follicular lymphoma,[4,5] Hodgkin lymphomas,[5,11] and rarely T-cell lymphomas have been reported in the literature as a PTL, the vast majority (70–90%) of PTL are of the DLBCL, MALT lymphoma, or combined features of DLBCL and MALT lymphoma histology.[4,5]

Histologically, DLBCL and MALT lymphomas of the thyroid are indistinguishable from lymphomas of the same histologic type involving other sites. Although by no means specific, morphologic features including prominent, destructive lymphoepithelial lesions, prominent plasmacytic differentiation, and lymphocyte "stuffing" of the glandular lumen can be seen in MALT lymphomas involving the thyroid.[12] Generally, MALT lymphomas of the thyroid show a nodular lymphoid infiltrate of predominantly small lymphocytes

J.L. Hunt (ed.), *Molecular Pathology of Endocrine Diseases*, Molecular Pathology Library 3,
DOI 10.1007/978-1-4419-1707-2_13,

with slightly irregular nuclei, mature chromatin, and moderate clear cytoplasm, so-called "monocytoid" morphology (Figure 13.1). Although it is not unusual for plasma cell differentiation or plasmacytoid morphology to be present, MALT lymphomas can rarely show extreme plasma cell differentiation, mimicking an extramedullary plasmacytoma. In cases with prominent plasmacytic differentiation, Dutcher bodies and cytoplasmic immunoglobulin accumulations can be seen (Figure 13.2). Thus, diagnosis of plasmacytoma at this site should only be made after exclusion of even a minor component of MALT lymphoma and should be reserved for resection specimens.

DLBCL of the thyroid can be seen concurrently with MALT lymphomas (Figure 13.3) as single or multiple foci, or

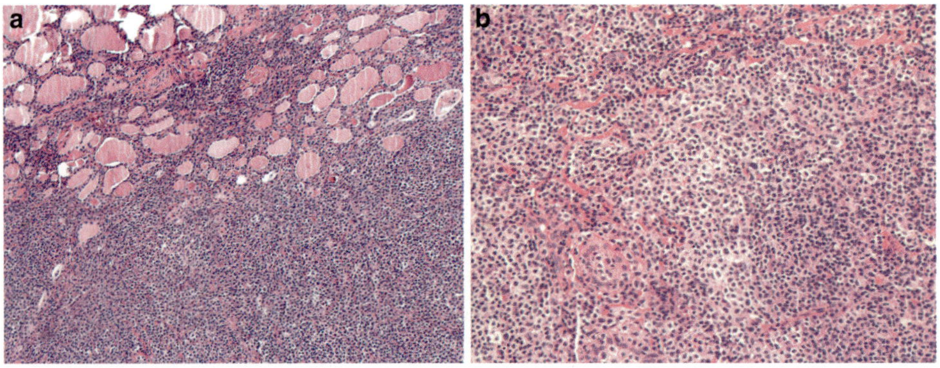

FIG. 13.1. Low grade MALT lymphoma of the thyroid. (**a**) Lymphoid proliferation showing destructive infiltration of thyroid follicular architecture (H&E, ×100). (**b**) The lymphoid proliferation consists of small lymphocytes with irregular nuclei, mature chromatin, and scant to moderate clear cytoplasm, consistent with monocytoid morphology. Occasional scattered larger lymphocytes can be present (H&E, ×200).

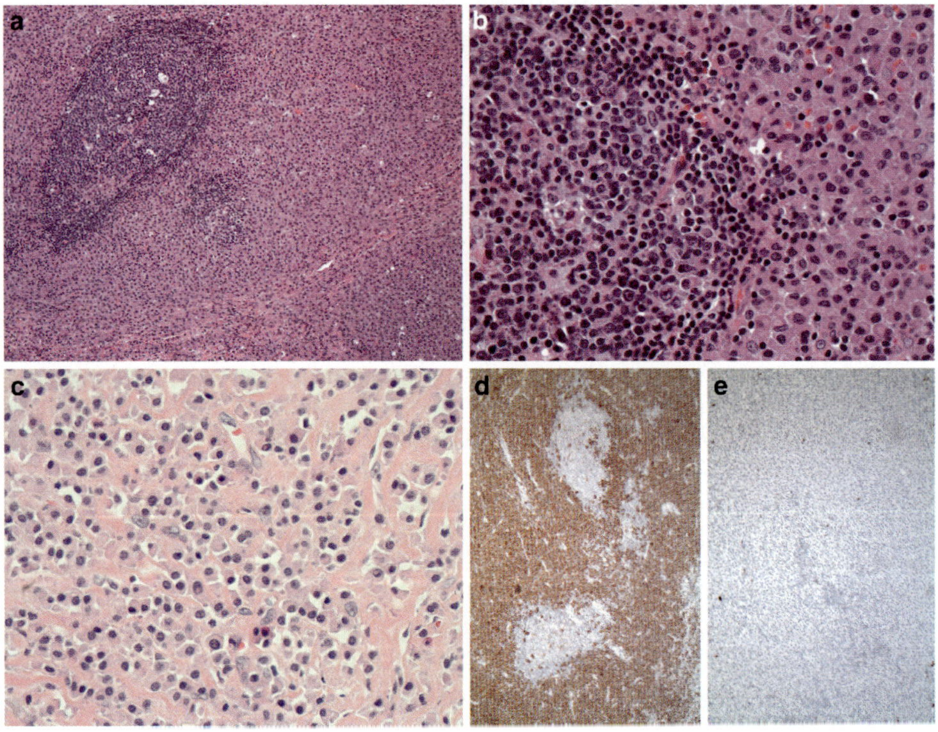

FIG. 13.2. Low grade MALT lymphoma of the thyroid with prominent plasma cell differentiation. (**a**) Lymphoid aggregates of small lymphocytes with prominent plasma cell proliferation. No identifiable residual thyroid architecture is present (H&E, ×100). (**b**) There is a distinct interface between the lymphocytes and plasma cells, but gradual interfaces with plasmacytoid lymphocytes can also be seen (H&E, ×400). (**c**) Prominent plasma cell differentiation can mimic plasma cell neoplasms. Dutcher bodies are present (H&E, ×400). (**d, e**) Plasma cell differentiation can be highlighted with immunohistochemistry for kappa and lambda light chains. The plasma cells in this case are kappa light chain restricted (**d**, kappa IHC; **e**, lambda IHC).

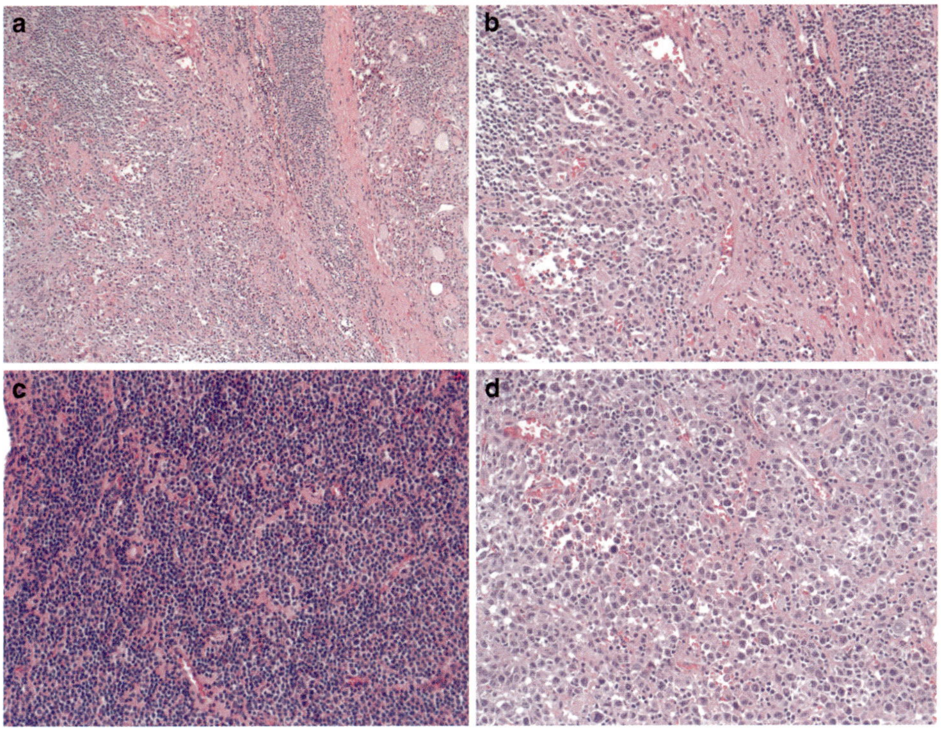

FIG. 13.3. Low grade MALT lymphoma with DLBCL component in thyroid. (**a**) Interface between low grade MALT (*right*) and DLBCL (*left*) in thyroid (H&E, ×100). (**b**) Higher magnification shows large transformed cells intermixed with small mature lymphocytes (H&E, ×200). (**c, d**) In other areas, there is predominantly low grade MALT lymphoma or DLCBL (H&E, ×200).

as the predominant histologic type. Cytologically, DLBCL of the thyroid are large transformed cells with irregular nuclei, vesicular chromatin, prominent nucleoli, and scant cytoplasm (Figure 13.3). Morphologic variants including centroblastic, immunoblastic, and anaplastic can be seen either focally or as the predominant histology. Focally, Burkitt morphology with intermediate-sized cells and regular to slightly irregular nuclei, fine chromatin, and scant basophilic cytoplasm can be present. When large areas are present, DLBCL need to be differentiated from Burkitt lymphoma, which can rarely present involving thyroid (Figure 13.4). Burkitt lymphomas should show the characteristic phenotype (CD20+, CD10+, BCL-2–, and Ki-67 proliferation index >95%) with translocation of the *MYC* gene and the absence of other translocations (i.e., *BCL2* or *BCL6*). Lymphoepithelial lesions are frequently present especially in cases with concurrent areas of MALT lymphoma. In some cases, large transformed cells are seen infiltrating epithelium and glands (Figure 13.5).

DLBCL, MALT lymphoma, and combined DLBCL and MALT lymphomas of the thyroid will all frequently show concurrent chronic lymphocytic thyroiditis. In these cases, follicular hyperplasia with or without colonization by neoplastic cells can be present. In some cases, the follicular hyperplasia can be so extensive as to mimic follicular lymphoma.

Morphology and immunophenotyping are the diagnostic mainstays for PTL. Flow cytometric analysis is the preferred method for phenotyping, but is limited by availability and the requirement for fresh tissue. In the absence of fresh samples, immunohistochemical staining using formalin fixed, paraffin embedded tissue can be used as an alternative. Primary thyroid DLBCL and MALT lymphomas are phenotypically similar to DLBCL and extranodal MALT lymphomas of other sites. Table 13.1 shows the characteristic phenotype of the various common histologic types of PTL.

Genetics

The molecular pathogenesis of PTL, as previously mentioned, is dependent on the specific histologic and phenotypic subtype. For many subtypes of PTL (i.e., Burkitt lymphoma, follicular lymphoma, etc.), the molecular changes, although not well-characterized in thyroid, are identical to their systemic counterparts. However, the two most common PTL, primary MALT lymphoma, and DLBCL of the thyroid have different clinical and molecular findings. Most importantly, unlike MALT lymphomas of other sites including gastric, pulmonary, and orbital, primary MALT lymphomas of the thyroid gland rarely show abnormalities involving the *MALT1* or *BCL10* gene.[13,14] Primary thyroid MALT lymphomas, however, show a close association to chronic lymphocytic thyroiditis including Hashimoto thyroiditis and Sjogren syndrome.[15–17] Similar to the association of gastric MALT lymphomas to *Helicobacter* infection, chronic antigen stimulation appears

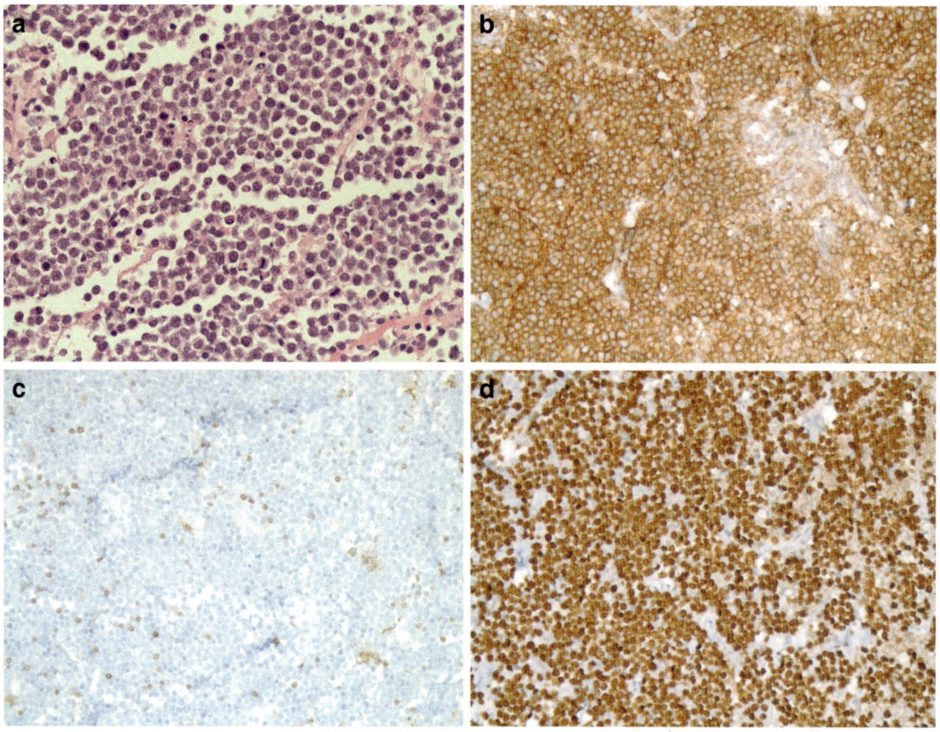

FIG. 13.4. Burkitt lymphoma of thyroid. (**a**) There is a monomorphic proliferation of intermediate lymphoid cells with round nuclei, homogenous chromatin, and scant cytoplasm. No identifiable underlying thyroid architecture is present. Numerous mitotic figures and apoptotic bodies are present. Macrophages impart a "starry sky" appearance (H&E, ×200). (**b**) The lymphocytes are B-cells expressing CD20, CD10, and BCL-6 (CD20 IHC, ×100). (**c**) There is no coexpression of BCL-2 (BCL-2 IHC, ×100). (**d**) The Ki-67 proliferation index approaches 100% (Ki-67 IHC, ×100).

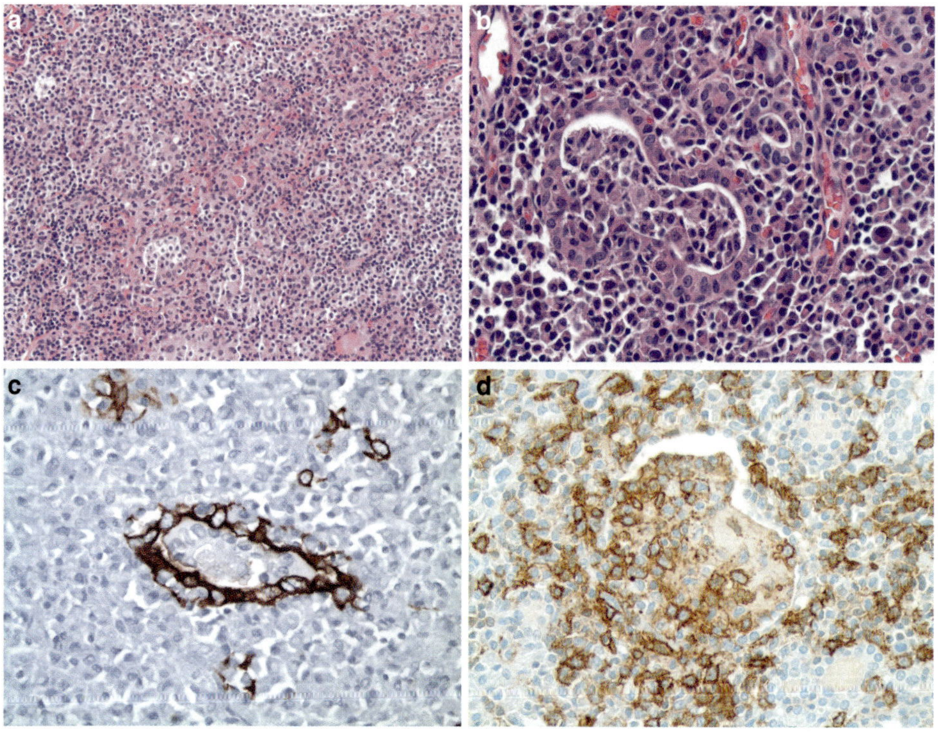

FIG. 13.5. Lymphoepithelial lesions. (**a**) Low power view of lymphoepithelial lesions with predominantly small lymphocytes infiltrating and disrupting thyroid follicles (H&E, ×100). (**b**) Higher power view of a thyroid follicle "stuffed" with larger transformed lymphocytes (H&E, ×200). (**c**) Cytokeratin stain highlights residual thyroid follicular epithelium disrupted by the lymphoma cells (CK IHC, ×200). (**d**) CD20 stain shows the large lymphocytes infiltrating and filling the lumen of a thyroid follicle (CD20 IHC, ×200).

TABLE 13.1. Key characteristics of some common lymphomas presenting as primary thyroid lymphomas.

Lymphoma type	Morphologic features	Characteristic phenotype	Characteristic molecular features
DLBCL	Intermediate to large transformed cells. Centroblastic, immunoblastic, anaplastic, T-cell/histiocyte rich variants	CD19+, CD20+, CD79a+, BCL-2+/–, Ki-67 index 40–90% Germinal center: CD10+, BCL-6+, LMO2+ Activated B-cell: MUM-1+	t(14;18)(q32;q21): IGH/BCL-2 3q27: BCL-6 abnormalities
MALT lymphoma	Small cells with "monocytoid" morphology. Lymphoepithelial lesions present. Prominent plasma cell differentiation. Presence of increased large cells in high grade and mixed DLBCL and MALT lymphoma type	CD19+, CD20+, CD79a+, CD5–, CD10–, CD23–, CD43+/–, cyclin-D1– Plasma cell differentiation: CD138+, Kappa/Lambda restricted	Varies with site. Refer to Table-13.3.
Follicular lymphoma	Nodular architecture with mixed small cleaved cells and large centroblasts. Increased centroblasts correspond with higher grade.	CD19+, CD20+, CD79a+, CD10+, BCL-6+, BCL-2+	t(14;18)(q32;q21): IGH/BCL2 3q27: BCL-6 abnormalities
Classical Hodgkin lymphoma	Reed-Sternberg or Hodgkin cells in a mixed inflammatory background	Reed-Sternberg and Hodgkin cells: CD30+, CD15+/–, PAX5+, CD45–, CD20–, OCT21+, BOB11+	None
Small lymphocytic leukemia	Diffuse small round lymphocytes with clumped chromatin and scant cytoplasm	CD19+, CD20+, CD5+, CD23+, FMC-7–, CD10–, BCL6–, cyclin-D1–	13q14 Trisomy 12 11q22-23: ATM 17p13: P53
Burkitt lymphoma	Diffuse, monomorphic intermediate sized cells with basophilic cytoplasm. High apoptotic and mitotic rate with "starry-sky" appearance.	CD19+, CD20+, CD10+, BCL-6+, Ki-67 index (100%), BCL-2–	8q24: MYC abnormality

to play a role in the lymphomagenesis of MALT lymphomas of the thyroid. The molecular changes of DLBCL in thyroid are not well understood, but an association with underlying MALT lymphomas of the thyroid and chronic lymphocytic thyroiditis has been noted.[4–6] Studies have suggested numerous molecular pathways, including cytokine induced proliferation,[18,19] inhibition of apoptosis,[20–23] and loss of cell cycle regulation,[23–27] might be involved in the pathogenesis of these lymphomas.

MALT Lymphomas

The association between MALT lymphoma and chronic antigenic stimulation is seen in the prototypic gastric MALT lymphoma and *Helicobacter* infection.[28–31] Infections by other organisms have been suggested in MALT lymphomas arising at other sites (Table 13.2). In recent studies, the molecular changes of MALT lymphomas have been further elucidated. These studies have implicated the activation of the NF-kB pathway as the common pathway in the pathogenesis of MALT lymphomas.[32–35] Translocations of the *MALT1* and *BCL10* genes have been characterized in a subset of MALT lymphomas (Table 13.3).[13,14] The most common *API2–MALT1* translocation results in upregulation of MALT1 and has been shown to participate in the activation of NF-kB pathway upon antigen stimulation.[36] However, MALT lymphomas of the thyroid rarely show translocation of *BCL10* and *MALT1*. The t(3;14)(p13;q32) translocation of *FOXP1* gene results in its deregulation. FOXP1 belongs to the Forkhead box (Fox)

TABLE 13.2. Epidemiological associations between MALT lymphomas and microorganisms.

MALT lymphoma site	Organism	Response to antibiotics
Gastric	*Helicobacter pylori*[29–31]	Yes[28]
	Helicobacter heilmannii[41]	Yes[41]
Intestinal (IPSID)[a]	*Campylobacter jejuni*[42]	Unknown
Skin	*Borrelia burgdorferi*[43,44]	Yes[45]
Ocular	*Chlamydia psittaci*[b]	Yes[46]
Thyroid	Unknown	Unknown

[a]IPSID, immunoproliferative small intestinal disease.
[b]Geographic variation of association seen.[47–49]

TABLE 13.3. Common translocations of MALT lymphomas of specific sites.

Translocation	Gene	Common MALT lymphoma sites[13,50]
t(11;18)(q21;q21)	*API2–MALT1*	Lung, gastrointestinal, ocular
t(1;14)(q22;q32)	*BCL10–MALT1*	Lung, gastric, ocular
t(14;18)(q32;q21)	*IGH–MALT1*	Lung, ocular, skin[51]
t(3;14)(p14.1;q32)	*FOXP1–IGH*	Ocular, skin, thyroid[37]

family of transcription factors and is involved in the regulation of B-cell development. This translocation was initially found in a significant proportion of MALT lymphomas of the thyroid.[37] However, subsequent studies have not confirmed this to be a significant molecular change in MALT lymphomas of the thyroid.

The close association between chronic lymphocytic thyroiditis and MALT lymphomas of the thyroid has implicated chronic antigen stimulation as a factor in the lymphomagenesis of MALT lymphomas in the thyroid. Patients with PTL will frequently have serum antibodies directed toward the thyroid.[5] The relative risk of MALT lymphoma in patients with Hashimoto thyroiditis is estimated to be as high as 67.[38] Molecular analysis of the immunoglobulin heavy chain (IGH) by PCR have identified clonal B-cell populations in a small subset of Hashimoto thyroiditis.[16] These B-cell clones are frequently seen in a background of polyclonal B-cells or as multiple clones, and are believed to be localized.[16] When cases of Hashimoto thyroiditis are compared with sub sequent MALT lymphomas, sequencing of the IGH gene shows homology between the B-cell clones seen in Hashimoto thyroiditis and the lymphoma, suggesting that the lymphoma arises from clones within the Hashimoto thyroiditis.[15] In addition, analysis of VH immunoglobulin gene usage shows a preference for VH3 and VH4 families, and may provide clues to the antigens that may be responsible for the development of MALT lymphoma. In one study, 89% of MALT lymphomas of the thyroid showed usage of VH3 (50%) or VH4 (38%) families. A subset of the VH genes in the MALT lymphomas showed sequence homology to the antibody of thyroglobulin and thyroid peroxidase, suggesting these lymphomas are derived from lymphocytes associated with antithyroid antibodies as seen in Hashimoto thyroiditis.[39]

Although chronic antigenic stimulation is likely to be an important initiating factor in the lymphogenesis of MALT lymphomas of the thyroid, secondary molecular changes are believed to be necessary. Studies comparing chronic lymphocytic thyroiditis with MALT lymphomas of the thyroid have suggested secondary molecular changes involving apoptosis signal transduction may be involved. In one study examining the Fas gene, an accumulation of Fas gene mutations was identified in PTL, especially MALT lymphomas.[22] These Fas mutations were most frequently frameshift mutations resulting in truncated forms of Fas protein with reduced response to Fas ligand (FasL) and apoptotic signal transduction. Death-associated protein-kinase (DAP-kinase) gene, a serine/threonine kinase involved in apoptosis induced by interferon-gamma, tumor necrosis factor-gamma (TNF-gamma), and FasL, was shown to have increased methylation in MALT lymphomas versus chronic lymphocytic thyroiditis.[21] Survivin, another protein belonging to a family of antiapoptotic proteins, has been reported to be highly expressed in PTL, including MALT lymphomas.[20] Molecular changes resulting in increased proliferation have also been suggested. One study found increased mRNA transcripts of IL-7, a stimulatory cytokine, in PTL.[18]

One can see that the molecular pathogenesis of primary MALT lymphoma of the thyroid is not well-understood. The close association with chronic lymphocytic thyroiditis suggests that chronic antigenic stimulation probably plays the role of an initiating factor. Although there is data suggesting additional secondary molecular genetic changes, these are currently not well characterized. However, a defect of apoptosis signal transduction pathways appears to be involved.

Diffuse Large B-Cell Lymphoma

At least a subset of DLBCL of the thyroid is believed to arise from preexisting MALT lymphomas of the thyroid. In one study of 108 cases of thyroid lymphoma, up to one-third of the cases morphologically showed DLBCL with areas of MALT lymphoma.[4] In some cases, there is not always a distinct separation between the areas of DLBCL and MALT lymphoma.[6] Although morphologically there appears to be close association between DLBCL and MALT lymphomas of the thyroid, the few molecular studies examining these lymphomas have shown, as expected, molecular heterogeneity between DLBCL and MALT lymphomas. The usage of the VH gene family has been evaluated and showed a preferential usage of VH4 immunoglobulin gene in MALT lymphomas of the thyroid, while the majority (89%) of the DLBCL of the thyroid used the VH3 immunoglobulin gene, suggesting that at least a subset of the DLBCL of the thyroid is de novo and develops in the absence of a preexisting MALT lymphoma.[39]

The molecular progression of MALT lymphomas to DLBCL of the thyroid is an area of interest. However, the current understanding of this progression is limited. Microsatellite instability suggests genetic instability may play a role, but data is limited to small studies.[23] Mutations in oncogenes and tumor suppressor genes including *KRAS* and *p53* have also been implicated.[23] Dysregulation of the cell cycle appears to play some role. Most studies evaluating expression by immunohistochemical techniques suggest dysregulation of cell cycle regulators in PTL correlate with the aggressiveness of the lymphoma.[24–27,40] However, most of the data is limited to small studies and have not been adequately reproduced.

Special Techniques

Morphology and immunophenotyping by flow cytometry or immunohistochemistry remain standard diagnostic procedures for PTL. However, molecular techniques can be helpful in difficult cases.

Immunoglobulin Heavy Chain

PCR analysis of the *IGH* gene rearrangement is a well established technique for identifying clonal B-cell populations. *IGH* gene rearrangement analysis can be helpful in differentiating reactive infiltrates of chronic lymphocytic thyroiditis from the low grade MALT lymphomas. However, *IGH* gene rearrangements can be absent in up to 30% of DLBCL and MALT lymphomas of the thyroid.[39] In addition, as previously discussed, minor clonal populations can be seen in chronic lymphocytic thyroiditis. These minor clones are infrequent, not reproducible, and are usually minor populations within a polyclonal background.[15,16] Currently, determining VH gene usage and sequencing are diagnostically unnecessary.

Fluorescent In Situ Hybridization

The utility of fluorescent in situ hybridization (FISH) varies with the type of PTL. In PTL types with characteristic molecular changes (Table 13.1), FISH can be diagnostically useful. For example, FISH for the *BCL2/IGH* translocation can be useful for differentiating follicular lymphoma of the thyroid from a follicular hyperplasia. However, in types of PTL lacking specific molecular genetics detectable by FISH, like MALT lymphomas, the utility of FISH is limited.

Cytogenetics

Cytogenetic karyotyping is helpful, but has limitations as a diagnostic test. Karyotyping can identify clonal population that may show specific or nonspecific genetic changes. Generally, the presence of clonal genetic abnormalities is evidence supportive of a neoplastic process. However, cytogenetic karyotyping requires fresh tissue sampled from involved areas. In addition, karyotyping is a time and labor intensive procedure with delayed results. Low grade lymphoproliferative disorders are not always detected by karyotyping and when detected, can show only nonspecific changes not helpful for subclassification. The yield and utility of cytogenetic karyotyping in PTL varies with the availability of FISH and specific histologic type.

Summary

The term "primary thyroid lymphoma" refers to a heterogeneous group of lymphomas of predominantly B-cell lineage, although rare T-cell lymphomas have been reported. PTL are rare entities and current data has been limited to predominantly small studies. The difficulty in differentiating PTL from systemic lymphomas involving thyroid further complicate studies in the area. Although it includes a wide spectrum of entities with widely disparate clinical, morphologic, and phenotypic features, the vast majority fall into DLBCL and MALT lymphoma histological types. The molecular changes of most PTL are unknown, but seem to correspond with their systemic counterparts. However, there is evidence that MALT lymphomas and DLBCL of the thyroid follow alternative paths of lymphomagenesis. Additional studies are necessary as the molecular pathogenesis of the most common histologic types of PTL, MALT lymphoma and DLBCL, are still largely unknown.

References

1. Freeman C, Berg JW, Cutler SJ. Occurrence and prognosis of extranodal lymphomas. *Cancer*. 1972;29:252–260.
2. Staunton MD, Greening WP. Clinical diagnosis of thyroid cancer. *Br Med J*. 1973;4:532–535.
3. Aozasa K, Tsujimoto M, Sakurai M, et al. Non-Hodgkin's lymphomas in Osaka, Japan. *Eur J Cancer Clin Oncol*. 1985;21:487–492.
4. Derringer GA, Thompson LD, Frommelt RA, Bijwaard KE, Heffess CS, Abbondanzo SL. Malignant lymphoma of the thyroid gland: a clinicopathologic study of 108 cases. *Am J Surg Pathol*. 2000;24:623–639.
5. Thieblemont C, Mayer A, Dumontet C, et al. Primary thyroid lymphoma is a heterogeneous disease. *J Clin Endocrinol Metab*. 2002;87:105–111.
6. Skacel M, Ross CW, Hsi ED. A reassessment of primary thyroid lymphoma: high-grade MALT-type lymphoma as a distinct subtype of diffuse large B-cell lymphoma. *Histopathology*. 2000;37:10–18.
7. Belal AA, Allam A, Kandil A, et al. Primary thyroid lymphoma: a retrospective analysis of prognostic factors and treatment outcome for localized intermediate and high grade lymphoma. *Am J Clin Oncol*. 2001;24:299–305.
8. DiBiase SJ, Grigsby PW, Guo C, Lin HS, Wasserman TH. Outcome analysis for stage IE and IIE thyroid lymphoma. *Am J Clin Oncol*. 2004;27:178–184.
9. Ha CS, Shadle KM, Medeiros LJ, et al. Localized non-Hodgkin lymphoma involving the thyroid gland. *Cancer*. 2001;91:629–635.
10. Niitsu N, Okamoto M, Nakamura N, Nakamine H, Bessho M, Hirano M. Clinicopathologic correlations of stage IE/IIE primary thyroid diffuse large B-cell lymphoma. *Ann Oncol*. 2007;18:1203–1208.
11. Wang SA, Rahemtullah A, Faquin WC, Roepke J, Harris NL, Hasserjian RP. Hodgkin's lymphoma of the thyroid: a clinicopathologic study of five cases and review of the literature. *Mod Pathol*. 2005;18:1577–1584.
12. Rawal A, Finn WG, Schnitzer B, Valdez R. Site-specific morphologic differences in extranodal marginal zone B-cell lymphomas. *Arch Pathol Lab Med*. 2007;131:1673–1678.
13. Remstein ED, Dogan A, Einerson RR, et al. The incidence and anatomic site specificity of chromosomal translocations in primary extranodal marginal zone B-cell lymphoma of mucosa-associated lymphoid tissue (MALT lymphoma) in North America. *Am J Surg Pathol*. 2006;30:1546–1553.
14. Joao C, Farinha P, da Silva MG, Martins C, Crespo M, Cabecadas J. Cytogenetic abnormalities in MALT lymphomas and their

precursor lesions from different organs. A fluorescence in situ hybridization (FISH) study. *Histopathology*. 2007;50:217–224.
15. Moshynska OV, Saxena A. Clonal relationship between Hashimoto thyroiditis and thyroid lymphoma. *J Clin Pathol*. 2008;61:438–444.
16. Saxena A, Alport EC, Moshynska O, Kanthan R, Boctor MA. Clonal B cell populations in a minority of patients with Hashimoto's thyroiditis. *J Clin Pathol*. 2004;57:1258–1263.
17. Dong L, Masaki Y, Takegami T, et al. Clonality analysis of lymphoproliferative disorders in patients with Sjogren's syndrome. *Clin Exp Immunol*. 2007;150:279–284.
18. Takakuwa T, Nomura S, Matsuzuka F, Inoue H, Aozasa K. Expression of interleukin-7 and its receptor in thyroid lymphoma. *Lab Invest*. 2000;80:1483–1490.
19. Ohshima K, Suefuji H, Karube K, et al. Expression of chemokine receptor CXCR3 and its ligand, mig, in gastric and thyroid marginal zone lymphomas. Possible migration and autocrine mechanism. *Leuk Lymphoma*. 2003;44:329–336.
20. Sugawara M, Matsuzuka F, Fukata S, Kuma K, Moatamed F, Haugen BR. Excessive survivin expression in thyroid lymphomas. *Hum Pathol*. 2002;33:524–527.
21. Nakatsuka S, Takakuwa T, Tomita Y, Miwa H, Matsuzuka F, Aozasa K. Role of hypermethylation of DAP-kinase CpG island in the development of thyroid lymphoma. *Lab Invest*. 2000;80:1651–1655.
22. Takakuwa T, Dong Z, Takayama H, Matsuzuka F, Nagata S, Aozasa K. Frequent mutations of Fas gene in thyroid lymphoma. *Cancer Res*. 2001;61:1382–1385.
23. Takakuwa T, Hongyo T, Syaifudin M, et al. Microsatellite instability and k-ras, p53 mutations in thyroid lymphoma. *Jpn J Cancer Res*. 2000;91:280–286.
24. Ito Y, Yoshida H, Matsuzuka F, et al. Jun activation domain-binding protein 1 expression in malignant lymphoma of the thyroid: its linkage to degree of malignancy and p27 expression. *Anticancer Res*. 2003;23:4121–4125.
25. Ito Y, Yoshida H, Matsuzuka F, et al. Expression of the components of the Cip/Kip family in malignant lymphoma of the thyroid. *Pathobiology*. 2004;71:164–170.
26. Ito Y, Yoshida H, Matsuzuka F, et al. Cdc25A and cdc25B expression in malignant lymphoma of the thyroid: correlation with histological subtypes and cell proliferation. *Int J Mol Med*. 2004;13:431–435.
27. Ito Y, Yoshida H, Matsuzuka F, et al. Cdc2 expression in primary thyroid lymphoma: its relationship with biological aggressiveness and G2 cyclins. *Pathol Res Pract*. 2003;199:533–538.
28. Wotherspoon AC, Doglioni C, Diss TC, et al. Regression of primary low-grade B-cell gastric lymphoma of mucosa-associated lymphoid tissue type after eradication of *Helicobacter pylori*. *Lancet*. 1993;342:575–577.
29. Hussell T, Isaacson PG, Crabtree JE, Spencer J. The response of cells from low-grade B-cell gastric lymphomas of mucosa-associated lymphoid tissue to *Helicobacter pylori*. *Lancet*. 1993;342:571–574.
30. Parsonnet J, Hansen S, Rodriguez L, et al. *Helicobacter pylori* infection and gastric lymphoma. *N Engl J Med*. 1994; 330:1267–1271.
31. Wotherspoon AC, Ortiz-Hidalgo C, Falzon MR, Isaacson PG. *Helicobacter pylori*-associated gastritis and primary B-cell gastric lymphoma. *Lancet*. 1991;338:1175–1176.
32. Ruland J, Duncan GS, Wakeham A, Mak TW. Differential requirement for Malt1 in T and B cell antigen receptor signaling. *Immunity*. 2003;19:749–758.
33. Ruland J, Duncan GS, Elia A, et al. Bcl10 is a positive regulator of antigen receptor-induced activation of NF-kappaB and neural tube closure. *Cell*. 2001;104:33–42.
34. Ruefli-Brasse AA, French DM, Dixit VM. Regulation of NF-kappaB-dependent lymphocyte activation and development by paracaspase. *Science*. 2003;302:1581–1584.
35. Xue L, Morris SW, Orihuela C, et al. Defective development and function of Bcl10-deficient follicular, marginal zone and B1 B cells. *Nat Immunol*. 2003;4:857–865.
36. Gaide O, Favier B, Legler DF, et al. CARMA1 is a critical lipid raft-associated regulator of TCR-induced NF-kappa B activation. *Nat Immunol*. 2002;3:836–843.
37. Streubel B, Vinatzer U, Lamprecht A, Raderer M, Chott A. T(3;14)(p14.1;q32) involving IGH and FOXP1 is a novel recurrent chromosomal aberration in MALT lymphoma. *Leukemia*. 2005;19:652–658.
38. Holm LE, Blomgren H, Lowhagen T. Cancer risks in patients with chronic lymphocytic thyroiditis. *N Engl J Med*. 1985;312:601–604.
39. Sato Y, Nakamura N, Nakamura S, et al. Deviated VH4 immunoglobulin gene usage is found among thyroid mucosa-associated lymphoid tissue lymphomas, similar to the usage at other sites, but is not found in thyroid diffuse large B-cell lymphomas. *Mod Pathol*. 2006;19:1578–1584.
40. Ito Y, Yoshida H, Matsuzuka F, et al. Polo-like kinase 1 (PLK1) expression is associated with cell proliferative activity and cdc2 expression in malignant lymphoma of the thyroid. *Anticancer Res*. 2004;24:259–263.
41. Morgner A, Lehn N, Andersen LP, et al. *Helicobacter heilmannii*-associated primary gastric low-grade MALT lymphoma: complete remission after curing the infection. *Gastroenterology*. 2000;118:821–828.
42. Lecuit M, Abachin E, Martin A, et al. Immunoproliferative small intestinal disease associated with *Campylobacter jejuni*. *N Engl J Med*. 2004;350:239–248.
43. Garbe C, Stein H, Dienemann D, Orfanos CE. *Borrelia burgdorferi*-associated cutaneous B cell lymphoma: clinical and immunohistologic characterization of four cases. *J Am Acad Dermatol*. 1991;24:584–590.
44. Cerroni L, Zochling N, Putz B, Kerl H. Infection by *Borrelia burgdorferi* and cutaneous B-cell lymphoma. *J Cutan Pathol*. 1997;24:457–461.
45. Kutting B, Bonsmann G, Metze D, Luger TA, Cerroni L. *Borrelia burgdorferi*-associated primary cutaneous B cell lymphoma: complete clearing of skin lesions after antibiotic pulse therapy or intralesional injection of interferon alfa-2a. *J Am Acad Dermatol*. 1997;36:311–314.
46. Ferreri AJ, Ponzoni M, Guidoboni M, et al. Regression of ocular adnexal lymphoma after *Chlamydia psittaci*-eradicating antibiotic therapy. *J Clin Oncol*. 2005;23:5067–5073.

47. Ferreri AJ, Guidoboni M, Ponzoni M, et al. Evidence for an association between *Chlamydia psittaci* and ocular adnexal lymphomas. *J Natl Cancer Inst*. 2004;96:586–594.
48. Rosado MF, Byrne GE Jr, Ding F, et al. Ocular adnexal lymphoma: a clinicopathologic study of a large cohort of patients with no evidence for an association with *Chlamydia psittaci*. *Blood*. 2006;107:467–472.
49. Vargas RL, Fallone E, Felgar RE, et al. Is there an association between ocular adnexal lymphoma and infection with *Chlamydia psittaci*? The University of Rochester experience. *Leuk Res*. 2006;30:547–551.
50. Streubel B, Simonitsch-Klupp I, Mullauer L, et al. Variable frequencies of MALT lymphoma-associated genetic aberrations in MALT lymphomas of different sites. *Leukemia*. 2004;18: 1722–1726.
51. Streubel B, Lamprecht A, Dierlamm J, et al. T(14;18)(q32;q21) involving IGH and MALT1 is a frequent chromosomal aberration in MALT lymphoma. *Blood*. 2003;101:2335–2339.

Section 3
Parathyroid Diseases

14
Clinical Detection and Treatment of Parathyroid Diseases

Michael T. Stang and Sally E. Carty

Introduction

Parathyroid pathology is usually manifested clinically as hyperparathyroidism (HPT), resulting from parathormone (PTH) excess. PTH is the chief hormone product of the parathyroid glands and can be overproduced in several complexly interrelated settings, termed primary (PHPT), secondary (SHPT), and tertiary hyperparathyroidism (THPT). PHPT can arise sporadically or from inherited syndromes that include multiple endocrine neoplasia type 1 (MEN1), multiple endocrine neoplasia type 2A (MEN2A), isolated familial hyperparathyroidism (FHPT), and familial hyperparathyroidism-jaw tumor syndrome (FHJT). SHPT is secondary to hypocalcemia, renal insufficiency, and/or severe vitamin D deficiency. THPT by definition occurs with a history of renal failure and long-standing SHPT.[1]

The disease processes governing PTH excess can be the result of a solitary enlarged gland (adenoma), two enlarged glands (double adenomata), diffuse enlargement of all glands (hyperplasia), or malignant growth (carcinoma). The rate of multiglandular disease varies widely by HPT disease type, namely 5–33% for sporadic PHPT,[2–7] 20–100% for inherited PHPT,[8] 100% for SHPT, and about 97% for THPT.[9] The rate of parathyroid carcinoma is uniformly low (<1%), and multiglandular carcinoma is exceedingly rare.[10]

The number and the locations of parathyroid glands can also vary widely. Anatomically most people have 4 glands, but supernumerary glands are common, in fact up to 13% of people have 5–9 parathyroid glands.[11] Derived embryologically from the third and fourth branchial pouches, enlarged parathyroid glands can reside in many locations in the neck and upper mediastinum. Although surgery is usually the best treatment for PHPT and for selected patients with SHPT and THPT, its success depends upon locating the enlarged, hyperfunctional gland(s). The dual complexities of HPT treatment, therefore, lie in correct identification of the HPT type, which determines the likelihood of gland heterogeneity, and in correct surgical management to achieve biochemical cure of the disease process.

Diagnosis

Inappropriate or unregulated overproduction of PTH leads to abnormal calcium homeostasis. Persistently high levels of PTH in patients with normal renal function cause an increase in renal resorption of calcium, phosphaturia, increased resorption of bone, and increased synthesis of 1, 25-dihydroxyvitamin D_3 (1,25 $(OH)_2D_3$).[12] The elevated 1,25 $(OH)_2D_3$ in turn augments intestinal calcium absorption.[12] The evident symptoms of longstanding excess PTH are directly related to these physiologic actions and to the effects of consequent hypercalemia on neuron and muscle function.

Nephrolithiasis still complicates PHPT, but less frequently than in prior decades. Earlier studies reported renal stones in up to 40% of PHPT patients,[13] but with the advent of routine screening for hypercalcemia this percentage has declined to 15–20%.[14,15] Hypercalciuria results from mismatch of the filtered and reabsorbed calcium and is one of several causative factors for renal stones, which in PHPT are usually composed of calcium oxalate or calcium phosphate.[16] Longstanding hypercalcemia and hypercalciuria can lead to calcific disease of the renal parynchema (nephrocalcinosis), and if left uncorrected ultimately results in a decreased glomerular filtration rate and renal insufficiency.[16] The deleterious effect on renal function is not reversed by curative parathyroid resection.[16]

PTH and calcium independently affect cardiovascular function.[17] PTH is vasodilatory, and has chronotropic and inotropic effects on the heart, while hypercalcemia is associated with vascular and valvular calcifications, hypertension and left ventricular hypertrophy.[17] In recent European series describing PHPT patients with high mean serum calcium, 82% had left ventricular hypertrophy, 46% had aortic valve calcifications, 39% had mitral calcifications, and with surgical correction of HPT the ventricular hypertrophy improved with concurrent stabilization of valvular sclerosis.[18,19] In other European studies, there is a well demonstrated increased risk of cardiovascular related mortality[20] and myocardial infarction[21] in PHPT which normalizes within 1 year following

J.L. Hunt (ed.), *Molecular Pathology of Endocrine Diseases*, Molecular Pathology Library 3,
DOI 10.1007/978-1-4419-1707-2_14, © Springer Science+Business Media, LLC 2010

curative resection. However, such findings are not yet replicated in US populations.[17]

PTH excess causes abnormally high bone turnover. Although the dramatic PHPT sequelae of brown tumors, fractures, and osteitis fibrosa cystica are uncommon now in industrialized countries,[22] dual-energy X-ray absorptiometry (DEXA) bone scans routinely show reduced cortical bone density in mild PHPT.[23,24] In PHPT, there is a decrease in bone density at sites rich in cortical bone, such as the distal radius, which is in contrast to the deficiencies of vertebral spine cancellous bone seen in postmenopausal women with osteoporosis. The resultant diminished bone density of PHPT does predispose to fracture of the distal forearm, vertebrae, ribs, and pelvis.[25] Following curative surgery for PHPT, patients demonstrate improvement in vertebral and hip bone mineral density of 12–20%.[15,26]

Patients with PHPT may have considerable sensation of early fatigue. Classically, advanced PHPT disease was associated with proximal muscle weakness affecting the lower extremities and characterized by neuropathic atrophy of type-2 muscle fibers.[27] In the modern era, this degree of neuromuscular dysfunction is rare, yet over half of PHPT patients will report some degree of muscle cramping or paresthesia.[28]

There is robust evidence not only for an increased prevalence of neuropsychiatric symptoms in PHPT, including depression, anxiety, malaise, and impaired cognition, but also that these symptoms demonstrably improve with normalization of PTH and calcium levels.[29–33] As yet, there is no universally accepted instrument to evaluate the neuropsychiatric symptoms of PHPT in relation to the degree of biochemical disease or to prove a cause and effect relationship.[17,34]

Historically, patients with advanced PHPT presented to physicians with nephrolithiasis, osteitis fibrosa cystica, muscle atrophy, hyperreflexia, and other overt symptoms including the extreme of coma.[35] In the modern era, the most common presentation of PHPT is the incidental finding of hypercalcemia first noted on routine biochemical screening, and usually termed "asymptomatic".[36] However, most patients with PHPT are by no means asymptomatic. In order of frequency, the subtler sequelae of HPT include bone mineralization deficits for 44% of patients (osteoporosis or osteopenia), neuromuscular complaints for 33% (fatigue, lethargy, muscle aches and bone aches), neuropsychiatric dysfunction for 15% of patients (insomnia, memory loss, depression, and mood disturbance), hypertension for 6%, gastrointestinal complaints for 4% (gastroesophageal reflux, peptic ulcer disease, dyspepsia and pancreatitis), and polyuria for <1%.[36] Because such symptoms were not noted to be among the "classic" sequelae described in early HPT literature, they have not always been described systematically and are still underreported in some studies today.[37]

Estimates of the incidence of PHPT have increased in previous decades, but this trend is certainly related to improvements in disease recognition. The most recent overall incidence rate for PHPT is 21–28 cases per 100,000 population annually in North America and England.[38–40] Of note, PHPT incidence rises to 190 cases per 100,000 population annually for Caucasian women greater than age 60.[41] PHPT is two to three times more common in women than men, and the incidence increases for both sexes with age.[42] Despite the relatively high frequency of PHPT in the general population, mortality is low accounting for an estimated 0.3 deaths per million per year in the United States.[42] The morbidity of PTHP and its impact on the US health care system remains less well described.

Biochemical Diagnosis of PHPT

Hyperfunctional parathyroid pathology is typically suggested by hypercalcemia, whether found by investigation of identified symptoms or incidentally on routine biochemical screening. Because hypercalcemia can also be caused by thiazide diuretic use, or spuriously by the ischemia of prolonged tourniquet time, PHPT diagnosis rests first on confirmation of hypercalcemia. Total serum calcium should be remeasured in the fasting state, off calcium supplements and after at least one week of discontinuation of thiazide diuretics.[43,44] Serum phosphorus is often low to low-normal in PHPT. Most patients have a normal albumin level thus measurement of ionized calcium offers minimal diagnostic advantage.[35]

After hypercalcemia is confirmed, the second step in PHPT diagnosis is the demonstration of an elevated or inappropriately high-normal serum PTH level.[43,44] Biologically active PTH circulates mostly as an 84 amino acid peptide but serum carboxyterminal degradation fragments of varying lengths are also present and may additionally be detected depending on the assay type used.[45] Accurate PTH measurement currently requires use of an immunoradiometric (IRMA) or immunochemiluminescent (ICMA) assay which measures "intact" PTH using antibodies directed simultaneously at both the amino- and carboxy-terminal regions.[46] The level of serum calcium is under sensitive feedback control via the calcium-sensing receptors in parathyroid glands. Hypercalcemia reduces PTH secretion; therefore, the concurrent elevation of serum calcium and PTH levels strongly suggests the diagnosis of PHPT (Figure 14.1).

Bisphosphonate use and chronic vitamin D deficiency are two common causes of secondary elevation in PTH, which may confound PHPT diagnosis. Low vitamin D levels indicate nutritional deficiency and should prompt medical correction. In this regard, many patients with PHPT have a subclinical initial presentation with normal or high-normal serum calcium level, becoming hypercalcemic only when vitamin D therapy is initiated.[47] Other conditions causing PHPT diagnostic uncertainty include hypercalcemia of malignancy, vitamin D toxicity, chronic granulomatous disease, and milk-alkali syndrome, and these can usually be identified on history with, if necessary, measurement of vitamin D levels and/or a PTH related-peptide level (PTHrp).[48]

Diagnostic dilemma may also be due to the rare, autosomal dominant disorder of familial benign hypocalciuric

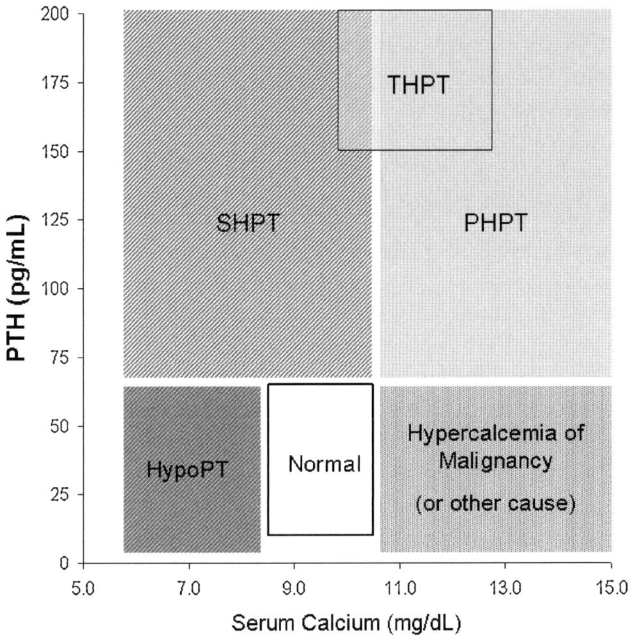

FIG. 14.1. Biochemical determination of HPT. This schematic illustrates the correlation of serum calcium levels and PTH with the corresponding clinical entities of primary hyperparathyroidism (PHPT), secondary hyperparathyroidism (SHPT), tertiary hyperparathyroidism (THPT), hypoparathyroidism (HypoPT), and hypercalcemia of malignancy or other chronic disease.

hypercalcemia (FBHH), which arises from an inactivating mutation in the calcium-sensing receptor of the parathyroid glands and kidneys.[49] This syndrome produces mild hypercalcemia, mild elevation, or lack of suppression in PTH level, low 24-h urine calcium excretion, and a Ca/Cr clearance ratio below 0.01.[44,50] FBHH has no known adverse sequelae other than unnecessary parathyroid surgery, which illustrates the importance of asking about family history of early onset asymptomatic hypercalcemia and measuring urine calcium excretion in patients with mild biochemical PHPT.

Biochemical Diagnosis of SHPT and THPT

SHPT typically arises in the setting of renal insufficiency but also can be due to any cause of chronic hypocalcemia and/or vitamin D deficiency. Most patients receiving dialysis for end-stage renal disease have some degree of SHPT especially if 1,25 dihydroxy vitamin D_3 is not adequately replaced or hyperphosphatemia is medically uncontrolled. SHPT is a complex, multifactorial process. One proximate cause is the significant loss of functional renal parenchyma in chronic renal disease leading to diminished production of 1,25-dihydroxy vitamin D_3 which results in diminished intestinal absorption of calcium.[51,52] Another factor is the hyperphosphatemia of renal failure.[51] The cumulative effect of low 1,25-dihydroxy vitamin D_3 and high phosphorus is a persistent hypocalcemic state.[51,52] These physiologic conditions combine to stimulate PTH production and parathyroid gland hyperplasia. The biochemical diagnosis of SHPT requires demonstration of normal or low-normal serum calcium levels, elevated PTH, and high phosphorus levels (Figure 14.1).[52]

As with PHPT, the spectrum of clinical SHPT has changed over time with more astute detection and with earlier treatment of patients on renal replacement therapy. Historically, symptoms of bone pain, myopathy, tendon rupture, and extraskeletal calcifications were common.[52] Today, most patients with SHPT are relatively asymptomatic, but some complications of SHPT persist and can require close attention including early coronary artery calcification, cardiomyopathy, pruritis, uremic calcific arteriolopathy (calciphylaxis), and neuropsychiatric issues.[52]

In the setting of prolonged SHPT, diffuse parathyroid gland hyperplasia can progress to nodular hyperplasia, which can ultimately transform from a polyclonal or oligoclonal process to a monoclonal parathyroid neoplasm with autonomous function.[53] This loss of feedback regulation is termed THPT, and is defined as hypercalcemia in a patient with a history of renal failure.[1] THPT can occur before renal transplantation, persist after transplantation, or can even arise de novo after transplantation.[54,55] As with primary hyperparathyroidism, THPT is marked biochemically by both elevated serum calcium and PTH levels (Figure 14.1).

Treatment

Surgery for PHPT

Once PHPT has been diagnosed biochemically, the current treatment standard rests on a distinction of whether symptoms are present. Although percutaneous alcohol ablation can temporarily palliate PHPT in selected high-risk patients,[56] surgery provides the only cure of PHPT. Parathyroid exploration is cost effective and is the current standard for symptomatic PHPT patients.[37,43,44,57] As detailed earlier, however, the definition of symptomatic has varied and is still incompletely defined. The goal of surgery for PHPT is to prevent progression to the more serious complications of renal failure, osteoporotic fracture, and cardiac mortality. Nonetheless, after curative surgery, even asymptomatic patients will enjoy a 60% increase in general health at 1 year with objectively measured improvements in fatigue, weakness, bone pain, joint pain, forgetfulness, mood swings, thirst, irritability, and depression among other PHPT disease-specific complaints.[30]

For asymptomatic PHPT patients, certain risk factors predict disease progression. The National Institutes of Health sponsored a consensus conference in 1990 to define guidelines for surgical intervention in asymptomatic PHPT. The panel recommended surgical treatment of PHPT for patients with any of the following: nephrolithiasis, osteitis fibrosis cystica, neuromuscular symptoms (documented proximal weakness, atrophy, hyperreflexia, gait disturbance), a life-threatening

TABLE 14.1. NIH criteria for parathyroid exploration.

Age	>50 year[a]
Serum level of calcium	>1.0 mg/dL above upper limit of normal
Creatinine clearance	Reduced by 30% compared to normal age-matched
24 h urinary calcium excretion	>400 mg
Bone mineral density	*t*-score <−2.5 at any site

[a]Or patients that are unable to provide consistent follow-up.

episode of hypercalcemia, age <50, serum calcium level 1–1.6 md/dL above the normal range, 30% reduction in creatinine clearance compared to age-matched controls, 24 h urine calcium excretion >400 mg, or forearm bone density reduced more than 2 standard deviations below the density of age-, gender-, and race-matched controls (*z* score).[43] The summary statement of a subsequent 2002 national workshop held to further discuss asymptomatic PHPT advised broader criteria for surgery, namely a calcium level 1.0 mg/dL above the normal range or a bone mineral density at any site reduced by more than 2.5 standard deviations over unmatched controls (*t*-score) (Table 14.1).[44] Both conferences advised careful long-term follow-up of patients being managed with observation and both cited patient unwillingness to participate in such follow-up to be a strong prompt for surgery.[43,44] For asymptomatic PHPT patients being observed, the NIH consensus conference advises twice-yearly physician evaluation and serum calcium level, as well as annual 24-h urine calcium, creatinine clearance, serum creatinine level, and bone density testing.[43]

Testing of the NIH criteria for surgery versus surveillance has not yet been systematically performed. We now know that during 15 years of surveillance, 37% of asymptomatic PHPT patients who do not originally meet NIH criteria will progress to meet criteria for surgery[58] and that progression is more likely for PHPT patients diagnosed at <50 years.[59] In an interesting 2004 report, Eigelberger et al objectively evaluated 178 surgically cured PHTP patients, 103 of whom met at least one of the NIH criteria for surgery, and also compared their outcomes to 63 nonPHPT patients who had thyroid surgery.[60] They observed that nonclassic PHPT symptoms including fatigue, bone pain, nocturia, and depression were indeed much more frequent in PHPT than in thyroid disease. Moreover, such symptoms occurred in PHPT regardless of whether the patient met NIH criteria for surgery and resolved postoperatively in many patients regardless of NIH criteria status. Multivariate analysis of practice patterns among endocrine surgeons show a lack of consensus on the threshold for surgery in asymptomatic patients[61] which is felt to lead to increased cost and burden on the health care system.[62] Cost efficacy studies also favor operative management for asymptomatic PHPT even for patients who do not meet NIH criteria for surgery.[63] In summary, based on multiple objective studies of symptom resolution after curative surgery,[29–33,60,64,65] we consider the subtler symptoms of PHPT including fatigue, musculoskeletal aches and pains, back pain, weakness, polydypsia, nocturia and memory loss, to be real, valid and potentially reversible. The emerging consensus nationally is that all patients with asymptomatic PHPT should consult with an experienced surgeon before selecting a treatment option.

Nonoperative Management of PHPT

Overall, medical management can achieve only partial, inconsistent reduction in calcium levels, and is not known to prevent the more dire sequelae of PHPT. Calcium restriction currently is not recommended for patients being observed since it can further raise PTH levels; daily replacement doses of 1,000–1,200 mg elemental calcium are suggested.[66] The antiresorptive properties of estrogens can decrease the effects of PTH on bone demineralization,[67] but the doses required are so high that exogenous estrogen treatment is not currently recommended.[68] Selective estrogen receptor modulators such as raloxifene are reported to reduce serum calcium and markers of bone turnover short-term, however the long term effects are not known.[69] Bisphosphonates such as alendronate can be associated with improvement in bone mineral density at the lumbar spine, femoral neck, and hip in patients with PHPT and osteoporosis but also can increase PTH levels, and the use of such agents in the medical treatment of PHPT is still under investigation.[70,71]

The extracellular calcium-sensing receptor (CaR) was identified and cloned in 1993 by Brown and colleagues and is a G-protein coupled membrane receptor that is activated by high extracellular Ca^{2+} to control PTH secretion.[72] Molecules that interact with parathyroid CaRs and mimic Ca^{2+} are termed calcimemetics and function to activate CaRs, suppress PTH secretion and/or block parathyroid gland hyperplasia.[73] The two distinct types of calcimemetics identified to date are termed type I and type II.[74] Type I calcimemetics are full agonists of CaRs and include various inorganic and organic polycations; this class lacks the specificity and safe therapeutic window to be used clinically.[75] Type II calcimemetics are small organic compounds that allosterically modulate the CaR to increase its sensitivity to activation in the presence of extracellular calcium.[75] The compound AMG 073 (cinacalcet HCl) may achieve normocalcemia and modest reduction of PTH levels in some patients with asymptomatic PHPT.[76–78] However, the longterm effects of cinacalcet in treating PHPT are unknown and cinacalcet HCl is not currently approved for the use in the treatment of PHPT except in an investigational setting.

Preoperative Localization

Parathyroid imaging does not play a role in the diagnosis of PHPT. Once the decision has been made for surgery, the routine use of preoperative imaging has been shown to increase the success rate, decrease the operative time, and decrease the major complications of parathyroid exploration. Because the anatomic location of parathyroid glands can

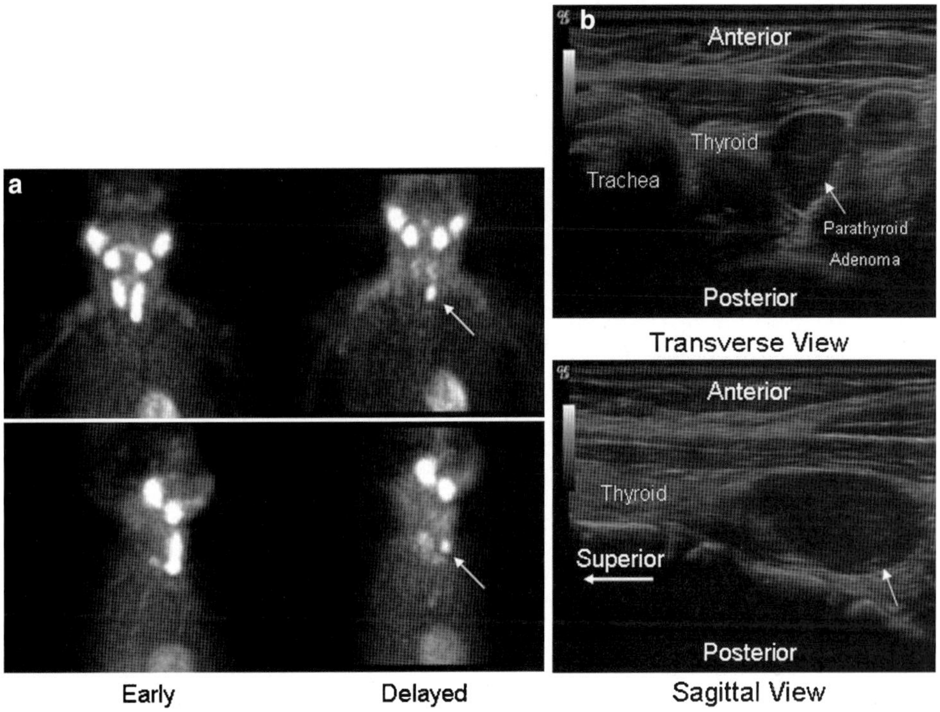

FIG. 14.2. Early and late SPECT ^{99m}Tc sestamibi images with corresponding cervical ultrasonography. (**a**) Shows a single strong focus of uptake by SPECT ^{99m}Tc sestamibi corresponding to an enlarged inferior/anterior parathyroid gland. (**b**) An enlarged inferior/anterior parathyroid gland illustrated by transverse and sagittal ultrasound images.

vary widely, hyperfunctioning glands can be difficult to locate intraoperatively and this is even truer with reoperation in a hostile surgical field. Among the imaging studies available, the most sensitive, specific, and cost-effective are ultrasonography and single photon emission computed tomography (SPECT) ^{99m}Technetium sestamibi.[79–81] Use of ^{99m}Tc-sestamibi nuclear imaging and ultrasound together can synergistically improve correct localization by 10–14% and are useful in operative planning (Figure 14.2).[80–82] Ultrasonography is now well-established to provide additional benefit in detecting concurrent thyroid pathology.[83] No current imaging test can reliably exclude multiglandular parathyroid disease, however,[79,84] and even a single bright focus on sestamibi SPECT imaging does not reliably exclude hyperplasia and is associated with multiglandular disease in 8% of patients undergoing initial exploration.[85]

Operative Strategy

Successful parathyroid surgery is defined as durable normalization of the serum calcium level, ie cure of PHPT. Operative failure is the most frequent risk of parathyroid exploration and carries a high morbidity and cost.[86] Because the therapeutic intent in PHPT is to remove the source(s) of PTH overproduction, the central issues in exploration are identifying the presence or absence of gland heterogeneity (adenoma versus hyperplasia) and locating the abnormal gland(s). Common locations for enlarged superior parathyroid glands include the tracheoesophageal groove, the retropharyngeal space, and the superior middle mediastinum; enlarged inferior glands can be intrathyroidal, undescended at the carotid bulb, within the thymus, or elsewhere in the superior anterior mediastinum.

Unfortunately, histologic criteria are not clinically reliable in distinguishing adenoma from multiglandular disease and in one recent study incorrectly predicted the number of abnormal parathyroid glands 62% of the time.[87] Intraoperative use of a gamma-probe for localization of abnormal parathyroid glands with ^{99m}Technectium has been examined but remains controversial. Currently, only two techniques are proven to reliably exclude multiglandular disease in PHPT. The first of these, bilateral 4-gland exploration, is the "gold standard" approach and involves dissection and visualization of all parathyroid glands. Normal parathyroid glands are 30–45 mg in size, while suppressed parathyroid glands in PHPT can be considerably smaller,[11] thus 4-gland exploration requires surgeon expertise in assessment of gland size. Enlarged parathyroid glands are resected and are weighed intraoperatively by the pathologist along with histopathologic confirmation that it is indeed parathyroid tissue (and not brown fat, lymph node, thymic, or thyroid tissue) that has been removed.[87] This information can be used intraoperatively to deduce the presence of missing or supranumery abnormal parathyroid glands. Should the patient have more than 2 enlarged glands (>double adenomata), they are considered to have hyperplasia, and a subtotal parathyroidectomy is performed, leaving a viable 50–100 mg remnant of one enlarged gland in situ and marked with a titanium clip.

The second technique validated to exclude multiglandular disease is intraoperative PTH monitoring, which is now widely used because it facilitates both focused dissection and shorter operative times. In this method, the serum PTH, which has a short half-life of 3–5 min in most patients, is measured just prior to and just after resection of an enlarged parathyroid gland using a modified rapid assay developed by Dr. Irvin at the University of Miami.[88–90] If the postresection PTH does not drop adequately, the presence of further hyperfunctional parathyroid glands is deduced, and further exploration is performed.[90–92] Although nationally the most widely used criterion for an adequate PTH drop is a simple 50% decrease at 10 min postresection, stricter criteria are in use in several centers; we require that PTH also drop into the normal range, to diagnose an appropriate response to parathyroid resection.[90,93] Intraoperative PTH monitoring facilitates a safe, successful focused dissection,[92,94] allows optimization of the postoperative calcium supplementation, and is particularly useful in successfully managing reexploration, double adenomata, hyperplasia, intrathyroidal adenoma, or supranumery adenoma, and in patients with a history of lithium use.[95] To summarize the operative strategy with PTH monitoring, "the localization tells you where to start looking and the PTH drop says you can stop looking."

Surgical Cure

As stated earlier, cure after parathyroid exploration for PHPT is defined as durable normalization of the serum calcium (>6 months after surgery). Operative failure is usefully categorized as either persistent or recurrent HPT. In *persistent* HPT, there is an elevated serum calcium and PTH within 6 months postoperatively, and this usually represents a missed adenoma, while in *recurrent* HPT hypercalcemia arises >6 months after initial exploration, and the situation generally indicates multiglandular disease that was unrecognized, or rarely parathyromatosis and/or parathyroid carcinoma.

Immediately after successful surgery for PHPT, many patients will show elevation of PTH despite correction to normal serum calcium levels. This phenomenon is well described, common (estimated occurrence of about 30% (8–40%) postoperatively),[96–103] in our recent experience occurs much less frequently when patients routinely take calcium and vitamin D supplements for 6 months postoperatively,[103] and thus is likely to be secondary to chronic dietary deficiency in calcium and vitamin D. All normocalcemic patients are thus recommended to receive maintenance calcium and vitamin D supplementation for 6 months after surgical cure of PHPT.[103] In a small proportion of patients (0.7%), a normocalcemic elevation in PTH at 6 months postoperatively can be the first indicator of recurrent PHPT, and such patients should thus be followed long-term.[103]

Reoperation

The causes of failed initial parathyroid exploration include surgeon inexperience, ectopic or supernumery parathyroid gland location, multiglandular disease, and parathyroid carcinoma.[104,105] The indications for initial and reoperative exploration differ. The risks of initial exploration for PHPT are few and are generally limited to operative failure (1–5%), permanent hypoparathyroidism (0.5–2%), permanent recurrent laryngeal nerve injury (1% or less), and cervical hematoma (0.3%) (reviewed in[106]). Because the risks of reoperation are higher across the board, and include bilateral recurrent nerve paralysis, surgery is usually reserved for clearly symptomatic patients or those with nephrolithiasis, osteoporosis, calcium level >12 mg/dL, or hypercalciuria.[43,107] After initial failed surgery, the first step is biochemical reconfirmation of the PHPT diagnosis including 24 h urinary calcium excretion. Histologic reexamination of the tissues removed at the initial exploration, review of prior records, precise localization, DEXA bone mineralization testing, laryngoscopy, careful family history, and a frank discussion of the risks and benefits with the patient are also necessary prior to reexploration.

Parathyroid Surgery in Inherited Syndromes

Hereditary syndromes resulting in HPT require special attention since the setting of the genetic defect involved can have a significant impact on both surgical approach and outcome. Further, hereditary HPT patients require screening for other clinical manifestations of the respective syndrome.

In MEN1, the penetrance of PHPT is close to 100%, and the associated pancreatic islet and pituitary tumors occur much less frequently.[108] The syndrome is secondary to genetic alteration of the MEN1 gene on chromosome 11q13, a tumor suppressor gene that encodes the ubiquitously expressed nuclear protein product *menin*.[109] Multiglandular parathyroid disease is assumed in all patients. If MEN1 is missed on family history, or in a patient who represents a new mutation, persistent HPT is likely and recurrent HPT is certain. The successful diagnosis of MEN1 in patients presenting with apparent sporadic PHPT is greatly facilitated by use of a simple 6-question panel, which focuses on a personal or family history of neck surgery, nephrolithiasis, brain tumors, peptic ulcer disease, high calcium levels and/or pancreatic tumors.[110] MEN1 accounts for about 26% of patients found to have parathyroid hyperplasia at exploration for presumed sporadic PHPT and is more likely in patients who are young and male.[110] MEN1 PHPT is currently treated either by total parathyroidectomy with nondominant forearm autotransplantation, or by subtotal parathyroidectomy, and patients require counseling preoperatively to assist in decision-making because these operations have differing morbidity rates. Cryopreservation of parathyroid tissue resected during parathyroid surgery should be performed to allow future treatment with preserved grafts in the event of hypoparathyroidism.

MEN2A is a hereditary syndrome expressed as medullary thyroid cancer (MTC), pheochromocytoma and PHPT, and arising from mutations in the tyrosine kinase RET.[8] The penetrance of PHPT in MEN 2A is approximately 30%, and it usually results in mild HPT presenting in mid adulthood.[111] Because the degree of parathyroid gland enlargement can be asymmetrical in MEN2A, surgical management is yet controversial and not all patients will require subtotal parathyroidectomy.[112,113] The unique feature of MEN2A is that 90% of patients will develop MTC prior to PHPT; total thyroidectomy for MTC thus can be followed decades later by difficult reoperative parathyroid exploration. If not already performed, total thyroidectomy is mandated at the time of parathyroid exploration.

Familial hyperparathyroidism-jaw tumor syndrome (FHJT or HPT-JT) arises from mutation of the tumor suppressor gene *HRPT2* which encodes the *parafibromin* protein product.[114] The primary clinical features are HPT, fibro-osseus lesions of the mandible and maxilla, and renal lesions including cysts, hamartoma, and Wilms tumor.[115] HPT is expressed in 80% of adults and tends to present at a relatively young age (mean 32 years).[115] Parathyroid gland enlargement is often asymmetric and glands may also be cystic in nature.[111,116] The surgical approach is the same as that for MEN2A with resection of all enlarged glands. An interesting and important feature of HPT-JT management is that parathyroid carcinoma may be present in as many as 15% of cases.[114]

Parathyroid Cysts and Parathyroid Cancer

Parathyroid cysts are uncommon lesions of the neck and mediastinum and may present as a symptomatic neck mass or be identified during evaluation of PHPT.[117] As many as 2.7% of patients with PHPT will have a cystic parathyroid gland. For patients with functional cysts, surgical excision should be performed in conjunction with intraoperative PTH monitoring to insure adequate resection and allow identification of concordant adenoma in another location or multiglandular disease.[117]

Parathyroid carcinoma (PC) is a rare malignancy but warrants special mention here because the diagnosis can be made intraoperatively, histologically, or by both methods[118–123]. Preoperative features which raise suspicion of malignancy include serum calcium level >14 mg/dL, PTH level >5 times normal, the presence of a palpable neck mass, or hoarseness (signifying involvement of the recurrent laryngeal nerve.) At exploration, features which suggest parathyroid carcinoma include: white color, firm consistency, gritty texture, and adherence to surrounding structures, and the alert surgeon needs to recognize these signs because en bloc resection of the lesion is then mandated. In the event of local recurrence, resection and neck dissection is best treatment. Palliative medical management with cinacalcet may be warranted; in a recent preliminary study examining 29 patients with inoperable parathyroid carcinoma, cinacalcet was able to modestly control hypercalcemia and reduce serum calcium by at least 1 mg/dL in 62% of patients, without significant decrease in serum PTH.[118]

Treatment of SHPT and THPT

Medical Management of SHPT and THPT

Overall, it is easier to prevent SHPT than to treat it. The aim of medical management is to abate the progression of diffuse to nodular hyperplasia by reducing serum phosphorus and appropriately replacing activated vitamin D, which lowers serum PTH.[119] Obsolete phosphate binding medications included aluminum (which was toxic) or calcium (which resulted in hypercalcemia). Currently, it is recommended that patients with hyperphosphatemia use calcium- and aluminum-free phosphate binders such as sevelamer HCl and lanthanum carbonate in addition to limiting dietary phosphate intake. Treatment with these agents is effective in lowering serum phosphorus but has little effect in reducing PTH levels.[120,121] Calcitriol (1,25-dihydroxy vitamin D_3) is used in SHPT to lower PTH levels but can induce hypercalcemia and hyperphosphatemia.[122] Newer vitamin D analogs such as paricalcitol and doxercalciferol have been shown to reduce PTH levels with less toxicity.[122] These analogs are designed to activate the vitamin D receptor selectively at the level of the parathyroid gland while minimizing the hypercalcemic and hyperphosphatemic effect seen with calcitriol.[122]

The Kidney Disease Outcomes Quality Initiative (KDOQI) has issued guidelines with respect to the clinical practice goals of medical therapy for patients on renal replacement therapy. Serum calcium should be maintained between 8.4 and 9.5 md/dL and serum phosphorus kept between 3.5 and 5.5 md/dL.[123] Together, the calcium phosphate product (Ca × P) should be less than 55. PTH levels should be controlled between 150 and 300 pg/mL,[123] In general, standard treatment with phosphate binders and vitamin D sterols is only able to achieve target serum PTH levels in 26% of hemodialysis patients, and achieves all four KDOQI parameters for only 6% of patients.[124]

The best treatment for SHPT is restoration of normal renal function by renal transplantation. When this is not possible or is delayed, the aforementioned strategies in addition to the calcimemetic agent cinacalcet can be used in treatment. Pooled data from phase III clinical studies of cinacalcet in combination with best standard care demonstrate a reduction in both serum PTH and phosphorus levels when compared to placebo.[125] The addition of cinacalcet achieves a serum PTH target ≤300 pg/mL in 56% of patients compared with 10% of placebo-treated controls. Further, 41% of patients treated with cinacalcet are able to achieve both PTH and Ca × P parameters as opposed to 6% of those receiving placebo.[126] The improved efficacy of cinacalcet in managing SHPT also translates into improved outcomes with a decreased risk of need for parathyroidectomy, bone fracture and cardiovascular hospitalization.[127] Treatment with cinacalcet is generally well tolerated with the most common adverse side effects being nausea, vomiting, or diarrhea which may limit its use.[128]

Surgery for SHPT and THPT

In SHPT, parathyroidectomy is indicated when medical management fails to meet the above stated goals. In addition, the KDOQI guidelines recommend parathyroidectomy for patients with PTH >800 pg/mL and hyperphosphatemia, extraosseus calcifications (calciphylaxis) with PTH >500 pg/mL, and progressive renal osteodystrophy or intractable pruritis.[123]

The presence of hypercalcemia in patients with longstanding SHPT indicates autonomous progression to THPT, which can occur in patients who remain dialysis dependent as well as those who have received renal transplantation. For those who will remain dialysis dependent indefinitely, the development of THPT indicates medical failure and parathyroid surgery is indicated.[123] The majority of patients (69–83%) who undergo renal transplantation with THPT, however, will demonstrate slow correction in serum calcium and PTH to near normal levels over the first year posttransplant[129,130] with only 12.4% remaining hypercalcemic at 48 months posttransplant.[130] Thus, when possible, THPT patients who have recently received or who anticipate renal transplantation should be managed nonoperatively for at least 12 months following transplantation, and surgery is usually reserved for patients with very severe disease.[129]

There are two varieties of parathyroidectomy in the treatment of SHPT/THPT: total parathyroidectomy (with or without autotransplantation) and subtotal parathyroidectomy. These procedures have been equally validated and choice is largely left to the discretion and outcomes of the endocrine surgeon.[9,131–135] In general, a balance needs to be struck between removing enough parathyroid tissue to achieve a normal PTH level, while guarding against hypoparathyroidism. All parathyroid glands should be identified and enough tissue resected to leave the patient with a tissue remnant weighing about 40–80 mg either in situ or at the site of autotransplantation.[9]

Conclusion

Parathyroid disease is common and its complications are related to its chief hormone product, PTH. The biochemical diagnosis of hyperparathyroidism is determined by concurrent assessment of fasting serum calcium and PTH levels. The role of parathyroid imaging, by ultrasound and/or sestamibi nuclear scintigraphy, is to aid in the conduct of a planned exploration. Ultimately, exploration by an experienced endocrine surgeon is the most proven and effective treatment for patients with primary hyperparathyroidism or persisting tertiary hyperparathyroidism. The first parathyroid exploration is the safest and best chance for disease cure. Recently developed molecular therapies targeting the calcium sensing receptor offer promise in treating patients with secondary hyperparathyroidism.

References

1. McPhaul JJ Jr, McIntosh DA, Hammond WS, et al. Autonomous secondary (renal) parathyroid hyperplasia. *N Engl J Med*. 1964;271:1342–1345.
2. van Heerden JA, Grant CS. Surgical treatment of primary hyperparathyroidism: an institutional perspective. *World J Surg*. 1991;15(6):688–692.
3. Kaplan EL, Yashiro T, Salti G. Primary hyperparathyroidism in the 1990s. Choice of surgical procedures for this disease. *Ann Surg*. 1992;215(4):300–317.
4. Weber CJ, Sewell CW, McGarity WC. Persistent and recurrent sporadic primary hyperparathyroidism: histopathology, complications, and results of reoperation. *Surgery*. 1994;116(6):991–998.
5. Molinari AS, Irvin GL 3rd, Deriso GT, et al. Incidence of multiglandular disease in primary hyperparathyroidism determined by parathyroid hormone secretion. *Surgery*. 1996;120(6):934–936.
6. Kebebew E, Clark OH. Parathyroid adenoma, hyperplasia, and carcinoma: localization, technical details of primary neck exploration, and treatment of hypercalcemic crisis. *Surg Oncol Clin N Am*. 1998;7(4):721–748.
7. Lee NC, Norton JA. Multiple-gland disease in primary hyperparathyroidism: a function of operative approach? *Arch Surg*. 2002;137(8):896–899.
8. Brandi ML, Gagel RF, Angeli A, et al. Guidelines for diagnosis and therapy of MEN type 1 and type 2. *J Clin Endocrinol Metab*. 2001;86(12):5658–5671.
9. Kebebew E, Duh QY, Clark OH. Tertiary hyperparathyroidism: histologic patterns of disease and results of parathyroidectomy. *Arch Surg*. 2004;139(9):974–977.
10. Sahasranam P, Tran MT, Mohamed H, Friedman TC. Multiglandular parathyroid carcinoma: a case report and brief review. *South Med J*. 2007;100(8):841–844.
11. Akerström G, Malmaeus J, Bergström R. Surgical anatomy of human parathyroid glands. *Surgery*. 1984;95(1):14–21.
12. Brown EM. The pathophysiology of primary hyperparathyroidism. *J Bone Miner Res*. 2002;17(suppl 2):N24–N29.
13. Bilezikian JP, Potts JT Jr. Asymptomatic primary hyperparathyroidism: new issues and new questions – bridging the past with the future. *J Bone Miner Res*. 2002;17(suppl 2):N57–N67.
14. Silverberg SJ, Shane E, Jacobs TP, et al. Nephrolithiasis and bone involvement in primary hyperparathyroidism. *Am J Med*. 1990;89(3):327–334.
15. Silverberg SJ, Shane E, Jacobs TP, Siris E, Bilezikian JP. A 10-year prospective study of primary hyperparathyroidism with or without parathyroid surgery. *N Engl J Med*. 1999;341(17):1249–1255.
16. Peacock M. Primary hyperparathyroidism and the kidney: biochemical and clinical spectrum. *J Bone Miner Res*. 2002;17 (suppl 2):N87–N94.
17. Silverberg SJ. Non-classical target organs in primary hyperparathyroidism. *J Bone Miner Res*. 2002;17(suppl 2):N117–N125.
18. Stefenelli T, Abela C, Frank H, et al. Cardiac abnormalities in patients with primary hyperparathyroidism: implications for follow-up. *J Clin Endocrinol Metab*. 1997;82(1):106–112.
19. Piovesan A, Molineri N, Casasso F, et al. Left ventricular hypertrophy in primary hyperparathyroidism. Effects of successful parathyroidectomy. *Clin Endocrinol (Oxf)*. 1999;50(3):321–328.
20. Leifsson BG, Ahrén B. Serum calcium and survival in a large health screening program. *J Clin Endocrinol Metab*. 1996;81(6):2149–2153.

21. Vestergaard P, Mollerup CL, Frøkjaer VG, Christiansen P, Blichert-Toft M, Mosekilde L. Cardiovascular events before and after surgery for primary hyperparathyroidism. *World J Surg*. 2003;27(2):216–222.
22. Parisien M, Silverberg SJ, Shane E, Dempster DW, Bilezikian JP. Bone disease in primary hyperparathyroidism. *Endocrinol Metab Clin North Am*. 1990;19(1):19–34.
23. Silverberg SJ, Shane E, de la Cruz L, et al. Skeletal disease in primary hyperparathyroidism. *J Bone Miner Res*. 1989;4(3):283–291.
24. Miller PD, Bilezikian JP. Bone densitometry in asymptomatic primary hyperparathyroidism. *J Bone Miner Res*. 2002;17(suppl 2):N98–N102.
25. Khosla S, Melton LJ 3rd, Wermers RA, Crowson CS, O'Fallon W, Riggs B. Primary hyperparathyroidism and the risk of fracture: a population-based study. *J Bone Miner Res*. 1999;14(10):1700–1707.
26. Silverberg SJ, Locker FG, Bilezikian JP. Vertebral osteopenia: a new indication for surgery in primary hyperparathyroidism. *J Clin Endocrinol Metab*. 1996;81(11):4007–4012.
27. Patten BM, Bilezikian JP, Mallette LE, Prince A, Engel WK, Aurbach GD. Neuromuscular disease in primary hyperparathyroidism. *Ann Intern Med*. 1974;80(2):182–193.
28. Turken SA, Cafferty M, Silverberg SJ, et al. Neuromuscular involvement in mild, asymptomatic primary hyperparathyroidism. *Am J Med*. 1989;87(5):553–557.
29. Chan AK, Duh QY, Katz MH, Siperstein AE, Clark OH. Clinical manifestations of primary hyperparathyroidism before and after parathyroidectomy. A case–control study. *Ann Surg*. 1995;222(3):402–412.
30. Pasieka JL, Parsons LL. Prospective surgical outcome study of relief of symptoms following surgery in patients with primary hyperparathyroidism. *World J Surg*. 1998;22(6): 513–518.
31. Talpos GB, Bone HG 3rd, Kleerekoper M, et al. Randomized trial of parathyroidectomy in mild asymptomatic primary hyperparathyroidism: patient description and effects on the SF-36 health survey. *Surgery*. 2000;128(6):1013–1020.
32. Sywak MS, Knowlton ST, Pasieka JL, Parsons LL, Jones J. Do the National Institutes of Health consensus guidelines for parathyroidectomy predict symptom severity and surgical outcome in patients with primary hyperparathyroidism? *Surgery*. 2002;132(6):1013–1019.
33. Pasieka JL, Parsons LL, Demeure MJ, et al. Patient-based surgical outcome tool demonstrating alleviation of symptoms following parathyroidectomy in patients with primary hyperparathyroidism. *World J Surg*. 2002;26(8):942–949.
34. Kleerekoper M, Bilezkian JP. A cure in search of a disease: parathyroidectomy for nontraditional features of primary hyperparathyroidism. *Am J Med*. 1994;96(2):99–100.
35. Silverberg SJ, Bilezikian JP. Evaluation and management of primary hyperparathyroidism. *J Clin Endocrinol Metab*. 1996;81(6):2036–2040.
36. Mazzaglia PJ, Berber E, Kovach A, Milas M, Esselstyn C, Siperstein AE. The changing presentation of hyperparathyroidism over 3 decades. *Arch Surg*. 2008;143(3):260–266.
37. Clark OH. "Asymptomatic" primary hyperparathyroidism: is parathyroidectomy indicated? *Surgery*. 1994;116(6):947–953.
38. Heath H 3rd, Hodgson SF, Kennedy MA. Primary hyperparathyroidism. Incidence, morbidity, and potential economic impact in a community. *N Engl J Med*. 1980;302(4):189–193.
39. Wermers RA, Khosla S, Atkinson EJ, Hodgson SF, O'Fallon WM, Melton LJ 3rd. The rise and fall of primary hyperparathyroidism: a population-based study in Rochester, Minnesota, 1965–1992. *Ann Intern Med*. 1997;126(6):433–440.
40. Mundy GR, Cove DH, Fisken R. Primary hyperparathyroidism: changes in the pattern of clinical presentation. *Lancet*. 1980;1(8182):1317–1320.
41. Heath H 3rd. Primary hyperparathyroidism: recent advances in pathogenesis, diagnosis, and management. *Adv Intern Med*. 1992;37:275–293.
42. Melton LJ 3rd. The epidemiology of primary hyperparathyroidism in North America. *J Bone Miner Res*. 2002;17(suppl 2):N12–N17.
43. National Institutes of Health Consensus Development Conference. Diagnosis and management of asymptomatic primary hyperparathyroidism. *Consens Statement*. October 29–31, 1990;8:1–18.
44. Bilezikian JP, Potts JT Jr, Fuleihan Gel-H, et al. Summary statement from a workshop on asymptomatic primary hyperparathyroidism: a perspective for the 21st century. *J Clin Endocrinol Metab*. 2002;87(12):5353–5361.
45. Jüppner H, Potts JT Jr. Immunoassays for the detection of parathyroid hormone. *J Bone Miner Res*. 2002;17(suppl 2): N81–N86.
46. Endres DB, Villanueva R, Sharp CF Jr, Singer FR. Immunochemiluminometric and immunoradiometric determinations of intact and total immunoreactive parathyrin: performance in the differential diagnosis of hypercalcemia and hypoparathyroidism. *Clin Chem*. 1991;37(2):162–168.
47. Silverberg SJ. Vitamin D deficiency and primary hyperparathyroidism. *J Bone Miner Res*. 2007;22(suppl 2):V100–V104.
48. Burtis WJ, Fodero JP, Gaich G, Debeyssey M, Stewart AF. Preliminary characterization of circulating amino- and carboxy-terminal fragments of parathyroid hormone-related peptide in humoral hypercalcemia of malignancy. *J Clin Endocrinol Metab*. 1992;75(4):1110–1114.
49. Pollak MR, Brown EM, Chou YH, et al. Mutations in the human Ca(2+)-sensing receptor gene cause familial hypocalciuric hypercalcemia and neonatal severe hyperparathyroidism. *Cell*. 1993;75(7):1297–1303.
50. Fuleihan Gel-H. Familial benign hypocalciuric hypercalcemia. *J Bone Miner Res*. 2002;17(suppl 2):N51–N56.
51. Slatopolsky E, Delmez JA. Pathogenesis of secondary hyperparathyroidism. *Am J Kidney Dis*. 1994;23(2):229–236.
52. Llach F, Velasquez Forero F. Secondary hyperparathyroidism in chronic renal failure: pathogenic and clinical aspects. *Am J Kidney Dis*. 2001;38(5 suppl 5):S20–S33.
53. Tominaga Y. Mechanism of parathyroid tumourigenesis in uraemia. *Nephrol Dial Transplant*. 1999;14(suppl 1):63–65.
54. Alfrey AC, Jenkins D, Groth CG, Schorr WS, Gecelter L, Ogden DA. Resolution of hyperparathyroidism, renal osteodystrophy and metastatic calcification after renal homotransplantation. *N Engl J Med*. 1968;279(25):1349–1356.
55. Latimer RG, Renning J, Stevens LE, Northway JD, Reemtsma K. Tertiary hyperparathyroidism following successful renal allografting. *Ann Surg*. 1970;172(1):137–141.
56. Karstrup S, Hegedüs L, Holm HH. Ultrasonically guided chemical parathyroidectomy in patients with primary hyperparathyroidism: a follow-up study. *Clin Endocrinol (Oxf)*. 1993;38(5):523–530.

57. AACE/AAES Task Force on Primary Hyperparathyroidism. The American Association of Clinical Endocrinologists and the American Association of Endocrine Surgeons position statement on the diagnosis and management of primary hyperparathyroidism. *Endocr Pract*. 2005;11(1):49–54.
58. Rubin MR, Bilezikian JP, McMahon DJ, et al. The natural history of primary hyperparathyroidism with or without parathyroid surgery after 15 years. *J Clin Endocrinol Metab*. 2008;93(9):3462–3470.
59. Silverberg SJ, Brown I, Bilezikian JP. Age as a criterion for surgery in primary hyperparathyroidism. *Am J Med*. 2002;113(8):681–684.
60. Eigelberger MS, Cheah WK, Ituarte PH, Streja L, Duh QY, Clark OH. The NIH criteria for parathyroidectomy in asymptomatic primary hyperparathyroidism: are they too limited? *Ann Surg*. 2004;239(4):528–535.
61. Sosa JA, Powe NR, Levine MA, Udelsman R, Zeiger MA. Profile of a clinical practice: thresholds for surgery and surgical outcomes for patients with primary hyperparathyroidism: a national survey of endocrine surgeons. *J Clin Endocrinol Metab*. 1998;83(8):2658–2665.
62. Sosa JA, Powe NR, Levine MA, Bowman HM, Zeiger MA, Udelsman R. Cost implications of different surgical management strategies for primary hyperparathyroidism. *Surgery*. 1998;124(6):1028–1035.
63. Zanocco K, Angelos P, Sturgeon C. Cost-effectiveness analysis of parathyroidectomy for asymptomatic primary hyperparathyroidism. *Surgery*. 2006;140(6):874–881.
64. Burney RE, Jones KR, Coon JW, Blewitt DK, Herm AM. Assessment of patient outcomes after operation for primary hyperparathyroidism. *Surgery*. 1996;120(6):1013-1018.
65. Burney RE, Jones KR, Peterson M, Christy B, Thompson NW. Surgical correction of primary hyperparathyroidism improves quality of life. *Surgery*. 1998;124(6):987–991.
66. Bilezikian JP, Silverberg SJ. Clinical practice. Asymptomatic primary hyperparathyroidism. *N Engl J Med*. 2004;350(17): 1746–1751.
67. Cosman F, Shen V, Xie F, Seibel M, Ratcliffe A, Lindsay R. Estrogen protection against bone resorbing effects of parathyroid hormone infusion. Assessment by use of biochemical markers. *Ann Intern Med*. 1993;118(5):337–343.
68. Marcus R. The role of estrogens and related compounds in the management of primary hyperparathyroidism. *J Bone Miner Res*. 2002;17(suppl 2):N146–N149.
69. Rubin MR, Lee KH, McMahon DJ, Silverberg SJ. Raloxifene lowers serum calcium and markers of bone turnover in postmenopausal women with primary hyperparathyroidism. *J Clin Endocrinol Metab*. 2003;88(3):1174–1178.
70. Rossini M, Gatti D, Isaia G, Sartori L, Braga V, Adami S. Effects of oral alendronate in elderly patients with osteoporosis and mild primary hyperparathyroidism. *J Bone Miner Res*. 2001;16(1):113–119.
71. Chow CC, Chan WB, Li JK, et al. Oral alendronate increases bone mineral density in postmenopausal women with primary hyperparathyroidism. *J Clin Endocrinol Metab*. 2003;88(2):581–587.
72. Brown EM, Gamba G, Riccardi D, et al. Cloning and characterization of an extracellular Ca(2+)-sensing receptor from bovine parathyroid. *Nature*. 1993;366(6455):575–580.
73. Nemeth EF, Steffey ME, Hammerland LG, et al. Calcimimetics with potent and selective activity on the parathyroid calcium receptor. *Proc Natl Acad Sci USA*. 1998;95(7):4040–4045.
74. Nemeth EF, Fox J. Calcimimetic compounds: a direct approach to controlling plasma levels of parathyroid hormone in hyperparathyroidism. *Trends Endocrinol Metab*. 1999;10(2):66–71.
75. Antoniucci DM, Shoback D. Calcimimetics in the treatment of primary hyperparathyroidism. *J Bone Miner Res*. 2002;17(suppl 2):N141–N145.
76. Shoback DM, Bilezikian JP, Turner SA, McCary LC, Guo MD, Peacock M. The calcimimetic cinacalcet normalizes serum calcium in subjects with primary hyperparathyroidism. *J Clin Endocrinol Metab*. 2003;88(12):5644–5649.
77. Peacock M, Bilezikian JP, Klassen PS, Guo MD, Turner SA, Shoback D. Cinacalcet hydrochloride maintains long-term normocalcemia in patients with primary hyperparathyroidism. *J Clin Endocrinol Metab*. 2005;90(1):135–141.
78. Sajid-Crockett S, Singer FR, Hershman JM. Cinacalcet for the treatment of primary hyperparathyroidism. *Metabolism*. 2008;57(4):517–521.
79. Siperstein A, Berber E, Mackey R, et al. Prospective evaluation of sestamibi scan, ultrasonography, and rapid PTH to predict the success of limited exploration for sporadic primary hyperparathyroidism. *Surgery*. 2004;136(4):872–880.
80. Arici C, Cheah WK, Ituarte PH, et al. Can localization studies be used to direct focused parathyroid operations? *Surgery*. 2001;129(6):720–729.
81. Quiros RM, Alioto J, Wilhelm SM, et al. An algorithm to maximize use of minimally invasive parathyroidectomy. *Arch Surg*. 2004;139(5):501–506.
82. Berri RN, Lloyd LR. Detection of parathyroid adenoma in patients with primary hyperparathyroidism: the use of office-based ultrasound in preoperative localization. *Am J Surg*. 2006;191(3):311–314.
83. Solorzano CC, Carneiro-Pla DM, Irvin GL 3rd. Surgeon-performed ultrasonography as the initial and only localizing study in sporadic primary hyperparathyroidism. *J Am Coll Surg*. 2006;202(1):18–24.
84. Yip L, Pryma DA, Yim JH, et al. Sestamibi SPECT intensity scoring system in sporadic primary hyperparathyroidism. *World J Surg*. 2009;33(3):426–433.
85. Yip L, Pryma DA, Yim JH, et al. Can a lightbulb sestamibi SPECT accurately predict single-gland disease in sporadic primary hyperparathyroidism? *World J Surg*. 2008;32(5):784–792.
86. Doherty GM, Weber B, Norton JA. Cost of unsuccessful surgery for primary hyperparathyroidism. *Surgery*. 1994;116(6):954–957.
87. Irvin GL 3rd, Carneiro DM, Solorzano CC. Progress in the operative management of sporadic primary hyperparathyroidism over 34 years. *Ann Surg*. 2004;239(5):704–708.
88. Irvin GL 3rd, Sfakianakis G, Yeung L, et al. Ambulatory parathyroidectomy for primary hyperparathyroidism. *Arch Surg*. 1996;131(10):1074–1078.
89. Boggs JE, Irvin GL 3rd, Molinari AS, Deriso GT. Intraoperative parathyroid hormone monitoring as an adjunct to parathyroidectomy. *Surgery*. 1996;120(6):954–958.
90. Carty SE, Worsey J, Virji MA, Brown ML, Watson CG. Concise parathyroidectomy: the impact of preoperative SPECT 99mTc sestamibi scanning and intraoperative quick parathormone assay. *Surgery*. 1997;122(6):1107–1114.
91. Molinari AS, Irvin GL 3rd, Deriso GT, Bott L. Incidence of multiglandular disease in primary hyperparathyroidism determined by parathyroid hormone secretion. *Surgery*. 1996;120(6):934–936.
92. Udelsman R. Six hundred fifty-six consecutive explorations for primary hyperparathyroidism. *Ann Surg*. 2002;235(5):665–670.

93. Karakousis GC, Han D, Kelz RR, et al. Interpretation of intra-operative PTH changes in patients with multi-glandular primary hyperparathyroidism (pHPT). *Surgery*. 2007;142(6):845–850.
94. Miura D, Wada N, Arici C, Morita E, Duh QY, Clark OH. Does intraoperative quick parathyroid hormone assay improve the results of parathyroidectomy? *World J Surg*. 2002;26(8):926–930.
95. Carchman E, Ogilvie J, Holst J, Yim J, Carty S. Appropriate surgical treatment of lithium-associated hyperparathyroidism. *World J Surg*. 2008;32(10):2195–2199.
96. Duh QY, Arnaud CD, Levin KE, Clark OH. Parathyroid hormone: before and after parathyroidectomy. *Surgery*. 1986;100(6):1021–1031.
97. Koivunen DG, Buick MK, Seaton JF, Harrison TS. Early postoperative function of suppressed parathyroid glands with microscopic hyperplasia. *Surgery*. 1986;100(6):1011–1020.
98. Lundgren E, Rastad J, Ridefelt P, Juhlin C, Akerström G, Ljunghall S. Long-term effects of parathyroid operation on serum calcium and parathyroid hormone values in sporadic primary hyperparathyroidism. *Surgery*. 1992;112(6):1123–1129.
99. Bergenfelz A, Valdemarsson S, Tibblin S. Persistent elevated serum levels of intact parathyroid hormone after operation for sporadic parathyroid adenoma: evidence of detrimental effects of severe parathyroid disease. *Surgery*. 1996;119(6):24–633.
100. Tisell LE, Jansson S, Nilsson B, Lundberg PA, Lindstedt G. Transient rise in intact parathyroid hormone concentration after surgery for primary hyperparathyroidism. *Br J Surg*. 1996;83(5):665–669.
101. Mandal AK, Udelsman R. Secondary hyperparathyroidism is an expected consequence of parathyroidectomy for primary hyperparathyroidism: a prospective study. *Surgery*. 1998;124(6):1021–1026.
102. Denizot A, Pucini M, Chagnaud C, Botti G, Henry JF. Normocalcemia with elevated parathyroid hormone levels after surgical treatment of primary hyperparathyroidism. *Am J Surg*. 2001;182(1):15–19.
103. Carty SE, Roberts MM, Virji MA, Haywood L, Yim JH. Elevated serum parathormone level after "concise parathyroidectomy" for primary sporadic hyperparathyroidism. *Surgery*. 2002;132(6):1086–1092.
104. Bruining HA, Birkenhäger JC, Ong GL, Lamberts SW. Causes of failure in operations for hyperparathyroidism. *Surgery*. 1987;101(5):562–565.
105. Boggs JE, Irvin GL 3rd, Carneiro DM, Molinari AS. The evolution of parathyroidectomy failures. *Surgery*. 1999;126(6):998–1002.
106. Carty SE. Prevention and management of complications in parathyroid surgery. *Otolaryngol Clin North Am*. 2004;37(4):897–907.
107. Wells SA Jr, Debenedetti MK, Doherty GM. Recurrent or persistent hyperparathyroidism. *J Bone Miner Res*. 2002;17(suppl 2):N158–N162.
108. Carty SE, Helm AK, Amico JA, et al. The variable penetrance and spectrum of manifestations of multiple endocrine neoplasia type 1. *Surgery*. 1998;124(6):1106–1113.
109. Chandrasekharappa SC, Guru SC, Manickam P, et al. Positional cloning of the gene for multiple endocrine neoplasia-type 1. *Science*. 1997;276(5311):404–407.
110. Yip L, Ogilvie JB, Challinor SM, et al. Identification of multiple endocrine neoplasia type 1 in patients with apparent sporadic primary hyperparathyroidism. *Surgery*. 2008;144(6):1002–1006.
111. Marx SJ, Simonds WF, Agarwal SK, et al. Hyperparathyroidism in hereditary syndromes: special expressions and special managements. *J Bone Miner Res*. 2002;17(suppl 2):N37–N43.
112. O'Riordain DS, O'Brien T, Grant CS, Weaver A, Gharib H, van Heerden JA. Surgical management of primary hyperparathyroidism in multiple endocrine neoplasia types 1 and 2. *Surgery*. 1993;114(6):1031–1037.
113. Kraimps JL, Duh QY, Demeure M, Clark OH. Hyperparathyroidism in multiple endocrine neoplasia syndrome. *Surgery*. 1992;112(6):1080–1086.
114. Carpten JD, Robbins CM, Villablanca A, et al. HRPT2, encoding parafibromin, is mutated in hyperparathyroidism-jaw tumor syndrome. *Nat Genet*. 2002;32(4):676–680.
115. Simonds WF, James-Newton LA, Agarwal SK, et al. Familial isolated hyperparathyroidism: clinical and genetic characteristics of 36 kindreds. *Medicine (Baltimore)*. 2002;81(1):1–26.
116. Jackson CE, Norum RA, Boyd SB, et al. Hereditary hyperparathyroidism and multiple ossifying jaw fibromas: a clinically and genetically distinct syndrome. *Surgery*. 1990;108(6):1006–1012.
117. McCoy KL, Yim JH, Zuckerbraun BS, et al. Cystic parathyroid lesions: functional and nonfunctional parathyroid cysts. *Arch Surg*. 2009;144(1):52–56.
118. Silverberg SJ, Rubin MR, Faiman C, et al. Cinacalcet hydrochloride reduces the serum calcium concentration in inoperable parathyroid carcinoma. *J Clin Endocrinol Metab*. 2007;92(10):3803–3808.
119. Indridason OS, Quarles LD. Comparison of treatments for mild secondary hyperparathyroidism in hemodialysis patients. Durham Renal Osteodystrophy Study Group. *Kidney Int*. 2000;57(1):282–292.
120. Sturtevant JM, Hawley CM, Reiger K, et al. Efficacy and side-effect profile of sevelamer hydrochloride used in combination with conventional phosphate binders. *Nephrology*. 2004;9(6):406–413.
121. Joy MS, Finn WF, LAM-302 Study Group. Randomized, double-blind, placebo-controlled, dose-titration, phase III study assessing the efficacy and tolerability of lanthanum carbonate: a new phosphate binder for the treatment of hyperphosphatemia. *Am J Kidney Dis*. 2003;42(1):96–107.
122. Martin KJ, González EA. Vitamin D analogues for the management of secondary hyperparathyroidism. *Am J Kidney Dis*. 2001;38(5 suppl 5):S34–S40.
123. National Kidney Foundation. K/DOQI clinical practice guidelines for bone metabolism and disease in chronic kidney disease. *Am J Kidney Dis*. 2003;42(4 suppl 3):S1–S201.
124. Young EW, Akiba T, Albert JM, et al. Magnitude and impact of abnormal mineral metabolism in hemodialysis patients in the Dialysis Outcomes and Practice Patterns Study (DOPPS). *Am J Kidney Dis*. 2004;44(5 suppl 2):34–38.
125. Block GA, Martin KJ, de Francisco AL, et al. Cinacalcet for secondary hyperparathyroidism in patients receiving hemodialysis. *N Engl J Med*. 2004;350(15):1516–1525.
126. Moe SM, Chertow GM, Coburn JW, et al. Achieving NKF-K/DOQI bone metabolism and disease treatment goals with cinacalcet HCl. *Kidney Int*. 2005;67(2):760–771.
127. Cunningham J, Danese M, Olson K, et al. Effects of the calcimimetic cinacalcet HCl on cardiovascular disease, fracture, and health–related quality of life in secondary hyperparathyroidism. *Kidney Int*. 2005;68(4):1793–1800.
128. Schaefer RM, Bover J, Dellanna F, et al. Efficacy of cinacalcet administered with the first meal after dialysis: the SENSOR Study. *Clin Nephrol*. 2008;70(2):126–134.

129. D'Alessandro AM, Melzer JS, Pirsch JD, et al. Tertiary hyperparathyroidism after renal transplantation: operative indications. *Surgery*. 1989;106(6):1049–1055.
130. Evenepoel P, Claes K, Kuypers D, et al. Natural history of parathyroid function and calcium metabolism after kidney transplantation: a single-centre study. *Nephrol Dial Transplant*. 2004;19(5):1281–1287.
131. Kerby JD, Rue LW, Blair H, et al. Operative treatment of tertiary hyperparathyroidism: a single-center experience. *Ann Surg*. 1998;227(6):878–886.
132. Rothmund M, Wagner PK, Schark C. Subtotal parathyroidectomy versus total parathyroidectomy and autotransplantation in secondary hyperparathyroidism: a randomized trial. *World J Surg*. 1991;15(6):745–750.
133. Lorenz K, Ukkat J, Sekulla C, et al. Total parathyroidectomy without autotransplantation for renal hyperparathyroidism: experience with a qPTH-controlled protocol. *World J Surg*. 2006;30(5):743–751.
134. Triponez F, Dosseh D, Hazzan M, et al. Subtotal parathyroidectomy with thymectomy for autonomous hyperparathyroidism after renal transplantation. *Br J Surg*. 2005;92(10):1282–1287.
135. Takagi H, Tominaga Y, Uchida K, et al. Subtotal versus total parathyroidectomy with forearm autograft for secondary hyperparathyroidism in chronic renal failure. *Ann Surg*. 1984;200(1):18–23.

15
Nonneoplastic Parathyroid Diseases

Lori A. Erickson

Introduction

The parathyroid glands are involved in regulating serum calcium concentrations and bone metabolism by the secretion of parathyroid hormone (PTH). Low concentrations of serum calcium are sensed by a calcium-sensing receptor (CASR) on the surface of parathyroid cells and result in stimulation of PTH secretion, while high serum calcium concentrations inhibit PTH secretion. The parathyroid glands are derived from the endodermal third and fourth branchial pouches. The normal parathyroid glands each measures 4–6 mm in length and weighs 20–40 mg. Generally, a parathyroid gland greater than 50–60 mg is considered abnormal.

Parathyroid glands are composed of chief cells, transitional cells, oxyphil cells, and adipose tissue. Chief cells measure 8–10 µm have amphophilic to eosinophilic cytoplasm with intracytoplasmic glycogen and lipid. Oxyphilic cells are 12–20 µm and have prominent cytoplasmic mitochondria accounting for the granular eosinophilic cytoplasm. Oxyphilic cells are not usually identified in children. Transitional oxyphilic cells are smaller and have less cytoplasm. The cellularity of parathyroid glands is variable and distributed unevenly in the gland. Cellularity also differs with constitutional factors and age; cellularity is high in infants and children and decreases with age.

Sporadic Hyperparathyroidism

Clinical

Hyperparathyroidism is an increase in PTH which often results in increased serum calcium levels. Sporadic primary hyperparathyroidism is caused by parathyroid hyperplasia, adenoma, or carcinoma. The neoplastic conditions will be dicussed in chapter 16. Parathyroid hyperplasia accounts for 15% of primary hyperparathyroidism.[1] Parathyroid hyperplasia is more common in women than in men (2:1) and often occurs in the fifth decade, but may occur over a wide age range. The incidence of primary hyperparathyroidism increased in the early 1970s with the onset of screening serum calcium.

The clinical presentation has changed over time. While patients used to present with nephrocalcinosis and osteopenia, today they usually present with weakness and lethargy or, even more commonly, patients are asymptomatic with elevated screening serum calcium. One percent of women who undergo thyroidectomy have diffusely enlarged or nodular parathyroid glands, possibly representing an early normocalcemic subclinical form of hyperparathyroidism.[2,3] Parathyroid hyperplasia has been associated with neck irradiation and drugs such as lithium.[4,5]

Patients with secondary hyperparathyroidism have increased PTH because of low serum calcium caused by disorders of vitamin D (Rickets, vitamin D deficiency or malabsorption), disorders of phosphate metabolism (malnutrition or malabsorption, renal disease, aluminum toxicity), tissue resistance to vitamin D, pseudohypoparathyroidism, hypomagnesemia, and calcium deficiency. Chronic renal failure is the most common cause of secondary hyperparathyroidism. Tertiary hyperparathyroidism is a rare condition, in which patients with secondary hyperparathyroidism develop an autonomously functioning parathyroid gland.

Histologic Features

Primary hyperparathyroidism caused by hyperplasia results in enlargement of multiple parathyroid glands. Sporadic and hereditary forms of primary parathyroid hyperplasia are histologically indistinguishable. Parathyroid glands usually show nodular hyperplastic areas but a diffuse increase in parenchymal cells can be seen (Figure 15.1). A study of sporadic primary hyperplasia showed diffuse hyperplasia was usually associated with moderately enlarged glands with little variability in gland size and morphologic patterns and was more prevalent in young patients with moderate hypercalcaemia.[6] In nodular hyperplasia, the glands were more asymmetric in size, showed variable cellularity with more oxyphil cells, and were more frequent in elderly patients. Parathyroid glands in primary hyperplasia can show an increase in chief, clear, oxyphil, transitional cells, or a mixture of cell types. The cells can show sheet like growth, palisading, glandular formations, cribriforming,

J.L. Hunt (ed.), *Molecular Pathology of Endocrine Diseases*, Molecular Pathology Library 3,
DOI 10.1007/978-1-4419-1707-2_15, © Springer Science+Business Media, LLC 2010

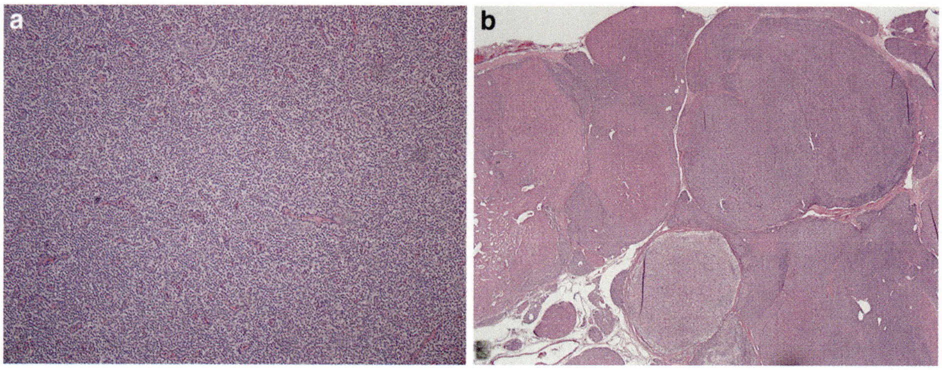

FIG. 15.1. Parathyroid hyperplasia. (**a**) Diffuse hyperplasia of chief cells. (**b**) Nodular hyperplasia with nodules of oxyphil cells, chief cells and transitional cells.

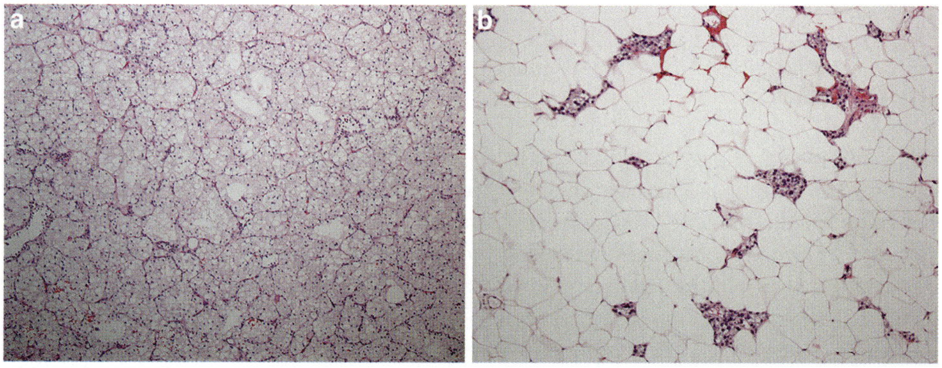

FIG. 15.2. Unusual variants of parathyroid hyperplasia. (**a**) Clear cell hyperplasia. (**b**) Lipohyperplasia.

papillary areas, microcystic formations, and cystic change. Surgeons and pathologists must be cautious in evaluating parathyroid glands in relation to size and cellularity as these parameters can vary greatly within a single patient with parathyroid hyperplasia. An asymmetrically enlarged gland can be misinterpreted as a parathyroid adenoma. Primary water-clear cell hyperplasia shows a diffuse increase in clear cells rather than nodular growth (Figure 15.2). Lipohyperplasia is rare and can occur both as a sporadic form and with familial benign hypocalciuric hypercalcemia (Figure 15.2).[6,7]

The parathyroid glands in secondary hyperplasia usually show more diffusely hyperplastic changes than in primary hyperparathyroidism. The glands usually show diffuse hyperplasia of chief cells. Oxyphilic cells can form nodular areas, as can chief cells, and nodularity may increase with increasing renal failure making the glands indistinguishable from primary or tertiary hyperplasia.

Immunohistochemical Studies

Hyperplastic parathyroid glands show immunoreactivity for the same markers and normal parathyroid tissue: chromogranin A, synaptophysin, low molecular weight keratins, and PTH. The expression of p27, a cyclin-dependent kinase inhibitor that helps regulate the transition from the G1 to the S phase of the cell cycle, is the highest normal parathyroid, followed by hyperplasia, adenomas, and carcinomas.[8] In situ hybridization showed no differences in p27 mRNA, indicating that the expression of the p27 gene is controlled at a posttranslational level in parathyroid tissues.[8] Ki67 expression is higher in carcinomas than in hyperplasia and adenomas.[8] Hyperplastic parathyroid glands overexpress fatty acid synthase.[9] A study evaluating angiogenic factors endoglin, vascular endothelial growth factor (VEGF), and VEGF-R2 differentiated hyperplastic parathyroid tissues from neoplastic parathyroids.[10]

Genetics

Unlike neoplastic causes of primary hyperparathyroidism, parathyroid hyperplasia is usually polyclonal although areas of monoclonality can be identified in nodular areas. Specific genetic abnormalities in idiopathic primary parathyroid hyperplasia have not been as well defined as in hereditary forms of hyperparathyroidism.

Hereditary Hyperparathyroidism

Clinical

Hereditary hyperparathyroidism is less common than primary sporadic hyperparathyroidism. The most common types of hereditary hyperparathyroidism are multiple endocrine neoplasia (MEN) type 1, MEN2A, familial hypocalciuric hypercalcemia, neonatal severe primary hyperparathyroidism,

hyperparathyroidism-jaw tumor syndrome (HP-JT), and familial isolated hyperparathyroidism (FIHP). MEN1 equally affects females and males and does not show ethnic or geographic differences. Parathyroid hyperplasia is the most common manifestation of MEN1, although parathyroid adenomas and carcinomas can occur. MEN1 associated hyperparathyroidism has an onset of 20–25 years of age which is four decades earlier than sporadic primary hyperparathyroidism.[11] Other features of MEN 1 include pituitary adenomas, neuroendocrine tumors of the pancreas, duodenum, thymus and lung, gastrinomas, adrenal cortical adenomas and hyperplasia, facial angiofibromas, collagenomas, café au lait macules, lipomas, gingival papules, meningiomas, ependymomas, and leiomyomas.[12,13]

MEN2A is associated with parathyroid hyperplasia and or adenomas in 20–30% of cases. MEN2A is diagnosed clinically by the occurrence of at least two specific endocrine tumors (medullary thyroid carcinoma, pheochromocytoma, or parathyroid hyperplasia/adenoma).

Familial hypocalciuric hypercalcemia is caused by an autosomal dominant mutation in the *CASR* gene causing lifelong hypercalcemia without hypercalciuria.[14–16] Neonatal primary hyperparathyroidism is a life-threatening disorder caused by homozygous inactivating mutation of the *CASR* gene. The parathyroid glands become hyperplasic, and infants are symptomatically hypercalcemic.

HP-JT is an autosomal dominant disorder of hyperparathyroidism, fibro-osseus jaw tumors, kidney cysts, hamartomas, and Wilms tumors. The parathyroids show hyperplasia or adenoma, and there is an increased risk of parathyroid carcinoma.[17] FIHP, an autosomal dominant disorder, accounts for 1% of primary hyperparathyroidism.[18] The cause of FIHP remains unknown in most families, but it has been thought to be a unique entity or possibly a subset may be variant of MEN1 or HP-JT syndrome.[18–22] This disorder is also associated with an increased risk of parathyroid carcinoma.[20,23]

TABLE 15.1. Hereditary hyperparathyroidism.

Disorder	GGen Genetics
Multiple endocrine neoplasia type 1	*MEN1* germline mutation (11q13) *MEN1* encodes menin, a 610 amino acid protein Autosomal dominant
Multiple endocrine neoplasia type 2A	*RET* proto-oncogene (10q21) Autosomal dominant
Familial hypocalciuric hypercalcemia	Heterozygous inactivating calcium-sensing receptor (*CASR*) mutation (3q13.3–q21) Autosomal dominant
Neonatal severe hyperparathyroidism	Homozygous inactivating *CASR* mutation (3q13.3–q21) Autosomal recessive
Hyperparathyroidism-jaw tumor syndrome	*HRPT2* gene (1q21–q31) Autosomal dominant
Familial isolated hyperparathyroidism	Unknown, possibly variant of MEN1 or HP-JT syndrome Autosomal dominant

Genetics

Although many genes associated with hereditary hyperparathyroidism have been identified, the exact mechanisms are still being elucidated (Table 15.1). *MEN1* is a tumor suppressor gene on chromosome 11q13 which encodes menin, a 610 amino acid protein.[24–26] Menin is truncated or absent with most germline or somatic mutations in *MEN1*.[24–26] Menin is mainly nuclear, relatively ubiquitous, and may function in tumor suppression by interacting with proteins regulating the cell cycle and proliferation.[27] *MEN1* is the only gene known to be associated with MEN1 syndrome. MEN1 is an autosomal dominant disorder with high penetrance, but it can occur sporadically from new mutations. Over 1,000 different mutations have been identified, the majority of which result in truncation of menin.[27] Germline *MEN1* mutations are identified in 80–94% of patients with familial MEN1 and 65–88% of patients with sporadic MEN1.[12,25,28] The detection rate of *MEN1* mutation increases with the number of MEN1 related tumors and family history of MEN1, as sporadic cases can be caused by somatic mosaicism.[29,30]

RET proto-oncogene (10q21) encodes a plasma membrane tyrosine kinase involved in cell growth and differentiation. Approximately 95% of MEN2A families have an *RET* mutation in exon 10 or 11.[31–33] The majority of mutations involve codon 634, with the other mutations identified mainly in codons 609, 611, 618, 612.[31,33,34] Mutations in codon 634 are associated with high penetrance.[34] Risk stratification by mutation status has been suggested as a basis for surgical decisions such that patients with the highest risk mutations would undergo prophylactic thyroidectomy at the youngest age.[34]

The CASR is present in parathyroid, kidney, thyroid C-cells, intestine, and bone.[35,36] CASRs sense extracellular calcium levels which inversely regulates the release of PTH.[37] An inactivating mutation in the *CASR* gene (3q13.3–21) results in decreased calcium sensitivity of the cells and excess PTH secretion. Heterozygous inactivating *CASR* mutations occur in familial hypocalciuric hypercalcemia, and homozygous inactivating mutations occur in neonatal severe hyperparathyroidism (Table 15.2). Hypocalciuric hypercalcemia is caused autoantibodies directed at CASR and can simulate familial hypocalciuric hypercalcemia.[38]

The *HRPT2* gene mapped to 1q25–q32 encodes parafibromin.[39,40] *HRPT2* is a putative tumor-suppressor gene, the inactivation of which is involved in HP-JT syndrome and some sporadic parathyroid tumors.[39]

Sporadic Hypoparathyroidism

Clinical

Hypoparathyroidism is characterized by hypocalcemia and hyperphosphatemia because of insufficient PTH secretion or when PTH is not able to function appropriately in target tissues

TABLE 15.2. Calcium-sensing receptor (CASR) abnormalities in nonneoplastic parathyroid disease.

Parathyroid disease	Genetic	Clinical
Familial hypocalciuric hypercalcemia	Inactivating (heterozygous loss-of-function) *CASR* mutation (3q13.3–q21)	Hyperparathyroidism
Neonatal severe hyperparathyroidism	Inactivating (homozygous loss-of-function) *CASR* mutation (3q13.3–q21)	Hyperparathyroidism
Familial isolated hypoparathyroidism	Various genes have reportedly been associated including *CASR* (3q13.3–q21)	Hypoparathyroidism
Sporadic idiopathic hypoparathyroidism	Unknown cause, but antibodies to calcium-sensing receptor in some cases	Hypoparathyroidism
Autoimmune polyglandular syndrome 1	Mutations in the *APECED* (autoimmune polyendocrinopathy-candidiasis-ectodermal-dystrophy) or *AIRE* (autoimmune regulator) gene (21q22.3) Autoantigens to calcium-sensing receptor	Hypoparathyroidism

despite adequate circulating levels. Hypoparathyroidism can result from removal or damage to parathyroid glands during surgery, developmental disorders, autoimmune hypoparathyroidism, PTH defects, and defective regulation of PTH secretion.[22] Sporadic idiopathic hypoparathyroidism is a common cause of hypoparathyroidism. Antibodies against the CASR have been identified in some cases, but the pathogenesis remains unclear.[41] DiGeorge syndrome is characterized by congenital aplasia of the thymus resulting in deficiency of T-cells, parathyroid aplasia resulting in hypocalcemia, cardiac outflow tract defects, characteristic facies, and short stature.[42,43] Kearns–Sayre syndrome is a rare neuromuscular disorder caused by abnormalities of mitochondrial DNA with an onset by young adulthood, hypoparathyroidism, eye movement limitation and pigmentation, weakness, cardiac conduction defects, hearing loss, ataxia, cognitive problems, and diabetes.[44]

Genetics

The genetic basis of sporadic idiopathic hypoparathyroidism is not known, although antibodies against the CASR have been identified in some cases.[41] DiGeorge syndrome is caused by hemizygous deletion of 22q11.2 with most abnormalities due to haploinsufficiency of the *TBX1* gene.[45] Kearns–Sayre syndrome is caused by abnormalities of mitochondrial DNA.[44]

Hereditary Hypoparathyroidism

Clinical

Hereditary hypoparathyroidism is relatively rare and encompasses a variety of syndromes. Sanjad–Sakati syndrome includes congenital hypoparathyroidism, mental retardation, and growth failure, while patients with Kenny–Caffey syndrome also have osteosclerosis and recurrent bacterial infections.[46] Both are chaperone diseases caused by a defect in tubulin physiology and parathyroid development.[46] Velocardiofacial syndrome is autosomal dominant condition typified by neonatal hypocalcemia, cleft palate, cardiac and ocular anomalies, learning disabilities, and T-cell dysfunction. Autoimmune polyglandular syndrome type 1 is an autoimmune disorder affecting endocrine glands and skin.[47] Familial isolated hypoparathyroidism is characterized by hypocalcemia and hyperphosphatemia because of inadequate PTH secretion. Jansen metaphyseal chondrodysplasia is a rare form of short-limbed dwarfism with hypercalcemia, hypophosphatemia, and normal to low PTH and PTH-related protein. Blomstrand chondrodysplasia is also associated with parathyroid disease.[48] Patients with pseudohypoparathyroidism type 1a (Albright's hereditary osteodystrophy) have short stature, short metacarpal and metatarsal bones, and round faces, while those with pseudohypoparathyroidism type 1b have hypocalcemia with PTH resistance confined to the kidney and lack other features of Albright's hereditary osteodystrophy.

Genetics

A variety of genes are associated with hereditary hypoparathyroidism (Table 15.3). The *TBCE* gene (tubulin-specific chaperone E) on chromosome 1q42–q43 encodes a chaperone protein required for folding of alpha-tubulin subunits and alpha-beta-tubulin heterodimers.[46] Mutations in *TBCE* cause Kenny–Caffey syndrome, which can have autosomal dominant or recessive transmission.[46] Velocardiofacial syndrome, like DiGeorge syndrome, is caused by hemizygous deletion of 22q11.2 with most abnormalities due to haploinsufficiency of the *TBX1* gene.[45] Mutations in the *APECED* (autoimmune polyendocrinopathy-candidiasis-ectodermal-dystrophy) or *AIRE* (autoimmune regulator) gene on chromosome 21q22.3, which codes for a putative transcription factor, have been identified in autoimmune polyglandular syndrome type 1 which has autoantigens against the CASR.[49] Activating *CASR* mutations occur in familial isolated hypoparathyroidism.[15,16] Familial isolated hypoparathyroidism, usually an autosomal dominant condition, can also be caused by mutation in *PTH* gene (11p15.3–p15.1)[50], mutation or polymorphism in the *GCM2* gene (6p24.2)[51,52] or mutation in the *GCMB* gene (6p23–24),[53] and there is an X-linked recessive (Xq26–q27)[54] form. In addition to familial isolated hypoparathyroidism, *PTH* mutations are identified in autosomal recessive hypoparathyroidism. Jansen chondrodysplasia is an autosomal dominant condition with activating mutations in PTH receptor type 1 (*PTHr1*) gene (3p22–p21.1), while Blomstrand chondrodysplasia is autosomal recessive with inactivating mutations in *PTHr1*.[48] Pseudohypoparathyroidism is caused by defects in stimulatory guanine nucleotide binding protein because of *GNAS1* mutation (Gsalpha1 protein of the adenyl cyclase complex). The *GNAS1* gene (20q13.11) encodes a stimulatory guanine nucleotide binding protein which is acted on by PTH receptor type 1. Patients with pseudohypoparathyroidism type 1a have an autosomal dominant trait caused by an inactivating mutation in *GNAS1*, while those with pseudohypoparathyroidism type 1b are associated with defective methylation in *GNAS1*.[55]

TABLE 15.3. Hypoparathyroid disorders with known genetic abnormalities.

Parathyroid disease	Genetic
DiGeorge syndrome	Sporadic 1.5–3.0 Hemizygous deletion of 22q11.2 (defects due to haploinsufficiency of *TBX1* gene)
Velocardiofacial syndrome	Autosomal dominant 1.5–3.0 Hemizygous deletion of 22q11.2 (defects due to haploinsufficiency of *TBX1* gene)
Kearns–Sayre syndrome	Mitochondrial DNA abnormalities
Kenny–Caffey syndrome	Autosomal dominant or autosomal recessive Mutations in gene encoding tubulin-specific chaperone E (*TBCE*) on 1q42–q43
Sporadic idiopathic hypoparathyroidism	Sporadic Unknown, but antibodies to calcium-sensing receptor in some cases
Autoimmune polyglandular syndrome type 1	Autosomal recessive Mutations in the *APECED* (autoimmune polyendocrinopathy-candidiasis-ectodermal-dystrophy) or *AIRE* (autoimmune regulator) gene (21q22.3) Autoantigens to calcium-sensing receptor
Familial isolated hypoparathyroidism	Usually autosomal dominant Various genes have reportedly been associated: *CASR* (3q13.3–21) mutation, *PTH* (11p15.3–p15.1) mutation, mutation or polymorphism in *GCM2* (6p24.2), mutation in *GCMB* (6p23–24), and X-linked form (Xq26–q27)
Autosomal recessive hypoparathyroidism	Autosomal recessive *PTH* (11p15.3–p15.1) point mutation
Jansen's chondrodystrophy	Autosomal dominant Activating *PTHr1* (3p22–p21.1) mutation
Blomstrand's chondrodystrophy	Autosomal recessive Inactivating *PTHr1* (3p22–p21.1) mutation
Pseudohypoparathyroidism type 1a (Albright's hereditary osteodystrophy)	Autosomal dominant Inactivating mutation in stimulatory guanine nucleotide binding protein (*GNAS1 gene*) (*GNAS1* mutation (Gsalpha1 protein of the adenyl cyclase complex))
Pseudohypoparathyroidism type 1b	Defects in methylation of stimulatory guanine nucleotide binding protein (*GNAS1 gene*) (*GNAS1* mutation (Gsalpha1 protein of the adenyl cyclase complex))
Pseudohypoparathyroidism type 2	Defective cAMP-dependent protein kinase

Miscellaneous Nonneoplastic Parathyroid Disorders

Parathyroid Cysts

Clinically apparent parathyroid cysts are relatively uncommon and can be functioning with hyperparathyroidism or nonfunctioning and present as a mass or mimicking a cystic thyroid nodule.[56] Functioning parathyroid cysts may represent cystic degeneration of a parathyroid adenoma. Parathyroid carcinoma has been reported in association with a parathyroid cyst.[57] Small microcysts are not uncommon incidental findings at autopsy, while macrocysts are often investigated clinically. The cysts may also be intrathyroidal or mediastinal.[58,59] Etiologies suggested for parathyroid cysts include developmental abnormalities, fluid accumulation in the parathyroid, coalescence of microcysts into clinical macrocysts, degeneration of a parathyroid neoplasm, and may from vestigial remnants of Kursteiner canals.[60] A literature review of 93 patients with parathyroid cysts identified parathyroid hyperparathyroidism in 39 cases (42%).[60] Over a 25-year period during which 22,009 thyroidectomies and 2,505 parathyroidectomies were performed, 38 nonfunctional parathyroid cysts were identified.[59] The cysts presented as incidental findings on chest X-ray, compressive symptoms, or an asymptomatic palpable neck mass.[59] Histologically, the cyst wall can contain a variety of elements including lymphoid, muscular, thymic, adipose, and mesenchymal tissues (Figure 15.3).[59]

Amyloid

Amyloid can involve both normal and diseased parathyroid glands and can be identified in patients with and without systemic amyloidosis.[61–64] Amyloid often shows an intrafollicular distribution in the parathyroid.[61] Amyloid in parathyroid glands shows uniform reactions with Congo red and Thioflavin T, but the pathogenesis of this amyloid remains uncertain.[63]

Parathyroiditis

Parathyroiditis can be autoimmune associated and may result in hypoparathyroidism or hyperparathyroidism.[65–68]

Glycogen Storage Diseases

Pompe's disease (type II glycogenosis) is a generalized glycogenosis caused deficiency of lysosomal acid alpha-1,4-glucosidase, which affects the central nervous system, heart, liver, muscle, and endocrine organs, including the parathyroids.[69,70]

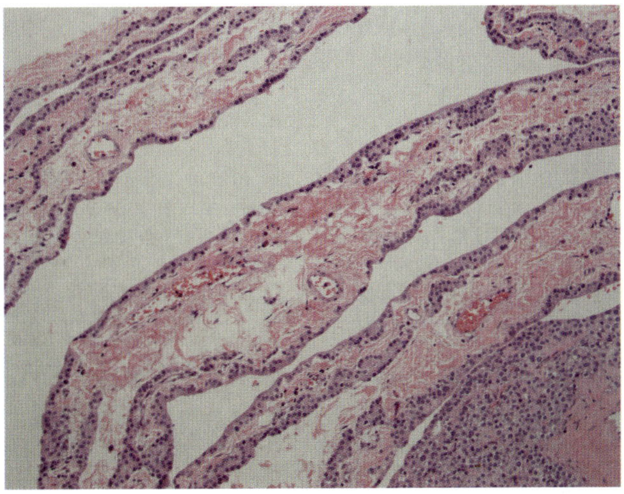

FIG. 15.3. Parathyroid cyst lined by parathyroid cells.

Conclusion

Nonneoplastic parathyroid disease encompasses a great variety of both sporadic and hereditary causes of hyperparathyroidism and hypoparathyroidism. The genetic basis for sporadic parathyroid disease is poorly understood. The genetic basis of hereditary parathyroid disorders is better understood, but the exact mechanisms still need to be further elucidated.

References

1. Castleman B, Schantz A, Roth S. Parathyroid hyperplasia in primary hyperparathyroidism: a review of 85 cases. *Cancer.* 1976;38:1668–1675.
2. Carnaille BM, Pattou FN, Oudar C, Lecomte-Houcke MC, Rocha JE, Proye CA. Parathyroid incidentalomas in normocalcemic patients during thyroid surgery. *World J Surg.* 1996;20:830–834. discussion 834.
3. Hellman P, Ohrvall U, Rudberg C, et al. Incidence, structure, and function of enlarged parathyroid glands discovered accidentally during thyroid surgery. *Surgery.* 1993;113:655–661.
4. Miller RW. Delayed effects of external radiation exposure: a brief history. *Radiat Res.* 1995;144:160–169.
5. Bendz H, Sjodin I, Toss G, Berglund K. Hyperparathyroidism and long-term lithium therapy – a cross-sectional study and the effect of lithium withdrawal. *J Intern Med.* 1996;240:357–365.
6. Tominaga Y, Grimelius L, Johansson H, et al. Histological and clinical features of non-familial primary parathyroid hyperplasia. *Pathol Res Pract.* 1992;188:115–122.
7. Yamauchi M, Sugimoto T, Yamaguchi T, et al. Familial hypocalciuric hypercalcemia caused by an R648stop mutation in the calcium-sensing receptor gene. *J Bone Miner Res.* 2002;17:2174–2182.
8. Erickson LA, Jin L, Wollan P, Thompson GB, van Heerden JA, Lloyd RV. Parathyroid hyperplasia, adenomas, and carcinomas: differential expression of p27Kip1 protein. *Am J Surg Pathol.* 1999;23:288–295.
9. Alo PL, Visca P, Mazzaferro S, et al. Immunohistochemical study of fatty acid synthase, Ki67, proliferating cell nuclear antigen, and p53 expression in hyperplastic parathyroids. *Ann Diagn Pathol.* 1999;3:287–293.
10. Lazaris AC, Tseleni-Balafouta S, Papathomas T, et al. Immunohistochemical investigation of angiogenic factors in parathyroid proliferative lesions. *Eur J Endocrinol.* 2006;154: 827–833.
11. Uchino S, Noguchi S, Sato M, et al. Screening of the Men1 gene and discovery of germ-line and somatic mutations in apparently sporadic parathyroid tumors. *Cancer Res.* 2000;60:5553–5557.
12. Marx SJ, Agarwal SK, Kester MB, et al. Multiple endocrine neoplasia type 1: clinical and genetic features of the hereditary endocrine neoplasias. *Recent Prog Horm Res.* 1999;54: 397–438. discussion 438–439.
13. Brandi ML, Gagel RF, Angeli A, et al. Guidelines for diagnosis and therapy of MEN type 1 and type 2. *J Clin Endocrinol Metab.* 2001;86:5658–5671.
14. Aida K, Koishi S, Inoue M, Nakazato M, Tawata M, Onaya T. Familial hypocalciuric hypercalcemia associated with mutation in the human Ca(2+)-sensing receptor gene. *J Clin Endocrinol Metab.* 1995;80:2594–2598.
15. Pearce SH, Williamson C, Kifor O, et al. A familial syndrome of hypocalcemia with hypercalciuria due to mutations in the calcium-sensing receptor. *N Engl J Med.* 1996;335:1115–1122.
16. Cole DE, Janicic N, Salisbury SR, Hendy GN. Neonatal severe hyperparathyroidism, secondary hyperparathyroidism, and familial hypocalciuric hypercalcemia: multiple different phenotypes associated with an inactivating Alu insertion mutation of the calcium-sensing receptor gene. *Am J Med Genet.* 1997; 71:202–210.
17. Cetani F, Pardi E, Borsari S, et al. Genetic analyses of the HRPT2 gene in primary hyperparathyroidism: germline and somatic mutations in familial and sporadic parathyroid tumors. *J Clin Endocrinol Metab.* 2004;89:5583–5591.
18. Warner JV, Nyholt DR, Busfield F, et al. Familial isolated hyperparathyroidism is linked to a 1.7 Mb region on chromosome 2p13.3–14. *J Med Genet.* 2006;43:e12.
19. Teh BT, Farnebo F, Twigg S, et al. Familial isolated hyperparathyroidism maps to the hyperparathyroidism-jaw tumor locus in 1q21–q32 in a subset of families. *J Clin Endocrinol Metab.* 1998;83:2114–2120.
20. Wassif WS, Moniz CF, Friedman E, et al. Familial isolated hyperparathyroidism: a distinct genetic entity with an increased risk of parathyroid cancer. *J Clin Endocrinol Metab.* 1993;77:1485–1489.
21. Villablanca A, Wassif WS, Smith T, et al. Involvement of the MEN1 gene locus in familial isolated hyperparathyroidism. *Eur J Endocrinol.* 2002;147:313–322.
22. Marx SJ. Hyperparathyroid and hypoparathyroid disorders. *N Engl J Med.* 2000;343:1863–1875.
23. Simonds WF, Robbins CM, Agarwal SK, Hendy GN, Carpten JD, Marx SJ. Familial isolated hyperparathyroidism is rarely caused by germline mutation in HRPT2, the gene for the hyperparathyroidism-jaw tumor syndrome. *J Clin Endocrinol Metab.* 2004;89:96–102.
24. Agarwal SK, Lee Burns A, Sukhodolets KE, et al. Molecular pathology of the MEN1 gene. *Ann N Y Acad Sci.* 2004;1014: 189–198.
25. Agarwal SK, Kester MB, Debelenko LV, et al. Germline mutations of the MEN1 gene in familial multiple endocrine neoplasia type 1 and related states. *Hum Mol Genet.* 1997;6:1169–1175.
26. Chandrasekharappa SC, Guru SC, Manickam P, et al. Positional cloning of the gene for multiple endocrine neoplasia-type 1. *Science.* 1997;276:404–407.
27. Lemos MC, Thakker RV. Multiple endocrine neoplasia type 1 (MEN1): analysis of 1336 mutations reported in the first decade following identification of the gene. *Hum Mutat.* 2008;29:22–32.
28. Guo SS, Sawicki MP. Molecular and genetic mechanisms of tumorigenesis in multiple endocrine neoplasia type-1. *Mol Endocrinol.* 2001;15:1653–1664.
29. Ellard S, Hattersley AT, Brewer CM, Vaidya B. Detection of an MEN1 gene mutation depends on clinical features and supports current referral criteria for diagnostic molecular genetic testing. *Clin Endocrinol (Oxf).* 2005;62:169–175.
30. Klein RD, Salih S, Bessoni J, Bale AE. Clinical testing for multiple endocrine neoplasia type 1 in a DNA diagnostic laboratory. *Genet Med.* 2005;7:131–138.
31. Oishi S, Sato T, Takiguchi-Shirahama S, Nakamura Y. Mutations of the RET proto-oncogene in multiple endocrine neoplasia type 2A (Sipple's syndrome). *Endocr J.* 1995;42:527–536.

32. Mulligan LM, Marsh DJ, Robinson BG, et al. Genotype–phenotype correlation in multiple endocrine neoplasia type 2: report of the International RET Mutation Consortium. *J Intern Med*. 1995;238:343–346.
33. Mulligan LM, Eng C, Attie T, et al. Diverse phenotypes associated with exon 10 mutations of the RET proto-oncogene. *Hum Mol Genet*. 1994;3:2163–2167.
34. Machens A, Dralle H. Genotype–phenotype based surgical concept of hereditary medullary thyroid carcinoma. *World J Surg*. 2007;31:957–968.
35. Aida K, Koishi S, Tawata M, Onaya T. Molecular cloning of a putative Ca(2+)-sensing receptor cDNA from human kidney. *Biochem Biophys Res Commun*. 1995;214:524–529.
36. Hauache OM. Extracellular calcium-sensing receptor: structural and functional features and association with diseases. *Braz J Med Biol Res*. 2001;34:577–584.
37. Hellman P, Carling T, Rask L, Akerstrom G. Pathophysiology of primary hyperparathyroidism. *Histol Histopathol*. 2000;15: 619–627.
38. Kifor O, Moore FD Jr, Delaney M, et al. A syndrome of hypocalciuric hypercalcemia caused by autoantibodies directed at the calcium-sensing receptor. *J Clin Endocrinol Metab*. 2003;88:60–72.
39. Carpten JD, Robbins CM, Villablanca A, et al. HRPT2, encoding parafibromin, is mutated in hyperparathyroidism-jaw tumor syndrome. *Nat Genet*. 2002;32:676–680.
40. Szabo J, Heath B, Hill VM, et al. Hereditary hyperparathyroidism-jaw tumor syndrome: the endocrine tumor gene HRPT2 maps to chromosome 1q21–q31. *Am J Hum Genet*. 1995;56:944–950.
41. Goswami R, Brown EM, Kochupillai N, et al. Prevalence of calcium sensing receptor autoantibodies in patients with sporadic idiopathic hypoparathyroidism. *Eur J Endocrinol*. 2004;150:9–18.
42. Kretschmer R, Say B, Brown D, Rosen FS. Congenital aplasia of the thymus gland (DiGeorge's syndrome). *N Engl J Med*. 1968;279:1295–1301.
43. Kirkpatrick JA Jr, DiGeorge AM. Congenital absence of the thymus. *Am J Roentgenol Radium Ther Nucl Med*. 1968;103:32–37.
44. Maceluch JA, Niedziela M. The clinical diagnosis and molecular genetics of Kearns–Sayre syndrome: a complex mitochondrial encephalomyopathy. *Pediatr Endocrinol Rev*. 2006;4: 117–137.
45. Yagi H, Furutani Y, Hamada H, et al. Role of TBX1 in human del22q11.2 syndrome. *Lancet*. 2003;362:1366–1373.
46. Parvari R, Hershkovitz E, Grossman N, et al. Mutation of TBCE causes hypoparathyroidism-retardation-dysmorphism and autosomal recessive Kenny–Caffey syndrome. *Nat Genet*. 2002;32:448–452.
47. Schumann C, Faust M, Gerharz M, Ortmann M, Schubert M, Krone W. Autoimmune polyglandular syndrome associated with idiopathic giant cell myocarditis. *Exp Clin Endocrinol Diabetes*. 2005;113:302–307.
48. Karaplis AC, He B, Nguyen MT, et al. Inactivating mutation in the human parathyroid hormone receptor type 1 gene in Blomstrand chondrodysplasia. *Endocrinology*. 1998;139:5255–5258.
49. Obermayer-Straub P, Manns MP. Autoimmune polyglandular syndromes. *Baillieres Clin Gastroenterol*. 1998;12:293–315.
50. Arnold A, Horst SA, Gardella TJ, Baba H, Levine MA, Kronenberg HM. Mutation of the signal peptide-encoding region of the preproparathyroid hormone gene in familial isolated hypoparathyroidism. *J Clin Invest*. 1990;86:1084–1087.
51. Baumber L, Tufarelli C, Patel S, et al. Identification of a novel mutation disrupting the DNA binding activity of GCM2 in autosomal recessive familial isolated hypoparathyroidism. *J Med Genet*. 2005;42:443–448.
52. Maret A, Ding C, Kornfield SL, Levine MA. Analysis of the GCM2 gene in isolated hypoparathyroidism: a molecular and biochemical study. *J Clin Endocrinol Metab*. 2008;93(4):1426–1432.
53. Ding C, Buckingham B, Levine MA. Familial isolated hypoparathyroidism caused by a mutation in the gene for the transcription factor GCMB. *J Clin Invest*. 2001;108:1215–1220.
54. Trump D, Dixon PH, Mumm S, et al. Localisation of X linked recessive idiopathic hypoparathyroidism to a 1.5 Mb region on Xq26–q27. *J Med Genet*. 1998;35:905–909.
55. Shapira H, Friedman E, Mouallem M, Farfel Z. Familial Albright's hereditary osteodystrophy with hypoparathyroidism: normal structural Gs alpha gene. *J Clin Endocrinol Metab*. 1996;81:1660–1662.
56. Mc GD, Cooley DA. Parathyroid cyst: an unusual cervical tumor; report of three cases. *Surgery*. 1951;30:725–732.
57. Vazquez FJ, Aparicio LS, Gallo CG, Diehl M. Parathyroid carcinoma presenting as a giant mediastinal retrotracheal functioning cyst. *Singapore Med J*. 2007;48:e304–e307.
58. Capezzone M, Morabito E, Bellitti P, Giannasio P, de Santis D, Bruno R. Ectopic intrathyroidal nonfunctioning parathyroid cyst. *Endocr Pract*. 2007;13:56–58.
59. Ippolito G, Palazzo FF, Sebag F, Sierra M, De Micco C, Henry JF. A single-institution 25-year review of true parathyroid cysts. *Langenbecks Arch Surg*. 2006;391:13–18.
60. Shields TW, Immerman SC. Mediastinal parathyroid cysts revisited. *Ann Thorac Surg*. 1999;67:581–590.
61. Lieberman A, DeLellis RA. Intrafollicular amyloid in normal parathyroid glands. *Arch Pathol*. 1973;95:422–423.
62. Koelmeyer TD. Generalised amyloidosis with involvement of the parathyroids: case report. *N Z Med J*. 1977;85:372–373.
63. Anderson TJ, Ewen SW. Amyloid in normal and pathological parathyroid glands. *J Clin Pathol*. 1974;27:656–663.
64. Keven K, Oztas E, Aksoy H, Duman N, Erbay B, Erturk S. Polyglandular endocrine failure in a patient with amyloidosis secondary to familial Mediterranean fever. *Am J Kidney Dis*. 2001;38:E39.
65. Van de Casseye M, Gepts W. Case report: primary (autoimmune?) parathyroiditis. *Virchows Arch A Pathol Pathol Anat*. 1973;361:257–261.
66. Furuto-Kato S, Matsukura S, Ogata M, et al. Primary hyperparathyroidism presumably caused by chronic parathyroiditis manifesting from hypocalcemia to severe hypercalcemia. *Intern Med*. 2005;44:60–64.
67. Chetty R, Forder MD. Parathyroiditis associated with hyperparathyroidism and branchial cysts. *Am J Clin Pathol*. 1991;96:348–350.
68. Boyce BF, Doherty VR, Mortimer G. Hyperplastic parathyroiditis – a new autoimmune disease? *J Clin Pathol*. 1982;35:812–814.
69. Hui KS, Williams JC, Borit A, Rosenberg HS. The endocrine glands in Pompe's disease. Report of two cases. *Arch Pathol Lab Med*. 1985;109:921–925.
70. Soejima K, Landing BH, Roe TF, Swanson VL. Pathologic studies of the osteoporosis of Von Gierke's disease (glycogenosis 1a). *Pediatr Pathol*. 1985;3:307–319.

16 Neoplastic Parathyroid Diseases

Raja R. Seethala

Introduction

The understanding of parathyroid diseases, particularly neoplastic processes, has advanced tremendously in the past century and a quarter since the original description of parathyroid glands by Sandström in 1880.[1] Parathyroid diseases are classically stratified into two major groups: single gland (and perhaps more controversially, double gland) disease; and multigland disease. Both processes manifest as physiologically, macroscopically and microscopically abnormal parathyroid gland proliferations resulting in enlargement. However, single gland disease is considered neoplastic, consisting of adenomas and more uncommonly, carcinomas, while multigland disease is considered to be nonneoplastic, hence the term hyperplasia.

This grouping is of practical importance as the approach to clinical management differs based on categorization. However, as the understanding of the histologic spectrum of abnormal parathyroid morphology has grown, it has become readily apparent that when examining one gland alone, there are no histological features that reliably separate adenoma from hyperplasia. The distinction is contextual, based on the reference point of the findings of the other glands, clinical history, and more recently the intraoperative parathyroid hormone (PTH) levels. Conversely, molecular findings have suggested that in some cases of multigland disease, particularly in the multiple endocrine neoplasia setting and even in some cases of tertiary hyperparathyroidism, enlarged parathyroids are actually mono or oligoclonal rather than polyclonal as expected in nonneoplastic processes. Ultimately, pragmatism prevails and the current definition of parathyroid neoplasms also incorporates the functional status of the disease gland and other glands.

Parathyroid adenoma is defined as a benign neoplastic proliferation of a single parathyroid gland that upon removal results in long-term cure.[2] Parathyroid carcinoma is a neoplastic parathyroid proliferation that fulfills clinical and/or histologic criteria for malignancy.[3] These criteria are controversial and will be discussed in further detail subsequently. Advances in the understanding of molecular alterations in adenomas and carcinomas have resulted in an improved understanding of the similarities and differences from the hyperplasia categories. And from a practical standpoint, molecular testing shows promise particularly in the distinction between adenoma and carcinoma when traditional clinicopathologic parameters are inconclusive.

Sporadic Parathyroid Adenoma and Carcinoma

Clinical

Parathyroid adenomas are the most common cause of primary hyperparathyroidism, comprising 85% of this group. By comparison, parathyroid carcinomas contribute to less than 1% of all primary hyperparathyroidism.[4] The annual incidence of adenoma in North America is 20–30 per 100,000 people. Parathyroid adenomas and carcinomas typically occur in the sixth to eighth decade with a female predilection of 2–3:1.[5,6] The vast majority of adenomas are indeed sporadic without any identifiable etiologic factors. Adenomas have been epidemiologically linked with radiation exposure.[7–9]

Clinical manifestations of adenomas are the result of hypercalcemia in the setting of an elevated PTH. With the frequent testing of serum calcium as part of screening metabolic serum chemistry panels, many patients with adenomas have no complaints at initial discovery, though if a thorough clinical history is taken, signs and symptoms of hypercalcemia are found.[10] Common clinical findings include nonspecific symptoms of fatigue, musculoskeletal or abdominal aches and pains, constipation, polydipsia, polyuria, and cognitive dysfunction. Other more severe complications rarely occur today, including osteitis fibrosa cystica, pathologic fractures, nephrolithiasis, nephrocalcinosis, renal insufficiency, peptic ulcer disease, hypertension, gout and pancreatitis. Parathyroid carcinomas are more likely to have extreme symptomatology and more often present with osteoporosis

J.L. Hunt (ed.), *Molecular Pathology of Endocrine Diseases*, Molecular Pathology Library 3,
DOI 10.1007/978-1-4419-1707-2_16, © Springer Science+Business Media, LLC 2010

and nephrolithiasis. They are also more likely to present with a palpable neck mass, and are characteristically "adherent" to surrounding soft tissue and the thyroid because of their local infiltration.[11,12] Parathyroid carcinoma patients tend to have much higher serum calcium and PTH levels than seen in adenomas. These clinical findings are described in more detail along with preoperative localization and surgical approach in Chap. 14. With current treatment modalities, durable normocalcemia can be attained in 98–100% of patients with parathyroid adenomas.[13,14] Age, gender, and presence of metastatic disease are considered important prognosticators.[15]

Gross and Histologic Features

Grossly, parathyroid adenomas are enlarged by size and by weight (on average 500 mg) and have a deeper red-brown appearance as compared to normal parathyroid tissue, which reflects a decrease in stromal fat and hyperemia.[16,17] Cystic change may be present in up to 10% of sporadic adenomas.[18,19] A rim of paler normal may be noted as well. Oxyphil adenomas (see below) may be mahogany brown[20], while lipoadenomas (see below) may be pale yellow.[21] Carcinomas are typically larger (2,000–10,000 mg) and may be paler and more fibrotic.[3]

Histologically, the prototypical parathyroid adenoma consists of an encapsulated solid, nested and corded proliferation of chief cells with minimal to no intervening fatty stroma surrounded by a rim of normal parathyroid tissue. However, these features may be occasionally seen in the glands of hyperplasia, and are thus not reliable alone. Practically speaking, any histology with increased parenchymal mass is acceptable as an adenoma if it is the only gland that is abnormal. Variant histologies include oxyphil rich adenomas, comprised of cells with mitochondria rich abundant granular eosinophilic modified chief cells (oxyphils)[20], and lipoadenomas which show a paradoxic increase in fatty stroma along with cell mass.[21] Parathyroid adenomas of all types generally have small round nuclei with only rare if any mitoses. The atypia present is often random, similar to that seen in most endocrine organ sites.

Minimal histologic criteria for defining parathyroid malignancy, and whether or not to incorporate clinical findings as criteria for malignancy (i.e., marked hypercalcemia and adherence to surrounding tissue) are up for debate. Histologically, parathyroid carcinomas tend to have broad fibrous bands and a trabecular growth pattern. Elevated mitotic counts are more frequent. Paradoxically, carcinomas may be more monomorphic than adenomas. However, these features may be seen in noninvasive parathyroid tumors that behave in a benign fashion, as well. Definitive criteria for malignancy that are generally accepted without argument are: vascular invasion, soft tissue/extracapsular invasion, thyroid invasion, perineural invasion, and nodal or distant metastatic disease.[22,23] Parathyroid neoplasms that are clinically worrisome, and/or have fibrosis, trabecular growth or elevated mitotic rates, but do not have definitive criteria for malignancy are labeled as "atypical adenomas."

Histochemistry and Immunohistochemistry

Histochemical and immunohistochemical features of parathyroid neoplasms are summarized in Table 16.1. Histochemical stains for lipid such as Oil red O may prove the hyperfunctional status in adenomas and carcinomas by demonstrating depleted or absent intracytoplasmic lipid.[24,25] Immunohistochemistry is usually of little value in parathyroid adenomas, except occasionally in the distinction between carcinoma. Here, a Ki-67 proliferative index greater than 6% is suggestive of a carcinoma, though many carcinomas have a proliferation index of less than 1%.[26,27] Other immunostains used to distinguish adenoma from carcinoma are often surrogates for molecular markers. Losses of pRB1, p27, parafibromin protein immunoexpression in carcinomas are reflective of alterations at the corresponding gene loci that are more frequently seen in carcinomas as compared to adenomas (see below).[28–30] More recently, galectin-3 has been observed to be preferentially expressed in carcinomas.[31] Cyclin D1, while frequently overexpressed in parathyroid neoplasia, does not discriminate between adenoma and carcinoma.[22] Additionally, mechanisms (see below) for overexpression in these two entities may be different. Immunostains may also

TABLE 16.1. Histochemical and immunohistochemical characteristics of parathyroid neoplasms.

	Normal parathyroid	Adenoma	Carcinoma
Lipid stain (Oil Red O, Sudan IV)	Abundant coarse globules	Depleted	Depleted
Vitamin D receptor	Strong and diffuse	Decreased	Decreased
Calcium sensing receptor	Strong and diffuse	Decreased	Markedly decreased
Cyclin D1	Rare cells positive	Positive (20–40%)	Positive (60%)
P27	Diffusely positive	Decreased	Markedly decreased
pRB	Diffusely positive	Positive (but heterogeneous)	Absent (50–100%)
Parafibromin	Diffusely positive	Diffusely positive (absent in FHJTS associated adenomas and <5% of sporadic adenomas)	Absent (70–100%)
Galectin-3	Negative	Negative (<5% positive)	Positive (>90%)
Ki-67	Mean LI=<1%	Mean LI=2%	Mean LI=8% (diagnostic if >6%)

FHJTS familial hyperparathyroidism jaw tumor syndrome, *LI* labeling index.

be used to suggest hyperfunctioning status in a similar fashion to Oil red O stains. Calcium sensing receptor (CaSR) and vitamin D receptor (VDR) immunostains show a lower staining intensity in adenomas and an even lower intensity in carcinomas as compared to normal since these PTH modulators are decreased in response to the persistently elevated serum calcium levels.[32,33]

Important Pathways

In sporadic parathyroid neoplasms, adenomas and carcinomas, there are three different genes that define the important known pathways of tumorigenesis: *CCND1/PRAD1*, *MEN1*, and *HRPT2*. It is important to note that these alterations do not define separate carcinogenesis pathways, as more than one mutation can be seen in a parathyroid neoplasm.

Genetics

Commonly altered genes in parathyroid neoplasia, sporadic, and familial (see below) are summarized in Table 16.2.

Oncogenes

Among the first, and the major gene implicated in parathyroid adenoma development is *CCND1/PRAD1* (chromosome 11q13) which encodes cyclin D1. Cyclin D1 functions by binding to the cyclin dependent kinases (Cdk4 and Cdk6) kinase complex that phosphorylates retinoblastoma protein (RB). RB represses the E2F transcription factor, but on phosphorylation, this repression is lost. Through a series of transcription events, this ultimately facilitates the transition of a cell from the G1 to the S-phase. Cyclin D1 thus promotes cell growth and can function as an oncogene. The most common known mechanism for overexpression of cyclin D1 is a pericentromeric gene rearrangement that brings the regulatory sequences of the *PTH* gene (on chromosome 11p15) in close proximity to the *CCND1/PRAD1* gene.[34,35] The simplest form of this would be a chromosomal inversion – inv(11) (p15; q13). However, breakpoints vary resulting in a distance between the *PTH* regulatory element and *CCNR/PRAD1* that ranges from 15 to 200 kb.[36] Additionally, not all cyclin D1 overexpression adenomas have this inversion – other mechanisms may exist for this overexpression. Nonetheless, cyclin D1 is overexpressed in 20–40% in sporadic adenomas, supporting an integral role in tumorigenesis.[37] Furthermore, transgenic mouse models with this PTH directed cyclin D1 overexpression develop primary hyperparathyroidism.[38]

The original methodology used to assess for this rearrangement was restriction enzyme digestion and southern blot with a radiolabeled PTH probes.[39,40] The ease and convenience of immunohistochemical staining of tissue sections has supplanted the approach to identify the gene rearrangement, particularly because of the variety and complexity of breakpoints.[37] Another common mechanism of cyclin D1 overexpression seen in other tumors, namely via *CCND/PRAD1* gene amplification has not been described in parathyroid adenomas. By immunohistochemistry, parathyroid carcinomas overexpress

TABLE 16.2. Genes commonly altered in parathyroid neoplasia.

	Adenoma	Carcinoma
Oncogenes		
CCND1/PRAD1 Ch. 11q13 Encodes cyclin D1	Overexpression Pericentromeric inversion placing *PTH* promoter near *CCND1/PRAD1* gene (5–10%) Other mechanisms unknown	Overexpression Mechanism unknown possibly secondary
RET Ch. 10q11 Encodes receptor tyrosine kinase	Not seen in sporadic cases Seen only in familial syndromes (MEN-2A) (20–30%) Germline mutation typically in codon 634 resulting in constitutive activation	Not described
Tumor suppressor genes		
MEN Ch. 11q13 Encodes Menin	Somatic mutations (sporadic cases ~20%) leading to loss of function LOH inactivation of second allele (20–30%) Biallelic mutations rare	Somatic mutations in almost 15% (sporadic) <Carcinomas in MEN-1 syndrome are exceptionally rare>
HRPT2 Ch. 1q21-23 Encodes parafibromin	Somatic mutations leading to loss of function uncommon (sporadic cases <10%, sporadic cystic tumors 20%) Germline mutations characteristic of adenomas in FHJTS LOH inactivation of second allele	Somatic mutations common (sporadic cases 66–100%) Germline mutations characteristic of carcinomas in FHJTS LOH inactivation of second allele Rare cases with hypermethylation
RB1 Ch. 13q14 Encodes RB protein	LOH in up to 30% Other mutations not described	LOH in up to 100% Other mutations not described
BRCA2 Ch. 13q12-14 Encodes Brca2 protein	–	LOH in up to 85% Other mutations not described

cyclin D1 in up to 60% of cases.[32] The molecular mechanism for this is not well studied, but may be related to alterations of parafibromin (see below).

While the germline mutations in the *RET* proto-oncogene define the multiple endocrine neoplasia syndrome 2 (MEN-2), somatic mutations have not been seen in sporadic parathyroid adenomas or carcinomas.[41]

Tumor Suppressor Genes

The *MEN1* gene is also located on chromosome 11q13, but functions as a putative tumor suppressor gene. While this gene is typically associated, as its name implies, with multiple endocrine neoplasia 1, this gene is commonly altered in sporadic adenomas. This gene encodes menin, a protein that interacts with the TGF-β/activin signaling pathway.[42] TGF-β inhibits the growth of most cells via interaction with type I and II serine–threonine kinase receptors. TGF-β binds to the constitutively phosphorylated type II receptor which in turn transphosphorylates a type I receptor. This results in the phosphorylation of the SMAD complex which then translocates to the nucleus to initiate transcription. Menin normally binds to SMAD-3 in the nucleus and facilitates transcription. Thus, when menin is altered, the TGF-β mediated inhibition is weakened facilitating cell growth. Loss of heterozygosity (LOH) at the *MEN1* gene locus can be observed in 20–30% of parathyroid adenomas, by FISH and or PCR based microsatellite analysis.[43-45] A fraction of these cases will have demonstrable mutations of the other allele.[44,46] These mutations span exons 2–10 of the *MEN1* gene.[47] To date, 203 of the 1,336 mutations noted to date are described in somatic disease.[48] There do not appear to be any mutational hotspots in sporadic or familial disease.[49] But somatic mutations are more likely to involve exon 2, though the significance of this finding is unclear.[48]

The standard method for detection of these mutations include direct sequencing of the gene, occasionally preceded by screening for mutations by single strand conformation polymorphism (SSCP) or dideoxy fingerprinting (ddF).[49] Since several different mutations have been described, a directed test such as restriction site based analysis or amplification of a limited portion of the gene will not reliably detect a large percentage of mutations. In rare instances, instead of LOH and a mutation of the remaining allele, parathyroid adenomas may show biallelic inactivating mutations.[50] While initially only reported rarely, somatic *MEN1* mutations may be seen in almost 15% of parathyroid carcinomas based on recent studies.[32,45]

Another relatively more recently characterized gene is *HRPT2*, which is mapped to chromosome 1q21–23 and is also an important gene in parathyroid tumorigenesis, particularly in carcinomas. *HRPT2* mutations may be noted in 66–100% of sporadic parathyroid carcinomas, but are only detected in about 8% of sporadic adenomas.[3,32,45,51] Tumors with this alteration are often cystic, and in sporadic cystic adenomas the prevalence of LOH in the 1q region is as high as 20%.[19] *HRPT2* is composed of 17 exons and encodes a 531 amino acid protein parafibromin which is involved in the RNA polymerase/Paf-1 complex and thus has a presumed histone deacetylation role.[52] This tumor has a presumed tumor suppressor function in parathyroid glands, since the described mutations in *HRPT2* lead to impaired parafibromin function. But the specific mechanism of growth inhibition by wild-type parafibromin is unclear. One study indicates that parafibromin normally inhibits cyclin D1 expression.[53] Thus, a potential model of neoplasia is the loss of this repression with *HRPT2* mutations. But whether the effect of parafibromin on cyclin D1 is direct or mediated through other steps has not been resolved.

Similar to *MEN1* mutations of *HRPT2* are detected by direct sequencing, often preceded by a screening procedure such as SSCP. Mutations that have been described span all 17 exons, thus detection strategies would have to be fairly comprehensive. The mechanism for inactivation of the second allele is usually LOH, which can be assessed via amplification of microsatellite markers that span this gene locus.[45] Loss of parafibromin protein expression by immunohistochemistry may serve as a surrogate for gene alterations.[54] Interestingly, parathyroid carcinomas arising in the background of secondary/tertiary hyperparathyroidism (which are exceptionally rare) do not show loss of parafibromin stain suggesting a different pathogenesis.[55]

The gene *RB1* on chromosome 13q14 encodes RB protein which as mentioned earlier interacts with the cyclin D1/Cdk 4/6 complex to direct the transition from the G1 to S phase. Inactivation of this gene has been linked not only to retinoblastoma, but to several other malignancies as well. Up to 100% of parathyroid carcinomas show LOH at *RB1*, but this alteration is not specific for malignancy as it may be seen in up to 30% of adenomas as well. The role of *RB1* in parathyroid carcinogenesis is debated.[30,56] Despite the high frequency of LOH, *RB1* point mutations, deletions, and insertions have not been described suggesting the possibility that another gene in this region may be responsible for tumorigenesis with *RB1* loss being an epiphenomenon.

The gene *BRCA2*, on chromosome 13q12–14 has also been implicated in parathyroid carcinogenesis. LOH at this gene locus has been reported in up to 85% of carcinomas in one small set of cases. It is often found in conjunction with loss of *RB1*, and similarly, point mutations, insertions, and deletions at this gene locus have not been described in parathyroid tumors raising doubts about its contribution to tumorigenesis.[56]

Epigenetics

Understanding of epigenetic alterations contributing to parathyroid tumorigenesis is sparse. One study has indicated that in a few cases, hypermethylation of *HRPT2* as assessed by methylation specific PCR is also a mechanism for inactivation in parathyroid carcinoma.[57]

Special Techniques

One fundamental biologically relevant question is the validity of clinicopathologic classification of parathyroid disease – is single gland disease truly monoclonal with multigland disease (hyperplasia) being a reactive polyclonal proliferation? Studies using various X-linked inactivation based methodologies generally support the notion that single gland disease is indeed monoclonal with at least 75% of adenomas showing a monoclonal pattern of hybridization. However, clonal patterns of X-linked inactivation may be demonstrated in hyperplasias as well particularly in the nodular form.[46,58,59] One caveat is that the X-inactivation patch size in parathyroid is not well described, and if similar to thyroid,[60] the apparent clonality in multigland disease may simply reflect a large patch size.

Only a handful of genes involved in parathyroid tumorigenesis are well characterized (see above). However, genomic profiling has been performed on these tumors with the potential to identify additional candidate genes. In addition to losses at chromosome 11q13 (where MEN1 resides), losses at chromosomes 1, 6q, 11q23, 13q and 15q are frequent as noted by comparative genomic hybridization (CGH) suggesting the presence of additional candidate tumor suppressor genes in this region.[61–63]

Emerging gene array data has suggested the capability of distinguishing adenoma from hyperplasia. One custom designed array demonstrated differential kinase expression profiles between adenomas and hyperplasia.[64] In a comprehensive survey by Haven et al,[65] parathyroid disease was resolved into three basic categories based on gene expression profile: (1) hyperplasia, (2) adenomas, MEN associated hyperplasias, and tertiary hyperplasias, and (3) carcinomas and HRPT associated adenomas. The implications are that MEN associated hyperplasias may be more accurately considered "adenomatoses," and that most adenomas are not precursors to carcinoma, which requires a specialized pathogenesis. Adenoma size may also be a determinant of gene expression, with a variety of calcium ion binding proteins being overexpressed in larger adenomas.[66]

Panel based microsatellite assessment at several known tumor suppressor gene loci for LOH is a popular, clinically available methodology that has been applied to several tumor types. Since the known biology of parathyroid disease is replete with tumor suppressor genes, some of which are selectively expressed in carcinomas, an LOH panel can help distinguish between adenoma and carcinoma in clinicopathologically challenging cases. In addition to specific gene loci, a panel can generate a fractional allelic loss (FAL) value that is to some extent an estimate of genetic abnormalities. Hunt et al[67] demonstrated that the FAL for a small set of parathyroid carcinomas was significantly higher than for adenomas and hyperplasias.

Hereditary

Background

Clinical

Single gland disease in the setting of familial hyperparathyroidism is less common than multigland disease. As such, the MEN syndromes are discussed in more detail in Chap. 11. However, as noted previously, by gene expression profile, MEN associated multigland disease may be more aptly considered an adenomatosis rather than a hyperplasia.[65] Parathyroid disease in MEN-1 syndrome is invariably multigland disease. MEN-2 syndrome on the other hand may present with less than four gland involvement or even with only one enlarged gland, but should be treated as a disease state with potential multigland involvement.[68] FHJTS is one familial hyperparathyroidism syndrome, in which single gland disease, i.e., adenomas are fairly common. With this syndrome, up to 15% of patients develop parathyroid carcinoma. Up to 30% will also develop ossifying fibromas of the mandible.[69] Other extra parathyroid manifestations include renal lesions including simple cysts, mixed epithelial stromal tumors, and Wilms tumors, and more recently uterine mesenchymal neoplasms including leiomyomas and adenomyomas.[70]

Gross and Histologic Features, Histochemistry and Immunohistochemistry

Grossly, parathyroid neoplasms in MEN syndromes are similar in appearance to their sporadic counterparts. Parathyroid tumors in FHJTS on the other hand are notoriously cystic.[19] The histologic spectrum and immunophenotype of familial parathyroid tumors is similar to sporadic tumors. One caveat is that even histologically normal appearing parathyroid tissue in MEN patients may be physiologically abnormal.

Important Pathways

As with sporadic parathyroid disease, *MEN1* and *HRPT2* are important genes in the pathogenesis of familial hyperparathyroidism. Here, however, mutations in the *RET* proto-oncogene also play a role in pathogenesis.

Genetics

Oncogenes

RET is a 20 exon gene located on chromosome 10q11 and encodes a receptor tyrosine kinase required for cell growth and differentiation. Common mutations in MEN-2A result in the disruption of cysteine residues that are normally involved disulfide bonding. This disruption leads to homodimerization with another unpaired mutant RET molecule resulting in constitutive activation. Parathyroid involvement in MEN-2A is more variable than MEN-1 with only 20–30% of patients manifesting with parathyroid disease. Mutations tend to cluster around exons 10–16, and point mutations of codon 634 result in a higher likelihood of parathyroid disease involvement.[71]

Tumor Suppressor Genes

HRPT2 shows germline mutations in FHJTS as opposed to the somatic mutations seen in sporadic adenomas and carcinomas (see detailed discussion above). The relatively high risk of carcinoma in FHJTS kindreds supports its role in malignant transformation.[52,65,69] In contrast, MEN-1 syndrome does not appear to have an increased risk of carcinomatosis,[45] even though somatic mutations of the *MEN* gene are not uncommon in sporadic carcinomas.

Epigenetics

While genomic imprinting has been known to effect certain phenotypes of familial hypoparathyroidism/pseudohypoparathyroidism, such phenomena have not been described in familial hyperparathyroidism states.

Special Techniques

As noted earlier, parathyroid proliferations in the setting of MEN are mono or oligoclonal rather than polyclonal as expected in a truly hyperplastic process. It is also interesting to note that parathyroid disease in the setting of MEN syndromes, whether single or multigland disease, clusters by gene array with adenomas (see above). Gene expression profiling lends credence to the notion that HRPT2 related parathyroid neoplasms represent a distinct tumorigenesis pathway. All tumors that harbor these mutations, including FHJTS adenomas, parathyroid carcinomas, and tumors arising in familial isolated hyperparathyroidism appear to form one main cluster.

Summary

Parathyroid neoplasms are traditionally considered to be represented by single (and rarely double) gland disease, namely adenomas and carcinomas. For sporadic adenomas, key gene alterations include: cyclin D1 overexpression, prototypically secondary to a pericentromeric inversion of chromosome 11 that places the *PTH* gene promoter adjacent to *CCND1/PRAD1* gene; and somatic *MEN* mutations. For sporadic carcinomas, mutations on *HRPT2* are the most common and significant, though they may be seen a subset of adenomas as well. LOH at the *RB1* and *BRCA2* loci are common, but not restricted to carcinoma, but other mutations (insertions, deletions, etc.) have not been described raising doubts about the primary significance of these particular alterations. Chromosomal losses at 1, 6q, 11q23, 13q, and 15q suggest the presence of additional tumor suppressor genes at these loci. Evaluation of LOH across multiple loci may be clinically useful in cases where the distinction between adenoma and carcinoma is particularly challenging.

Familial parathyroid proliferations are generally multigland disease and grouped with hyperplasias. However, clonality studies and gene expression profiling suggest that these hyperplasias are, from a biologic standpoint, "adenomatoses." Unlike sporadic parathyroid neoplasms, activating mutations of the RET proto-oncogene do have a role in familial hyperparathyroidism with mutations of the codon 634 being most commonly associated with hyperparathyroidism. FHJTS is defined by germline mutations on *HRPT2*, and predispose affected patients to a relatively high risk of carcinoma, while MEN syndrome patients do not. Genotypically, all HRPT2 associated parathyroid neoplasms (both benign and malignant) cluster separately from other parathyroid disease, suggesting a fundamentally unique pathogenesis.

References

1. Sandström I. Om en ny körtel hos menniskan och àtskilliga däggdjur. *Ups Läk Forh*. 1880;15:441–471.
2. Elliott DD, Monroe DP, Perrier ND. Parathyroid histopathology: is it of any value today? *J Am Coll Surg*. 2006;203(5):758–765.
3. Rodgers SE, Perrier ND. Parathyroid carcinoma. *Curr Opin Oncol*. 2006;18(1):16–22.
4. Hundahl SA et al. Two hundred eighty-six cases of parathyroid carcinoma treated in the U.S. between 1985–1995: a National Cancer Data Base Report. The American College of Surgeons Commission on Cancer and the American Cancer Society. *Cancer*. 1999;86(3):538–544.
5. Wermers RA et al. Incidence of primary hyperparathyroidism in Rochester, Minnesota, 1993–2001: an update on the changing epidemiology of the disease. *J Bone Miner Res*. 2006;21(1): 171–177.
6. Heath H 3rd, Hodgson SF, Kennedy MA. Primary hyperparathyroidism. Incidence, morbidity, and potential economic impact in a community. *N Engl J Med*. 1980;302(4):189–193.
7. Fujiwara S et al. Hyperparathyroidism among atomic bomb survivors in Hiroshima. *Radiat Res*. 1992;130(3):372–378.
8. Mihailescu D et al. Multiple neoplasms in an irradiated cohort: pattern of occurrence and relationship to thyroid cancer outcome. *J Clin Endocrinol Metab*. 2002;87(7):3236–3241.
9. Rao SD et al. Hyperparathyroidism following head and neck irradiation. *Arch Intern Med*. 1980;140(2):205–207.
10. Lundgren E et al. Case-control study on symptoms and signs of "asymptomatic" primary hyperparathyroidism. *Surgery*. 1998; 124(6):980-985. discussion 985–986.
11. Shane E. Clinical review 122: parathyroid carcinoma. *J Clin Endocrinol Metab*. 2001;86(2):485–493.
12. Wynne AG et al. Parathyroid carcinoma: clinical and pathologic features in 43 patients. *Medicine (Baltimore)*. 1992;71(4): 197–205.
13. Ambrogini E et al. Surgery or surveillance for mild asymptomatic primary hyperparathyroidism: a prospective, randomized clinical trial. *J Clin Endocrinol Metab*. 2007;92(8): 3114–3121.
14. Pasieka JL et al. Patient-based surgical outcome tool demonstrating alleviation of symptoms following parathyroidectomy

in patients with primary hyperparathyroidism. *World J Surg*. 2002;26(8):942–949.
15. Lee PK et al. Trends in the incidence and treatment of parathyroid cancer in the United States. *Cancer*. 2007;109(9):1736–1741.
16. Apel RL, Asa SL. The parathyroid glands. In: Barnes EL, ed. *Surgical Pathology of the Head and Neck*. New York: Marcel Dekker; 2000:1719–1792.
17. DeLellis RA. Tumors of the parathyroid glands. In: Rosai J, ed. *Atlas of Tumor Pathology*. 3rd ed. Bethesda: Armed Forces Institute of Pathology; 1993.
18. Gough IR. Parathyroid cysts. *Aust N Z J Surg*. 1999;69(5):404–406.
19. Villablanca A et al. Genetic and clinical characterization of sporadic cystic parathyroid tumours. *Clin Endocrinol (Oxf)*. 2002;56(2):261–269.
20. Bedetti CD, Dekker A, Watson CG. Functioning oxyphil cell adenoma of the parathyroid gland: a clinicopathologic study of ten patients with hyperparathyroidism. *Hum Pathol*. 1984;15(12):1121–1126.
21. Chow LS et al. Parathyroid lipoadenomas: a rare cause of primary hyperparathyroidism. *Endocr Pract*. 2006;12(2):131–136.
22. Stojadinovic A et al. Parathyroid neoplasms: clinical, histopathological, and tissue microarray-based molecular analysis. *Hum Pathol*. 2003;34(1):54–64.
23. Schantz A, Castleman B. Parathyroid carcinoma. A study of 70 cases. *Cancer*. 1973;31(3):600–605.
24. Dufour DR, Durkowski C. Sudan IV stain. Its limitations in evaluating parathyroid functional status. *Arch Pathol Lab Med*. 1982;106(5):224–227.
25. Kasdon EJ et al. Surgical pathology of hyperparathyroidism. Usefulness of fat stain and problems in interpretation. *Am J Surg Pathol*. 1981;5(4):381–384.
26. Lloyd RV et al. Immunohistochemical analysis of the cell cycle-associated antigens Ki-67 and retinoblastoma protein in parathyroid carcinomas and adenomas. *Endocr Pathol*. 1995;6(4):279–287.
27. Abbona GC et al. Proliferative activity in parathyroid tumors as detected by Ki-67 immunostaining. *Hum Pathol*. 1995;26(2):135–138.
28. Gill AJ et al. Loss of nuclear expression of parafibromin distinguishes parathyroid carcinomas and hyperparathyroidism-jaw tumor (HPT-JT) syndrome-related adenomas from sporadic parathyroid adenomas and hyperplasias. *Am J Surg Pathol*. 2006;30(9):1140–1149.
29. Erickson LA et al. Parathyroid hyperplasia, adenomas, and carcinomas: differential expression of p27Kip1 protein. *Am J Surg Pathol*. 1999;23(3):288–295.
30. Cetani F et al. A reappraisal of the Rb1 gene abnormalities in the diagnosis of parathyroid cancer. *Clin Endocrinol (Oxf)*. 2004;60(1):99–106.
31. Bergero N et al. Galectin-3 expression in parathyroid carcinoma: immunohistochemical study of 26 cases. *Hum Pathol*. 2005;36(8):908–914.
32. Haven CJ et al. Differential expression of the calcium sensing receptor and combined loss of chromosomes 1q and 11q in parathyroid carcinoma. *J Pathol*. 2004;202(1):86–94.
33. Yano S et al. Decrease in vitamin D receptor and calcium-sensing receptor in highly proliferative parathyroid adenomas. *Eur J Endocrinol*. 2003;148(4):403–411.
34. Arnold A et al. Molecular pathogenesis of primary hyperparathyroidism. *J Bone Miner Res*. 2002;17(suppl 2):N30–N36.
35. Mallya SM, Arnold A. Cyclin D1 in parathyroid disease. *Front Biosci*. 2000;5:D367–D371.
36. Hosokawa Y, Arnold A. Cyclin D1/PRAD1 as a central target in oncogenesis. *J Lab Clin Med*. 1996;127(3):246–252.
37. Hsi ED et al. Cyclin D1/PRAD1 expression in parathyroid adenomas: an immunohistochemical study. *J Clin Endocrinol Metab*. 1996;81(5):1736–1739.
38. Imanishi Y et al. Primary hyperparathyroidism caused by parathyroid-targeted overexpression of cyclin D1 in transgenic mice. *J Clin Invest*. 2001;107(9):1093–1102.
39. Arnold A et al. Molecular cloning and chromosomal mapping of DNA rearranged with the parathyroid hormone gene in a parathyroid adenoma. *J Clin Invest*. 1989;83(6):2034–2040.
40. Arnold A et al. The putative oncogene PRAD1 encodes a novel cyclin. *Cold Spring Harb Symp Quant Biol*. 1991;56:93–97.
41. Uchino S et al. Absence of somatic RET gene mutation in sporadic parathyroid tumors and hyperplasia secondary to uremia, and absence of somatic Men1 gene mutation in MEN2A-associated hyperplasia. *Biomed Pharmacother*. 2000;54(suppl 1):100s–103s.
42. Shattuck TM et al. Mutational analysis of Smad3, a candidate tumor suppressor implicated in TGF-beta and menin pathways, in parathyroid adenomas and enteropancreatic endocrine tumors. *J Clin Endocrinol Metab*. 2002;87(8):3911–3914.
43. Cetani F et al. MEN1 gene alterations do not correlate with the phenotype of sporadic primary hyperparathyroidism. *J Endocrinol Invest*. 2002;25(6):508–512.
44. Dwight T et al. Loss of heterozygosity in sporadic parathyroid tumours: involvement of chromosome 1 and the MEN1 gene locus in 11q13. *Clin Endocrinol (Oxf)*. 2000;53(1):85–92.
45. Haven CJ et al. Identification of MEN1 and HRPT2 somatic mutations in paraffin-embedded (sporadic) parathyroid carcinomas. *Clin Endocrinol (Oxf)*. 2007;67(3):370–376.
46. Miedlich S et al. Frequency of somatic MEN1 gene mutations in monoclonal parathyroid tumours of patients with primary hyperparathyroidism. *Eur J Endocrinol*. 2000;143(1):47–54.
47. Pannett AA, Thakker RV. Multiple endocrine neoplasia type 1. *Endocr Relat Cancer*. 1999;6(4):449–473.
48. Lemos MC, Thakker RV. Multiple endocrine neoplasia type 1 (MEN1): analysis of 1336 mutations reported in the first decade following identification of the gene. *Hum Mutat*. 2008;29(1):22–32.
49. Balogh K et al. Genetic screening methods for the detection of mutations responsible for multiple endocrine neoplasia type 1. *Mol Genet Metab*. 2004;83(1–2):74–81.
50. Tanaka C et al. Biallelic inactivation by somatic mutations of the MEN1 gene in sporadic parathyroid tumors. *Cancer Lett*. 2002;175(2):175–179.
51. Juhlin C et al. Loss of parafibromin expression in a subset of parathyroid adenomas. *Endocr Relat Cancer*. 2006;13(2):509–523.
52. Carpten JD et al. HRPT2, encoding parafibromin, is mutated in hyperparathyroidism-jaw tumor synrome. *Nat Genet*. 2002;32(4):676–680.
53. Woodard GE et al. Parafibromin, product of the hyperparathyroidism-jaw tumor syndrome gene HRPT2, regulates cyclin D1/PRAD1 expression. *Oncogene*. 2005;24(7):1272–1276.

54. Cetani F et al. Should parafibromin staining replace HRTP2 gene analysis as an additional tool for histologic diagnosis of parathyroid carcinoma? *Eur J Endocrinol.* 2007;156(5): 547–554.
55. Tominaga Y et al. Expression of parafibromin in distant metastatic parathyroid tumors in patients with advanced secondary hyperparathyroidism due to chronic kidney disease. *World J Surg.* 2008;32(5):815–821.
56. Shattuck TM et al. Mutational analyses of RB and BRCA2 as candidate tumour suppressor genes in parathyroid carcinoma. *Clin Endocrinol (Oxf).* 2003;59(2):180–189.
57. Hewitt KM et al. Aberrant methylation of the HRPT2 gene in parathyroid carcinoma. *Ann Otol Rhinol Laryngol.* 2007;116(12):928–933.
58. Arnold A et al. Monoclonality of parathyroid tumors in chronic renal failure and in primary parathyroid hyperplasia. *J Clin Invest.* 1995;95(5):2047–2053.
59. Tominaga Y et al. Clonal analysis of nodular parathyroid hyperplasia in renal hyperparathyroidism. *World J Surg.* 1996;20(7):744-750. discussion 750–752.
60. Jovanovic L et al. Thyroid gland clonality revisited: the embryonal patch size of the normal human thyroid gland is very large, suggesting X-chromosome inactivation tumor clonality studies of thyroid tumors have to be interpreted with caution. *J Clin Endocrinol Metab.* 2003;88(7): 3284–3291.
61. Hemmer S et al. Deletion of 11q23 and cyclin D1 overexpression are frequent aberrations in parathyroid adenomas. *Am J Pathol.* 2001;158(4):1355–1362.
62. Agarwal SK et al. Comparative genomic hybridization analysis of human parathyroid tumors. *Cancer Genet Cytogenet.* 1998;106(1):30–36.
63. Palanisamy N et al. Novel chromosomal abnormalities identified by comparative genomic hybridization in parathyroid adenomas. *J Clin Endocrinol Metab.* 1998;83(5):1766–1770.
64. Schachter PP et al. Differential expression of kinase genes in primary hyperparathyroidism: adenoma versus normal and hyperplastic parathyroid tissue. *Arch Pathol Lab Med.* 2007;131(1): 126–130.
65. Haven CJ et al. Gene expression of parathyroid tumors: molecular subclassification and identification of the potential malignant phenotype. *Cancer Res.* 2004;64(20):7405–7411.
66. Rosen JE et al. Gland size is associated with changes in gene expression profiles in sporadic parathyroid adenomas. *Ann Surg Oncol.* 2005;12(5):412–416.
67. Hunt JL et al. Allelic loss in parathyroid neoplasia can help characterize malignancy. *Am J Surg Pathol.* 2005;29(8):1049–1055.
68. Carling T, Udelsman R. Parathyroid surgery in familial hyperparathyroid disorders. *J Intern Med.* 2005;257(1):27–37.
69. Mizusawa N et al. Genetic analyses in patients with familial isolated hyperparathyroidism and hyperparathyroidism-jaw tumour syndrome. *Clin Endocrinol (Oxf).* 2006;65(1):9–16.
70. Bradley KJ et al. Uterine tumours are a phenotypic manifestation of the hyperparathyroidism-jaw tumour syndrome. *J Intern Med.* 2005;257(1):18–26.
71. Machens A, Dralle H. Genotype–phenotype based surgical concept of hereditary medullary thyroid carcinoma. *World J Surg.* 2007;31(5):957–968.

Section 4
Pituitary Diseases

17 Clinical Detection and Treatment of Benign and Malignant Pituitary Diseases

Dima L. Diab and Amir H. Hamrahian

Introduction

Anatomy and Physiology of the Pituitary Gland

The pituitary gland weighs about 0.5–1 g and is divided into an anterior and a posterior lobe. The pituitary gland sits in the sella turcica immediately behind and superior to the sphenoid sinus. Cavernous sinuses are located laterally on each side of the sella and include the internal carotid artery and cranial nerves III, IV, V1, V2, and VI. Magnetic resonance imaging (MRI) is the best method for visualization of hypothalamic–pituitary anatomy (Figure 17.1).

Anterior pituitary hormones are regulated by hypothalamic releasing and inhibitory hormones as well as negative feedback action of the target glandular hormones at both the pituitary and hypothalamic levels (Table 17.1). Among the pituitary hormones, only secretion of prolactin is increased in the absence of hypothalamic influence since it is mainly under tonic suppression by dopamine, the main prolactin inhibitory factor.[1] Antidiuretic hormone (ADH, Vasopressin) is produced by the supraoptic and paraventricular nuclei of the hypothalamus and travels in axons through the pituitary stalk to the posterior pituitary gland.

Benign Diseases: Pituitary Adenomas

Definition and Prevalence

Pituitary adenomas arise from adenohypophyseal cells and are almost always benign (Table 17.2). They are arbitrarily designated as microadenomas (<10 mm in diameter) and macroadenomas (≥10 mm in diameter) (Figure 17.2). The true incidence and prevalence of pituitary adenomas is difficult to establish; however, autopsy studies suggest that up to 20% of normal individuals may harbor pituitary microadenomas.[2] Those that are discovered by CT or MRI examination, in the absence of any symptoms or clinical findings suggestive of a pituitary disease, are referred to as pituitary incidentalomas.[3] Recent advances in molecular biology have confirmed that most pituitary adenomas are monoclonal in origin. Some possible underlying mechanisms include overexpression of pituitary oncogenes, inactivation of tumor suppressor genes, hypersecretion of hypothalamic-releasing hormones and/or hyposecretion of inhibitory hormones.[4,5]

Pituitary adenomas are rarely associated with parathyroid and neuroendocrine hyperplasia or neoplasia as part of the multiple endocrine neoplasia type I (MEN I) syndrome. Other rare genetic disorders associated with pituitary tumors include Carney syndrome, MacCune–Albright syndrome, and familial pituitary disorders such as familial acromegaly.

Signs and Symptoms

Pituitary tumors may present with signs and symptoms related to mass effect (Table 17.3), including pituitary insufficiency and/or hormonal hypersecretion. Pituitary adenomas are the most common cause of hypopituitarism, but other causes include parasellar diseases, pituitary surgery, radiation therapy, inflammatory and granulomatous diseases, and head injury. The sequential loss of pituitary hormones deficiency secondary to a mass effect is in the following order: GH, LH/FSH, TSH, ACTH, and prolactin.[1] Isolated deficiency of various anterior pituitary hormones may occur. In general, pituitary microadenomas are rarely associated with hypopituitarism. Diabetes insipidus is almost never seen in patients with pituitary adenomas during initial presentation, except in those with very large tumors extending superiorly, affecting the hypothalamus.

Impingement on the chiasm or its branches by a pituitary tumor may result in visual field defects, most commonly as bitemporal hemianopsia. Lateral extension of the pituitary mass to the cavernous sinuses may result in diplopia, ptosis, or altered facial sensation. Among the cranial nerves, the third nerve is the most commonly affected. There is no specific headache pattern associated with pituitary tumors except SUNCT (short lasting unilateral neuralgiform headache with conjunctival injection and tearing). In some patients, the headache is unrelated to the pituitary adenoma.

J.L. Hunt (ed.), *Molecular Pathology of Endocrine Diseases*, Molecular Pathology Library 3,
DOI 10.1007/978-1-4419-1707-2_17, © Springer Science+Business Media, LLC 2010

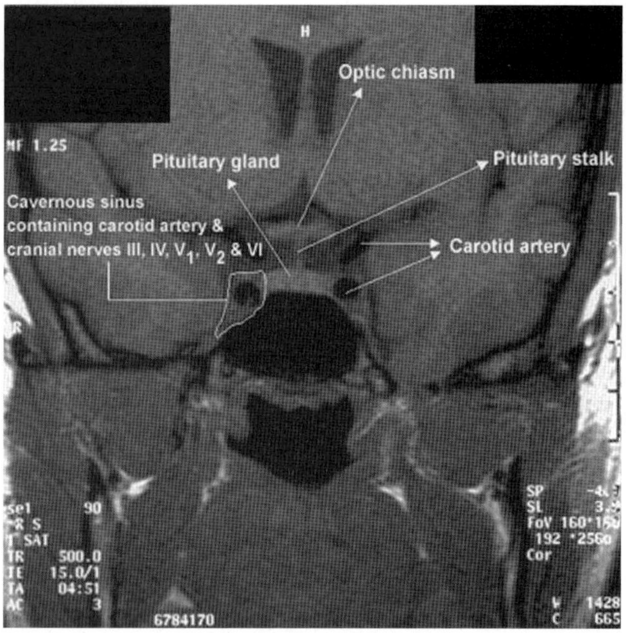

FIG. 17.1. MRI image of normal pituitary gland and perisellar structures.

TABLE 17.1. *Pituitary*: relationship among hypothalamic, pituitary, target glands, and feedback hormones.

Hypothalamic regulatory hormone	Pituitary hormone	Target gland	Feedback hormone
TRH	TSH	Thyroid gland	T4, T3
LHRH	LH	Gonad	E_2, T
LHRH	FSH	Gonad	Inhibin, E_2, T
GHRH, SMS	GH	Multiorgans	IGF-1
PIF	Prolactin	Breast	?
CRH, ADH	ACTH	Adrenal	Cortisol

ADH antidiuretic hormone; *CRH* corticotropin-releasing hormone; E_2 estradiol; *GHRH* growth hormone-releasing hormone; *LHRH* luteinizing hormone-releasing hormone; *PIF* prolactin release-inhibitory factor; *SMS* somatostatin; *T* testosterone; *TRH* thyrotropin-releasing hormone.

TABLE 17.2. *Pituitary*: prevalence of pituitary adenomas.

Adenoma type	Prevalence (%)
GH cell adenoma	15
PRL cell adenoma	30
GH and PRL cell adenoma	7
ACTH cell adenoma	10
Gonadotroph cell adenoma	10
Nonfunctioning adenoma	25
TSH cell adenoma	1
Unclassified adenoma	2

GH growth hormone; *PRL* prolactin; *ACTH* adrenocorticotropic hormone; *TSH* thyroid-stimulating hormone.

Diagnosis

Pituitary MRI is the preferred diagnostic imaging technique in patients suspected to have pituitary pathology including pituitary adenomas (Figure 17.2). Once a pituitary adenoma is found, it is necessary to assess its type (functional vs. nonfunctional), pituitary function, and the presence of mass effect such as visual field defects, especially in those with macroadenomas. Hormonal evaluation can be usually performed on an outpatient basis.

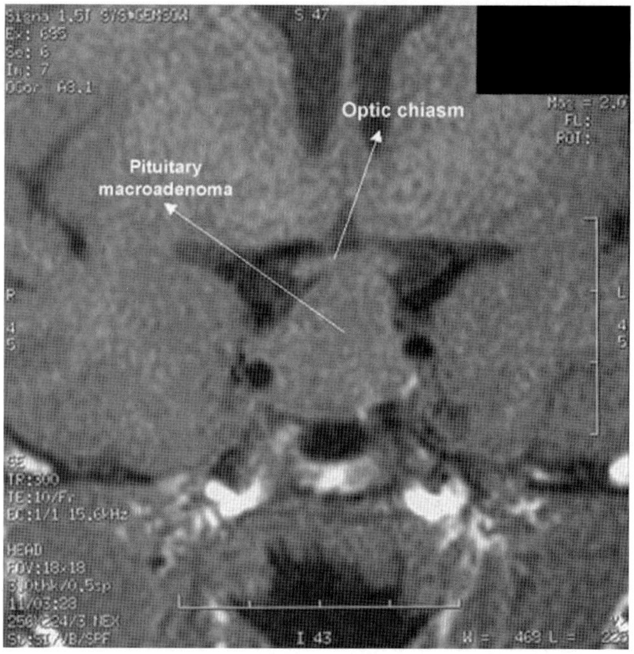

FIG. 17.2. Pituitary macroadenoma with minimal pressure on optic chiasm.

TABLE 17.3. *Pituitary*: clinical manifestations of pituitary tumors secondary to mass effect.

Headache
Chiasmal syndrome
Cranial nerves III, IV, V1, V2 and VI dysfunction
Hypothalamic syndrome*
Disturbances of thirst, appetite, satiety, sleep, and temperature
Diabetes insipidus
SIADH (syndrome of inappropriate ADH secretion)
Obstructive hydrocephalus*
Frontal and temporal lobe syndromes*
CSF rhinorrhea

ADH antidiuretic hormone; *CSF* cerebrospinal fluid.
*Very rare and may only be associated with giant pituitary tumors with significant superior extension.

Treatment

The goals for treatment of a pituitary tumor include reduction or complete removal of the tumor, elimination of mass effect if present, normalization of hormonal hypersecretion, and restoration of normal pituitary function. Some patients, especially those with large tumors, may require several therapeutic modalities including medical, surgical, and radiation therapy. The most important factor in pituitary surgery is availability of a good neurosurgeon. In general, once a patient has been diagnosed with a pituitary tumor, lifelong medical follow-up is necessary to detect early recurrence, to monitor hormone replacement, and to treat any complication related to the tumor.

Prolactinoma

Clinical features of prolactinomas may be related to excess prolactin and associated secondary hypogonadism or mass effect. All patients with macroprolactinomas and most patients with microprolactinomas require treatment. Some indications for treatment of patients with microprolactinomas include bothersome galactorrhea, oligomenorrhea/amenorrhea, infertility, and sexual dysfunction. Medical therapy with dopamine agonists is the therapy of choice for most patients, since medical therapy is effective in decreasing adenoma size and restoration of normal prolactin level in majority of patients.[6] Dopamine agonists usually restore visual field defects to an extent similar to surgery. Therefore, visual field defects associated with prolactinomas are not a neurosurgical emergency. Cabergoline and bromocriptine are potent inhibitors of PRL secretion and often result in tumor shrinkage. Dopamine agonists should be initiated slowly, since side effects often occur at the beginning of treatment. The most common side effects of dopamine agonists include nausea, headache, dizziness, nasal congestion, and constipation. Bromocriptine is the drug of choice in women who want to become pregnant due to considerable worldwide experience with the drug. Cabergoline is more potent, may be taken only twice a week, and is better tolerated by most patients. There have been some reports about association of high dose ergot-derived dopamine agonists, such as cabergoline and pergolide, with valvular heart disease, especially in patients with Parkinson's disease.[7] Considering the superior efficacy and tolerability of cabergoline, routine switching of patients on cabergoline to bromocriptine is not indicated at this point. However, periodic echocardiogram surveillance in patients on long-term therapy with cabergoline is recommended until further studies involving patients on low dose therapy are available.

Surgery is reserved for patients who are intolerant of or refractory to medical therapy. Radiation therapy may be considered for patients who poorly tolerate dopamine agonists and can not be cured by surgery (e.g., tumor invasion of cavernous sinuses).

Acromegaly

Clinical features of acromegaly may be related to excess GH/IGF-1 or associated mass effect including hypopituitarism, since most patients present with pituitary macroadenomas (Table 17.4). Measurement of IGF-1 is the initial screening test of choice (Figure 17.3).[8] Acromegaly is associated with increased morbidity and mortality if untreated. The goal of therapy for most patients is to achieve a normal sex and age-adjusted IGF-1 and GH < 1 ng/mL. Surgery is the treatment of choice for most patients presenting with acromegaly even if a cure cannot be achieved. Even a subtotal resection of the tumor will improve the efficacy of subsequent adjuvant therapy. Conventional fractionated radiotherapy is very effective for tumor size control but multiple studies have shown poor long-term results in regard to normalization of IGF-1 level.[9] Radiosurgery (Gamma knife) achieves remission faster and is more effective in normalization of IGF-1 compared to fractionated radiotherapy, but the rate of hypopituitarism seems to be similar.

TABLE 17.4. *Pituitary*: clinical features in patients with Acromegaly.

Acral enlargement
Arthralgias, neuropathic joints
Carpal tunnel syndrome
Coarsening of facial features
Excessive sweating
Goiter
Hypertension, congestive heart failure
Impaired glucose tolerance, diabetes mellitus
Macroglossia
Malocclusion and tooth gaps
Pituitary mass effect including headache and visual field defect
Pituitary insufficiency
Sensory and motor peripheral neuropathy
Snoring, sleep apnea
Symptoms associated with hyperprolactinemia
Thick and course skin, skin tags

Medical treatment of acromegaly has gained significance since the limitations of radiations and surgical therapy have become evident. Somatostatin analogues inhibit GH secretion mainly by binding to somatostatin receptors type 2 and 5 and result in normalization of IGF-1 in up to 65% of patients. The most common side effects are gastrointestinal, including diarrhea, abdominal pain, and nausea. Gallbladder sludge and cholelithiasis have been reported in up to 25% of patients on long-term therapy with somatostatin analogues but the majority are asymptomatic. Dopamine agonists have been reported to have variable efficacy in patients with acromegaly but may be an attractive first line medical therapy especially in those with cosecretion of prolactin and GH. Pegvisomant has increased affinity to GH receptors as compared to native GH but inhibits its dimerization, which is necessary for the action of GH. It is administered once daily and is usually reserved for those not responding to other medical therapies. It is very effective, with normalization of IGF-1 seen in up to 95% of patients. Due to its mechanism of action and associated increase in GH during therapy, the tumor size needs to be monitored during therapy. Liver function test needs to be monitored during therapy and the drug to be discontinued if liver enzymes increase to more than three times the upper limit of normal. During therapy with Pegvisomant, IGF-1 should be used to monitor therapy.[10,11] Recently, it was shown that activation of the Ret receptor blocked somatotroph tumor growth in mice, providing a novel potential therapeutic target for treating GH-cell adenomas.[12]

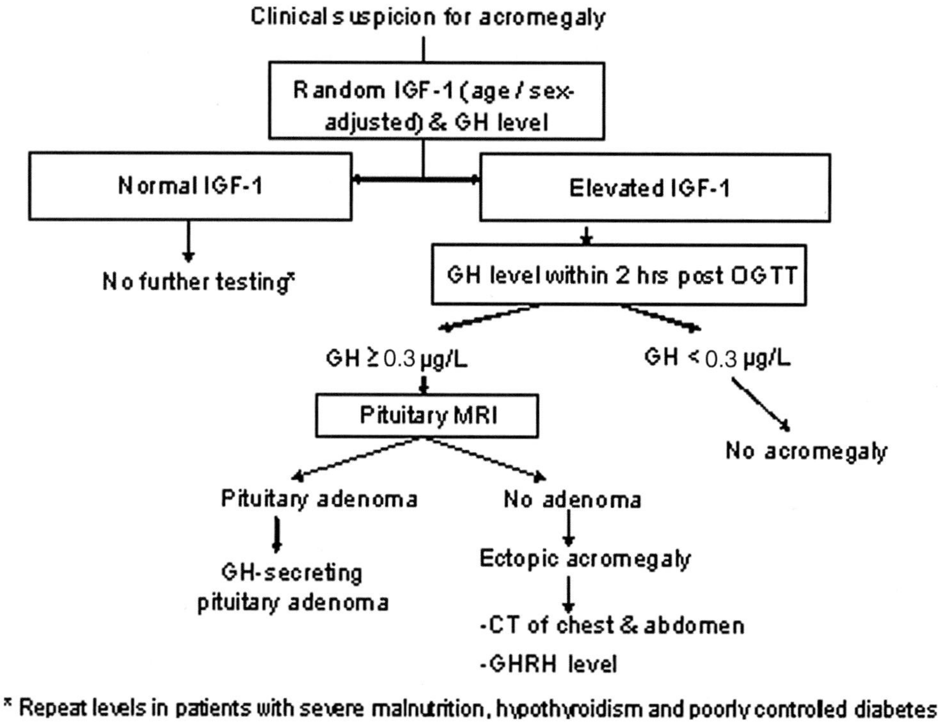

Fig. 17.3. Diagnostic work up of acromegaly.

Cushing's Disease

Clinical features of Cushing's syndrome is shown in Table 17.5. Once the diagnosis is established (Figure 17.4), surgical removal of the ACTH-secreting pituitary tumor is the treatment of choice.[13] Availability of an experienced neurosurgeon is crucial with upto 80% long-term remission rate following surgery. A low (<3 µg/dL) or undetectable cortisol level postoperatively off glucocorticoids is considered to be a good marker for long-term cure. For those not cured by the surgery, other options include reoperation and radiotherapy. Bilateral adrenalectomy is reserved for those who continue to be hypercortisolemic. Medical therapy for Cushing's syndrome has limited value because of the associated toxicity and gradual decrease in efficacy. It is mainly used for short-term symptomatic control or preparation of patients prior to surgery. Among the available agents, ketoconazole and metyrapone are the most commonly used. During therapy, liver function tests need to be closely monitored. Some reports indicate that the use of cabergoline may be effective in at least a subpopulation of patients with CS, which may be worth a trial before initiating ketoconazole. Mifepristone a cortisol receptor antagonist is currently undergoing clinical trials with promising results. Finally, a novel target for Cushing's disease therapy has been proposed, whereby bone morphogenetic protein-4 (BMP-4), which is induced by the retinoic acid pathway, was shown to inhibit corticotroph cell tumor growth in mice.[14]

Table 17.5. *Pituitary:* clinical features suggestive of Cushing's syndrome.

Central obesity
Unexplained osteoporosis
Proximal myopathy
Wide purplish striae (>1 cm)
Facial plethora
Spontaneous bruising
Hypokalemia
Serial photographs

TSH-Secreting Adenoma (TSHoma)

Patients usually present with clinical and biochemical evidence of hyperthyroidism without suppressed TSH. In patients with TSH-secreting adenomas, surgery is the primary therapeutic approach. Radiation is generally used for those with residual tumor. Somatostatin analogues are effective in most patients for control of excess TSH production leading to improvement in hyperthyroidism and possibly to a decrease in tumor size.[15] Beta blockers should be initiated in patients with uncontrolled hyperthyroidism and antithyroid medications may be used only for a short period prior to surgery (if somatostatin analogs cannot be used) since long-term usage may result in stimulation of tumor growth.

Nonfunctional/Glycoprotein-Secreting Pituitary Adenoma

Patients with small nonfunctional pituitary adenomas are usually observed; however, the standard treatment for those with mass effect is surgery mainly through the transsphenoidal approach. Radiotherapy is indicated in those with

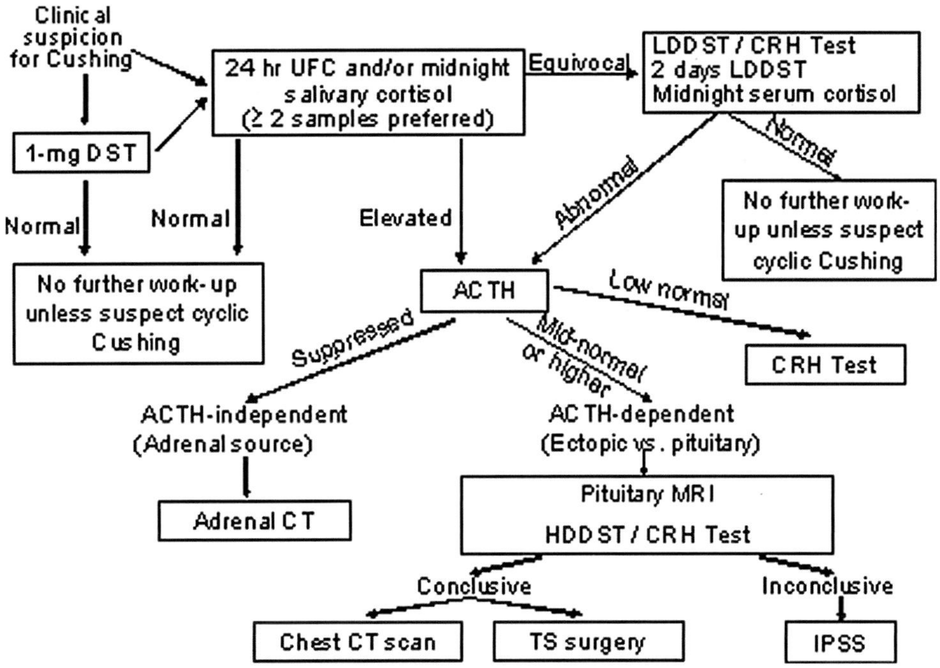

FIG. 17.4. Diagnostic work up algorithm for Cushing's syndrome.

residual pituitary tumor following surgical debulking or in those who may not be surgical candidates. The use of high-dose dopamine agonists has been associated with a decrease in tumor size in about 10% of such patients.[16]

Malignant Diseases

Pituitary carcinomas are extremely rare,[17] comprising about 0.2% of all pituitary tumors. These usually arise from invasive pituitary adenomas. Current therapeutic modalities are mainly palliative and the prognosis of these tumors is relatively poor. Additional research delineating the underlying molecular mechanisms in the pathogenesis of these tumors would hopefully lead to the development of targeted molecular therapies, including drugs based on growth factor and kinase inhibitors, potentially improving the outcome of these patients.[18]

Pituitary metastases from other malignancies can occur. These are found in up to 3.5% of patients with cancer.[19] The posterior pituitary is the preferred site for metastatic spread, since its vascular supply is derived directly from the carotid arterial circulation, as opposed to the anterior lobe, which has an indirect supply from the portal circulation.[1,5] Carcinomas that metastasize to the pituitary include breast, lung, prostate, renal cell, and gastrointestinal tract cancers.[3,20] Hemopoietic malignancies that may present with posterior lobe metastases include plasmacytomas, lymphomas, and leukemias. Although the majority of metastases occur in the context of advanced malignancy, symptomatic posterior lobe metastases, mainly diabetes insipidus, may be the presenting sign of occult malignancy. Pituitary imaging may not clearly distinguish metastatic deposits from a pituitary adenoma, and diagnosis is mostly made by histologic study of the resected specimen.[21] When the diagnosis is clear-cut in the presence of a primary cancer, low-dose pituitary radiation may be sufficient to shrink the metastasis and decrease morbidity. Depending on the responsiveness of the primary tumor and the clinical status of the patient, chemotherapy may be considered.

Summary

In summary, pituitary adenomas are essentially benign tumors, which may cause signs and symptoms of space occupation, hypopituitarism, or hormone excess. With the exception of prolactinomas, surgery remains the most appropriate initial treatment to relieve optic chiasmal compression and to reduce hormone hypersecretion. Persistent hormone elevation may be successfully treated with medical therapy and/or radiotherapy. Regular surveillance is necessary to monitor for recurrence as well as to detect development of hypopituitarism. Pituitary carcinomas are very rare and are associated with a poor outcome. It is hoped that further studies of the molecular pathogenesis of these tumors will allow for precise molecular targeting and improve the overall response rates in such cases.

References

1. Melmed S, Kleinberg D. Anterior pituitary. In: Larsen PR, Kronenberg HM, Melmed S, Polonsky KS, eds. *Williams Textbook of Endocrinology*. 10th ed. Philadelphia: Saunders; 2003:177–279.
2. Ezzat S, Asa SL, Couldwell WT, et al. The prevalence of pituitary adenomas: a systematic review. *Cancer*. 2004;101:613-619.

3. Gopan T, Toms SA. Symptomatic pituitary metastases from renal cell carcinoma. *Pituitary*. 2007;10(3):251–259.
4. Melmed S. Update in pituitary disease. *J Clin Endocrinol Metab*. 2008;93:331–338.
5. Powell M, Lightman S, Laws E. *Management of Pituitary Tumors the Clinician's Practical Guide*. 2nd ed. Totowa: Humana; 2003.
6. Casanueva FF, Molitch ME, Schlechte JA, et al. Guidelines of the Pituitary Society for the diagnosis and management of prolactinomas. *Clin Endocrinol (Oxf)*. 2006;65:265–273.
7. Schade R, Andersohn F, Suissa S, Haverkamp W, Garbe E. Dopamine agonists and the risk of cardiac-valve regurgitation. *N Engl J Med*. 2007;356:29–38.
8. Freda PU, Reyes CM, Nuruzzaman AT, Sundeen RE, Bruce JN. Basal and glucose-suppressed GH levels less than 1 microg/L in newly diagnosed acromegaly. *Pituitary*. 2003;6:175–180.
9. Powell JS, Wardlaw SL, Post KD, Freda PU. Outcome of radiotherapy for acromegaly using normalization of insulin-like growth factor I to define cure. *J Clin Endocrinol Metab*. 2000;85:2068–2071.
10. Bonadonna S, Doga M, Gola M, Mazziotti G, Giustina A. Diagnosis and treatment of acromegaly and its complications: consensus guidelines. *J Endocrinol Invest*. 2005;28:43–47.
11. Ezzat S, Serri O, Chik CL, et al. Canadian consensus guidelines for the diagnosis and management of acromegaly. *Clin Invest Med*. 2006;29:29–39.
12. Canibano C, Rodriguez NL, Saez C, et al. The dependence receptor Ret induces apoptosis in somatotrophs through a Pit-1/p53 pathway, preventing tumor growth. *EMBO J*. 2007;26:2015–2028.
13. Findling JW, Raff H. Cushing's Syndrome: important issues in diagnosis and management. *J Clin Endocrinol Metab*. 2006;91:3746–3753.
14. Giacomini D, Paez-Pereda M, Theodoropoulou M, et al. Bone morphogenetic protein-4 inhibits corticotroph tumor cells: involvement in the retinoic acid inhibitory action. *Endocrinology*. 2006;147:247–256.
15. Ness-Abramof R, Ishay A, Harel G, et al. TSH-secreting pituitary adenomas: follow-up of 11 cases and review of the literature. *Pituitary*. 2007;10:307–310.
16. Vance ML. Treatment of patients with a pituitary adenoma: one clinician's experience. *Neurosurg Focus*. 2004;16:E1.
17. Lubke D, Saeger W. Carcinomas of the pituitary: definition and review of the literature. *Gen Diagn Pathol*. 1995;141:81–92.
18. Kaltsas GA, Nomikos P, Kontogeorgos G, Buchfelder M, Grossman AB. Clinical review: diagnosis and management of pituitary carcinomas. *J Clin Endocrinol Metab*. 2005;90:3089–3099.
19. Max MB, Deck MD, Rottenberg DA. Pituitary metastasis: incidence in cancer patients and clinical differentiation from pituitary adenoma. *Neurology*. 1981;31:998–1002.
20. Serhal D, Weil RJ. Evaluation and management of pituitary incidentalomas. *Cleve clin J Med*. 2008;75(11):793–801.
21. Schubiger O, Haller D. Metastases to the pituitary – hypothalamic axis. An MR study of 7 symptomatic patients. *Neuroradiology*. 1992;34:131–134.

18 Nonneoplastic and Neoplastic Pituitary Diseases

Christine B. Warren Baran and Richard A. Prayson

Introduction

The role of molecular testing in the routine evaluation of pituitary disease is in its infancy. There is currently a very limited role for such testing in the routine clinical evaluation of pituitary lesions. Research studies using molecular techniques is augmenting our understanding of pituitary disease and particularly neoplastic lesions. This chapter provides an overview of the interface between molecular pathology and both nonneoplastic and neoplastic conditions of the pituitary gland.

Inflammatory Lesions

A variety of inflammatory lesions can affect the pituitary gland. Infectious diseases in the form of abscess can rarely involve the gland itself (Figures 18.1–18.3). Special stains for microorganisms can be useful sometimes in identifying the etiologic agent. The abscess may be associated with granulomatous inflammation (granulomatous hypophysitis). The most common etiologic agents associated with granulomatous inflammation include tuberculosis, fungal infections, and syphilis. The diagnostic yield in tissue sections is relatively low for some of these agents, particularly tuberculosis; use of Ziehl–Neelsen or FITE stains may allow for early identification of the organism and a more directed treatment. Occasionally, sarcoidosis may also affect the pituitary gland; typically, the granulomatous inflammation in the setting of sarcoidosis is not associated with necrosis[1] (Figure 18.4). Rare cases of inflammatory pseudotumor marked by prominent chronic inflammation and fibrosis have also been reported to involve the sellar and parasellar region.[2] Patients may present with hypopituitarism and imaging studies can show a lesion which mimicks a tumor.

Perhaps, the most well-known inflammatory condition to involve the pituitary gland is lymphocytic hypophysitis. The disorder is thought to have an immunologic basis and is associated with other autoimmune disorders including thyroiditis, adrenalitis, atrophic gastritis, and parathyroiditis.[3,4] The vast majority of patients are female, and commonly, this disorder presents during late pregnancy or in the postpartum period.[5] The affected pituitary gland is typically enlarged, and patients may present with symptoms related to mass effect including headaches and visual field problems. Most patients also manifest with endocrine abnormalities related to hypofunctioning of the adenohypophysis, secondary to destruction of the gland by the inflammation. An enlargement of the gland can be observed on imaging studies, and occasionally, the imaging findings may resemble that of a pituitary adenoma, often resulting in the patient being biopsied for evaluation.

Microscopically, lymphocytic hypophysitis is marked by a prominent lymphoplasmacytic infiltrate (Figure 18.5). Occasional lymphoid aggregates and variable numbers of neutrophils and eosinophils may be observed. Destruction of the adenohypophysis accompanied by variable degrees of fibrosis are also common (Figure 18.6). Immunohistochemistry confirms that the inflammatory infiltrate consists of a mixture of benign appearing B and T lymphocytes. Ancillary molecular testing is usually not required to arrive at the proper diagnosis.

The clinical course of the disease is variable. Some patients develop progressive and permanent hypopituitarism; whereas, others show a partial or total return of function to the pituitary gland in their recovery process. Most patients require some treatment, particularly during the course of the disease, in order to quell the inflammatory response and prevent further destruction. A frozen section diagnosis is useful in patients who undergo surgical intervention. Identification of the pathology may prevent a more radical resection of the gland and help preserve future residual pituitary function.

Sheehan's Syndrome

Sheehan's syndrome is a rare condition resulting in pituitary infarction; it may be associated with postpartum uterine hemorrhage. The syndrome usually manifests as hypopituitarism and primarily affects the adenohypophysis with relative

J.L. Hunt (ed.), *Molecular Pathology of Endocrine Diseases*, Molecular Pathology Library 3,
DOI 10.1007/978-1-4419-1707-2_18,

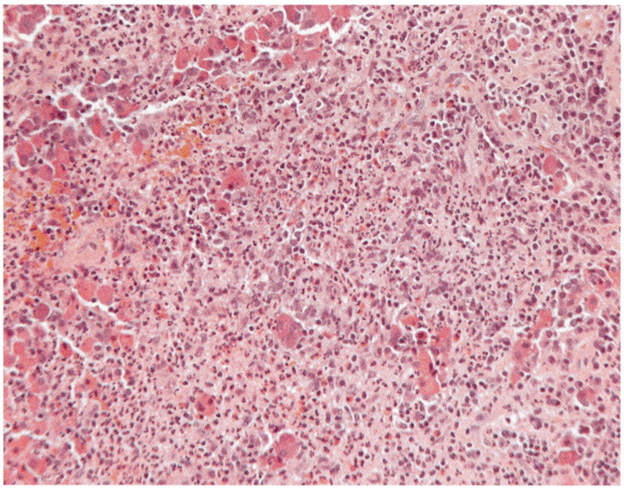

FIG. 18.1. Acute inflammation associated with an abscess in the adenohypophysis (hematoxylin and eosin, original magnification 200×).

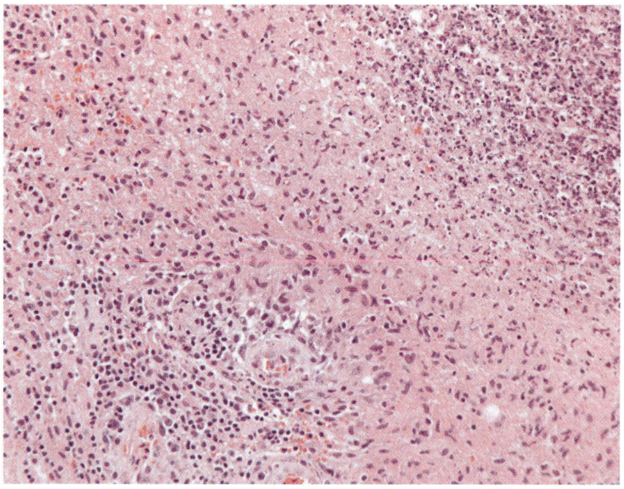

FIG. 18.2. Organizing abscess in the pituitary gland (hematoxylin and eosin, original magnification 200×).

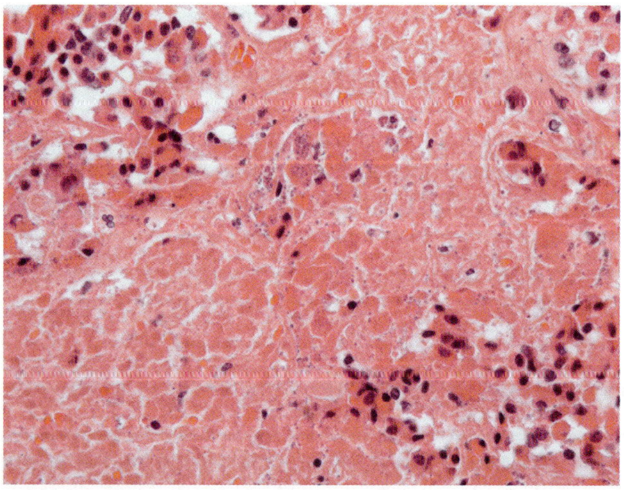

FIG. 18.3. Toxoplasma gondii organisms in a pituitary abscess; the patient was severely immunocompromised (hematoxylin and eosin, original magnification 400×).

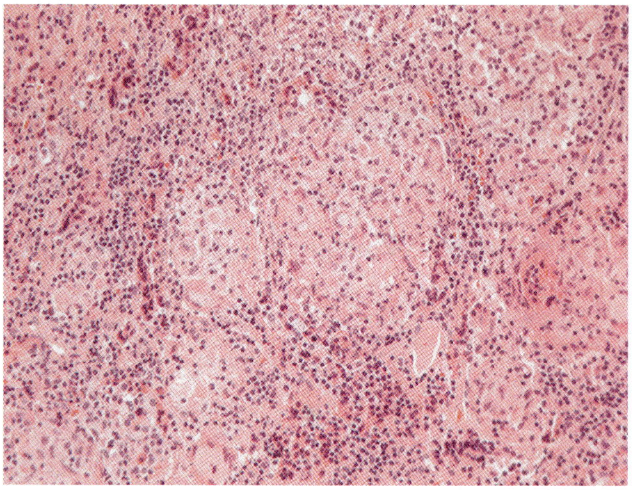

FIG. 18.4. Sarcoidosis with non-necrotizing granulomatous inflammation (hematoxylin and eosin, original magnification 200×).

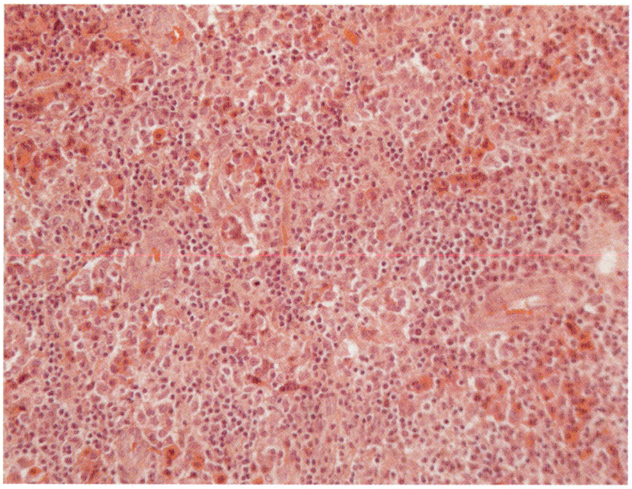

FIG. 18.5. Prominent lymphoplasmacytic infiltrate in lymphocytic hypophysitis (hematoxylin and eosin, original magnification 200×).

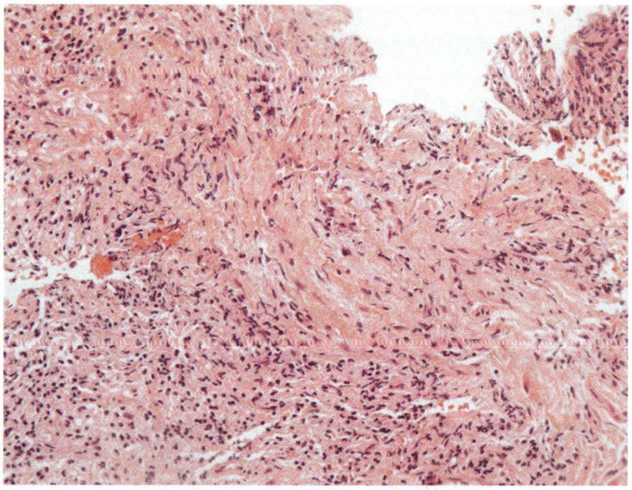

FIG. 18.6. Fibrosis and chronic inflammation in lymphocytic hypophysitis (hematoxylin and eosin, original magnification 200×).

sparing of the neurohypophysis. Necrotic tissue is eventually replaced by scar. Patients typically require replacement hormonal therapy.

Empty Sella Syndrome

Empty sella syndrome is marked by a decrease in the volume of the sellar contents because of extension of the subarachnoid space into the sella turcica.[6,7] The condition may present in a primary form because of an incomplete or incompetent sellar diaphragm with downward herniation of the arachnoid membrane, resulting in compression of the pituitary gland. This form is more commonly encountered in women. Secondary forms of empty sella syndrome may be associated with a variety of causes including radiation, hemorrhagic necrosis, and previous surgery. Middle-aged women with histories of hypertension and obesity are at higher risk. Occasionally, an adenoma may be observed in association with secondary forms of the disease.

Cysts of Pituitary Gland

Four major types of cystic lesions may be encountered in the region of the pituitary gland: Rathke's cleft cysts, dermoid cysts, epidermoid cysts, and cystic craniopharyngiomas. Craniopharyngiomas will be discussed later in this chapter.

Rathke's cleft cysts are derived from remnants of the Rathke's pouch and typically are situated between the anterior and intermediate lobes of the pituitary gland.[8–11] A commonly encountered finding, it may be seen in up to 20% of patients at the time of autopsy. There is no gender predilection. Lesions are most commonly observed in adults. Large cysts may be symptomatic because of mass effect, resulting in compression of the optic chiasm or pituitary gland. Pathologically, the cysts are typically lined by a single layer of ciliated cuboidal or columnar epithelium with scattered mucous secretory type cells (Figure 18.7). Focal squamous metaplasia may be observed. The cyst lining will stain with antibodies to cytokeratin and epithelial membrane antigen. When the squamous metaplasia component is prominent, confusion of this lesion with other squamous-lined cysts may occur.

Dermoid cysts arising in the sellar region may develop from inclusion of epithelial elements during the closure of the neural tube.[12] Cysts usually present in childhood with no gender predilection. A CT scan may show a low density mass; whereas on MRI imaging, heterogeneous signal intensity due to the presence of hair or sebaceous material may be present. Microscopically, the cysts resemble their counterparts elsewhere in the body. The cysts are lined by squamous epithelium with associated adnexal structures including hair follicles, sebaceous glands, eccrine glands, and apocrine glands (Figure 18.8). Rarely, mature bone may be seen.

Epidermoid cysts can also arise in the sellar or parasellar region.[13] In contrast to the dermoid cysts, epidermoid cysts lacks adnexal structures. Rupture and leakage of cysts may elicit an inflammatory giant cell reaction. The squamous cell epithelial lining often demonstrates evidence of maturation with a surface granular layer (Figure 18.9), a feature that is typically not observed in the squamous metaplasia of the Rathke's cleft cyst and in cystic craniopharyngiomas. Molecular genetic studies currently play no role in the differentiation of cystic lesions in the sellar and pituitary gland region.

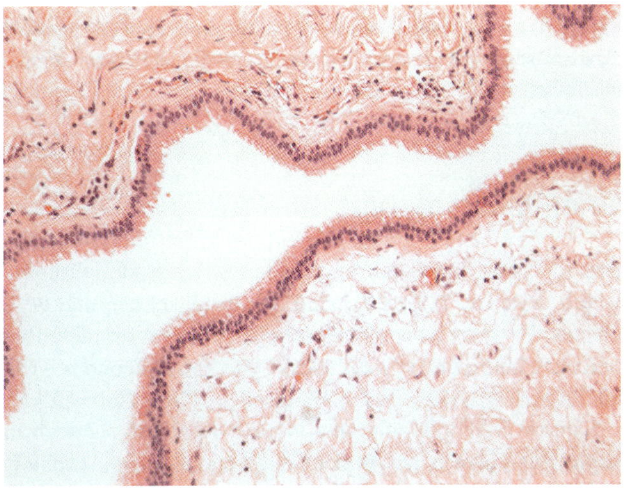

FIG. 18.7. Rathke's cleft cyst lined by ciliated columnar epithelium (hematoxylin and eosin, original magnification 200×).

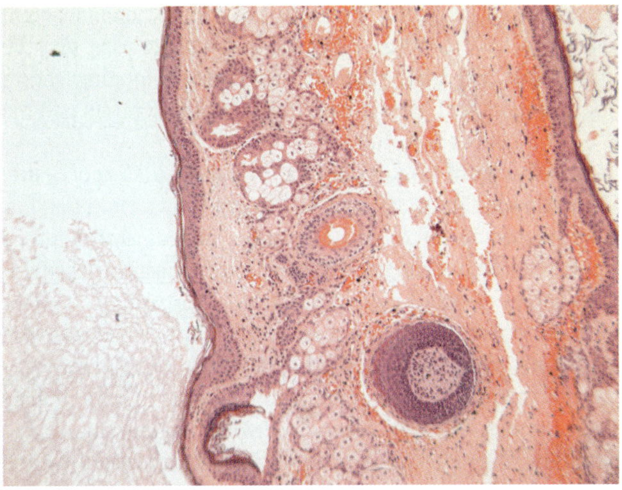

FIG. 18.8. A dermoid cyst lined by squamous epithelium with subjacent adnexal structures (hematoxylin and eosin, original magnification 100×).

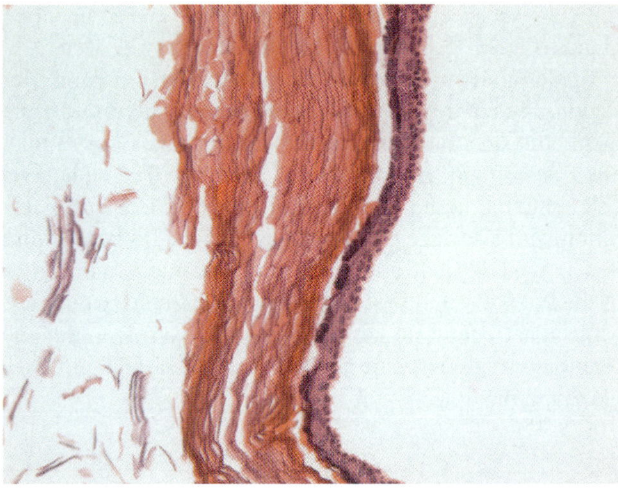

FIG. 18.9. An epidermoid cyst lined by squamous epithelium with a clearly discernable granular layer (hematoxylin and eosin, original magnification 200×).

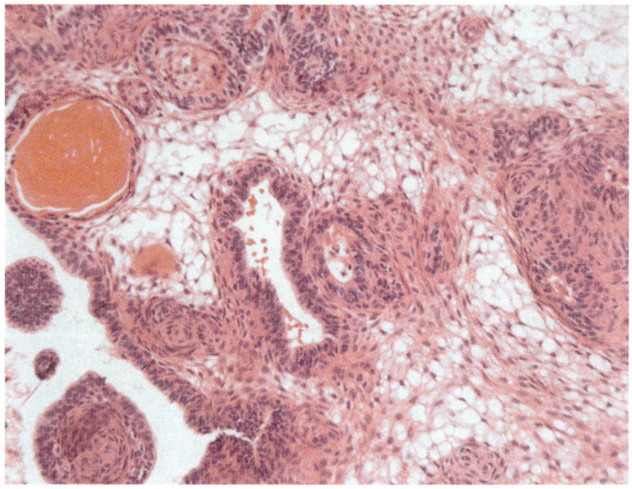

FIG. 18.10. Adenomantinous variant of a craniopharyngioma marked by squamoid epithelium with peripheral columnar epithelium and a loose stellate reticulin (hematoxylin and eosin, original magnification 200×).

Craniopharyngioma

Craniopharyngiomas are low grade (WHO grade I) tumors which comprise between 1 and 5% of all intracranial neoplasms.[14,15] They have a bimodal age presentation including one peak in the first two decades of life and a second peak in adults during the fifth and sixth decades of life. The papillary variant of craniopharyngioma is almost exclusively seen in adults.[16,17] There is no gender predilection. The vast majority of these tumors arise in the suprasellar compartment, although rare cases of tumors situated in other locations, such as the sphenoid sinus, have been reported. The clinical presentation most commonly includes visual disturbances, endocrine abnormalities related to pituitary dysfunction, diabetes insipidus, and cognitive impairment. On CT imaging, these tumors frequently demonstrate contrast enhancement and often have a cystic component. Calcifications may be identifiable. On MRI studies, T1-weighted imaging shows homogeneously intense areas corresponding to cysts and the solid component is isointense.

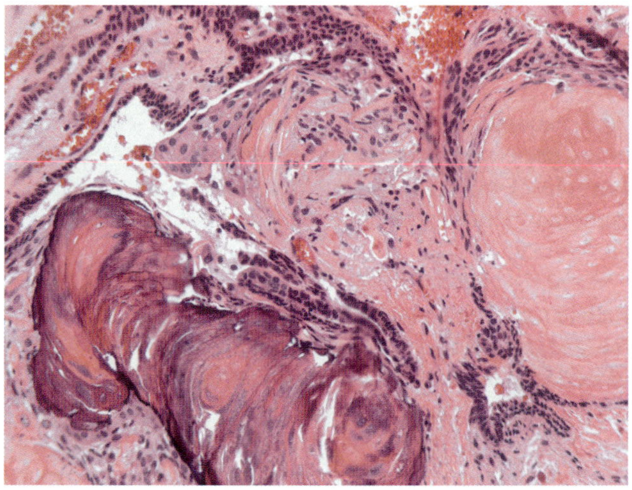

FIG. 18.11. Craniopharyngioma with keratin nodule and calcification (hematoxylin and eosin, original magnification 200×).

Grossly, these tumors may be variably solid and cystic. On sectioning, the cysts contain a green-brown fluid that has been likened to motor oil. The tumor and its surroundings frequently show changes of fibrosis, calcification, ossification, and cholesterol cleft formations. The papillary variant of craniopharyngioma often is well-circumscribed and less commonly cystic and calcified.

Microscopically, there are two variants of craniopharyngioma that are well-recognized: adamantinomatous and papillary. The adamantinomatous variant is marked by the presence of squamoid epithelium arranged in lobules and trabeculae separated by dense connective tissue. The perimeter of the squamoid islands is often lined by palisaded columnar epithelium. The centers of the epithelial islands often have a loosely cohesive appearance and has been referred to as stellate reticulum (Figure 18.10). Nodules of keratin material and calcification are commonly seen (Figure 18.11). Cystic cavities may be lined by a flattened squamoid-type epithelium which lacks a granular layer (Figure 18.12). The adjacent tissue frequently shows a granulomatous reaction with cholesterol cleft formations (Figure 18.13). Prominent gliosis, sometimes accompanied by Rosenthal fiber formations (Figure 18.14), is a fairly common finding around the perimeter of the lesion.

The papillary craniopharyngioma is characterized by squamous-type epithelium lining fibrovascular cores (Figure 18.15). In contrast to epidermoid cysts, there is no obvious maturation of the squamous epithelium as one progresses

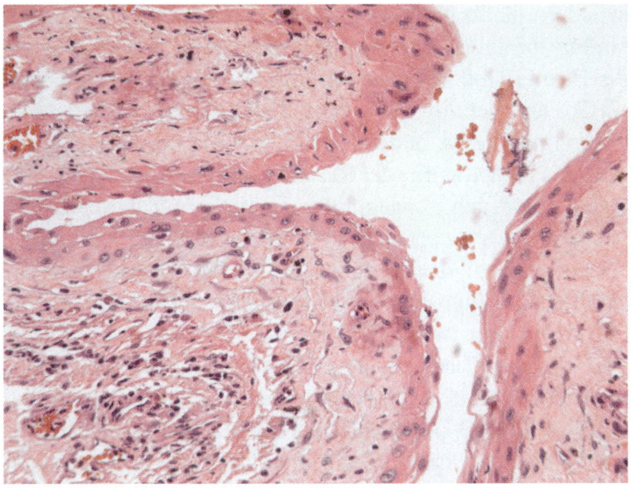

Fig. 18.12. Cystic craniopharyngioma lined by squamous-type epithelium devoid of a granular layer (hematoxylin and eosin, original magnification 200×).

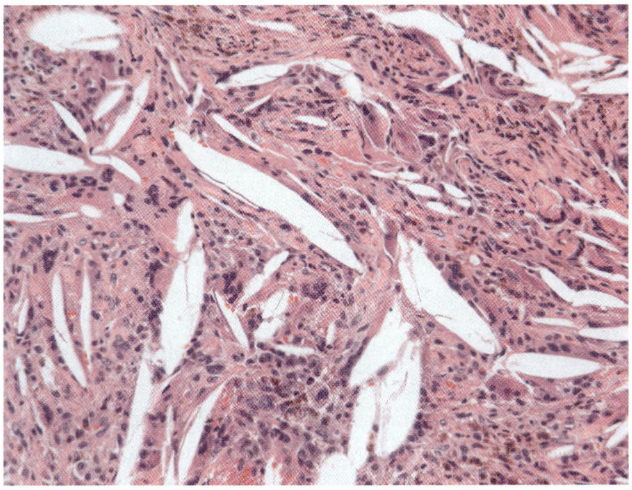

Fig. 18.13. Abundant cholesterol cleft formation and giant cell reaction related to cyst fluid extravasation in a craniopharyngioma (hematoxylin and eosin, original magnification 200×).

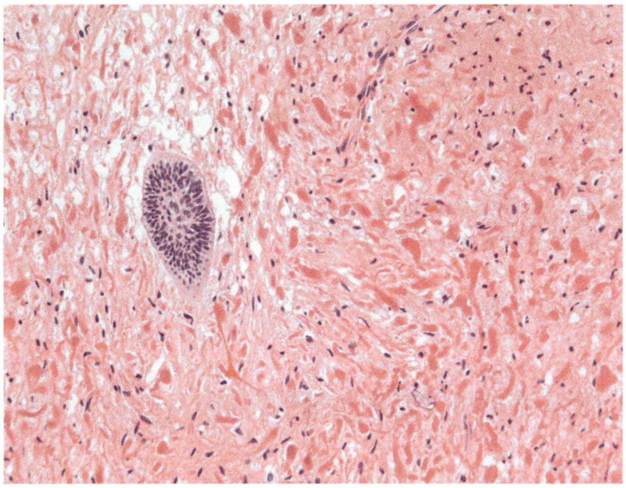

Fig. 18.14. Abundant Rosenthal fibers with gliosis in tissue adjacent to a craniopharyngioma (hematoxylin and eosin, original magnification 200×).

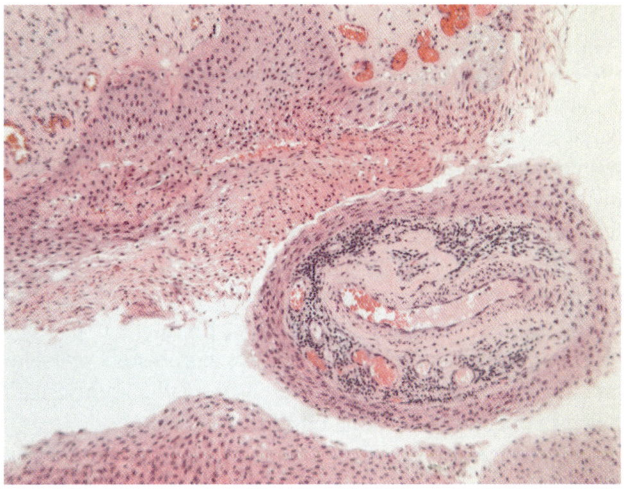

Fig. 18.15. Papillary variant of a craniopharyngioma marked by fibrovascular cores lined by squamous-type epithelium (hematoxylin and eosin, original magnification 100×).

from the base to the surface. Occasionally, ciliated cells or goblet cells may be intermixed with the squamous epithelium. Microcalcifications and abundant cholesterol cleft formations and granulomatous responses are unusual in this variant. The epithelial component of both variants will stain with a variety of cytokeratin markers.

Examination of these tumors with cell proliferation markers, such as Ki-67 or MIB-1, shows immunoreactivity primarily located around the periphery of the squamoid nests in the adamantinomatous variant.[18] Cell proliferation marker immunoreactivity is more homogeneously distributed in the papillary variant. No relationship between labeling indices and tumor recurrence or behavior has been documented reliably in the literature.

There is currently no role for the routine evaluation of these tumors from a molecular or genetic perspective. Multiple chromosomal abnormalities have been documented in the few cases that have been studied.[19] Mutation of the beta-catenin gene has been noted in the majority of adamantinomatous craniopharyngiomas.[20,21] This results in an accumulation of nuclear beta-catenin protein which can be demonstrated by immunohistochemistry. In a few cases, similar beta-catenin mutations were identified in mesenchymal cells situated between the squamous epithelioid cells, suggesting a biphasic nature for this neoplasm. Interestingly, beta-catenin mutations have not been demonstrated in papillary craniopharyngiomas. Although comparative genomic hybridization studies have demonstrated genomic alterations in the majority of adamantinomatous craniopharyngiomas, significant chromosomal imbalances have not been identified in these tumors.

A significant factor associated with tumor recurrence is the extent of surgical excision. Generally, tumors greater than 5 cm in diameter are associated with a worse prognosis, as are incompletely resected neoplasms. The literature is mixed with regard to prognosis associated with histologic subtype with some papers reporting a better prognosis for the papillary variant, while other papers failing to demonstrate a significant difference. Rare cases of malignant transformation to squamous cell carcinoma, particularly following radiation therapy, have been documented.

Pituitary Hyperplasia

Pituitary hyperplasia can be physiological or pathological and clinically indistinguishable from an adenoma. Radiological imaging can sometimes distinguish hyperplasia from normal: in hyperplasia, the proliferation is diffuse, and there is no normal rim that enhances with gadolinium.[22] A reticulin stain can also help differentiate these entities. In hyperplasia, the acinar architecture is maintained and the reticulin network is preserved, but the acini are increased in size.[23] In contrast, pituitary adenomas are characterized by complete disruption of the reticulin fiber network. Immunohistochemical stains for hormones are required to determine the secretory nature of the hyperplastic cell population.

Pituitary hyperplasia can be diffuse or nodular, unifocal or multifocal.[24,25] In the diffuse type, the number of cells increases without a major change in the morphology or acinar architecture. In the focal type, there is a small circumscribed increase of cell type without clinical significance.

Cell proliferation indices, though higher than the normal adenohypophysis, are not high enough to be used as a reliable marker.[24,25] Similarly, molecular techniques, such as in situ hybridization, PCR, and blotting studies have contributed little to the diagnosis of pituitary hyperplasia.[25] Due to the difficulty in establishing the diagnosis, the incidence of pituitary hyperplasia in general and the frequency of its various patterns are not known.

Pituitary Adenoma

Recognizing molecular determinants in normal pituitary gland cytodifferentiation is important in determining the cytogenesis of pituitary adenomas, as well as providing a framework for classification.[26,27] Three main pathways of cell differentiation have been identified in the anterior pituitary. Adenohypophysial cells arise from Rathke's pouch stem cells, and the corticotrophs are the first cells to differentiate. This process is determined by the Tpit transcription factor[28] that works in concert with Ptx1 and neuroD1,[29,30] previously called corticotroph upstream transcription element (CUTE) binding proteins. The second line of differentiation is via Pit-1 expression, activating growth hormone (GH), prolactin (PRL), and beta-thyrotropin (b-TSH) genes.[31,32] The somatotroph phenotype is determined, and the expression of the estrogen receptor allows PRL and GH to be made in a bihormonal population of mammosomatotrophs.[33] Mature lactotrophs develop in the presence of a putative GH repressor, which has not yet been identified. Some of the Pit-1-expressing cells also make thyrotroph embryonic factor (TEF) and develop into thyrotrophs when GH repressor and GATA-2 are present.[34] Somatotrophs, mammosomatotrophs and lactotrophs transdifferentiate in a reversible fashion,[35] and all three cell types are Pit-1 dependent. The third line of differentiation is that of the gonadotrophs, which are determined by steroidogenic factor-1 (SF-1) and GATA-2 in the presence of estrogen receptor.[34,36] Commercially available antibodies exist for the nuclear transcription factors, Pit-1, and SF-1.[26]

The 2004 WHO Classification of Tumors report contains three accepted types of primary adenohypophysial lesions: typical pituitary adenoma, atypical pituitary adenoma, and pituitary carcinoma.[37] An atypical adenoma is an invasive tumor marked by an elevated mitotic index, a MIB-1 labeling index >3%, and an extensive nuclear immunostaining for p53.[37] Pituitary carcinoma is defined by metastasis or noncontiguous spread. The most important clinical and prognostic features of pituitary adenomas remain the hormonal profile and subtype classification, because specific subtypes (such as the sparsely granulated growth hormone adenoma) have a greater propensity for aggressive clinical behavior.[38]

Pituitary adenomas are classified clinically into functioning or nonfunctioning adenomas, according to whether or not an endocrine syndrome is present. The majority of adenomas are functioning; however, about a third of all pituitary adenomas lack clinical or biochemical evidence of hormone excess.[39] According to tumor size, adenomas are divided into microadenomas (<1 cm in diameter) and macroadenomas (>1 cm diameter). Macroadenomas possess a tendency for suprasellar extension, gross invasion, and recurrence. Staining characteristics of the tumor cells, such as acidophilic, basophilic, or chromophobe, are outdated as a primary means of classification, because they do not identify specific adenoma subtypes. Adenomas are histologically marked by a disruption of the normal nested pattern of the adenohypophysis (Figure 18.16). Growth patterns (diffuse, pseudopapillary, trabecular, etc.), are of no prognostic significance, but they may be helpful in the differential diagnosis of adenoma (Figures 18.17–18.19). Hormone content of the tumor can be assessed by immunohistochemistry; however, it does not always discriminate between specific subtypes of adenomas that have prognostic clinical significance.

Recently, a number of novel molecular techniques, such as in situ hybridization, have been applied to the experimental study of pituitary tumors. These methods are primarily regarded as

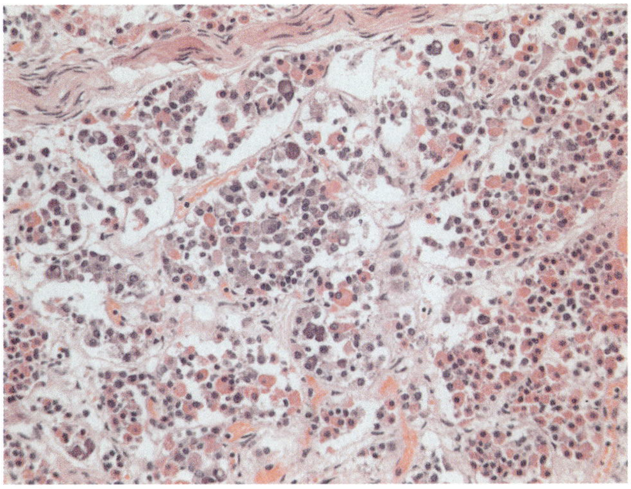

FIG. 18.16. Normal nested architecture of the adenohypophysis. Each nest shows a mixture of acidophilic, basophilic and chromophobe cells (hematoxylin and eosin, original magnification 200×).

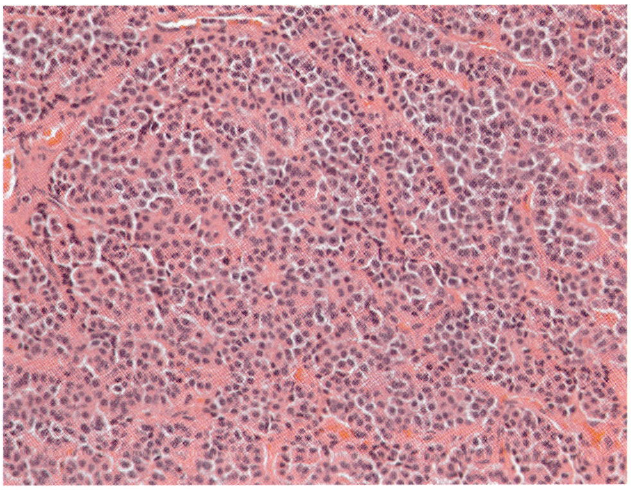

FIG. 18.17. Diffuse growth pattern in a pituitary adenoma; this is the most common pattern seen (hematoxylin and eosin, original magnification 200×).

research tools, but in the near future they may be used in routine diagnosis.

Prolactinomas comprise nearly 80% of functioning pituitary tumors and about 40–50% of all pituitary adenomas.[40,41] Most are microadenomas, occurring in reproductive-age women who present with amenorrhea, galactorrhea, and infertility. In men and elderly women, prolactinomas are usually macroadenomas and are commonly associated with headaches, neurological deficits, and visual loss. Impotence and decreased libido are common symptoms in men with hyperprolactinemia.

By light microscopy, tumor cells are medium-sized with chromophobic or slightly acidophilic cytoplasm and central, oval nucleus. Small nucleoli can be present (Figure 18.20). Approximately 10–20% of cases show variably prominent

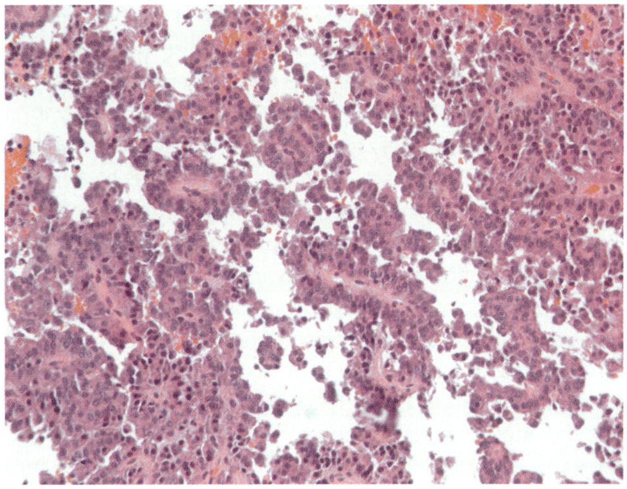

FIG. 18.18. A pseudopapillary architecture in a pituitary adenoma (hematoxylin and eosin, original magnification 200×).

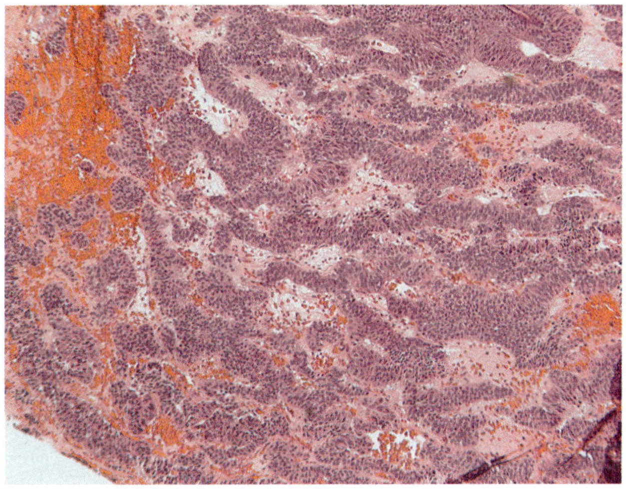

FIG. 18.19. A trabecular growth pattern in a pituitary adenoma (hematoxylin and eosin, original magnification 100×).

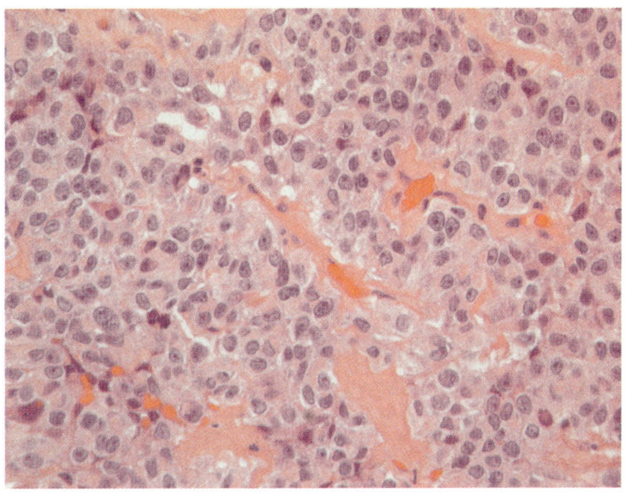

FIG. 18.20. Prolactin secreting adenoma with nucleolated tumor cells (hematoxylin and eosin, original magnification 400×).

microcalcifications. Nuclear pleomorphism may be evident but is not of any clinical significance (Figure 18.21). Immunohistochemistry shows nuclear prolactin (PRL) positivity in a "dot like" pattern, reflecting hormone localization in the Golgi complex (Figure 18.22). If previously treated with dopamine agonists, there is atrophy of lactotrophs with resultant tumor shrinkage and hyperchromasia of the nuclei.[42] Strong nuclear positivity for Pit-1 is seen. Ultrastructurally, lactotroph adenomas can be subclassified into sparsely and densely granulated variants. Sparsely granulated tumors are the most common and resemble normal, actively secreting lactrotrophs. Adenoma cells show a prominent rough endoplasmic reticulin (RER) network, conspicuous Golgi complex, and a sparse number of small (150–300 nm) secretory granules. The densely granulated variant is very rare and contains elongated acidophilic cells with elongated nuclei and increased chromatin. Reactivity for PRL is strong and diffuse. Electron microscopy reveals large, somewhat densely arranged secretory granules with exocytoses and a well developed RER.[43] Amyloid derived from PRL is seen in up to 48% of adenomas.[44] Cell proliferation indices are typically low.

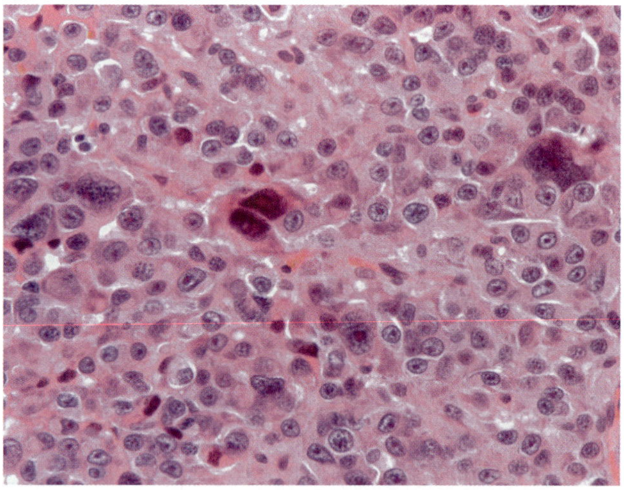

FIG. 18.21. Scattered pleomorphic nuclei in a prolactinoma (hematoxylin and eosin, original magnification 400×).

About 20% of pituitary adenomas are associated with evidence of growth hormone (GH) secretion, which can be accompanied by high serum GH and insulin-like growth factor I (IGF-I) levels.[45] Patients presenting with acromegaly or gigantism may rarely have somatotroph hyperplasia owing to ectopic production of growth hormone releasing hormone; therefore, the reticulin stain may be critical to exclude this possibility. Both genders are affected with a mean age of presentation of 40–45 years. Most acromegalic patients have macroadenomas when first diagnosed, often with suprasellar expansion and parasellar invasion.[46]

GH secreting adenomas are either eosinophilic or chromophobic. In eosinophilic adenomas, the cytoplasm shows considerable granularity. The oval nucleus tends to be central with a prominent nucleolus. Nuclear pleomorphism and multinucleation are common. GH reactivity is marked by diffuse cytoplasmic staining throughout the tumor (Figure 18.23). By electron microscopy, the densely granulated variant has adenomatous cells that resemble normal somatotrophs, having a well developed RER network, prominent Golgi complexes, and numerous large (300–600 nm) secretory granules. In sparsely granulated GH tumors, the cytoplasm is more chromophobic, the nucleus tends to be eccentric, and the cytoplasm contains a few small (100–250 nm) secretory and paranuclear eosinophilic structures called "fibrous bodies." These bodies are strongly positive for cytokeratin[47] and ultrastructurally, represent accumulations of intermediate filaments and tubular formations. GH immunostaining is focal

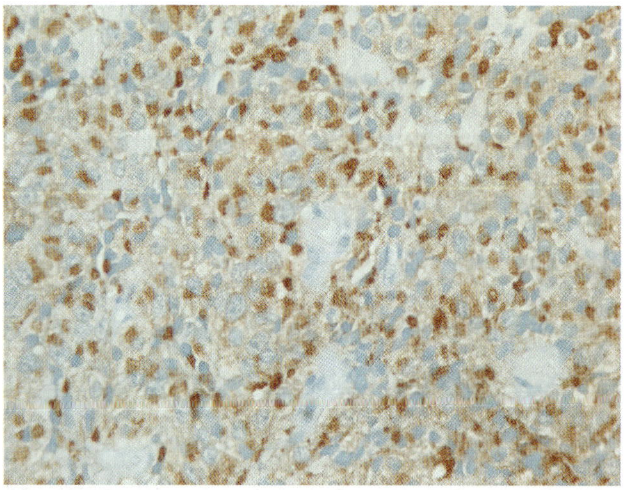

FIG. 18.22. Dot-like immunoreactivity in a prolactin positive adenoma – same tumor as Figure 18.20 (prolactin, original magnification 400×).

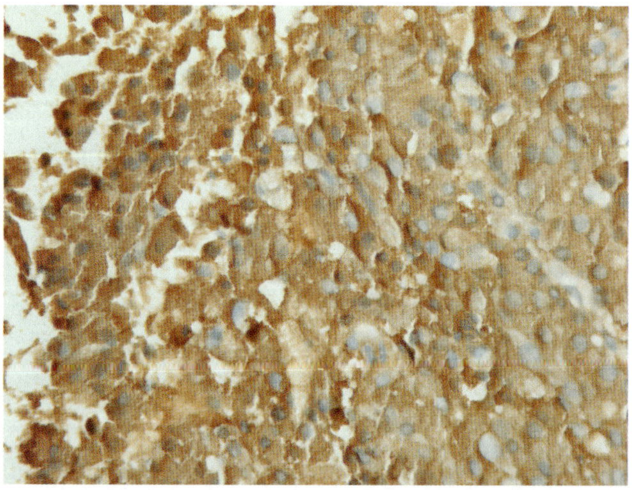

FIG. 18.23. Diffuse positive staining of an adenoma with growth hormone antibody (growth hormone, original magnification 400×).

within the tumor and tends to be localized in a paranuclear distribution. GH reactivity is weaker in the sparsely granulated variant, and may even be negative in some cases.[48] In situ hybridization may be used to detect GH mRNA, which will be positive in sparsely granulated GH cell adenomas.[49] CAM 5.2 identifies perinuclear keratin in densely granulated adenomas[50] and fibrous bodies in the sparsely granulated adenomas. Long-acting somatostatin analog may change the morphology, resulting in varying degrees of perivascular and interstitial fibrosis.[51] The clinical importance of distinguishing these two subtypes of GH cell adenomas is controversial, but the sparsely granulated GH cell adenomas appear to exhibit more aggressive biological behavior than the densely granulated tumors.[52,53]

Adrenocorticotropic hormone (ACTH) dependent Cushing's syndrome is caused by pituitary ACTH secreting adenomas in 80% of cases.[45] ACTH secreting adenomas constitute two major groups: endocrinologically active tumors associated with either Cushing's disease or Nelson's syndrome,[54] and tumors that are clinically nonfunctioning, also known as silent corticotroph adenomas.[55] Cushing's disease affects patients of varying ages, with a peak at 30–40 years, and it shows a female predominance.[45] On rare occasions, corticotroph cell hyperplasia may be the source of Cushing's disease (Figure 18.24).

Microadenomas associated with Cushing's disease are densely granulated with strongly basophilic cells and strong PAS positivity. Immunohistochemically, they express ACTH and usually react strongly with the CAM 5.2 antibody and cytokeratins 7 and 8. Crooke's hyaline change may also be present. In addition, other peptides related to the proopiomelanocortin (POMC) precursor molecule, including beta-lipotropin, beta-endorphin, and alpha-melanocyte-stimulating hormone, can be present.[56] The ultrastructural features are characterized by well-differentiated cells that resemble normal corticotrophs. Well developed organelles, including RER, smooth endoplasmic reticulum, and conspicuous Golgi are associated with numerous large (250–700 nm) secretory granules, which often are different shapes and vary in electron density. Sparsely granulated ACTH cell adenomas are only weakly basophilic and weakly PAS-positive or chromophobic. Cellular pleomorphism is more frequent. Immunostaining reactions, especially for ACTH, are weaker than the densely granulated variant, and may be negative (Figure 18.25). EM reveals less numerous and often smaller secretory granules than in the densely granulated ACTH cell adenomas, whereas the organelles structures are similar or slightly irregular. In adenomas from patients with Cushing's disease, bundles of intermediate filaments adjacent to the nucleus and/or forming large circles are easily identified. Histologic and immunohistochemical studies are sufficient for the right diagnosis.

Crooke's cell adenomas are very rare and the morphology can be quite atypical, with prominent nuclear pleomorphism and large cells that can resemble gangliocytoma or metastatic carcinoma. It is defined by PAS positivity and immunoreactivity for ACTH, as well as the dense ring of keratin that fills the tumor cell cytoplasm, and is identified with CAM 5.2 staining.[50] The clinical course is variable, with some tumors demonstrating an aggressive behavior, and others only being discovered as small incidental inactive adenomas in postmortem pituitaries.[57] In a recent study, invasiveness was found in 72% of these adenomas.[58]

The rare silent corticotroph cell adenoma demonstrates immunoreactivity for ACTH without clinical signs of Cushing's disease or serum levels reflecting excess. The majority are macroadenomas and present with signs of a mass lesion and show a high tendency to hemorrhage and necrosis (apoplexy) (Figure 18.26), which may be the presenting symptom in about a third of patients.[59]

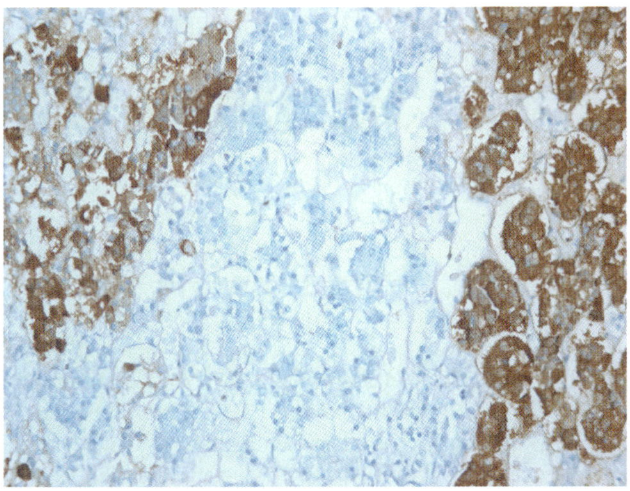

Fig. 18.24. Normal adenohypophysis stained with ACTH antibody. Regional variability of staining should not be misinterpreted as representing a hyperplasia (ACTH, original magnification 200×).

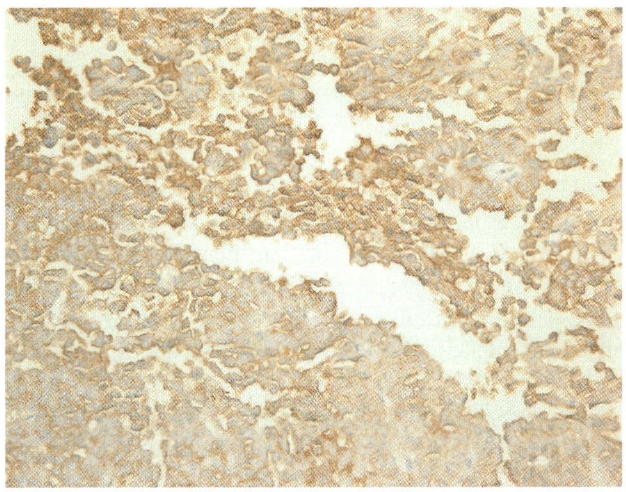

Fig. 18.25. Diffuse but weak staining of a ACTH secreting adenoma (ACTH, original magnification 200×).

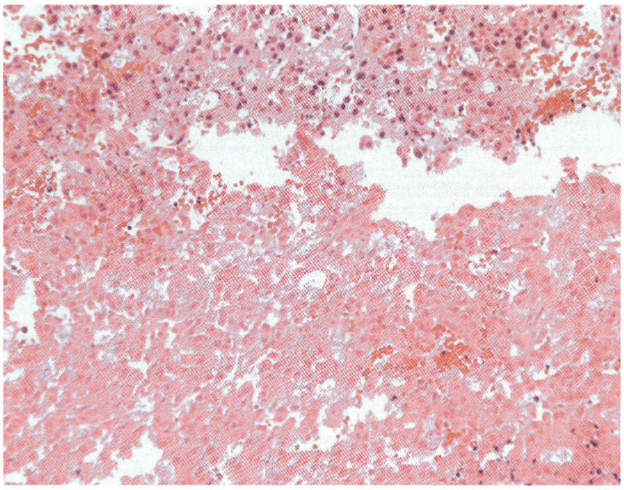

FIG. 18.26. Hemorrhagic necrosis (apoplexy) in a silent corticotroph cell adenoma (hematoxylin and eosin, original magnification 200×).

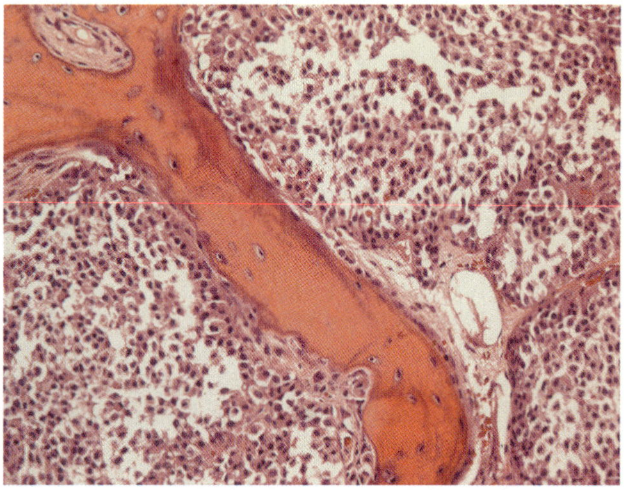

FIG. 18.27. A bone invasive TSH secreting adenoma (hematoxylin and eosin, original magnification 200×).

Thyroid stimulating hormone (TSH) cell adenomas are the least frequent of pituitary adenomas.[60] Most are invasive macroadenomas[61,62] (Figure 18.27). Light microscopy reveals medium-sized chromophobic cells. Globular PAS-positive inclusions representing lysosomes may be found. Immunostaining for TSH is variable and may be negative. The ultrastructure is characterized by similarities to normal TSH cells with often prominent RER, globoid Golgi complexes, and sparse small (150–250 nm), rod-shaped or spherical or irregular secretory granules.

Gonadotropin-secreting adenomas secrete follicle stimulating hormone (FSH) and/or leutinizing hormone (LH), and do not usually have a clinical syndrome related to hormone overproduction. They may present with symptoms related to mass effect. With modern lab techniques, a large number of pituitary adenomas previously classified as non-functioning adenomas have been found to produce gonadotropins or their subunits.[63] Hence, gonadotroph adenomas may account for a large proportion of clinically nonfunctioning adenomas and about 20% of all adenomas.[64] They occur most frequently in the sixth decade or older, showing a slight male predominance. By light microscopy, most cells have chromophobic cytoplasm and a nucleus with a fine chromatin pattern. The cells may be arranged in a diffuse pattern, but a distinct papillary arrangement is commonly seen. Immunohistochemistry demonstrates varying levels of reactivity for beta-FSH, beta-LH, alpha-SU, or a combination. Ultrastructurally, these adenomas are characterized by elongated polar cells containing scant numbers of small (50–200 nm) secretory granules. The secretory granules are distributed unevenly within the cytoplasm or along the cytoplasmic membrane.

Plurihormonal adenomas have unusual immunoreactivity for more than one type of pituitary hormone, which are unrelated by normal cytogenesis and development of anterior pituitary. Clinically, these patients present with symptoms attributable to mass effect. With improved methods of immunostaining and the increased use of monoclonal antibodies, the incidence of plurihormonal adenomas is lower than expected from former studies with polyclonal antibodies.[48] The most common combination is an adenoma secreting PRL and GH. Reports of adenomas expressing GH or PRL with gonadotropins are now recognized to reflect an aberration that was identified as non-specific cross-reactivity.[65] Plurihormonal adenomas can be monomorphous or plurimorphous in nature.

Approximately 20% of adenomas show neither clinical nor immunohistochemical evidence of hormone production[66,67] and are labeled as null cell adenomas. Most commonly, they arise in postmenopausal females and elderly males, presenting with signs and symptoms of mass effect. By light microscopy, they are mostly chromophobic and can be arranged in a diffuse pattern and/or in well-defined papillary arrangements. Oncocytic degeneration can be seen.

Pituitary adenomas without clinically active hypersecretion are characterized as non-functioning pituitary adenomas (NFPA). They represent about one quarter of all pituitary tumors and are often asymptomatic and manifest themselves only after they have grown to sufficient size to produce mass effect. Symptoms referable to hypopituitarism can often be elicited and verified by endocrine testing. Moderate prolactinemia from stalk compression may be present; sometimes these adenomas are erroneously diagnosed as prolactinomas. A subset of clinically inactive adenomas are silent adenomas, which are characterized by the insufficient secretion of active hormones into the circulation, despite their expression.[37] Most of these are ACTH cell adenomas.

Pituitary apoplexy is the rapid enlargement of an adenoma due to tumoral infarction and hemorrhage, presenting usually as an acute event and often neurosurgical emergency. All immunotypes of adenoma may present with apoplexy, but large nonfunctioning adenomas are particularly prone.

The majority of pituitary adenomas are sporadic, although some arise as a component of familial syndromes. Pituitary adenomas can occur in a familial setting in multiple endocrine neoplasia type I (MEN 1),[68] Carney complex (CNC)[69] and in the context of isolated, autosomal dominant acromegaly or gigantism. Less frequently, they can occur in the context of a familial predisposition to the development of pituitary tumors.[70] Another rare genetic disorder associated with GH and PRL producing tumors is McCune–Albright syndrome (MAS).[71]

So far, four genes have been identified that predispose to familial pituitary tumorigenesis.[72] Multiple endocrine neoplasia type I (MEN 1) (11q13) and protein kinase A regulatory subunit-1-alpha (PRKAR1A)(17q24) genes have been associated in multiple endocrine neoplasia type 1 (MEN1) and Carney complex (CNC), respectively. More recently, pituitary adenoma predisposition (PAP) genes, cyclin-dependent kinase inhibitor 1B (CDKN1B) (12p13), and aryl hydrocarbon receptor (AHR) interacting protein (AIP) (11q13) have been identified.[73] In addition, familial pituitary adenoma is seen in the isolated familial somatotropinomas (IFS) (linkage to 11q13) and familial isolated pituitary adenomas (FIPA),[74] the former probably in part allelic to PAP and caused by mutations in AIP gene, and in the FIPA phenotype. MEN1 is a tumor suppressor gene; the syndrome is inherited as an autosomal dominant trait. Pituitary adenomas affect 23–30% of MEN1 patients.[75] MEN1 mutations predispose to all major pituitary tumor subtypes, but the most common subtypes seen are those secreting PRL (60%) and GH (20%); ACTH secreting and nonfunctional adenomas represent less than 15%.[76]

Pituitary Carcinoma

Pituitary carcinomas are very rare neoplasms, representing fewer than 0.2% of all anterior pituitary tumors.[77] The definition of carcinoma depends on the demonstration of craniospinal and systemic metastases. The most common sites of metastases are subarachnoid space, cervical lymph nodes, bone, liver, and lungs. There appears to be an equal gender distribution and tumors present with a peak incidence in the fifth decade. The diagnosis of pituitary carcinoma cannot be based solely on histologic appearance, as invasion, cellular pleomorphism, nuclear abnormalities, mitotic activity, and necrosis can all be seen in adenomas. Tumors arise in the anterior lobe and depending on growth rate, spread to neighboring structures. Craniospinal space spread and systemic spread follows. The majority of cases are endocrinologically functioning tumors, most commonly secreting PRL or ACTH.[78,79] Carcinomas show a higher Ki-67 labeling index and increased p53 protein expression as compared with adenomas.[80] Ras mutations can be found in PRL cell carcinomas.[81] Nuclear p27 protein expression is significantly decreased in adenomas as compared with normal pituitary, and is much lower in pituitary carcinoma as compared to both normal and adenomas.[82,83] Using comparative genomic hybridization (CGH), chromosomal imbalances are common, with gains being more common than losses[84]; the most frequent changes are gains of chromosomes 5, 7p, and 14q. The prognosis of pituitary carcinomas is generally poor, although patients with long-term survival have been described.[85]

Tumor Proliferation Markers and Invasiveness in Adenomas and Carcinomas

The molecular mechanisms controlling cell proliferation and invasion in pituitary tumors are largely unknown. Studies of proliferative activity have been used as an adjuvant tool for distinguishing between aggressive and indolent, benign pituitary adenomas.[86-89] Clinically functioning adenomas have a significantly higher growth fraction than nonfunctioning tumors.[87] Growth fractions are also significantly higher among invasive adenomas and pituitary carcinomas when compared with noninvasive adenomas.[86,89-91]

Invasive adenomas may demonstrate p53-positive nuclei, which are found to be absent in regular adenomas.[92,93] p53 expression has been correlated significantly with the numbers of MIB-1 positive nuclei and PCNA positive nuclei.

Investigators have found that cyclooxygenase-2 (COX-2) expression correlates with patient age, but not with tumor size or invasiveness.[94] Galectin-3, a beta galactosidase binding protein implicated in cellular differentiation and proliferation as well as angiogenesis, tumor progression, and metastasis, may play a role in pituitary tumor progression.[95] The polypeptide insulin-like growth factor-1 (IGF-I) is demonstrable in most pituitary adenomas,[96] but a distinct correlation to adenoma growth could not be found. Parathormone (PTH)-related protein was demonstrated in normal pituitary and in pituitary adenomas, as well as overexpressed in a metastasis of GH secreting carcinoma.[97]

Oncogenes and Tumor Suppressor Genes in Pituitary Tumorigenesis

The mechanisms underlying human pituitary tumorigenesis and progression are largely unknown. X-chromosomal inactivation analyses in a large number of pituitary adenomas demonstrated that a majority of the tumors are monoclonal in origin.[98] Sporadic and low frequency mutations in oncogenes and tumor suppressor genes are observed in pituitary adenomas. Two well-characterized genetic abnormalities have been identified in pituitary adenomas. The first one is a putative tumor suppressor gene at 11q13, the genetic defect in multiple endocrine neoplasia 1 (MEN1).[99] In patients with MEN1 syndrome, loss of 11q13 is present in pituitary adenomas, but only 3% of pituitary adenomas occur in the context of MEN1. Loss of heterozygosity (LOH) at 11q13 has been demonstrated in 10–20% of sporadic pituitary adenomas, suggesting the presence of a tumor suppressor gene at this location,[100] but the somatic MEN1 mutation rate is very low (approximately 2%).[101] Therefore, the *MEN1* gene does not appear to play a major role in the pathogenesis of sporadic pituitary adenomas.

The second gene mutation described in pituitary adenomas is the *gsp* oncogene mutation of the alpha subunit of the G-protein.[102,103] The *gsp* mutation has been identified in about 40% of GH secreting adenomas, 10% of nonfunctioning pituitary adenomas, and 5% of corticotroph adenomas.[103-105] Although some clinical and biochemical differences are observed, these tumors do not differ morphologically from tumors without *gsp*. The activating mutation of *gsp* is demonstrated in McCune–Albright syndrome, which is characterized by somatotroph hyperplasia and polyostotic fibrous dysplasia of the bones.[106]

A number of other oncogenes and tumor suppressor genes have been identified as possible players in the pituitary tumorigenesis. The protein expressed by the pituitary transforming gene (PTTG) has roles in mitosis control, cell transformation, and DNA repair. Three homologue genes have been identified: (1) *PTTH1* located on chromosome 5q33, (2) *PTTG2* on chromosome 4p12; and (3) *PTTG3* on chromosome 8q22.[107] PTTG protein is expressed at low levels in the normal human pituitary, but at high levels in a variety of solid tumors, including pituitary adenomas.[108] Approximately 90% of pituitary adenomas overexpress PTTG, with the highest levels seen in ACTH secreting and nonfunctioning pituitary tumors. One study reported higher expression levels of PTTG, PTTG binding factor, and fibroblast growth factor 2 (FGF-2) and its FGF receptor FGFR1 mRNAs in pituitary adenomas as compared to normal tissue.[109] In the clinical setting, where other markers of tumor aggressiveness (such as expression of PCNA, Ki-67, etc.) have failed, PTTG and possibly FGF-2 and FGFR1 may be the best available markers of pituitary tumors. In addition, FGF-2 and -4 have been implicated in prolactinoma development. Expression of the pituitary tumor derived (ptd)-FGFR4 protein is more frequently found in macroadenomas than in microadenomas and correlated with the Ki-67 labeling index.

Mutation of the tumor suppressor gene *TP53* is the most common genetic event associated with human cancers. However, neither *TP53* gene mutations nor chromosome 17p deletions have been demonstrated in pituitary adenomas or carcinomas.[110,111] However, overexpression of *p53* protein has been shown in a number of highly invasive adenomas and carcinomas.[112] The expression of p27 is reduced in pituitary adenomas, mainly in ACTH producing tumors, and hypermethylation of p16 is detected in adenomas of gonadotroph lineage.[37] Cyclin D1 is sparsely demonstrated and more frequently found in nonfunctioning and aggressive adenomas than in other adenoma types.[113] Overexpression of cyclin D3 has been found in the nuclei of 68% of inactive adenomas and correlated with the Ki-67 labeling index.[113] Cyclins A, B, and E are expressed in all adenoma types and are significantly higher in macroadenomas when compared to microadenomas.[114] Screening of numerous adenomas failed to reveal mutations of the tumor suppressor gene *RB*[115]; however, allelic loss of *RB* has been demonstrated in some highly invasive adenomas and pituitary carcinomas.[116] Point mutations of the H-*ras* proto-oncogene have been identified in rare cases of distant metastases of pituitary carcinoma.[106,111]

A number of growth factors and hypothalamic trophic factors are also believed to participate in the maintenance of pituitary tumors by dysregulated autocrine and paracrine mechanisms.[37]

The vast majority of genetic alterations in pituitary adenomas seem to be due to promoter methylation or acetylation with silencing of tumor suppressors. The mRNA expression of *GADD45* gamma gene (growth arrest and DNA damage inducible gene family) is significantly reduced in clinically nonfunctioning pituitary adenomas using cDNA representational difference analysis.[37] This is believed to be due to promoter methylation.

Granular Cell Tumor

Granular cell tumors arising in the neurohypophysis are relatively rare lesions.[117–119] These tumors show a female predominance and most commonly present with symptoms related to visual field deficits secondary to compression of the optic nerve and chiasm. Occasionally, endocrine abnormalities may also be observed. Most of these tumors are slow growing and symptoms may develop gradually over a long period of time. On imaging, the tumor presents as a well circumscribed, suprasellar mass which demonstrates areas of contrast enhancement. In contrast to craniopharyngiomas which may arise in the region, calcification is unusual in these lesions. Necrosis, cystic degeneration, and hemorrhage are uncommon.

Morphologically, these tumors resemble their extra-pituitary counterparts in that they are marked by a proliferation of polygonal cells with abundant granular, eosinophilic cytoplasm (Figure 18.28). Ultrastructurally, the granular appearance of the cytoplasm correlates with an increased number of lysosomes. Cells may be arranged in nodules and focal spindling of cells may be evident. Perivascular chronic inflammation is relatively common. Mitotic activity is usually not observable. Tumors which show evidence of increased nuclear pleomorphism, prominent nucleolation, and increased mitotic activity are designated as atypical granular cell tumors by some; the significance of these lesions is uncertain. By immunohistochemistry, the tumor demonstrates positivity with antibodies to CD68, S-100 protein, cathepsin B, and alpha-1-antitrypsin.[120] Tumors do not stain with antibodies to neurofilaments, cytokeratins, synaptophysin, or chromogranin.

Anecdotal studies examining genetic alterations in these tumors have been performed. Utilizing comparative genomic

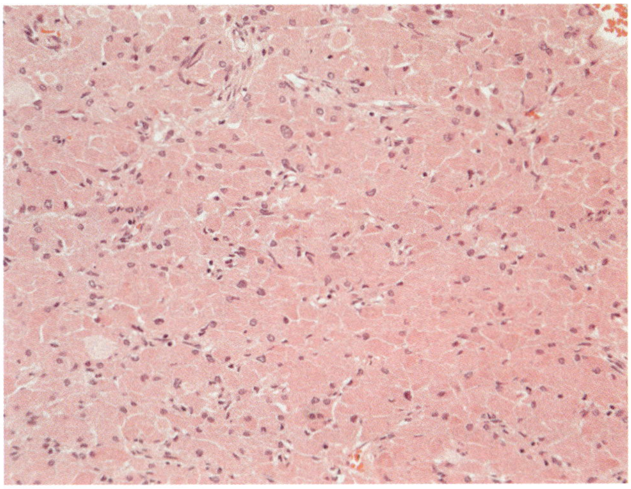

Fig. 18.28. Granular cell tumor characterized by polygonal cells with abundant granular, eosinophilic cytoplasm (hematoxylin and eosin, original magnification 200×).

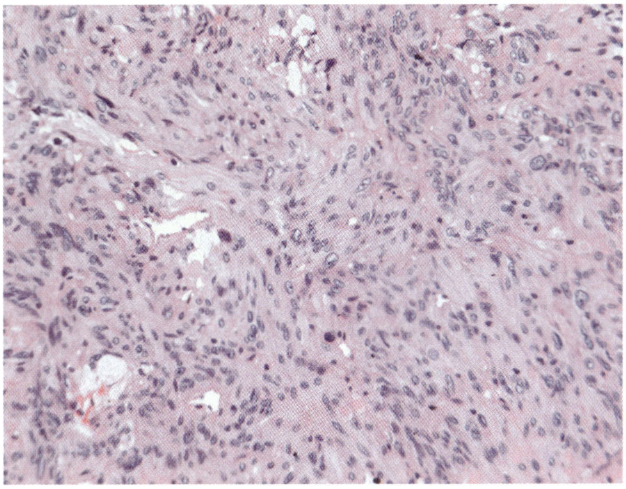

Fig. 18.29. Pituicytoma marked by spindled cells (hematoxylin and eosin, original magnification 200×).

hybridization, one tumor studied did not show any evidence of chromosomal imbalances.[121] In another case of atypical granular cell tumor, the majority of tumor cells demonstrated p53 accumulation.

The majority of these tumors behave in a benign fashion (WHO grade I). Because of their nodular architecture and their epithelioid appearance, they may be confused with pituitary adenoma, if one is not careful.

Pituicytoma

Pituicytomas are rare tumors arising in adults in the neurohypophysis.[122–124] In cases that have been thus far reported in the literature, there appears to be a slight male predominance. The clinical presentation usually involves symptoms related to a slowly expanding mass lesion in the sella and includes visual disturbances, headaches, and signs of hypopituitarism. On imaging, the lesions are typically well-demarcated and uniformly contrast-enhancing.

Pathologically, the pituicytoma is a solid, well-circumscribed lesion. The tumor consists of elongated bipolar spindled cells arranged in interlacing fascicles and a storiform pattern (Figure 18.29). Scattered tumor cells may be marked by abundant eosinophilic cytoplasm. Nuclear atypia or pleomorphism is not a salient feature of this tumor. Mitotic figures are unusual. Oncocytic features are not present.

In terms of immunohistochemistry, pituicytomas generally stain positively with antibodies to vimentin, GFAP, and S-100 protein. Markers of neural differentiation or neuroendocrine markers including synaptophysin, chromogranin as well as cytokeratins are negative. Occasional EMA immunoreactivity may be observed. Cell proliferation indices are low, in most cases less than 2%. Currently, there is a paucity of literature regarding molecular or genetic characteristic

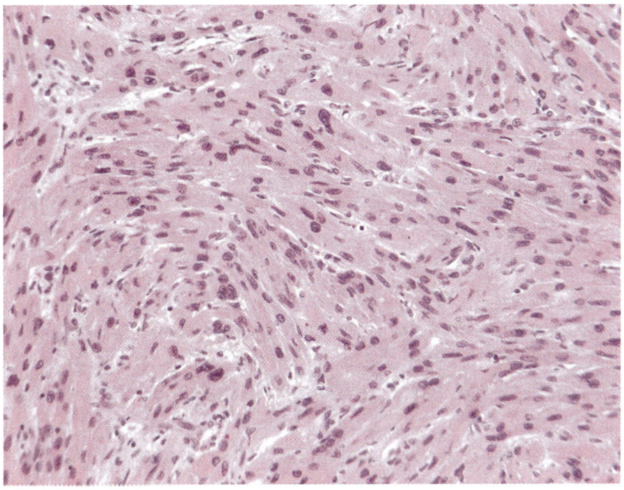

Fig. 18.30. Spindle cell oncocytoma marked by generally spindled cells with oncocytic cytoplasm (hematoxylin and eosin, original magnification 200×).

features of these tumors. Behaviorally, these are slow growing, low grade lesions (WHO grade I). Tumors which are subtotally resected may recur.

Spindled Cell Oncocytoma

This lesion is a new addition to the World Health Organization Classification of Tumors of the Central Nervous System and comprises less than 1% of all of sellar neoplasms.[125,126] Most of the tumors that have been reported thus far have occurred in adults. Clinical presentation and imaging studies are similar to nonsecreting pituitary adenomas.

Microscopically, the tumor is marked by a mixture of spindled and epithelioid cells with eosinophilic and oncocytic cytoplasm (Figure 18.30). Focal nuclear pleomorphism may be evident. Mitotic activity is generally low. Ultrastructurally, these tumors are marked by cytoplasm filled with mitochondria. In contrast to adenomas, these lesions lack cytoplasmic secretory granules. By immunohistochemistry, these tumors usually demonstrate immunoreactivity with antibodies to vimentin, S-100 protein, and EMA. Antibodies to pituitary hormones, GFAP, cytokeratins, synaptophysin, chromogranin, CD34, and muscle-related antibodies such as smooth muscle actin and desmin are negative. Cell proliferation indices are generally low. Most tumors behave in an apparently benign fashion, although tumor recurrence with an increased MIB-1 labeling index and necrosis has been documented.[125]

Metastatic Tumors

The incidence of metastases is variable in the literature, ranging as high as 25% in some autopsy series. In surgical pathology practice, however, a metastatic lesion to the pituitary gland is seldom the target of a surgical procedure. The clinical presentation may be asymptomatic or if the neurohypophysis is involved, diabetes insipidus may develop. There is no obvious gender predilection. Lung and gastric cancers are among the more frequent tumors to metastasize to the pituitary.[127-131] In addition, metastases from breast carcinoma in women and prostate carcinoma in men are also relatively common. Lymphomatous and leukemic involvement of the gland are relatively common in patients who have systemic disease.

Imaging studies are nonspecific. Destruction of adjacent bone, cavernous sinus invasion, development of cranial neuropathies, infundibular stalk invasion, and evidence of metastases elsewhere in the brain are possible clues on imaging that a lesion may be metastatic. Rare reports of metastasis to pituitary adenomas have been documented[132,133] (Figure 18.31). Microscopically, the morphology of the lesion is consistent with the tumor of origin. Similarly, the immunohistochemical profile is also consistent with the derivation of the lesion. Currently, there is no role for genetic testing in the evaluation of metastatic lesions to the central nervous system. Occasionally in patients with known breast carcinoma, evaluation of the metastasis for estrogen and progesterone receptors and Her2neu status may be warranted for therapeutic management.

Patients with metastatic disease to the pituitary gland usually have poor survival, and the tumor is often widespread at the time of diagnosis.

Miscellaneous Neoplasms

There are a variety of other tumors that rarely can be encountered in the pituitary gland and sellar regions. Germ cell tumors arising as primary neoplasms in the sellar region have been described[134,135]; the suprasellar region is the second most common site of involvement following the pineal gland. Most of these tumors present in the first two decades of life with a clear male predominance. Germ cell tumors may be associated with hypopituitarism, diabetes insipidus, and visual disturbances. Large lesions may cause symptoms related to hypertension, hydrocephalus, and altered mentation. The most common of these tumors is the germinoma, which on imaging presents as a well-demarcated lesion that has high signal intensity on a CT scan and enhances with contrast (Figure 18.32). Adipose tissue and calcifications which may be part of a teratoma can alter the imaging appearance. All types of germ cell tumors, including germinoma, teratomas, embryonal carcinoma, endodermal sinus tumor, and choriocarcinomas have been described, at one time or another, in this region. The morphologic appearance of these lesions and their immunohistochemical profile

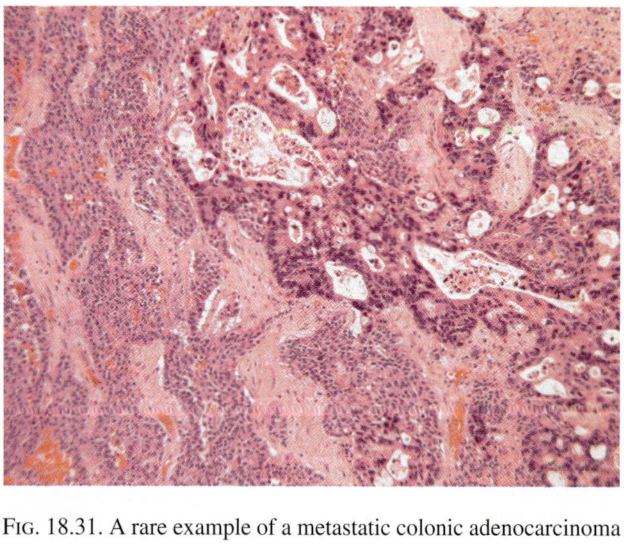

FIG. 18.31. A rare example of a metastatic colonic adenocarcinoma to a nonfunctioning pituitary adenoma (hematoxylin and eosin, original magnification 100×).

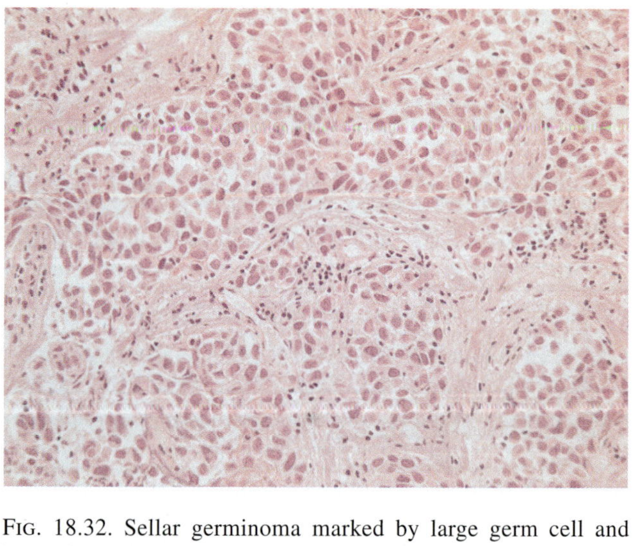

FIG. 18.32. Sellar germinoma marked by large germ cell and intermixed benign lymphocytes (hematoxylin and eosin, original magnification 200×).

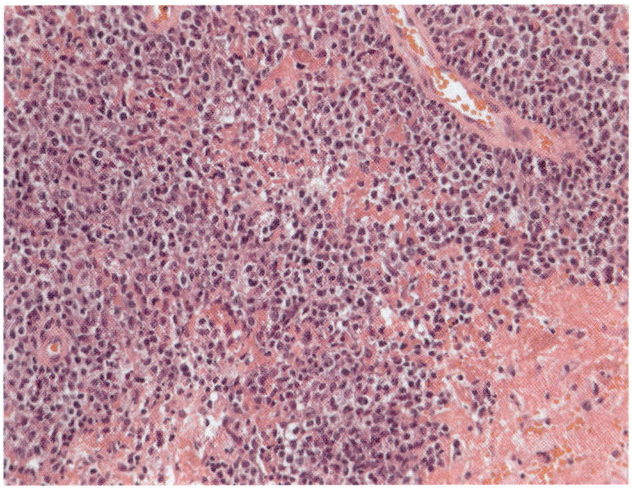

Fig. 18.33. Involvement of the pituitary gland by a diffuse large B cell lymphoma (hematoxylin and eosin, original magnification 200×).

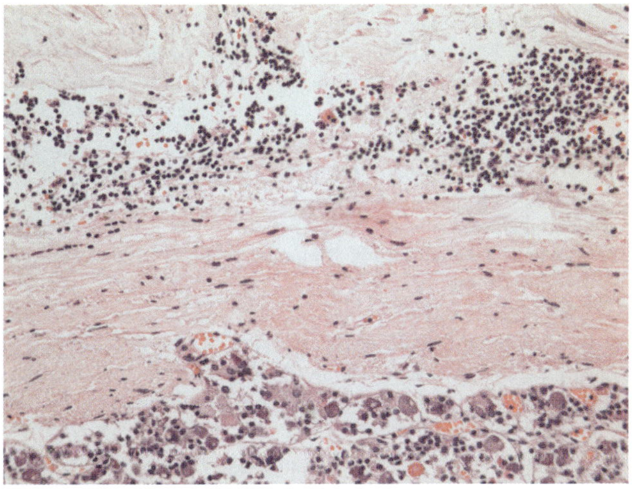

Fig. 18.34. Chronic lymphocytic leukemia (CLL) involving tissue adjacent to the adenohypophysis (hematoxylin and eosin, original magnification 200×).

are well established and can be useful in distinguishing these tumors from each other and from other primary tumors arising in the location. Molecular genetic testing is not routinely employed in the evaluation of these neoplasms in the central nervous system.

Rare cases of lymphoma, leukemia, or plasmacytoma arising as a primary lesion in the sellar area have been reported[136–139] (Figures 18.33 and 18.34). Presenting symptoms are those of a mass lesion or hypopituitarism. The histologic appearance of the lesions are similar to those arising elsewhere in the body. Antibodies typically employed in the evaluation of these disorders can be similarly applied to tumors in this location. Likewise, gene rearrangement studies may also be of utility in selected instances in demonstrating monoclonality.

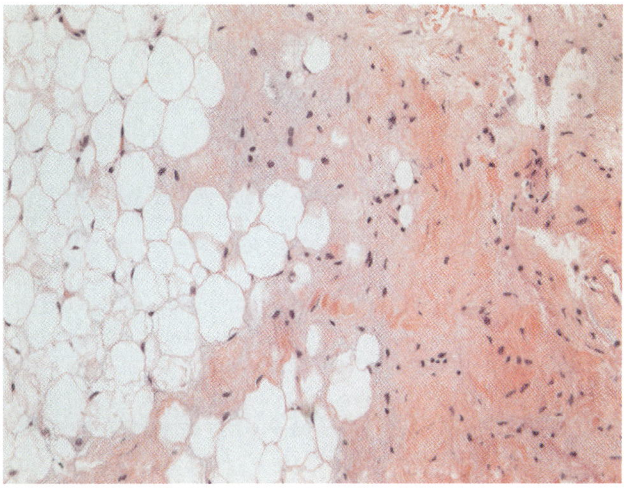

Fig. 18.35. Rare example of a sellar spindle cell lipoma (hematoxylin and eosin, original magnification 200×).

Cases of Langerhans cell histiocytosis or histiocytosis X have been rarely described in this location.[140,141] The symptoms of hypopituitarism and diabetes insipidus are the most common presentations. On imaging studies, CT scans show an ill-defined, contrast enhancing hypodense mass with areas of edema. Lesions may be hypointense and demonstrate slight increased T1 and contrast enhancement and increased T2 signal intensity on MRI studies. Microscopically, these lesions show the typical morphology of Langerhans cells characterized by kidney shaped nuclei with abundant cytoplasm. These cells are usually admixed with acute and chronic inflammatory cells including prominent numbers of eosinophils. CD1a and S-100 immunoreactivity may be helpful to confirm the diagnosis by immunohistochemistry. Ultrastructural examination for Birbeck granules may also be employed to confirm a diagnosis.

There are a variety of vascular and mesenchymal tumors that have been documented to arise in this location. These lesions include cavernous hemangiomas, glomangioma, hemangioblastomas, chondromyxoid chondromas, chondrosarcomas, lipomas, and alveolar soft part sarcomas or sarcomas have been variously described[142–149] (Figure 18.35).

References

1. Missler V, Mack M, Nowack G, et al. Pituitary sarcoidosis. *Klin Wochenschr*. 1990;68:342–345.
2. Gartman JJ Jr, Powers SK, Fortune M. Pseudotumor of the sellar and parasellar areas. *Neurosurgery*. 1989;24:896–901.
3. Thodou E, Asa SL, Kontogeorgos G, Kovacs K, Horvath E, Ezzat S. Clinical case seminar: lymphocytic hypophysitis: clinicopathological findings. *J Clin Endocrinol Metab*. 1995;80:2302–2311.
4. Pastell RG, Best JD, Alford FP. Lymphocytic hypophysitis. The clinical spectrum of the disorder and evidence for an autoimmune pathogenesis. *Clin Endocrinol*. 1990;33:457–466.

5. Beressi N, Beressi J-P, Cohen R, Modigliani E. Lymphocytic hypophysitis. A review of 145 cases. *Ann Med Interne (Paris)*. 1999;150:327–341.
6. Bergeron C, Kovacs K, Bilbao SM. Primary "empty sella". A histologic and immunologic study. *Arch Intern Med*. 1979;139:248–249.
7. Bergland RM, Ray BS, Torack RM. Anatomical variations in the pituitary gland and adjacent structures in 225 human autopsy cases. *J Neurosurg*. 1968;28:93–99.
8. Barrow DL, Spector RH, Takei Y, Tindall GT. Symptomatic Rathke's cleft cysts located entirely in the suprasellar region: review of diagnosis, management and pathogenesis. *Neurosurgery*. 1985;16:766–772.
9. Keyaki A, Hirano A, Llena JF. Asymptomatic and symptomatic Rathke's cleft cysts. Histological study of 45 cases. *Neurol Med Chir (Tokyo)*. 1989;29:88–93.
10. Steinberg GK, Koenig GH, Golden JB. Symptomatic Rathke's cleft cysts. Report of two cases. *J Neurosurg*. 1982;56:290–295.
11. Ikeda H, Yoshimoto T. Clinicopathological study of Rathke's cleft cysts. *Clin Neuropathol*. 2002;21:82–91.
12. Lundardi P, Missori P, Gagliardi FM, Fortuna A. Dermoid cysts of the posterior cranial fossa in children. Report of nine cases and review of the literature. *Surg Neurol*. 1990;34:39–42.
13. Yamakawa K, Shitara N, Genka S, Manaka S, Takakura K. Clinical course and surgical prognosis of 33 cases of intracranial epidermoid tumors. *Neurosurgery*. 1989;24:568–573.
14. Petito CK, DeGirolami U, Earle KM. Craniopharyngiomas: a clinical and pathological review. *Cancer*. 1976;37:1944–1952.
15. Van Effenterre R, Boch AL. Craniopharyngioma in adults and children: a study of 122 surgical cases. *J Neurosurg*. 2002;97: 3–11.
16. Giangaspero F, Burger PC, Osborne DR, Stein RB. Suprasellar papillary squamous epithelioma ("papillary craniopharyngioma"). *Am J Surg Pathol*. 1984;8:57–64.
17. Crotty TB, Scheithauer BW, Young WF Jr, et al. Papillary craniopharyngioma: a clinicopathological study of 48 cases. *J Neurosurg*. 1995;83:206–214.
18. Nishi T, Kuratsu J, Takeshima H, Saito Y, Kochi M, Ushio Y. Prognostic significance of the MIB-1 labeling index for patients with craniopharyngioma. *Int J Mol Med*. 1999;3:157–161.
19. Rickert CH, Paulus W. Lack of chromosomal imbalances in adamantinomatous and papillary craniopharyngiomas. *J Neurol Neurosurg Psych*. 2003;74:260–261.
20. Hofmann BM, Kreutzer J, Saeger W, et al. Nuclear beta-catenin accumulation as reliable marker for the differentiation between cystic craniopharyngiomas and Rathke cleft cells: a clinicopathologic approach. *Am J Surg Pathol*. 2006;30: 1595–1603.
21. Sekine S, Shibata T, Kokubu A, et al. Craniopharyngiomas of adamantinomatous type harbor beta-catenin gene mutations. *Am J Pathol*. 2002;161:1997–2001.
22. Ezzat S, Asa SL, Stefaneanu L, et al. Somatotroph hyperplasia without pituitary adenoma associated with a long standing growth hormone-releasing hormone-producing bronchial carcinoid. *J Clin Endocrinol Metab*. 1994;78:555–560.
23. Al-Gahtany M, Horvath E, Kovacs K. Pituitary hyperplasia. *Hormones (Athens)*. 2003;2:149–158.
24. Horvath E, Kovacs K, Scheithauer BW. Pituitary hyperplasia. *Pituitary*. 1999;1:169–179.
25. Scheithauer BW, Horvath E, Randall RV, Kovacs K. Pituitary hyperplasia. *Pathol Res Pract*. 1998;3:281–289.
26. Kleinschmidt-DeMasters BK. Subtyping does matter in pituitary adenomas. *Acta Neuropathol*. 2006;111:84–85.
27. Asa SL, Ezzat S. Molecular basis of pituitary development and cytogenesis. *Front Horm Res*. 2004;32:1–19.
28. Lamolet B, Pulichino AM, Lamonerie T, et al. A pituitary cell-restricted T box factor, Tpit, activates POMC transcription in cooperation with Pitx homeoproteins. *Cell*. 2001;104: 849–859.
29. Lamonerie T, Tremblay JJ, Lanctot C, Therrien M, Gauthier Y, Drouin J. Ptx1, a bicoid-related homeo box transcription factor involved in transcription of the pro-opiomelanocortin gene. *Genes Dev*. 1996;10:1284–1295.
30. Poulin G, Turgeon B, Drouin J. NeuroD1/beta2 contributes to cell-specific transcription of the proopiomelanocortin gene. *Mol Cell Biol*. 1997;17:6673–6682.
31. Mangalam HJ, Albert VR, Ingraham HA, et al. A pituitary POU domain protein, Pit-1, activates both growth hormone and prolactin promoters transcriptionally. *Genes Dev*. 1989;3: 946–958.
32. Simmons DM, Voss JW, Ingraham HA, et al. Pituitary cell phenotypes involve cell-specific Pit-1 mRNA translation and synergistic interactions with other classes of transcription factors. *Genes Dev*. 1990;4:695–711.
33. Day RN, Koike S, Sakai M, Muramatsu M, Maurer RA. Both Pit-1 and the estrogen receptor are required for estrogen responsiveness of the rat prolactin gene. *Mol Endocrinol*. 1990;4: 1964–1971.
34. Scully KM, Rosenfeld MG. Pituitary development: regulatory codes in mammalian organogenesis. *Science*. 2002;295: 2231–2235.
35. Frawley LS, Boockfor FR. Mammosomatotropes: presence and functions in normal and neoplastic pituitary tissue. *Endocr Rev*. 1991;12:337–355.
36. Asa SL, Bamberger AM, Cao B, Wong M, Parker KL, Ezzat S. The transcription activator steroidogenic factor-1 is preferentially expressed in the human pituitary gonadotroph. *J Clin Endocrinol Metab*. 1996;81:2165–2170.
37. Lloyd R. Tumors of the pituitary gland. In: DeLellis RA, Lloyd R, Heitz PU, eds. *World Health Organization Classification of Tumours. Pathology and Genetics. Tumors of Endocrine Organs*. Lyons: IARC; 2004:9–48.
38. Laws ER Jr, Lopes MB. The new WHO classification of pituitary tumors: highlights and areas of controversy. *Acta Neuropathol*. 2006;111:80–81.
39. Snyder PJ. Clinically nonfunctioning pituitary adenomas. *Endocrinol Metab Clin North Am*. 1993;22:163–175.
40. Serri O, Chik CL, Ur E, Ezzat S. Diagnosis and management of hyperprolactinemia. *CMAJ*. 2003;169:575–581.
41. Horvath E, Kovacs K. Pathology of prolactin cell adenomas of the human pituitary. *Semin Diagn Pathol*. 1986;3:4–17.
42. Kovacs K, Stefaneanu L, Horvath E, et al. Effect of dopamine agonist medication on prolactin producing pituitary adenomas. A morphological study including immunocytochemistry, electron microscopy and in situ hybridization. *Virchows Arch A Pathol Anat Histopathol*. 1991;418:439–446.
43. Asa SL. *Tumors of the Pituitary Gland*. Washington, DC: Armed Forces Institute of Pathology; 1998.
44. Rocken C, Uhlig H, Saeger W, Linke RP, Fehr S. Amyloid deposits in pituitaries and pituitary adenomas: immunohistochemistry and in situ hybridization. *Endocr Pathol*. 1995;6: 135–143.

45. Thorner MO. The anterior pituitary. In: Wilson JD, Foster DW, Kronenberg HM, eds. *Williams Textbook of Endocrinology*. Philadelphia: WB Saunders; 1998:249–340.
46. Kovacs K, Scheithauer BW, Horvath E, Lloyd RV. The World Health Organization classification of adenohypophysial neoplasms. A proposed five-tier scheme. *Cancer*. 1996;78: 502–510.
47. Neumann PE, Goldman JE, Horoupian DS, Hess MA. Fibrous bodies in growth hormone-secreting adenomas contain cytokeratin filaments. *Arch Pathol Lab Med*. 1985;109:505–508.
48. Saeger W, Wilczak W, Ludecke DK, Buchfelder M, Fahlbusch R. Hormone markers in pituitary adenomas: changes within last decade resulting from improved method. *Endocr Pathol*. 2003;14(1):49–54.
49. Tallen G, Fehr S, Saeger W, Uhlig H, Ludecke DK. Detection of growth hormone, prolactin and human beta-chorionic gonadotropin mRNA in growth hormone-secreting pituitary adenomas and in prolactin-secreting pituitary adenomas by in situ hybridization using a non-isotopic detection method. *Acta Endocrinol*. 1993;128:411–417.
50. Al-Brahim NY, Asa SL. My approach to pathology of the pituitary gland. *J Clin Pathol*. 2006;59:1245–1253.
51. Ezzat S, Horvath E, Harris AG, Kovacs K. Morphological effects of octreotide on growth hormone-producing pituitary adenomas. *J Clin Endocrinol Metab*. 1994;79:113–118.
52. Kovacs K, Horvath E. Pathology of growth hormone-producing tumors of the human pituitary. *Semin Diagn Pathol*. 1986;3: 18–33.
53. Yamada S, Aiba T, Sano T, et al. Growth hormone-producing pituitary adenomas: correlations between clinical characteristics and morphology. *Neurosurgery*. 1993;33:20–27.
54. Kemink SA, Wesseling P, Pieters GF, Verhofstad AA, Hermus AR, Smals AG. Progression of a Nelson's adenoma to pituitary carcinoma; a case report and review of the literature. *J Endocrinol Invest*. 1999;22:70–75.
55. Scheithauer BW, Jaap AJ, Horvath E, et al. Clinically silent corticotroph tumors of the pituitary gland. *Neurosurgery*. 2000;47:723-729. discussion 729–730.
56. Stefaneanu L, Kovacs K, Horvath E, Lloyd RV. In situ hybridization study of pro-opiomelanocortin (POMC) gene expression in human pituitary corticotrophs and their adenomas. *Virchows Arch A Pathol Anat Histopathol*. 1991;419: 107–113.
57. Kurosaki M, Saeger W, Ludecke DK. Pituitary tumors in the elderly. *Pathol Res Pract*. 2001;197:493–497.
58. George DH, Scheithauer BW, Kovacs K, et al. Crooke's cell adenoma of the pituitary: an aggressive variant of corticotroph adenoma. *Am J Surg Pathol*. 2003;27:1330–1336.
59. Webb KM, Laurent JJ, Okonkwo DO, Lopes MB, Vance ML, Laws ER Jr. Clinical characteristics of silent corticotrophic adenomas and creation of an internet-accessible database to facilitate their multi-institutional study. *Neurosurgery*. 2003;53:1076-1084. discussion 1084–1075.
60. Mindermann T, Wilson CB. Thyrotropin-producing pituitary adenomas. *J Neurosurg*. 1993;79:521–527.
61. Scheithauer BW, Kovacs KT, Laws ER Jr, Randall RV. Pathology of invasive pituitary tumors with special reference to functional classification. *J Neurosurg*. 1986;65:733–744.
62. Sanno N, Teramoto A, Osamura RY. Long-term surgical outcome in 16 patients with thyrotropin pituitary adenoma. *J Neurosurg*. 2000;93:194–200.
63. Young WF Jr, Scheithauer BW, Kovacs KT, Horvath E, Davis DH, Randall RV. Gonadotroph adenoma of the pituitary gland: a clinicopathologic analysis of 100 cases. *Mayo Clin Proc*. 1996;71:649–656.
64. Lopes B. Tumors of the pituitary gland. In: Fletcher CDM, ed. *Diagnostic Histopathology of Tumors*, vol. 2. Philadelphia: Churchill Livingstone Elsevier; 2007:971–996.
65. Labat-Moleur F, Trouillas J, Seret-Begue D, Kujas M, Delisle MB, Ronin C. Evaluation of 29 monoclonal and polyclonal antibodies used in the diagnosis of pituitary adenomas. A collaborative study from pathologists of the Club Francais de l'Hypophyse. *Pathol Res Pract*. 1991;187:534–538.
66. Asa SL, Kovacs K. Clinically non-functioning human pituitary adenomas. *Can J Neurol Sci*. 1992;19:228–235.
67. Losa M, Mortini P, Barzaghi R, Franzin A, Giovanelli M. Endocrine inactive and gonadotroph adenomas: diagnosis and management. *J Neurooncol*. 2001;51:16–177.
68. Zhuang Z, Ezzat SZ, Vortmeyer AO, et al. Mutations of the MEN1 tumor suppressor gene in pituitary tumors. *Cancer Res*. 1997;57:5446–5451.
69. Boikos SA, Stratakis CA. Pituitary pathology in patients with Carney Complex: growth-hormone producing hyperplasia or tumors and their association with other abnormalities. *Pituitary*. 2006;9:203–209.
70. Daly AF, Jaffrain-Rea ML, Beckers A. Clinical and genetic features of familial pituitary adenomas. *Horm Metab Res*. 2005;37:347–354.
71. Akintoye SO, Chebli C, Booher S, et al. Characterization of gsp-mediated growth hormone excess in the context of McCune-Albright syndrome. *J Clin Endocrinol Metab*. 2002;87: 5104–5112.
72. Karhu A, Aaltonen LA. Susceptibility to pituitary neoplasia related to MEN-1, CDKN1B and AIP mutations: an update. *Hum Mol Genet*. 2007;16:R73–R79.
73. Vierimaa O, Georgitsi M, Lehtonen R, et al. Pituitary adenoma predisposition caused by germline mutations in the AIP gene. *Science*. 2006;312:1228–1230.
74. Daly AF, Jaffrain-Rea ML, Ciccarelli A, et al. Clinical characterization of familial isolated pituitary adenomas. *J Clin Endocrinol Metab*. 2006;91:3316–3323.
75. Burgess JR, Greenaway TM, Shepherd JJ. Expression of the MEN-1 gene in a large kindred with multiple endocrine neoplasia type 1. *J Intern Med*. 1998;243:465–470.
76. Thakker RV. Multiple endocrine neoplasia – syndromes of the twentieth century. *J Clin Endocrinol Metab*. 1998;83:2617–2620.
77. Lopes MB, Scheithauer BW, Schiff D. Pituitary carcinoma: diagnosis and treatment. *Endocrine*. 2005;28:115–121.
78. Lubke D, Saeger W. Carcinomas of the pituitary: definition and review of the literature. *Gen Diagn Pathol*. 1995;141:81–92.
79. Saeger W, Lubke D. Pituitary carcinomas. *Endocr Pathol*. 1996;7:21–35.
80. Gaffey TA, Scheithauer BW, Lloyd RV, et al. Corticotroph carcinoma of the pituitary: a clinicopathological study. Report of four cases. *J Neurosurg*. 2002;96:352–360.
81. Cai WY, Alexander JM, Hedley-Whyte ET, et al. Ras mutations in human prolactinomas and pituitary carcinomas. *J Clin Endocrinol Metab*. 1994;78:89–93.
82. Korbonits M, Chahal HS, Kaltsas G, et al. Expression of phosphorylated p27(Kip1) protein and Jun activation domain-binding protein 1 in human pituitary tumors. *J Clin Endocrinol Metab*. 2002;87:2635–2643.

83. Musat M, Vax VV, Borboli N, et al. Cell cycle dysregulation in pituitary oncogenesis. *Front Horm Res*. 2004;32:34–62.
84. Rickert CH, Scheithauer BW, Paulus W. Chromosomal aberrations in pituitary carcinoma metastases. *Acta Neuropathol*. 2001;102:117–120.
85. Landman RE, Horwith M, Peterson RE, Khandji AG, Wardlaw SL. Long-term survival with ACTH-secreting carcinoma of the pituitary: a case report and review of the literature. *J Clin Endocrinol Metab*. 2002;87:3084–3089.
86. Thapar K, Kovacs K, Scheithauer BW, et al. Proliferative activity and invasiveness among pituitary adenomas and carcinomas: an analysis using the MIB-1 antibody. *Neurosurgery*. 1996;38:99-106. discussion 106–107.
87. Jaffrain-Rea ML, Di Stefano D, Minniti G, et al. A critical reappraisal of MIB-1 labelling index significance in a large series of pituitary tumours: secreting versus non-secreting adenomas. *Endocr Relat Cancer*. 2002;9:103–113.
88. Hentschel SJ, McCutcheon E, Moore W, Durity FA. P53 and MIB-1 immunohistochemistry as predictors of the clinical behavior of nonfunctioning pituitary adenomas. *Can J Neurol Sci*. 2003;30:215–219.
89. Schreiber S, Saeger W, Ludecke DK. Proliferation markers in different types of clinically non-secreting pituitary adenomas. *Pituitary*. 1999;1:213–220.
90. Mastronardi L, Guiducci A, Spera C, Puzzilli F, Liberati F, Maira G. Ki-67 labelling index and invasiveness among anterior pituitary adenomas: analysis of 103 cases using the MIB-1 monoclonal antibody. *J Clin Pathol*. 1999;52:107–111.
91. Saeger W. Pituitary tumors: prognostic indicators. *Endocrine*. 2005;28:57–66.
92. Pizarro CB, Oliveira MC, Coutinho LB, Ferreira NP. Measurement of Ki-67 antigen in 159 pituitary adenomas using the MIB-1 monoclonal antibody. *Braz J Med Biol Res*. 2004;37:235–243.
93. Oliveira MC, Marroni CP, Pizarro CB, Pereira-Lima JF, Barbosa-Coutinho LM, Ferreira NP. Expression of p53 protein in pituitary adenomas. *Braz J Med Biol Res*. 2002;35:561–565.
94. Vidal S, Kovacs K, Bell D, Horvath E, Scheithauer BW, Lloyd RV. Cyclooxygenase-2 expression in human pituitary tumors. *Cancer*. 2003;97:2814–2821.
95. Riss D, Jin L, Qian X, et al. Differential expression of galectin-3 in pituitary tumors. *Cancer Res*. 2003;63:2251–2255.
96. Spada A. Growth factors and human pituitary adenomas. *Eur J Endocrinol*. 1998;138:255–257.
97. Ito M, Enomoto H, Usa T, et al. Expression of parathyroid hormone related peptide in human pituitary tumours. *J Clin Pathol*. 1993;46:682–683.
98. Clayton RN, Farrell WE. Clonality of pituitary tumours: more complicated than initially envisaged? *Brain Pathol*. 2001;11: 313–327.
99. Bystrom C, Larsson C, Blomberg C, et al. Localization of the MEN1 gene to a small region within chromosome 11q13 by deletion mapping in tumors. *Proc Natl Acad Sci USA*. 1990;87:1968–1972.
100. Bale AE, Norton JA, Wong EL, et al. Allelic loss on chromosome 11 in hereditary and sporadic tumors related to familial multiple endocrine neoplasia type 1. *Cancer Res*. 1991;51: 1154–1157.
101. Wrocklage C, Gold H, Hackl W, Buchfelder M, Fahlbusch R, Paulus W. Increased menin expression in sporadic pituitary adenomas. *Clin Endocrinol*. 2002;56:589–594.
102. Vallar L, Spada A, Giannattasio G. Altered Gs and adenylate cyclase activity in human GH-secreting pituitary adenomas. *Nature*. 1987;330:566–568.
103. Clementi E, Malgaretti N, Meldolesi J, Taramelli R. A new constitutively activating mutation of the Gs protein alpha subunit-gsp oncogene is found in human pituitary tumours. *Oncogene*. 1990;5:1059–1061.
104. Lania A, Mantovani G, Spada A. Genetics of pituitary tumors: focus on G-protein mutations. *Exp Biol Med*. 2003;228: 1004–1017.
105. Boggild MD, Jenkinson S, Pistorello M, et al. Molecular genetic studies of sporadic pituitary tumors. *J Clin Endocrinol Metab*. 1994;78:387–392.
106. Weinstein LS, Yu S, Warner DR, Liu J. Endocrine manifestations of stimulatory G protein alpha-subunit mutations and the role of genomic imprinting. *Endocr Rev*. 2001;22:675–705.
107. Pei L, Melmed S. Isolation and characterization of a pituitary tumor-transforming gene (PTTG). *Mol Endocrinol*. 1997;11: 433–441.
108. Zhang X, Horwitz GA, Heaney AP, et al. Pituitary tumor transforming gene (PTTG) expression in pituitary adenomas. *J Clin Endocrinol Metab*. 1999;84:761–767.
109. Heaney AP, Horwitz GA, Wang Z, Singson R, Melmed S. Early involvement of estrogen-induced pituitary tumor transforming gene and fibroblast growth factor expression in prolactinoma pathogenesis. *Nat Med*. 1999;5:1317–1321.
110. Levy A, Hall L, Yeudall WA, Lightman SL. p53 gene mutations in pituitary adenomas: rare events. *Clin Endocrinol*. 1994; 41:809–814.
111. Herman V, Drazin NZ, Gonsky R, Melmed S. Molecular screening of pituitary adenomas for gene mutations and rearrangements. *J Clin Endocrinol Metab*. 1993;77:50–55.
112. Thapar K, Scheithauer BW, Kovacs K, Pernicone PJ, Laws ER Jr. p53 expression in pituitary adenomas and carcinomas: correlation with invasiveness and tumor growth fractions. *Neurosurgery*. 1996;38:765-770. discussion 770–761.
113. Jordan S, Lidhar K, Korbonits M, Lowe DG, Grossman AB. Cyclin D and cyclin E expression in normal and adenomatous pituitary. *Eur J Endocrinol*. 2000;143:R1–R6.
114. Turner HE, Nagy Z, Sullivan N, Esiri MM, Wass JA. Expression analysis of cyclins in pituitary adenomas and the normal pituitary gland. *Clin Endocrinol*. 2000;53: 337–344.
115. Cryns VL, Alexander JM, Klibanski A, Arnold A. The retinoblastoma gene in human pituitary tumors. *J Clin Endocrinol Metab*. 1993;77:644–646.
116. Pei L, Melmed S, Scheithauer B, Kovacs K, Benedict WF, Prager D. Frequent loss of heterozygosity at the retinoblastoma susceptibility gene (RB) locus in aggressive pituitary tumors: evidence for a chromosome 13 tumor suppressor gene other than RB. *Cancer Res*. 1995;55:1613–1616.
117. Cohen-Gadol AA, Pichelmann MA, Link MJ, et al. Granular cell tumor of the sellar and suprasellar region: clinicopathologic study of 11 cases and literature review. *Mayo Clinic Proc*. 2003;78:567–573.
118. Luse SA, Kernohan JW. Granular cell tumors of the stalk and posterior lobe of the pituitary gland. *Cancer*. 1955;8: 616–622.
119. Vogelgesang S, Junge MH, Pahnke J, Gaab MR, Warzok RW. Sellar/suprasellar mass in a 59-year-old woman. *Brain Pathol*. 2002;12:136–139.

120. Nishioka H, Ii K, Llena JF, Hirano A. Immunohistochemical study of granular cell tumors of the neurophypophysis. *Virchow Arch.* 1991;60:413–417.
121. Rickert CH, Paulus W. Genetic characterization of granular cell tumours. *Acta Neuropathol.* 2002;103:309–312.
122. Figarella-Branger D, Dufour H, Fernandez C, Boyvier-Labbit C, Grisoli F, Pellissier JF. Pituicytoma, a mis-diagnosed benign tumor of the neurohypophysis: report of three cases. *Acta Neuropathol.* 2002;104:313–319.
123. Brat DJ, Scheithauer BW, Staugaitis SM, Cortez SC, Brecher K, Burger PC. Pituicytoma: a distinctive low-grade gloma of the neurohypophysis. *Am J Surg Pathol.* 2000;24:362-368.
124. Kowalski RJ, Prayson RA, Mayberg MR. Pituicytoma. *Ann Diagn Pathol.* 2004;8:290–294.
125. Kloub O, Perry A, Tu PH, Lipper M, Lopes MB. Spindle cell oncocytoma of the adenohypophysis: report of two recurrent cases. *Am J Surg Pathol.* 2005;29:247–253.
126. Roncaroli F, Scheithauer BW, Cenacchi G, et al. Spindle cell oncocytoma of the adenohypophysis: a tumor of folliculostellate cells. *Am J Surg Pathol.* 2002;26:1048–1055.
127. Aaberg TM Jr, Kay M, Sternau L. Metastatic tumor to the pituitary. *Am J Ophtalmol.* 1995;119:779–785.
128. Heshmati HM, Scheithauer BW, Young WF Jr. Metastases to the pituitary gland. *Endocrinologist.* 2002;12:45–49.
129. Max MB, Deck MD, Rottenberg DA. Pituitary metastasis: incidence in cancer patients and clinical differentiation from pituitary adenoma. *Neurology.* 1981;31:998–1002.
130. Teears RJ, Silverman EM. Clinicopathologic review of 88 cases of carcinoma metastatic to the pituitary gland. *Cancer.* 1975;36:216–220.
131. Kattah JC, Silgals RM, Manz H, Toro JG, Dritschilo A, Smith FP. Presentation and management of parasellar and suprasellar metastatic mass lesions. *J Neurol Neurosurg Psych.* 1985;48:44–49.
132. Molinatti PA, Scheithauer BW, Randall RV, Laws ER Jr. Metastases to pituitary adenoma. *Arch Pathol Lab Med.* 1985;109:287–289.
133. Noga C, Prayson RA, Kowalski R, Sweeney PJ, Mayberg M. Metastatic adenocarcinoma to a pituitary adenoma: a case report and review of the literature. *Ann Diagn Pathol.* 2001;5: 354–360.
134. Jennings MT, Gelman R, Hochberg F. Intracranial germ-cell tumors: natural history and pathogenesis. *J Neurosurg.* 1985;63: 155–167.
135. Poon W, Ng HK, Wong K, South JR. Primary intrasellar germinoma presenting with cavernous sinus syndrome. *Surg Neurol.* 1988;30:402–405.
136. Nemoto K, Ohnishi Y, Tsukada T. Chronic lymphocytic leukemia showing pituitary tumor with massive leukemic cell infiltration, and special reference to clinicopathological findings of CLL. *Acta Pathol Jpn.* 1978;28:797–805.
137. Samaratunga H, Perry-Keene D, Apel RL. Primary lymphoma of pituitary gland: a neoplasm of acquired MALT? *Endocr Pathol.* 1997;8:335–341.
138. Sanchez JA, Rahman S, Strauss RA, Kaye GI. Multiple myeloma masquerading as a pituitary tumor. *Arch Pathol Lab Med.* 1977;101:55–56.
139. Nishio S, Mizuno J, Barrow DL, Takei Y, Tindall GT. Isolated histiocytosis X of the pituitary gland: case report. *Neurosurgery.* 1987;21:718–721.
140. Ober KP, Alexander E Jr, Challa VR, Ferree C, Elster A. Histiocytosis X of the hypothalamus. *Neurosurgery.* 1989; 24:93–95.
141. Vaquero J, Areitio E, Martinez R. Intracranial parasellar plasmacytoma. *Arch Neurol.* 1982;39:738.
142. Angiari P, Torcia E, Botticelli RA, Villani M, Merli GA, Crisi G. Ossifying parasellar chondroma. Case report. *J Neurosurg Sci.* 1987;31:59–63.
143. Asa SL, Kovacs K, Horvath E, Ezrin C, Weiss MH. Sellar glomangioma. *Ultrastruct Pathol.* 1984;7:49–54.
144. Bots GT, Tijssen CC, Wijnalda D, Teepen JL. Alveolar soft part sarcoma of the pituitary gland with secondary involvement of the right cerebral ventricle. *Br J Neurosurg.* 1988;2:101–107.
145. Chang WH, Khosla VK, Radotra BD, Kak VK. Large cavernous hemangioma of the pituitary fossa: a case report. *Br J Neurosurg.* 1991;5:627–629.
146. Dan NG, Smith DE. Pituitary hemangioblastoma in a patient with von Hippel-Lindau disease. *J Neurosurg.* 1975;42:232–235.
147. Miki K, Kawamoto K, Kawamura Y, Matsumura H, Asada Y, Hamada A. A rare case of Maffucci's syndrome combined with tuberculum sella enchondroma, pituitary adenoma and thyroid adenoma. *Acta Neurochir.* 1987;87:79–85.
148. Sansone ME, Liwnicz BH, Mandybur TI. Giant pituitary cavernous hemangioma: case report. *J Neurosurg.* 1980;53:124-126.
149. Viswanathan R, Jegathraman AR, Ganapathy K, Bharati AS, Govindan R. Parasellar chondromyxofibroma with ipsilateral total internal carotid artery occlusion. *Surg Neurol.* 1987;28:141–144.

Section 5
Adrenal Diseases

19 Clinical Detection and Treatment of Adrenal Disease

Adrian M. Harvey, Allan A. Siperstein, and Eren Berber

Introduction

Diagnosis and treatment of patients with adrenal lesions is both challenging and fascinating owing to the wide range of biologically important compounds produced by these small glands. Tumors of the adrenal cortex may produce mineralocorticoids, glucocorticoids, sex steroids or in specific cases, combinations of these. Tumors of the adrenal medulla may produce catecholamines and other related compounds making them particularly challenging to diagnose and treat. Malignant disease of the adrenal glands may also be hormonally active.

In this chapter, we review the work-up and treatment of benign, functional masses and malignant diseases of the adrenal cortex and medulla. The appropriate application and interpretation of biochemical and imaging tests in the setting adrenal disease are explored. The role of laparoscopic and open surgery and the outcomes in benign and malignant disease are also presented. In addition, medical therapies and their role in the preoperative and postoperative setting or as primary treatment of adrenal disease are touched on.

Hypercortisolism: Work-Up

The clinical manifestations of Cushings Syndrome (CS) include centripetal obesity, rounded face, abdominal striae, and muscle weakness.[1] More recently however, the term Sub-Clinical Cushing's (SCC) has been used to describe patients with adrenal incidentalomas, autonomous cortisol production but more subtle clinical and laboratory abnormalities including hypertension, impaired glucose tolerance, osteoporosis, depression and renal stones.[2] If these patients are followed, approximately 12.5% will develop overt CS by 1 year.[3]

The differential diagnosis of endogenous CS can be divided into ACTH dependent and independent causes. Overall, 80% of the patients will have an ACTH dependent etiology.[1] Most of these will have a pituitary adenoma, (80%), producing ACTH with the remainder having an ectopic source.[1] Tumors associated with ectopic ACTH production include small cell lung cancer, thymic and bronchial carcinoids, medullary thyroid cancer, pheochromocytoma, and pancreatic islet cell tumors.[4] Those patients with ACTH independent CS have a primary adrenal source of cortisol production, with the two most common being unilateral adenoma, (60%) and adrenal cortical carcinoma, (40%).[4] Rare causes include bilateral macronodular hyperplasia, primary pigmented nodular adrenal disease, and McCune–Albright Syndrome.

The incidence of endogenous CS is 1–2 per million per year.[5] Patients with overt signs and symptoms of CS and those with adrenal incidentalomas should undergo screening tests. In addition, screening should be strongly considered in patients with osteoporosis, and poorly controlled diabetes as these populations are known to have a disproportionately high prevalence of this syndrome.

Commonly utilized screening methods include 24-h urinary free cortisol and dexamethasone suppression tests. Urinary measurements over four times the upper limit of normal are almost always indicative of CS.[6] Pseudo-Cushing's states such as depression, alcoholism, and chronic illness may produce lesser elevations. Other potential methods for the diagnosis of CS include an unsuppressed AM cortisol and late-night/midnight salivary. Salivary cortisol has received increasing attention because of its noninvasive nature and ease of repeating the test. Reference values are laboratory dependent, but the test has demonstrated sensitivity and specificity in excess of 90%.[1,7] This test can be repeated up to three times when the index of suspicion is high as intermittent over-production may be missed.[6]

Low dose dexamethasone suppression tests work on the principle that the hypothalamic–pituitary–adrenal (HPA) regulation is dysfunctional in patients with CS. Following administration of 1 mg of dexamethasone at 23:00, morning values less than 50 nmol/L, are considered normal.[6] A 2-day, 2 mg form of the low dose suppression test is also used for screening purposes in some centers. Once the diagnosis has been made, measurement of serum

J.L. Hunt (ed.), *Molecular Pathology of Endocrine Diseases*, Molecular Pathology Library 3,
DOI 10.1007/978-1-4419-1707-2_19, © Springer Science+Business Media, LLC 2010

ACTH with an assay capable of detecting concentrations below 2 pmol/L is the appropriate next step. Values below 1.1 pmol/L are indicative of ACTH independent CS, whereas values above 3.3 pmol/L suggest corticotrophin dependent disease.[1] Equivocal values may be repeated or a corticotrophin releasing hormone, (CRH) stimulation test may be utilized.[6]

In the majority of patients with ACTH independent CS, CT scan will demonstrate the abnormality, most commonly a unilateral adenoma or carcinoma.[8] Gadolinium enhanced, pituitary MRI should be performed in patients with ACTH dependent CS. The presence of a 6 mm or greater lesion on MRI with proven ACTH dependent CS is generally considered diagnostic. However, up to 40% of patients with Cushing's disease will have a normal appearing MRI.[9] High dose dexamethasone suppression and CRH stimulation tests are used in some centers. Patients with pituitary CS will not demonstrate suppression with the low dose test but will suppress with high dose dexamethasone. In contrast, patients with an ectopic or adrenal source of excess cortisol production will not suppress with either a high or low dose test. When MRI and biochemical testing are equivocal, bilateral inferior petrosal sinus sampling may be performed to determine the source of ACTH production. Excellent sensitivity and specificity have been demonstrated, but the procedure is technically demanding.[10] In cases of suspected ectopic ACTH production, CT and/or MRI of the neck, thorax, and abdomen should be performed.[4]

Hypercortisolism: Treatment

In patients with adrenal adenomas, laparoscopic adrenalectomy has become the "gold-standard" treatment.[11,12] A recent review identified 12 series of laparoscopic adrenalectomy's for CS.[13] Overall, conversion to open was required in 8.6%, complications occurred in 15% and length of postoperative stay was 3.9 days.[13] In this review, 10 of the 12 series reported a 100% rate of biochemical cure. Postoperatively, patients require glucocorticoid replacement until recovery of the Hypothalamic Pituitary Adrenal axis can occur which may take up to 18 months.[12]

Bilateral causes of ACTH independent CS may be treated medically or with bilateral adrenalectomy. Ketoconazole, metyrapone, and aminoglutethimide inhibit various steps of steroid synthesis through their action on cytochrome p450 enzymes.[14] Side effect may limit use and effectiveness may decrease with time. Mitotane, an adrenolytic drug inhibits steroid synthesis by causing selective destruction of the zona reticularis and fasciculate of the cortex. Unfortunately, a high percentage of patients have severe side effects limiting its use.[14]

Trans-sphenoidal pituitary microsurgery is the appropriate first line treatment for patients with Cushing's disease. Most patients develop transient hypopituitarism requiring short-term glucocorticoid and L-thyroxine replacement. Failed surgical therapy may be managed with re-operation or pituitary irradiation, but success rates are only around 50%. Medical therapy or bilateral adrenalectomies are also options following failed surgery. While relief from irradiation may take up to 12 months, bilateral adrenalectomy yields immediate results. Expansion of the pituitary neoplasm (Nelson's Syndrome) following bilateral adrenalectomy is seen in up to 30% of patients by 10 years.[15]

Hyperaldosteronism: Work-Up

Conn's syndrome is a constellation of hypertension and hypokalemia associated with elevated plasma aldosterone and suppressed plasma renin activity.[16] Recently, more widespread use of screening, with the plasma aldosterone concentration (PAC) to plasma renin activity (PRA) ratio has resulted in increased prevalence estimates from 0.5%[17,18] to 5–13% of patients with hypertension.[19,20] Common causes of primary hyperaldosteronism include aldosterone producing adenoma (APA) and idiopathic hyperaldosteronism from bilateral adrenal hyperplasia (IAH).[21] Less common causes include unilateral hyperplasia and familial forms.

Hypertensive patients with hypokalemia, medication resistant hypertension, a family history of hypertension and/or early stroke and those with incidentalomas should undergo initial screening with a serum PAC/PRA ratio.[22] Plasma aldosterone concentration >15 ng/dL and a ratio >20 ng/dL per ng/mL/h are generally considered positive.[21] A positive screening test is usually followed by confirmation with saline loading, captopril or fludrocortisone suppression testing.[23]

This search for a specific cause should begin with imaging. CT and MRI have similar diagnostic performance in the detection of APA's.[24] A unilateral macroadenoma (>1 cm) with a normal contralateral gland in a young (<40 years) patient may be enough to make the diagnosis of an APA and proceed to surgery.[25] In patients with bilateral adrenal nodules, adrenal venous sampling is required to localize the pathology to one side.[25-27] The major drawback of adrenal venous sampling lies in its technical difficulty. Radio cholesterol scintigraphy provides functional imaging of the adrenals and has been used at some centers.

Hyperaldosteronism: Treatment

Adrenalectomy is an appropriate treatment for unilateral adrenal adenoma. In properly selected patients, normalization of BP without medications can be expected in ~33%[28,29] with 80–90% experiencing improved BP control.[26,28,29] Factors associated with postop normalization of BP include young age, short duration of disease, and single agent therapy.[28] Bilateral hyperplasia should be treated medically with spironolactone as the primary agent.

Pheochromocytoma: Work-Up

Overall, the incidence of pheochromocytoma is 2 per million[30] and less than 0.2% in patients with hypertension.[31] The classical symptomatic triad is headache, cardiac palpitations, and diaphoresis. However, most patients do not present in the classical manner. Hypertension may be sustained, not episodic and some patients may present with an incidentaloma.[32] The classical "rule of tens," has been challenged in recently published literature.[33,34] In particular up to 25% may be extra-adrenal in location,[34] 15–35% of these extra-adrenal tumors are malignant,[33] and careful screening may reveal a germline mutation in up to 25%.[35] Hereditary pheochromocytoma is associated with Multiple Endocrine Neoplasia (MEN) 2A and 2B, von Hipple Lindau (VHL), neurofibromatosis (NF) 1, and paraganglioma syndromes (PGL) 1 and 4. Familial paragamglioma syndromes are related to mutations in various subunits of the succinate dehydrogenase gene. Screening should be performed in all patients with multifocal, extra-adrenal or malignant tumors and all those diagnosed under the age of 50.[33]

Biochemical testing is indicated in patients with the classical presentation, patients with adrenal incidentaloma, and those with resistant or early-onset hypertension.[36] Screening relies on the detection of excess catecholamines and/or their metabolites in plasma or urine.[37] Twenty-four hour urinary catecholamines and metanephrines have a sensitivity of 88–90% and a specificity of 99%.[38] While once a commonly ordered test, an isolated elevation of vanillyl mandelic acid lacks the sensitivity to serve as a screening test for these tumors.[39] Plasma free metanephrines have a high sensitivity but a specificity of only 85%.[40] Values below a threshold may be used to rule out pheochromocytoma, values more than four times above the upper limit of normal are nearly 100% specific and those values in the "gray area" require further testing (Figure 19.1).

Following biochemical diagnosis, imaging studies are appropriate. Both CT and MRI tests have high sensitivity, (90–95%) but limited specificity.[41] The use functional imaging with ^{123}I labeled metaiodobenzylguanidine (MIBG) scinitgraphy is somewhat controversial. In a recent review of patients with a unilateral lesion on CT or MRI and no family history or features suspicious of malignancy, MIBG scanning did not reveal any additional disease.[42]

Pheochromocytoma: Treatment

Preoperative treatment with alpha blockade is the standard care for these patients. Common agents include phenoxybenzamine and doxazosin. As prolonged vasoconstriction results in intravascular volume depletion, liberal use of fluids is also recommended. Control of hypertension, with some degree of orthostatic hypotension following volume replacement is the goal of preoperative alpha blockade. At our center, we are prepping outpatients with escalating doses of phenoxybenzamine for at least 3 weeks. In patients resistant to phenoxybenzamine, tyrosine hydroxylase inhibitors can be used. Calcium channel blockers have been advocated with patients in a few centers.[43] In one series, appropriate preoperative medication was credited for a reduction in mortality from 18 to 2%.[44] Beta blockade may be used in patients with adequate alpha blockade and tachycardia but should never be used alone as they may precipitate a hypertensive crisis.

Surgery is the mainstay of treatment for pheochromocytoma with laparoscopic surgery being the treatment of choice.

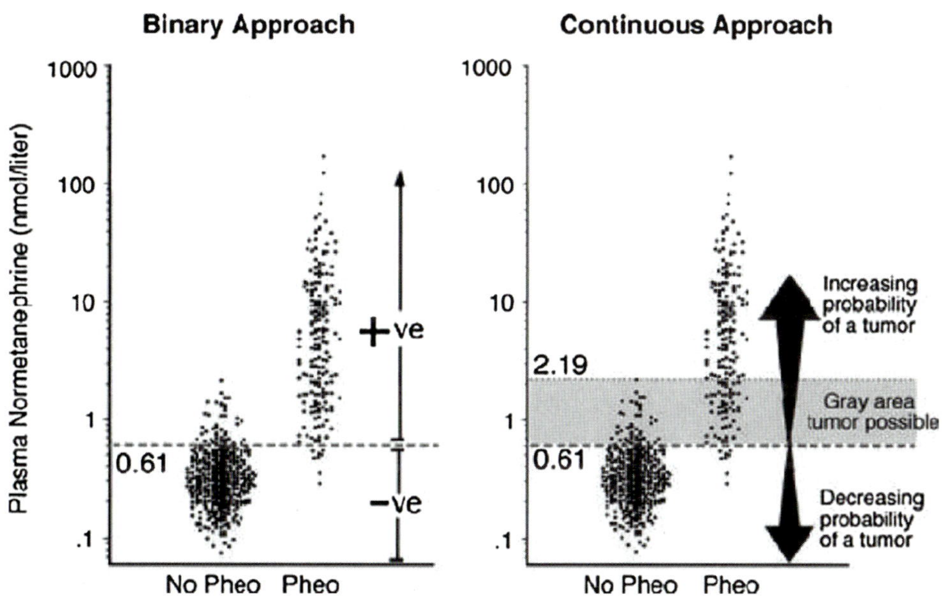

FIG. 19.1. Binary vs. continuous interpretation of plasma metanephrines for pheochromocytoma.

Sill, these patients need to be carefully managed as mortality of 2.4% and morbidity of 24% have been seen in several series.[44–46] Despite initial concerns, laparoscopic adrenalectomy has proven to be a safe approach for these patients.[45,47] Indications for open surgery include peri-adrenal fibrosis, evidence of local invasion, and recurrence.[31] Several series have documented comparable safety of laparoscopic adrenalectomy in large, (>6 cm) and small (<6 cm) tumors, and better intraoperative blood pressure control versus open surgery.[46,47]

In the immediate postoperative period, patients remain at risk for hypotension and hypoglycemia.[48] We follow patients closely with plasma metanephrines every 3 months and abdominal CT scans every 6 months for recurrence.[38,49] Histological features can not rule of malignancy and recurrence can occur even after normal initial biochemical testing, so long term follow-up is important.[38,49] In fact recurrences, both benign and malignant have been reported as long as 17 years following "successful" surgery.[50]

Malignant

Adrenocortical Carcinoma: Work-Up

Primary malignancy of the adrenal gland is a rare occurrence. Adrenocortical carcinoma (ACC) has an incidence of 1:1.7 million and accounts for just 0.02% of all malignancies.[51] Unfortunately, more than 20% have distant metastases at the time of diagnosis, and 20–30% have loco-regional disease.[52] In a series of 253 patients with ACC, overall 5-year actuarial survival was 38%, and 50% after surgery with curative intent.[52] Patients may present with a hypersecretion syndrome and/or a mass. Clinical evidence of hypersecretion, most commonly resulting in CS is seen in 60–70% of patients with ACC.[52,53] Other hormones including sex steroids and occasionally aldosterone may also be secreted. This tumor may present as a non-secretory mass as well. Finally, ACC may also be discovered on imaging done for an unrelated reason. A systematic review of more than 2,000 "incidentalomas" revealed that 4.7% were ACC's.[36]

Absolute criteria for malignancy are limited to metastases and local invasion. Risk of potential malignancy has also been linked to tumor size.[36,54] Lesions of 4 cm in size are associated with a 10% probability of malignancy, and at 8 cm the post-test probability is 47%. Many authors recommend removing all lesions above 4 cm as the risk of malignancy is doubled at this point.[54] Unfortunately, ACC in lesions smaller than 3 cm have been reported.[36,55] Other features, including heterogeneous tumors with necrosis, irregular margins, and patterns of contrast washout or signal intensity may be suggestive of malignancy.[36,56] Image guided biopsy has played a limited role in the work up of adrenal lesions because of concerns regarding tumor seeding and limited ability to distinguish adenoma from carcinoma.

Adrenocortical Carcinoma: Treatment

Outcome in most patients is poor with an overall 5-year survival of 40% or less.[52,57] Adrenalectomy provides the only chance for cure. In general, open adrenalectomy via an anterior transperitoneal approach is preferred. Laparoscopic surgery has generally been avoided in ACC because of concerns about rupturing the capsule and incomplete resection. However, some authors have suggested that laparoscopic resection of adrenal malignancy may be feasible if the principles of oncologic resections are respected.[58,59] In a recent series of 253 patients in France, operative mortality was found to be 5.5% and 5-year survival was 38%.[52] Factors affecting survival included stage, curative intent, and age <35 years.[52] Resection of metachronous isolated metastases may be beneficial in select cases. In a recent series, three of 15 patients with resected ACC liver metastases were alive at 5 years.[60] Similarly, complete resection of locoregional recurrence may result in 5-year survival rates of almost 30%.[57]

Adjuvant therapy for ACC has been disappointing. Mitotane is the most effective agent however, in one series a survival advantage was found, only in patients with stage 4 disease.[52] Unfortunately, mitotane is poorly tolerated with toxicity sufficiently severe to discontinue therapy is seen in 30–40% of patients.[61] In general, ACC is considered radiation resistant, but tumor bed radiation following resection may decrease the risk of recurrence.[62]

Metastases to the Adrenal Gland

The adrenal gland is a common site of metastases. A classic series of 1,000 autopsies on patients with known primary cancers revealed adrenal metastases in 27%.[63] Tumors that metastasize to the adrenal gland include non-small cell lung cancer, renal cell carcinoma, colorectal cancer, melanoma and others.[64] Image guided fine needle aspiration biopsy may be useful in confirming the diagnosis of metastatic disease in patients with known carcinoma and an adrenal mass. Resection of both synchronous and metachronous isolated adrenal metastases has been reported with 5-year actuarial survival rates of 25–30%.[65] As well, laparoscopic resection of isolated adrenal metastases appears to be feasible. Some authors have suggested that similar oncological outcomes with reduced morbidity can be achieved using laparoscopic resection.[58,59]

Adrenal Incidentaloma

Discovery of an "incidental" or "clinical inapparent" adrenal lesion has become a more frequent occurrence as the use of radiological modalities such as ultrasound, MRI, and CT has increased. Large autopsy series have found unexpected adrenal nodules in 6% of patients. A recent study from Italy found a 4.2% incidence of benign adrenal lesions on CT scan of patients enrolled in a lung cancer screening study.[66]

The differential diagnosis of these, "incidentalomas" or "adrenalomas" is broad, (Table 19.1). While the majority of these lesions are benign, nonfunctioning adenomas, a smaller but significant proportion are hormonally active and/or potentially lethal tumors. Thus, the work-up of these lesions must seek to answer two questions: (1) is this adrenal lesion hormonally active; and (2) could this lesion be malignant? As always the evaluation of any disease of the adrenal gland begins with a complete history and physical examination.

Approximately 5.4% of patients with adrenal incidentalomas are found to have SCC, making it the most common hormonal abnormality in this population.[36] All patients with incidentalomas should undergo biochemical screening with serum and urine 24-h catecholamines and metanephrines. Serum AM cortisol and 24-h urinary cortisol should be obtained and dexamethasone suppression testing may be required in selected cases. Serum potassium, aldosterone and rennin will complete the work-up.[36] Patients in whom metastatic disease is suspected can undergo FNA only after catecholamine secretion has been ruled out. Imaging phenotype may also help to guide treatment. Malignant tumors are typically larger with irregular margins.[36,67] A size cutoff of 4 cm is approximately 90% sensitive for ACC, however 76% above 4 cm are benign. Adrenal Cortical Carcinoma is usually hyperintense on T2 weighted MRI. As well incidentalomas with density greater than 15 Housfield units on non-contrast CT scan and delayed contrast wash-out are more likely malignant.[36] Overall, all hormonally active tumors should be removed. Currently, in the absence of hormonal secretion, laparoscopic adrenalectomy is recommended for lesions >3–4 cm, as those with other concerning features on imaging.

TABLE 19.1. Differential diagnosis of adrenal incidentalomas.

Benign nonfunctioning mass
Adenoma
Adrenolipoma
Amyloidosis
Cyst
Ganglioneuroma
Granuloma
Hamartoma
Hematoma
Hemangioma
Infection (fungal, tuberculosis, echinococcosis, cryptococcosis, nocardiosis, paragonimiasis)
Leiomyoma
Lipoma
Myelolipoma
Neurofibroma
Pseudocyst
Teratoma
Malignant nonfunctioning mass
Angiosarcoma
Ganglioneuroblastoma
Leiomyosarcoma
Malignant schwannoma
Metastatic carcinoma
Primary malignancy (adrenocortical carcinoma)
Primary malignant melanoma
Hyperfunctioning mass
Congenital adrenal hyperplasia
Masculinizing or feminizing tumor
Nodular hyperplasia
Pheochromocytoma
Subclinical Cushing syndrome
Primary aldosteronism
Primary malignancy
Pseudoadrenal mass
Mistaken vasculature
Liver
Lymph nodes
Pancreatic mass
Renal mass
Spleen
Stomach mass
Technical artifact

Conclusion

Evaluation of patients with adrenal disease begins with a thorough history and physical examination. Advances in imaging technology have resulted in increased detection of clinically in apparent adrenal masses on tests done for unrelated indications. Some of these patients will ultimately prove to have functional or malignant tumors. In all patients with adrenal lesions, efficient and appropriate use of biochemical testing and imaging is important. In the work up of all adrenal masses, the clinician should seek to answer two questions: (1) is this mass functional; and (2) could this lesion be malignant.

References

1. Newell-Price J, Bertagna X, Grossman AB, Nieman LK. Cushing's syndrome. *Lancet*. 2006;367(9522):1605–1617.
2. Charbonnel B, Chatal JF, Ozanne P. Does the corticoadrenal adenoma with "pre-Cushing's syndrome" exist? *J Nucl Med*. 1981;22(12):1059–1061.
3. Barzon L, Fallo F, Sonino N, Boscaro M. Development of overt Cushing's syndrome in patients with adrenal incidentaloma. *Eur J Endocrinol*. 2002;146(1):61–66.
4. Ilias I, Torpy DJ, Pacak K, Mullen N, Wesley RA, Nieman LK. Cushing's syndrome due to ectopic corticotropin secretion: twenty years' experience at the National Institutes of Health. *J Clin Endocrinol Metab*. 2005;90(8):4955–4962.
5. Lindholm J, Juul S, Jorgensen JO, et al. Incidence and late prognosis of Cushing's syndrome: a population-based study. *J Clin Endocrinol Metab*. 2001;86(1):117–123.
6. Arnaldi G, Angeli A, Atkinson AB, et al. Diagnosis and complications of Cushing's syndrome: a consensus statement. *J Clin Endocrinol Metab*. 2003;88(12):5593–5602.
7. Findling JW, Kehoe ME, Raff H. Identification of patients with Cushing's disease with negative pituitary adrenocorticotropin gradients during inferior petrosal sinus sampling: prolactin as an index of pituitary venous effluent. *J Clin Endocrinol Metab*. 2004;89(12):6005–6009.
8. Rockall AG, Babar SA, Sohaib SA, et al. CT and MR imaging of the adrenal glands in ACTH-independent Cushing syndrome. *Radiographics*. 2004;24(2):435–452.

9. Invitti C, Pecori GF, de Martin M, Cavagnini F. Diagnosis and management of Cushing's syndrome: results of an Italian multicentre study. Study Group of the Italian Society of Endocrinology on the Pathophysiology of the Hypothalamic-Pituitary-Adrenal Axis. *J Clin Endocrinol Metab*. 1999;84(2):440–448.
10. Lindsay JR, Nieman LK. Differential diagnosis and imaging in Cushing's syndrome. *Endocrinol Metab Clin North Am*. 2005;34(2):403–421, x.
11. Iacobone M, Mantero F, Basso SM, Lumachi F, Favia G. Results and long-term follow-up after unilateral adrenalectomy for ACTH-independent hypercortisolism in a series of fifty patients. *J Endocrinol Invest*. 2005;28(4):327–332.
12. Mishra AK, Agarwal A, Gupta S, Agarwal G, Verma AK, Mishra SK. Outcome of adrenalectomy for Cushing's syndrome: experience from a tertiary care center. *World J Surg*. 2007;31(7):1425–1432.
13. Gumbs AA, Gagner M. Laparoscopic adrenalectomy. *Best Pract Res Clin Endocrinol Metab*. 2006;20(3):483–499.
14. Sonino N, Boscaro M, Fallo F. Pharmacologic management of Cushing syndrome: new targets for therapy. *Treat Endocrinol*. 2005;4(2):87–94.
15. Sonino N, Zielezny M, Fava GA, Fallo F, Boscaro M. Risk factors and long-term outcome in pituitary-dependent Cushing's disease. *J Clin Endocrinol Metab*. 1996;81(7):2647–2652.
16. Conn JW, Louis LH. Primary aldosteronism: a new clinical entity. *Trans Assoc Am Physicians*. 1955;68:215–231.
17. Lim PO, Dow E, Brennan G, Jung RT, Macdonald TM. High prevalence of primary aldosteronism in the Tayside hypertension clinic population. *J Hum Hypertens*. 2000;14(5):311–315.
18. Rossi GP, Bernini G, Caliumi C, et al. A prospective study of the prevalence of primary aldosteronism in 1, 125 hypertensive patients. *J Am Coll Cardiol*. 2006;48(11):2293–2300.
19. Kaplan NM. Hypokalemia in the hypertensive patient, with observations on the incidence of primary aldosteronism. *Ann Intern Med*. 1967;66(6):1079–1090.
20. Sinclair AM, Isles CG, Brown I, Cameron H, Murray GD, Robertson JW. Secondary hypertension in a blood pressure clinic. *Arch Intern Med*. 1987;147(7):1289–1293.
21. Young WF Jr. Minireview: primary aldosteronism – changing concepts in diagnosis and treatment. *Endocrinology*. 2003; 144(6):2208–2213.
22. Gordon RD, Stowasser M. Primary aldosteronism: the case for screening. *Nat Clin Pract Nephrol*. 2007;3(11):582–583.
23. Mulatero P, Milan A, Fallo F, et al. Comparison of confirmatory tests for the diagnosis of primary aldosteronism. *J Clin Endocrinol Metab*. 2006;91(7):2618–2623.
24. Lingam RK, Sohaib SA, Rockall AG, et al. Diagnostic performance of CT versus MR in detecting aldosterone-producing adenoma in primary hyperaldosteronism (Conn's syndrome). *Eur Radiol*. 2004;14(10):1787–1792.
25. Young WF, Stanson AW, Thompson GB, Grant CS, Farley DR, van Heerden JA. Role for adrenal venous sampling in primary aldosteronism. *Surgery*. 2004;136(6):1227–1235.
26. Harvey A, Kline G, Pasieka JL. Adrenal venous sampling in primary hyperaldosteronism: comparison of radiographic with biochemical success and the clinical decision-making with "less than ideal" testing. *Surgery*. 2006;140(6):847–853.
27. Rossi GP, Sacchetto A, Chiesura-Corona M, et al. Identification of the etiology of primary aldosteronism with adrenal vein sampling in patients with equivocal computed tomography and magnetic resonance findings: results in 104 consecutive cases. *J Clin Endocrinol Metab*. 2001;86(3):1083–1090.
28. Sawka AM, Young WF, Thompson GB, et al. Primary aldosteronism: factors associated with normalization of blood pressure after surgery. *Ann Intern Med*. 2001;135(4):258–261.
29. Sywak M, Pasieka JL. Long-term follow-up and cost benefit of adrenalectomy in patients with primary hyperaldosteronism. *Br J Surg*. 2002;89(12):1587–1593.
30. Sheps SG, Jiang NS, Klee GG. Diagnostic evaluation of pheochromocytoma. *Endocrinol Metab Clin North Am*. 1988; 17(2):397–414.
31. Yeo H, Roman S. Pheochromocytoma and functional paraganglioma. *Curr Opin Oncol*. 2005;17(1):13–18.
32. Kudva YC, Sawka AM, Young WF Jr. Clinical review 164: the laboratory diagnosis of adrenal pheochromocytoma: the Mayo Clinic experience. *J Clin Endocrinol Metab*. 2003;88(10): 4533–4539.
33. Elder EE, Elder G, Larsson C. Pheochromocytoma and functional paraganglioma syndrome: no longer the 10% tumor. *J Surg Oncol*. 2005;89(3):193–201.
34. Madani R, Al Hashmi M, Bliss R, Lennard TW. Ectopic pheochromocytoma: does the rule of tens apply? *World J Surg*. 2007;31(4):849–854.
35. Neumann HP, Bausch B, McWhinney SR, et al. Germ-line mutations in nonsyndromic pheochromocytoma. *N Engl J Med*. 2002;346(19):1459–1466.
36. Young WF, Jr. Management approaches to adrenal incidentalomas. A view from Rochester, Minnesota. *Endocrinol Metab Clin North Am*. 2000;29(1):159–185, x.
37. Sawka AM, Jaeschke R, Singh RJ, Young WF Jr. A comparison of biochemical tests for pheochromocytoma: measurement of fractionated plasma metanephrines compared with the combination of 24-hour urinary metanephrines and catecholamines. *J Clin Endocrinol Metab*. 2003;88(2):553–558.
38. Pacak K, Eisenhofer G, Ahlman H, et al. Pheochromocytoma: recommendations for clinical practice from the First International Symposium. October 2005. *Nat Clin Pract Endocrinol Metab*. 2007;3(2):92–102.
39. Boyle JG, Davidson DF, Perry CG, Connell JM. Comparison of diagnostic accuracy of urinary free metanephrines, vanillyl mandelic Acid, and catecholamines and plasma catecholamines for diagnosis of pheochromocytoma. *J Clin Endocrinol Metab*. 2007;92(12):4602–4608.
40. Lenders JW, Pacak K, Walther MM, et al. Biochemical diagnosis of pheochromocytoma: which test is best? *JAMA*. 2002; 287(11):1427–1434.
41. Grossman A, Pacak K, Sawka A, et al. Biochemical diagnosis and localization of pheochromocytoma: can we reach a consensus? *Ann N Y Acad Sci*. 2006;1073:332–347.
42. Miskulin J, Shulkin BL, Doherty GM, Sisson JC, Burney RE, Gauger PG. Is preoperative iodine 123 meta-iodobenzylguanidine scintigraphy routinely necessary before initial adrenalectomy for pheochromocytoma? *Surgery*. 2003;134(6):918–922.
43. Lebuffe G, Dosseh ED, Tek G, et al. The effect of calcium channel blockers on outcome following the surgical treatment of phaeochromocytomas and paragangliomas. *Anaesthesia*. 2005;60(5):439–444.
44. Modlin IM, Farndon JR, Shepherd A, et al. Phaeochromocytomas in 72 patients: clinical and diagnostic features, treatment and long term results. *Br J Surg*. 1979;66(7):456–465.

45. Poulose BK, Holzman MD, Lao OB, Grogan EL, Goldstein RE. Laparoscopic adrenalectomy: 100 resections with clinical long-term follow-up. *Surg Endosc*. 2005;19(3):379–385.
46. Wilhelm SM, Prinz RA, Barbu AM, Onders RP, Solorzano CC. Analysis of large versus small pheochromocytomas: operative approaches and patient outcomes. *Surgery*. 2006;140(4): 553–559.
47. Dimas S, Roukounakis N, Kafetzis I, et al. Feasibility of laparoscopic adrenalectomy for large pheochromocytomas. *JSLS*. 2007;11(1):30–33.
48. Costello GT, Moorthy SS, Vane DW, Dierdorf SF. Hypoglycemia following bilateral adrenalectomy for pheochromocytoma. *Crit Care Med*. 1988;16(5):562–563.
49. Mannelli M. Management and treatment of pheochromocytomas and paragangliomas. *Ann N Y Acad Sci*. 2006;1073:405–416.
50. Nap RR, Meinardi JR, van den Berg G, Dullaart RP, de Vries J, Wolffenbuttel BH. [Long-term follow-up is indicated after surgery for a phaeochromocytoma]. *Ned Tijdschr Geneeskd*. 2006;150(19):1045–1049.
51. Vaughan ED Jr. Diseases of the adrenal gland. *Med Clin North Am*. 2004;88(2):443–466.
52. Icard P, Goudet P, Charpenay C, et al. Adrenocortical carcinomas: surgical trends and results of a 253-patient series from the French Association of Endocrine Surgeons study group. *World J Surg*. 2001;25(7):891–897.
53. Tauchmanova L, Colao A, Marzano LA, et al. Andrenocortical carcinomas: twelve-year prospective experience. *World J Surg*. 2004;28(9):896–903.
54. Sturgeon C, Shen WT, Clark OH, Duh QY, Kebebew E. Risk assessment in 457 adrenal cortical carcinomas: how much does tumor size predict the likelihood of malignancy? *J Am Coll Surg*. 2006;202(3):423–430.
55. Terzolo M, Ali A, Osella G, Mazza E. Prevalence of adrenal carcinoma among incidentally discovered adrenal masses. A retrospective study from 1989 to 1994. Gruppo Piemontese Incidentalomi Surrenalici. *Arch Surg*. 1997;132(8):914–919.
56. Fajardo R, Montalvo J, Velazquez D, et al. Correlation between radiologic and pathologic dimensions of adrenal masses. *World J Surg*. 2004;28(5):494–497.
57. Meyer A, Niemann U, Behrend M. Experience with the surgical treatment of adrenal cortical carcinoma. *Eur J Surg Oncol*. 2004;30(4):444–449.
58. Duh QY. Laparoscopic adrenalectomy for isolated adrenal metastasis: the right thing to do and the right way to do it. *Ann Surg Oncol*. 2007;14(12):3288–3289.
59. Porpiglia F, Fiori C, Tarabuzzi R, et al. Is laparoscopic adrenalectomy feasible for adrenocortical carcinoma or metastasis? *BJU Int*. 2004;94(7):1026–1029.
60. Weitz J, Blumgart LH, Fong Y, et al. Partial hepatectomy for metastases from noncolorectal, nonneuroendocrine carcinoma. *Ann Surg*. 2005;241(2):269–276.
61. Decker RA, Elson P, Hogan TF, et al. Eastern Cooperative Oncology Group study 1879: mitotane and adriamycin in patients with advanced adrenocortical carcinoma. *Surgery*. 1991;110(6):1006–1013.
62. Fassnacht M, Hahner S, Polat B, et al. Efficacy of adjuvant radiotherapy of the tumor bed on local recurrence of adrenocortical carcinoma. *J Clin Endocrinol Metab*. 2006;91(11):4501–4504.
63. Abrams HL, Spiro R, Goldstein N. Metastases in carcinoma; analysis of 1000 autopsied cases. *Cancer*. 1950;3(1):74–85.
64. Sarela AI, Murphy I, Coit DG, Conlon KC. Metastasis to the adrenal gland: the emerging role of laparoscopic surgery. *Ann Surg Oncol*. 2003;10(10):1191–1196.
65. Kim SH, Brennan MF, Russo P, Burt ME, Coit DG. The role of surgery in the treatment of clinically isolated adrenal metastasis. *Cancer*. 1998;82(2):389–394.
66. Bovio S, Cataldi A, Reimondo G, et al. Prevalence of adrenal incidentaloma in a contemporary computerized tomography series. *J Endocrinol Invest*. 2006;29(4):298–302.
67. Angeli A, Osella G, Ali A, Terzolo M. Adrenal incidentaloma: an overview of clinical and epidemiological data from the National Italian Study Group. *Horm Res*. 1997;47(4–6):279–283.

20
Benign and Malignant Pheochromocytomas and Paragangliomas

Ronald R.de Krijger and Francien H.van Nederveen

Introduction

Pheochromocytomas (PCC) and paragangliomas (PGL) are tumors arising from neural crest-derived chromaffin cells. PCC are located in the adrenal medulla and produce, with few exceptions, catecholamines. Sympathetic PGL (sPGL, previously also designated extraadrenal PCC) also produce catecholamines but arise in the chromaffin tissue of the sympathetic trunk that is situated along the proximal aorta reaching down to the abdominal aorta and the urinary bladder. In the developing embryo, the organs of Zuckerkandl, which serve as catecholamine-releasing organs during development of the fetal adrenals, can be identified in the sympathetic trunk, which is an important site for sPGL to occur, especially in young patients. Together, PCC and sPGL have an incidence that varies between 2 and 8 per million.[1]

The parasympathetic nervous tissue gives rise to small clusters of chief cells located in the head and neck region. Tumors arising from these cells are designated parasympathetic PGL (pPGL), although a wide range of terms has been applied for these tumors in the past (e.g., chemodectoma and glomus tumor), which should no longer be used. pPGL arise in the majority of cases in the carotid body and the jugulotympanic paraganglia, followed by vagal, laryngeal, and, in some cases, aorticopulmonary paraganglia. These tumors usually do not produce catecholamines. PCC, sPGL, and pPGL share many histological and immunohistochemical characteristics, but recent work has shown that they have distinct genetic aberrations, as will be specified later in this chapter.

Clinical Presentation, Histology, and Immunohistochemistry

In clinical practice, PCC and sPGL have a heterogeneous presentation and are therefore known as "the great mimic." The vast majority of patients present with continuously or paroxysmally increased blood pressure, with headaches, signs of flushing or palpitations, although a small number of patients will be asymptomatic. In the latter cases, the diagnosis is incidental, often in the context of diagnostic imaging procedures for other purposes; these tumors are known as "incidentalomas." One study of Mayo clinic patients demonstrated that 10% of the adrenal incidentalomas are in fact PCC.[2] pPGL, which do not produce catecholamines, usually present because of mass effect, which can cause symptomatic cranial nerve palsy.

PCC and PGL usually have a characteristic histological pattern. In the context of a typical clinical presentation, the diagnosis should be relatively straightforward. Occasionally, however, these tumors must be distinguished from a variety of other endocrine and nonendocrine tumors. The classical growth pattern shows so-called "Zellballen," formed by rounded nests of large uniform polygonal cells (Figure 20.1). These cells have granular amphophilic or basophilic cytoplasm. The cellular nests are surrounded by S100-positive sustentacular cells, which are nonneoplastic and can usually be seen with the help of immunohistochemical stains. Sometimes, the Zellballen pattern is not so clear, with a more diffuse architecture and cells arranged in large sheets. The variable degree of cytologic atypia of PCC may be impressive, to the extent of mimicking malignancy. pPGL may have more pronounced Zellballen and more eosinophilic cytoplasm, but overlap exists between the two types of tumor.

The best immunohistochemical marker currently used for PCC and PGL is chromogranin A (CgA), a major constituent of secretory granules.[3] Immunoreactivity for CgA will distinguish PCC and PGL from adrenocortical tumors and nonendocrine tumors. Staining of PCC for CgA is usually moderate to strong and diffuse. This marker is so consistent that the diagnosis of PCC should be reconsidered if CgA is negative. In contrast, the vast majority of adrenocortical tumors will show reactivity to inhibin and/or Melan A, which are rare to absent in PCC and PGL.

The issue of malignancy in PCC and PGL is one that has been extensively investigated but remains unresolved. Currently, the 2004 WHO definition states that malignancy

J.L. Hunt (ed.), *Molecular Pathology of Endocrine Diseases*, Molecular Pathology Library 3,
DOI 10.1007/978-1-4419-1707-2_20, © Springer Science+Business Media, LLC 2010

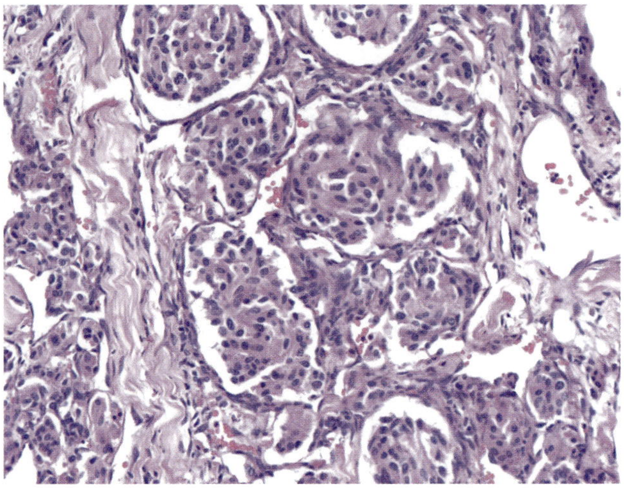

FIG. 20.1. Classical histology of pheochromocytomas and paragangliomas, showing nests of cells with amphophilic cytoplasm and moderately atypical nuclei, separated by fibrous septa containing numerous vessels.

can only be diagnosed when metastases are present in sites where chromaffin tissue does not normally occur.[4] This specific definition is used to prevent overdiagnosis of carcinoma in patients who have second primary tumors in the setting of hereditary syndromes (see below). From a clinical patient management perspective, other indicators of malignancy in the primary tumor would obviously be of great benefit. Though many studies have investigated differentiating benign from malignant tumors, most suffer from low numbers of tumors and poor adherence to the strict criteria as set out by the WHO. Three important studies have been based predominantly on histological criteria. A study by Linnoila et al in 1990 examined 120 sympathetic PGL and PCC and developed a statistical model according to which >70% of the tumors could be classified correctly with >95% probability on the basis of four criteria: extraadrenal location, coarse nodularity, confluent necrosis, and absence of hyaline globules.[5] Most malignant tumors had two or three of those features, while 89% of benign tumors had one or none.

In 2002, Thompson proposed the PASS system (*p*heochromocytoma of the *a*drenal *s*caled *s*core) specific to the adrenal gland. This system scores multiple microscopic findings to arrive at a total score that correlates with metastatic potential.[6] All tumors that metastasized had a score >4, but 17/50 with score >4 had not metastasized in a follow-up period of ~5 years. A recent study that investigated the applicability of the PASS by a group of five endocrine pathologists showed a large inter and intraobserver variation in a large set of PCC.[7] As there are no other validation studies, the practical use of the PASS is currently limited.

Numerous immunohistochemical markers have been reported to correlate with malignancy, but their usefulness is still limited to research purposes.[8–10] The marker most consistently reported to be correlated with malignancy is the proliferation marker Ki-67, which is performed on paraffin sections using monoclonal antibody MIB-1.[10–12] However, in some studies, MIB-1 labeling does not correlate with malignancy. Studies of MIB-1 labeling show a striking lack of methodological consistency, and many papers do not provide sufficient methodological detail to permit replication.

A 2005 scoring system proposed by Kimura for both PCC and extraadrenal sPGL combines histological, immunohistochemical, and biochemical characteristics to arrive at a score reported to predict both the metastatic potential of tumors and the prognosis for patients with tumors that metastasize.[11] However, of so-called low grade tumors, there was still a considerable proportion that metastasized, limiting the practical usefulness.

Molecular Abnormalities in Sporadic PCC and PGL

Over the past two decades, six candidate genes involved in the pathogenesis of hereditary PCC and PGL have been identified, including RET, VHL, SHDB, SDHC, SDHD, and NF1. Thus, the genetic basis for several hereditary tumor syndromes has been elucidated: MEN2 caused by RET, Von Hippel–Lindau disease caused by VHL, hereditary PCC/PGL caused by one of the SDH genes, and neurofibromatosis type 1 caused by NF1. Interestingly, in the absence of known hereditary disease, it has also been demonstrated that a substantial number of patients with apparently sporadic PCC and/or PGL carry germline mutations in one of the above genes.[13] Currently, it is estimated that 25–30% of PCC and PGL patients have germline mutations, whether they are from a known family or not. Consequently, truly sporadic PCC and PGL should be a diagnosis of exclusion, after genetic testing for the above genes and in the context of a negative family history.

After the identification of these important candidate genes, several studies have been performed to investigate the occurrence of somatic mutations in these genes as well. Although low frequencies of somatic RET and VHL mutations have been found, somatic mutations in SDHB and SDHD are exceedingly rare.[14,15] Many other candidate genes, including both oncogenes and tumor suppressor genes have also been investigated, including c-mos, p53, and PTEN, but no mutations have been detected.[16–18] The advent of techniques that allow genome-wide analysis of DNA in large series of tumors has confirmed and expanded previously known data from LOH analysis. It now appears that the majority of PCC is characterized by the loss of chromosomal regions 1p and 3q.[19–20] A more detailed analysis of the short arm of chromosome 1 has been investigated by several groups with the aim of finding candidate genes in the smallest region of overlap of the various losses, but these efforts have not been fruitful.[21] Likewise, other regions of chromosomal loss or gain have not yielded candidate genes, which could be further tested by mutation analysis. Recently, work from our own group has indicated that there are likely two groups of PCC and sPGL, one with the characteristic loss of 1p and 3q, and another with loss of 3p and 11p. The losses of the former group correspond to the genetic profile of MEN2-related PCC, whereas those of the latter group correspond to VHL-related PCC.[22,23] Other chromosomal regions that appear of interest in PCC tumorigenesis are 8p, 21q, and 22q.[24,25]

Only recently, gene expression profiling and proteomics studies have been reported in PCC and PGL research. Several of these have been employed in the context of hereditary tumors and will be discussed in the next session. Further, gene expression studies have been used in an attempt to distinguish benign from malignant PCC and PGL.[26,27] In a study of 18 PCC, 9 malignant and 9 benign, Thouënnon et al describe a set of differentially expressed genes that are predominantly downregulated in malignant PCC. In another study by Brouwers et al, a larger but more heterogeneous group of PCC and PGL was investigated. In agreement with Thouënnon et al, the majority of differentially expressed genes were downregulated in malignant PCC. While these studies are promising, it is not clear whether these findings may be used as the basis of a clinically useful discriminatory test. In addition, they need to be confirmed in larger validation studies in international consortia.

Molecular Abnormalities in Hereditary PCC and PGL

Multiple endocrine neoplasia syndromes are currently subdivided into MEN1 and MEN2. MEN1 is due to mutations in the *menin* tumor-suppressor gene (TSG) located on 11q13. The occurrence of PCC in this syndrome is very rare, with only seven patients with mutations in the *menin* gene described in the literature. Thus, the discussion will be limited to MEN2, which can be divided into MEN2A and MEN2B. In the past, MEN2B was also designated MEN3, but this term is no longer applied in current literature. Recently, an MEN4-syndrome has been described with mutations in the *CDKN1B* gene, with an MEN1-like phenotype, but the occurrence of PCC has only been documented only in animal models, not in humans.[28,29]

The incidence of MEN2 is not known, but it is estimated to be 1.25–7.5/10,000,000 per year.[4] The syndrome is due to activating mutations in the *RET* proto-oncogene, coding for a tyrosine kinase receptor, located on 10q11.2. In MEN2A, the mutations are mainly found in the exons coding for the extracellular domain (exon 10 and 11 of the *RET* gene), but exons 13–15 can be involved in some cases. Functional changes due to these mutations are ligand-independent dimerization of the RET receptor, with subsequent activation of the RET signaling pathway. MEN2A is clinically defined by the presence of parathyroid hyperplasia, C-cell hyperplasia/medullary thyroid carcinoma, and PCC. The disease can manifest early in life, usually with medullary thyroid carcinoma (MTC), and can also manifest with a hypertensive crisis due to a PCC. PCC occur in about 50% of all patients with MEN2-syndrome and are frequently bilateral.[30,31] In addition, as described by Carney et al, most contralateral adrenal glands show either diffuse or nodular hyperplasia, which represents a precursor for PCC. It should be noted that the absence of a characteristic family history is not sufficient to rule out the diagnosis of MEN2A, since de novo germline mutations have been reported.[32]

MEN2B is also due to activating mutations in the *RET* proto-oncogene, with mutations in the kinase domain of the receptor (coded by exon 16 of the *RET* gene, p.M918T in 95% of all cases). The functional consequences of this mutation are diverse with loss of kinase inhibition, dimerization, and autophosphorylation without substrate binding to the receptor, all of which lead to aberrant RET signaling.[33] Clinically, the syndrome has overlapping features with the MEN2A syndrome, with the exception of the parathyroid hyperplasia. Striking in this syndrome is the occurrence of mucosal ganglioneuromas, giving a peculiar facial appearance, and skeletal deformities as described by Carney et al[34] De novo mutations causing MEN2B syndrome occur frequently, up to 50%.[35] In addition to germline mutations, somatic *RET* mutations in PCC have been described (the exon 16 p.M918T), but these mutations are not clinically relevant, since they do not increase the risk for other tumors. For all MEN-syndromes, the occurrence of malignancy of PCC is rare. No pPGL and sPGL have been described in MEN2 in the literature.

Using comparative genomic hybridization (CGH), genomic alterations in PCC from patients with MEN2 syndrome have been analyzed. In MEN2A patients, there is a consistent pattern of 1p and 3q loss, indicating that not only the involvement of the RET-oncogene itself but also potential tumor suppressor genes located on 1p and 3q may be involved in the pathogenesis of MEN2-related PCC.

Von Hippel–Lindau (VHL) disease has an incidence ranging from 1/36,000 to 1/39,000.[36,37] The disease has been subdivided into VHL type 1 and VHL type 2 (2a, 2b, and 2c). PCC do not develop in VHL type 1, but a considerable risk (16–30%) in VHL type 2 mutation carriers has been reported. Overall, PCC develop in 10–20% of patients with VHL and are usually bilateral.[30,31] The VHL protein is involved in the regulation of HIF degradation in the presence of normal oxygen tension. The majority of mutations described in PCC are missense mutations that abrogate their ability to degrade HIF. The occurrence of sPGL and pPGL is rare but has been described in VHL patients.[38]

Apart from PCC, VHL type 2a patients present with hemangioblastomas. In VHL type 2b, the same tumors occur with the addition of clear cell renal cell carcinoma. Rarer are cystic adenomas and endocrine tumors of the pancreas, papillary cystadenomas of the broad ligament and epididymis as well as endolymphatic sac tumors. In VHL type 2c, there is isolated familial PCC. VHL disease is due to mutations and other genetic abnormalities in the *VHL* tumor suppressor gene, located on 3p25. De novo mutations occur in about 20% of clinically detected VHL-patients. Therefore, not only family history but also the clinical presentation is important in PCC. There is a slight correlation of *VHL* mutations and malignancy,[14] but the majority of VHL-related PCC is benign. In addition to germline mutations, somatic *VHL* mutations in PCC have been described, although these mutations do not appear to be clinically relevant.

PCC that occur in the context of either germline or somatic *VHL* mutations[22] also have consistent genomic alterations as shown by CGH or array-CGH. These mainly consist of loss of 3p and 11p, which matches the localization of the *VHL* tumor suppressor gene on 3p.

In neurofibromatosis type 1 (also known as von Recklinghausen's disease), there is a small proportion of patients (up to 5%) with PCC. Compared to the previously described PCC susceptibility syndromes, this syndrome occurs much more frequently, affecting 1:3,000 individuals. The hallmarks of this syndrome are the occurrence of multiple neurofibromas and the presence of café-au-lait pigmentations and Lisch-nodules of the iris. However, the spectrum is much more diverse with the occurrence of gastrointestinal stromal tumors (GIST), central nervous system malignancies, and an increased risk of breast cancer in young women.[39,40] NF1 syndrome is caused by mutations in the *neurofibromin* or *nf1* tumor suppressor gene located on 17q11. Because the gene is exceptionally large and there are no mutation hotspots, mutation analysis is not routinely performed, as the diagnosis can also be reliably made on clinical characteristics. Although autosomally dominant, the syndrome also arises de novo in almost half of the cases. In the literature, a subset of apparently sporadic PCC has been investigated, of which one patient turned out to have NF1 after clinical examination.[41] There is no relationship between the type of *neurofibromin* mutation and the occurrence of PCC in NF1 patients.[42] Thus far, no somatic mutations in PCC of NF1 patients have been described. Malignancy in NF1-related PCC is extremely rare.

In studies on genetic alterations, only few NF1-related PCC have been investigated. Only one was investigated in the study by Edström et al, which displayed loss of 1p and 3q. Interestingly, an NF1 mouse model was developed, with the same phenotype as human NF1.[43] The genetic profiles of the three cell lines derived from the mouse PCC resembled that of human PCC, also displaying loss of the mouse homologues of 1p and 3q.

The PCC–PGL syndrome is caused by mutations in three of four genes coding for the succinate–ubiquinone oxidoreductase complex II of the aerobic transport chain and the tricarboxylic acid cycle. These genes are all tumor suppressor genes and are named *SDHB*, *SDHC*, and *SDHD*, located on 1p36, 1q21, and 11q23, respectively. The fourth gene involved in complex II, *SDHA*, is known to be involved in Leigh syndrome, where both alleles are inactivated through mutations.[44] *SDHB*, *SDHC*, and *SDHD* are the genes in the chromosomal regions that had been designated PGL4, PGL3, and PGL1, respectively and that were linked to the occurrence of PGL. Recently, the *SDH5* gene has been discovered as the candidate gene in the PGL2 chromosomal region 11q13.1, and renamed to *SDHAF2*.[45] It was since shown that the gene is mutated in a limited number of families with head and neck PGL, but not in a large series of sporadic PCC and PGL.[46] The spectrum of the PCC–PGL syndrome is expanding but seems to comprise almost all patients with any combination of PCC, pPGL, and sPGL. Although a positive family history for PCC and/or PGL is indicative of the syndrome, a significant subset of apparently sporadic PGL has germline mutations in the genes involved in the PCC–PGL syndrome.[47,48] It has been hypothesized that the penetrance of the syndrome is low and is influenced by the oxygen tension of the patients' habitat.[49]

SDHB germline gene mutations are frequently involved in sPGL but have also been described in PCC and pPGL. In addition, *SHDB* mutations have been found in patients or families with the co-occurrence of GIST and PCC or PGL, reported as the Carney–Stratakis syndrome. Also, three patients have been described in the literature with pPGL and renal cell carcinoma that harbored a germline *SDHB* mutation. Mutations in *SDHC* are infrequently found and have been reported in sPGL and pPGL so far.[50–53] Also, the co-occurrence of GIST and PGL is found due to mutations in *SDHC*. Finally, mutations involving *SDHD* are not only frequently found in pPGL but have also been found in PCC and sPGL. Not only patients with a positive familial history but also a subset of "apparently" sporadic pPGL are due to germline mutations in this gene. Detection of genetic abnormalities in each of these three SDH genes is usually performed by direct sequence analysis of the entire coding region, but it must be noted that multiplex ligation-dependent probe amplification (MLPA) has shown larger gene deletions in a number of cases.[54]

Malignancy in SDHx-related PCC and PGL is more frequent than in the aforementioned syndromes. In SDHB-related PCC and sPGL, the risk of malignancy, defined as the presence of metastases, appears to be 30–50% and is suggested to be even higher by some.[55–58] Also *SDHB* germline mutations in pPGL give an increased risk of malignant behavior, as described by Boedeker et al in a large series of pPGL. There has been a single case of sPGL with malignant behavior with an *SDHC* mutation. Malignancy in patients with *SDHD* mutations has been described, and a possible correlation is found with the "Dutch founder mutation" of the *SDHD* gene D92Y. All five malignant *SDHD*-related tumors described by Havekes et al were PGL, including one sPGL and four pPGL that harbored the D92Y mutation. In the literature the occurrence of malignancy in *SDHD*-related PCC and PGL does not seem to be increased.[30,59] Somatic mutation of the *SDHx* genes are rare, with two cases that have been described, one *SDHD* mutation in a PCC and one *SDHB* mutations in an sPGL.[15,60]

Few tumors in the context of the PCC–PGL syndrome have been investigated by CGH. However, the series of pPGL as published by Dannenberg et al contained familial pPGL that turned out to be due to SDHD-related.[19,47] In this small series, the consistent feature was the small number of genomic alterations, where the hallmark of the familial tumors was loss of 11q, matching the location of the *SDHD* gene. The only *SDHB*-related sPGL CGH-analysis described in the literature showed distinct loss of chromosome 1, in accordance with the location of the *SDHB* gene.[15] However, this sPGL contained a somatic and not a germline mutation. In the small series investigated so far, it appears that PCC and sPGL in patients with germline *SDHB* and *SDHD* mutations show a distinct loss of 1p and 11q, respectively, with only few alterations throughout the genome, indicating the importance of the TSG in the tumorigenesis of these tumors.

Other Susceptibility Loci

Finally, it should be mentioned that other loci are found to be involved in familial pPGL and PCC. A study using linkage analysis in PCC has found 2 loci for familial PCC located at 2cen and 16p13.[61] However, the genes associated with these loci are not known.

Summary

Molecular markers play a crucial role in the diagnosis of hereditary tumor syndromes in whose context PCC and PGL may occur. To detect mutations and other genetic abnormalities, genetic screening is advocated for *RET*, *VHL*, *SDHB*, and *SDHD* in all PCC and PGL patients, at least under the age of 50. The frequency of *SDHC* mutations is too low to warrant investigation of this gene systematically. Likewise, the complexity of *NF1* precludes inclusion of this gene in routine screening. Analysis should predominantly consist of direct sequencing of the entire coding region of genes, with the exception of RET, for which selected exons[10,11,16] can be studied. However, it is evident that larger genetic abnormalities occur in several of these genes, which need other molecular approaches.

The detection of mutations has a profound effect on follow-up of the patient, depending on the specific syndrome. In addition, the detection of *SDHB* mutations not only has a diagnostic significance, but also a prognostic one, as they correlate strongly with malignant tumor behavior. Apart from an effect on the patient, the detection of germline mutations impinges also on family members and relatives, depending on the fact whether such mutations are de novo or inherited. Thus, genetic counseling of PCC and PGL patients and family members is imperative before embarking on genetic analyses.

Currently, there do not exist therapeutic molecular markers for PCC and PGL, but it is expected that with the gradual elucidation of tumorigenesis, these may be developed in the next decade. In this respect, it is interesting to note that recently a hypothesis has been put forward, unifying all PCC/PGL susceptibility genes in a single biochemic pathway.[62]

References

1. Harding JL, Yeh MW, Robinson BG, Delbridge LW, Sidhu SB. Potential pitfalls in the diagnosis of phaeochromocytoma. *Med J Aust*. 2005;182(12):637–640.
2. Thompson GB, Young WF Jr. Adrenal incidentaloma. *Curr Opin Oncol*. 2003;15(1):84–90.
3. Feldman SA, Eiden LE. The chromogranins: their roles in secretion from neuroendocrine cells and as markers for neuroendocrine neoplasia. *Endocr Pathol*. 2003;14:3–23.
4. DeLellis RA, Lloyd RV, Heitz PU, Eng C, eds. *Tumours of Endocrine Organs*. Lyon: IARC; 2004.
5. Linnoila RI, Keiser HR, Steinberg SM, Lack EE. Histopathology of benign versus malignant sympathoadrenal paragangliomas: clinicopathologic study of 120 cases including unusual histologic features. *Hum Pathol*. 1990;21:1168–1180.
6. Thompson LD. Pheochromocytoma of the Adrenal gland Scaled Score (PASS) to separate benign from malignant neoplasms: a clinicopathologic and immunophenotypic study of 100 cases. *Am J Surg Pathol*. 2002;26:551–566.
7. Wu D, Tischler AS, Lloyd RV, et al. Observer variation in the application of the Pheochromocytoma of the Adrenal Gland Scaled Score. *Am J Surg Pathol*. 2009;33(4):599–608.
8. Eisenhofer G, Bornstein SR, Brouwers FM, et al. Malignant pheochromocytoma: current status and initiatives for future progress. *Endocr Relat Cancer*. 2004;11:423–436.
9. Portela-Gomes GM, Stridsberg M, Grimelius L, Falkmer UG, Falkmer S. Expression of chromogranins A, B, and C (secretogranin II) in human adrenal medulla and in benign and malignant pheochromocytomas An immunohistochemical study with region-specific antibodies. *APMIS*. 2004;112: 663–673.
10. August C, August K, Schroeder S, et al. CGH and CD 44/ MIB-1 immunohistochemistry are helpful to distinguish metastasized from nonmetastasized sporadic pheochromocytomas. *Mod Pathol*. 2004;17:1119–1128.
11. Kimura N, Watanabe T, Noshiro T, Shizawa S, Miura Y. Histological grading of adrenal and extra-adrenal pheochromocytomas and relationship to prognosis: a clinicopatho-logical analysis of 116 adrenal pheochromocytomas and 30 extra-adrenal sympathetic paragangliomas including 38 malignant tumors. *Endocr Pathol*. 2005;16:23–32.
12. van der Harst E, Bruining HA, Jaap Bonjer H, et al. Proliferative index in phaeochromocytomas: does it predict the occurrence of metastases? *J Pathol*. 2000;191:175–180.
13. Neumann HP, Bausch B, McWhinney SR, et al. Germ-line mutations in nonsyndromic pheochromocytoma. *N Engl J Med*. 2002;346:1459–1466.
14. Dannenberg H, De Krijger RR, van der Harst E, et al. Von Hippel-Lindau gene alterations in sporadic benign and malignant pheochromocytomas. *Int J Cancer*. 2003;105:190–195.

15. van Nederveen FH, Korpershoek E, Lenders JW, de Krijger RR, Dinjens WN. Somatic SDHB mutation in an extraadrenal pheochromocytoma. *N Engl J Med*. 2007;357:306–308.
16. Eng C, Foster KA, Healey CS, et al. Mutation analysis of the c-mos proto-oncogene and the endothelin-B receptor gene in medullary thyroid carcinoma and phaeochromocytoma. *Br J Cancer*. 1996;74:339–341.
17. van Nederveen FH, Perren A, Dannenberg H, et al. PTEN gene loss, but not mutation, in benign and malignant phaeochromocytomas. *J Pathol*. 2006;209:274–280.
18. Petri BJ, Speel EJ, Korpershoek E, et al. Frequent loss of 17p, but no p53 mutations or protein overexpression in benign and malignant pheochromocytomas. *Mod Pathol*. 2008;21:407–413.
19. Dannenberg H, Speel EJ, Zhao J, et al. Losses of chromosomes 1p and 3q are early genetic events in the development of sporadic pheochromocytomas. *Am J Pathol*. 2000;157(2):353–359.
20. Edström E, Mahlamäki E, Nord B, et al. Comparative genomic hybridization reveals frequent losses of chromosomes 1p and 3q in pheochromocytomas and abdominal paragangliomas, suggesting a common genetic etiology. *Am J Pathol*. 2000;156:651–659.
21. Aarts M, Dannenberg H, deLeeuw RJ, et al. Microarray-based CGH of sporadic and syndrome-related pheochromocytomas using a 0.1-0.2 Mb bacterial artificial chromosome array spanning chromosome arm 1p. *Genes Chromosomes Cancer*. 2006; 45:83–93.
22. Lui WO, Chen J, Gläsker S, et al. Selective loss of chromosome 11 in pheochromocytomas associated with the VHL syndrome. *Oncogene*. 2002;21:1117–1122.
23. Horn IR, van den Berg BM, van der Meijden PZ, et al. Molecular analysis of ligand binding to the second cluster of complement-type repeats of the low density lipoprotein. Evidence for an allosteric component in receptor-associated protein-mediated inhibiton of ligand binding. *J Biol Chem*. 1997;272(21):13608–13613
24. Jarbo C, Buckley PG, Piotrowski A, et al. Detailed assessment of chromosome 22 aberrations in sporadic pheochromocytoma using array-CGH. *Int J Cancer*. 2006;118:1159–1164.
25. Cascón A, Ruiz-Llorente S, Rodríguez-Perales S, et al. A novel candidate region linked to development of both pheochromocytoma and head/neck paraganglioma. *Genes Chromosomes Cancer*. 2005;42:260–268.
26. Thouënnon E, Elkahloun AG, Guillemot J, et al. Identification of potential gene markers and insights into the pathophysiology of pheochromocytoma malignancy. *J Clin Endocrinol Metab*. 2007;92:4865–4872.
27. Brouwers FM, Elkahloun AG, Munson PJ, et al. Gene expression profiling of benign and malignant pheochromocytoma. *Ann N Y Acad Sci*. 2006;1073:541–556.
28. Pellegata NS, Quintanilla-Martinez L, Keller G, et al. Human pheochromocytomas show reduced p27Kip1 expression that is not associated with somatic gene mutations and rarely with deletions. *Virchows Arch*. 2007;451:37–46.
29. Pellegata NS, Quintanilla-Martinez L, Siggelkow H, et al. Germ-line mutations in p27Kip1 cause a multiple endocrine neoplasia syndrome in rats and humans. *Proc Natl Acad Sci USA*. 2006;103:15558–15563.
30. Amar L, Bertherat J, Baudin E, et al. Genetic testing in pheochromocytoma or functional paraganglioma. *J Clin Oncol*. 2005;23:8812–8818.
31. Korpershoek E, Petri BJ, van Nederveen FH, et al. Candidate gene mutation analysis in bilateral adrenal pheochromocytoma and sympathetic paraganglioma. *Endocr Relat Cancer*. 2007;14: 453–462.
32. Neumann HP, Eng C, Mulligan LM, et al. Consequences of direct genetic testing for germline mutations in the clinical management of families with multiple endocrine neoplasia, type II. *JAMA*. 1995;274:1149–1151.
33. Gujral TS, Singh VK, Jia Z, Mulligan LM. Molecular mechanisms of RET receptor-mediated oncogenesis in multiple endocrine neoplasia 2B. *Cancer Res*. 2006;66(22):10741–10749.
34. Carney JA, Go VL, Sizemore GW, Hayles AB. Alimentary-tract ganglioneuromatosis. A major component of the syndrome of multiple endocrine neoplasia, type 2b. *N Engl J Med*. 1976; 295(23):1287–1291.
35. Carlson KM, Bracamontes J, Jackson CE, et al. Parent-of-origin effects in multiple endocrine neoplasia type 2B. *Am J Hum Genet*. 1994;55(6):1076–1082.
36. Neumann HP, Wiestler OD. Clustering of features of von Hippel-Lindau syndrome: evidence for a complex genetic locus. *Lancet*. 1991;337(8749):1052–1054.
37. Maher ER, Iselius L, Yates JR, et al. Von Hippel-Lindau disease: a genetic study. *J Med Genet*. 1991;28:443–447.
38. Hes FJ, van der Luijt RB, Janssen AL, et al. Frequency of Von Hippel-Lindau germline mutations in classic and non-classic Von Hippel-Lindau disease identified by DNA sequencing, Southern blot analysis and multiplex ligation-dependent probe amplification. *Clin Genet*. 2007;72:122–129.
39. Walker L, Thompson D, Easton D, et al. A prospective study of neurofibromatosis type 1 cancer incidence in the UK. *Br J Cancer*. 2006;95:233–238.
40. Kramer K, Hasel C, Aschoff AJ, Henne-Bruns D, Wuerl P. Multiple gastrointestinal stromal tumors and bilateral pheochromocytoma in neurofibromatosis. *World J Gastroenterol*. 2007;13:3384–3387.
41. Bausch B, Koschker AC, Fassnacht M, et al. Comprehensive mutation scanning of NF1 in apparently sporadic cases of pheochromocytoma. *J Clin Endocrinol Metab*. 2006;91: 3478–3481.
42. Bausch B, Borozdin W, Mautner VF, et al. European-American Phaeochromocytoma Registry Study Group. Germline NF1 mutational spectra and loss-of-heterozygosity analyses in patients with pheochromocytoma and neurofibromatosis type 1. *J Clin Endocrinol Metab*. 2007;92:2784–2792.
43. Powers JF, Evinger MJ, Zhi J, Picard KL, Tischler AS. Pheochromocytomas in Nf1 knockout mice express a neural progenitor gene expression profile. *Neuroscience*. 2007;147: 928–937.
44. Baysal BE, Lawrence EC, Ferrell RE. Sequence variation in human succinate dehydrogenase genes: evidence for long-term balancing selection on SDHA. *BMC Biol*. 2007;5:12.
45. Hao HX, Khalimonchuk O, Schraders M, et al. SDH5, a gene required for flavination of succinate dehydrogenase, is mutated in paraganglioma. *Science*. 2009;325(5944):1139–1142.
46. Bayley JP, Kunst HP, Cascon A, et al. SDHAF2 mutations in familial and sporadic paraganglioma and phaeochromocytoma. *Lancet Oncol*. 2010.
47. Dannenberg H, Dinjens WN, Abbou M, et al. Frequent germline succinate dehydrogenase subunit D gene mutations in

patients with apparently sporadic parasympathetic paraganglioma. *Clin Cancer Res*. 2002;8:2061–2066.
48. Baysal BE, Willett-Brozick JE, Lawrence EC, et al. Prevalence of SDHB, SDHC, and SDHD germline mutations in clinic patients with head and neck paragangliomas. *J Med Genet*. 2002;39:178–183.
49. Baysal BE. Genomic imprinting and environment in hereditary paraganglioma. *Am J Med Genet C Semin Med Genet*. 2004; 129C:85–90.
50. Mannelli M, Ercolino T, Giachè V, Simi L, Cirami C, Parenti G. Genetic screening for pheochromocytoma: should SDHC gene analysis be included? *J Med Genet*. 2007;44:586–587.
51. Bayley JP, van Minderhout I, Weiss MM, et al. Mutation analysis of SDHB and SDHC: novel germline mutations in sporadic head and neck paraganglioma and familial paraganglioma and/or pheochromocytoma. *BMC Med Genet*. 2006;7:1.
52. Schiavi F, Boedeker CC, Bausch B, et al. European-American Paraganglioma Study Group. Predictors and prevalence of paraganglioma syndrome associated with mutations of the SDHC gene. *JAMA*. 2005;294:2057–2063.
53. Niemann S, Müller U. Mutations in SDHC cause autosomal dominant paraganglioma, type 3. *Nat Genet*. 2000;26: 268–270.
54. Cascón A, Montero-Conde C, Ruiz-Llorente S, et al. Gross SDHB deletions in patients with paraganglioma detected by multiplex PCR: a possible hot spot? *Genes Chromosomes Cancer*. 2006;45:213–219.
55. Amar L, Baudin E, Burnichon N, et al. Succinate dehydrogenase B gene mutations predict survival in patients with malignant pheochromocytomas or paragangliomas. *J Clin Endocrinol Metab*. 2007;92:3822–3828.
56. Timmers HJ, Kozupa A, Chen CC, et al. Superiority of fluorodeoxyglucose positron emission tomography to other functional imaging techniques in the evaluation of metastatic SDHB-associated pheochromocytoma and paraganglioma. *J Clin Oncol*. 2007;25:2262–2269.
57. Van Nederveen FH, Dinjens WN, Korpershoek E, De Krijger RR. The occurrence of SDHB gene mutations in pheochromocytoma. *Ann N Y Acad Sci*. 2006;1073:177–182.
58. Brouwers FM, Eisenhofer G, Tao JJ, et al. High frequency of SDHB germline mutations in patients with malignant catecholamine-producing paragangliomas: implications for genetic testing. *J Clin Endocrinol Metab*. 2006;91:4505–4509.
59. Benn DE, Gimenez-Roqueplo AP, Reilly JR, et al. Clinical presentation and penetrance of pheochromocytoma/paraganglioma syndromes. *J Clin Endocrinol Metab*. 2006;91:827–836.
60. Gimm O, Armanios M, Dziema H, Neumann HP, Eng C. Somatic and occult germ-line mutations in SDHD, a mitochondrial complex II gene, in nonfamilial pheochromocytoma. *Cancer Res*. 2000;60:6822–6825.
61. Dahia PL, Hao K, Rogus J, et al. Familial Pheochromocytoma Consortium. Novel pheochromocytoma susceptibility loci identified by integrative genomics. *Cancer Res*. 2005;65: 9651–9658.
62. Lee S, Nakamura E, Yang H, et al. Neuronal apoptosis linked to EglN3 prolyl hydroxylase and familial pheochromocytoma genes: developmental culling and cancer. *Cancer Cell*. 2005; 8:155–167.

21 Benign and Malignant Diseases of the Adrenal Cortex

Anne Marie McNicol

Introduction

Adrenal cortical diseases are relatively rare but are important to recognize and understand because of their significant morbidity and mortality. Developments in both molecular biology and molecular genetics have significantly increased our understanding of the process of steroidogenesis and steroid action. This in turn has allowed us to broaden our understanding of the various inherited diseases that affect this pathway. The main diseases and their pathogenesis will be presented in this chapter.

The investigation of the molecular pathways involved in the pathogenesis of adrenal cortical tumors has been hampered by the rarity of adrenal cortical carcinoma (ACC) and the fact that, until recently, adrenal cortical adenoma (ACA) was only identified during life if the tumor was secreting excess hormone. However, by learning lessons from other tumor types, from familial syndromes in which these tumors occur more frequently and by examining the signaling pathways involved in steroidogenesis and adrenal cortical growth, the molecular genetics of these tumors are being unraveled. Again, the current state of knowledge will be presented. Autoimmune adrenalitis also has molecular genetic aspects, but these are not dealt with here.

Normal Adrenal Structure and Function

The adrenal cortex has a critical role in homeostasis-producing glucocorticoids, mineralocorticoids, and sex steroids. It arises from the adrenogonadal primordium that develops from the urogenital ridge.[1] The Wilm's tumor gene (*WT-1*) and the *WNT4* gene play early roles in development. Other important regulators include the transcription factor, steroidogenic factor 1 (SF-1), and the nuclear receptor, dosage-sensitive sex reversal, adrenal hypoplasia critical region gene 1 (DAX-1).[2] The adult cortex comprises three zones. The outer zona glomerulosa (ZG) produces aldosterone, the main mineralocorticoid and is made up of small angular cells, dispersed focally under the capsule. The zona fasciculata (ZF) is the major component, formed of large lipid-laden cells arranged in columns from the capsule or ZG to the inner zona reticularis (ZR). It is thought to be the major source of glucocorticoids – cortisol in the human adrenal. The ZR is made up of eosinophilic (compact) cells arranged around branching vascular sinusoids. It is the source of adrenal androgens.[3]

Cholesterol is the precursor for all steroids and the enzymes involved are four members of the cytochrome P-450 family and a 3β-hydroxysteroid dehydrogenase (Figure 21.1). These are localized in the smooth endoplasmic reticulum and mitochondria, and the precursors move between the two during synthesis. Initially, cholesterol is transported to the inner mitochondrial membrane by steroid acute response (StAR) protein.[4] The production of aldosterone is mainly under the control of the renin–angiotensin system, although potassium, adrenocorticotrophic hormone (ACTH), catecholamines, and prostaglandins also play a role, and recent evidence suggests that endothelial cell-derived factors and adipokines are involved.[5] The production of aldosterone specifically by the ZG is because the enzyme aldosterone synthase is expressed only in this zone. The secretion of cortisol is controlled mainly by ACTH acting through the ACTH membrane receptor, a G protein-linked receptor. The G protein comprises three polypeptide subunits, (α, β and γ). On ligand binding, the α subunit (Gs) dissociates from the other subunits and when bound to guanosine triphosphate (GTP) activates adenylate cyclase, causing the production of cyclic AMP (cAMP). Cyclic AMP binds to the regulatory subunits of the tetrameric protein protein kinase A (PKA), allowing the catalytic subunits to be released, phosphorylated, and transferred to the nucleus where they influence gene transcription.[6] Other factors possibly involved include insulin-like growth factors (IGF-1 and IGF-2),[7] adrenomedullin,[8] transforming growth factor β and activin A that may have an inhibitory role.[9] Catecholamines may also have a role.[10,11]

J.L. Hunt (ed.), *Molecular Pathology of Endocrine Diseases*, Molecular Pathology Library 3,
DOI 10.1007/978-1-4419-1707-2_21, © Springer Science+Business Media, LLC 2010

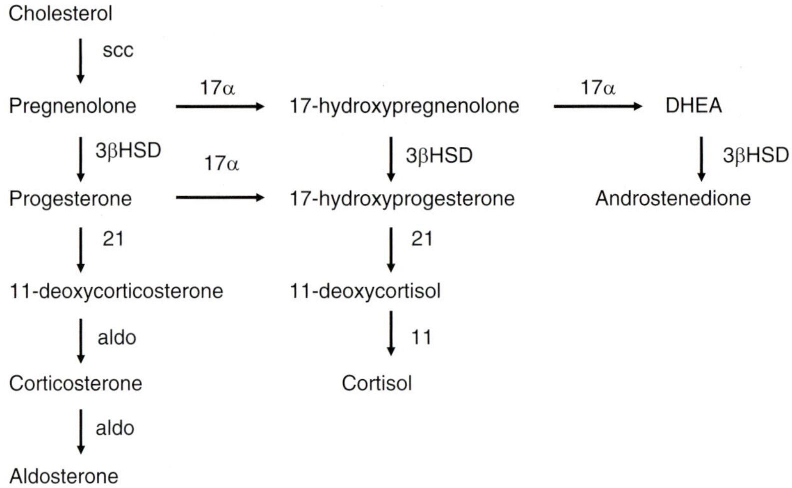

FIG. 21.1. Adrenal cortical steroidogenic pathway. *Scc* side chain cleavage enzyme; *3βHSD* 3β-hydroxysteroid dehydrogenase; *17* 17α-hydroxylase; *21* 21-hydroxylase; *11* 11β-hydroxylase; *aldo* aldosterone synthase; *DHEA* dehydroepiandrosterone.

Clinical Features of Adrenal Cortical Disease

Hypersecretion of Hormones

Diseases of the adrenal can present with signs and symptoms of excess or reduced hormone secretion or with evidence of an adrenal mass or metastases from a carcinoma. Three classical syndromes are associated with hypersecretion of steroids. These are primary hyperaldosteronism (including Conn syndrome), hypercortisolism (Cushing syndrome), and hypersecretion of sex steroids (adrenogenital syndrome).

Primary Hyperaldosteronism

This is now recognized as accounting for 5–13% of cases of hypertension, mostly sporadic. About one third are associated with an adrenal adenoma and a further 60% with bilateral idiopathic hyperplasia (IHA). Unilateral hyperplasia accounts for ~2% of cases.[12] Carcinomas are rare. Adenomas are often less than 2 cm in diameter and the cut surface is golden-yellow. Histologically, they comprise mainly cells resembling ZF, but some contain cells similar to ZG and hybrid cells sharing features of both (Figure 21.2). Focal compact cells are also found. The paraadenomatous gland may contain micronodules. The adjacent cortex may show hyperplasia of the ZG, but it is unclear whether this is related to pathogenesis or to the effects of treatment. In IHA, the ZG usually forms a continuous band rather than being focally dispersed. However, unless nodules are present, the glands in IHA may be of normal weight. Familial hyperaldosteronism is discussed later.

Cushing Syndrome

The clinical features of this syndrome are well recognized and include centripetal obesity, moon face, hypertension, striae, osteoporosis, and psychiatric symptoms. Two-thirds of cases are the result of hypersecretion of ACTH by the anterior pituitary gland, with 80–90% of patients having a corticotroph adenoma. Most have bilateral diffuse cortical hyperplasia (Figure 21.3) and the glands usually weigh 6–12 g, with broadening of the ZF and ZR and a relative prominence of ZR. Microscopic nodules are not uncommon, especially in the outer ZF. Ten to twenty percent of patients have bilateral nodular hyperplasia, with nodules visible to the naked eye. The intervening cortex is also hyperplastic. The relationship between the two is unclear, but they may be a continuum, with nodules developing in longer-standing disease.

Ectopic ACTH syndrome underlies about 15% of cases, around half associated with small-cell lung carcinoma or bronchial carcinoid. Other tumors causing the syndrome include thymic carcinoids, endocrine tumors of pancreas, medullary carcinoma of thyroid, and pheochromocytoma.

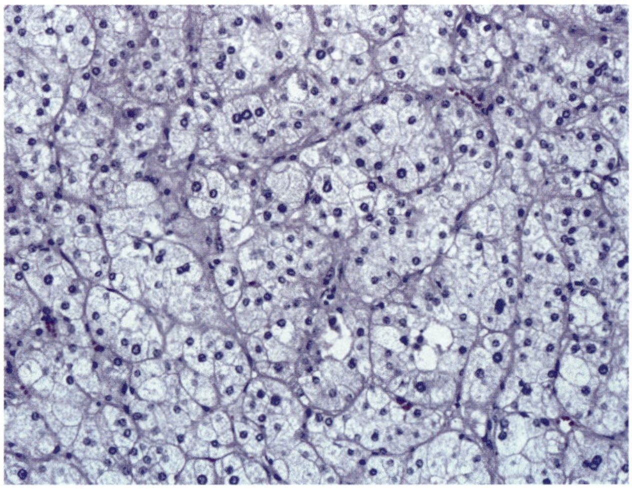

FIG. 21.2. Adrenal cortical adenoma causing Conn syndrome. There is a mixture of cell types, most of the cells resembling those of the zona fasciculata, large and lipid-laden. Scattered among these are smaller cells with a higher nuclear to cytoplasmic ratio, so-called hybrid cells.

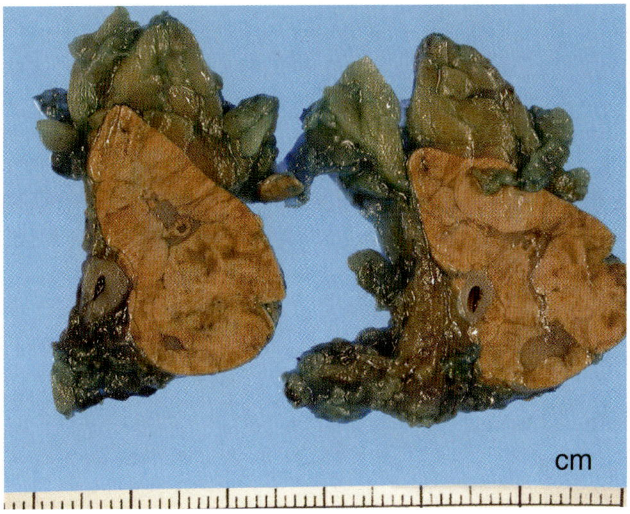

FIG. 21.3. Diffuse cortical hyperplasia in a patient with Cushing syndrome.

The adrenals usually show bilateral symmetrical hyperplasia, weighing an average of 15 g each. Nodules are rare. Compact cells extend out close to the capsule and pleomorphism, and mitotic figures are not infrequent.

Fifteen to twenty percent of adults have an adrenal tumor, equally split between benign and malignant. Females are more commonly affected. In children, more than half the cases are associated with tumor, the majority carcinoma. Because of the increased negative feedback to the pituitary, ACTH secretion is suppressed and the adjacent and opposite ZF and ZR are atrophic. Because of this, the ZG may appear more prominent.

ACTH-independent macronodular adrenal hyperplasia (AIMAH) is a rare variant of the syndrome.[13,14] The adrenal glands are often distorted and markedly enlarged. ACTH levels are suppressed. In many of these cases, the adrenal expresses inappropriate receptors and responds to ligands such as gastric inhibitory polypeptide (GIP), where the increase in cortisol secretion is related to food intake.[15] Other receptors identified include those for vasopressin, luteinizing hormone,[16] and serotonin.[17]

Adrenogenital Syndrome

Excess production of sex steroids causes virilization, feminization, or precocious puberty, depending on the age and sex of the patient and the nature of the steroids secreted. Congenital adrenal hyperplasia (CAH) is a group of autosomal recessive diseases associated with inherited defects in steroidogenesis.[18–23] Most present early in life. The lack of negative feedback by cortisol to the pituitary causes an increase in ACTH secretion and marked adrenal cortical hyperplasia. The clinical presentation depends on the enzyme involved and is related to the range of steroids produced. The details are discussed below. Adrenal cortical tumors can also produce sex steroids, usually androgens.

General Aspects of Adrenal Cortical Tumors

Adrenal cortical nodules can be found in up to 53% of adrenal glands at autopsy.[24,25] It is unclear exactly what proportion is neoplastic and what hyperplastic, but by using architectural and histological features, these studies suggested that adrenal cortical adenomas (ACA) were present in ~5%. This is similar to the 4% prevalence of adrenal lesions identified by computed tomography scan.[26] They are more common with increasing age, seen in 7% of those over 70 years.[27] Adenomas are usually single and unilateral, although bilateral lesions have been reported.[28] They are intraadrenal, may be unencapsulated or show a true capsule or pseudocapsule. They show an expansile pattern of growth. On slicing, they usually have a yellow color with brown foci. The majority comprise mainly lipid-laden cells resembling ZF in an alveolar pattern. Groups of compact cells may be scattered throughout and may predominate in tumors producing androgens.

Adrenal cortical carcinoma (ACC) is a rare tumor, with an estimated prevalence of between 4 and 12 per million[29] and accounts for 0.05–2% of all malignancies.[30–32] Women are more commonly affected.[33] There is a peak in early childhood and a second in the fifth to seventh decades.[34] The tumor is aggressive with 67–94% mortality, and median or mean survival is between 4 and 30 months. Many are locally invasive at time of presentation and up to two-thirds have metastasized. They commonly metastasize to liver, lung, retroperitoneum, and lymph nodes.[35] Between 26 and 76% of tumors are nonfunctional.[35] The commonest functional syndrome is Cushing syndrome, often also with androgen excess. Virilization may occur alone, but estrogen secretion is rare. There may also be nonhormonal symptoms such as abdominal fullness or pain, loin pain, fever, weight loss, or other malignancy-related features. Most respond poorly to treatment and surgery is the mainstay. Resistance to chemotherapy may be related to the expression of glutathione-*S*-transferases[36,37] and P-glycoprotein,[38,39] which have roles in conferring drug resistance.

The majority of carcinomas weigh over 100 g, but small tumors may also be malignant. They may be encapsulated, but many infiltrate adjacent tissues and there may be obvious vascular invasion. The cut surface is usually yellow to brown and is often lobulated with fibrous bands separating the lobules. Necrosis and hemorrhage are common (Figure 21.4) and cystic degeneration may be present. Histologically, trabecular and diffuse architectural patterns are usual; compact cells predominate, and pleomorphism (Figure 21.5) and mitotic activity are common. Vascular (Figure 21.6) and capsular invasion may be identified.

Most carcinomas are easy to diagnose, but even those without overt evidence of malignancy must be assessed for malignant potential. This is done by multifactorial analysis and a number of schemes have been proposed. Some combine

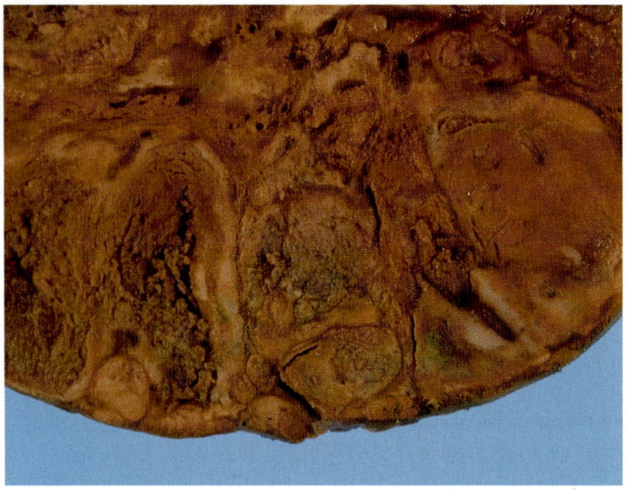

FIG. 21.4. Macroscopic appearance of an adrenal cortical carcinoma from a patient with Cushing syndrome. There is obvious lobulation and necrosis.

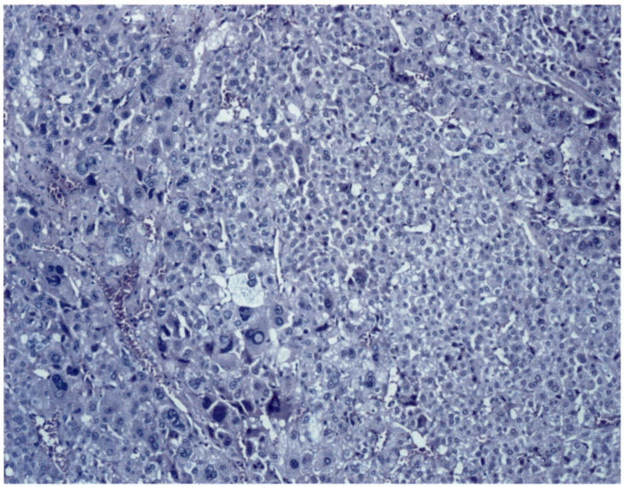

FIG. 21.5. Adrenal cortical carcinoma showing marked nuclear pleomorphism.

clinical and histologic features.[40,41] However, the most commonly used is still that of Weiss[42,43] where a series of nine histologic features are assessed (Table 21.1), the presence of three or more indicating malignant potential. This has been validated in a more recent study,[44] but the authors found poorer correlation over the assessment of nuclear pleomorphism and vascular invasion than of the other features and proposed that these should be omitted from the assessment and the others incorporated into a weighted numerical score (Table 21.2). This approach has been compared with the van Slooten and Weiss scores and has been shown to correlate with diagnosis and to survival in metastasizing carcinoma.[45] Occasional tumors with a Weiss score of 2 or less may behave in a malignant fashion.[46]

There is no formal staging system for adrenal cortical carcinoma from either the International Union against Cancer (UICC) or the American Joint Committee on Cancer (AJCC), but most use that of Macfarlane,[32] modified by Sullivan[47] (Table 21.3). Seventy percent of patients present with stage 3 or 4 disease.[48]

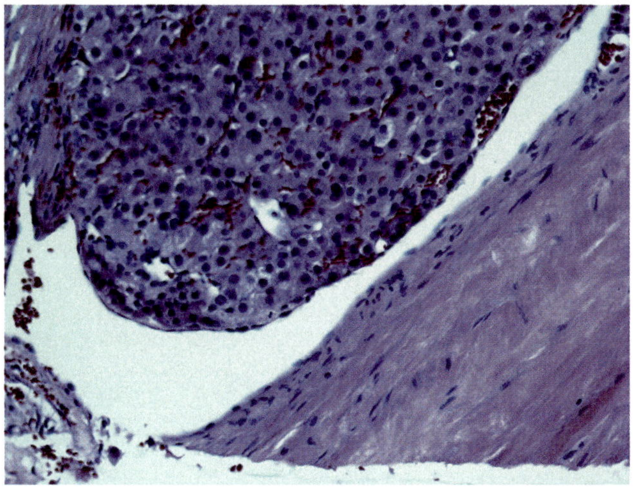

FIG. 21.6. Adrenal cortical carcinoma with obvious vascular invasion.

TABLE 21.1. Diagnosis of malignancy in adrenal cortical tumors according to the Weiss system.[42,43]

Histological features to be assessed
Diffuse architecture > 1/3rd
Clear cells ≤ 25% of total
Significant nuclear pleomorphism
Confluent necrosis
Mitotic count ≥ 6 per 50 HPF
Atypical mitoses
Capsular invasion
Sinusoidal invasion
Venous invasion

TABLE 21.2. Diagnosis of malignancy in adrenal cortical tumors according to the Aubert modification of the Weiss system.[44]

Histological features to be assessed
Mitotic count ≥ 6 per 50 HPF
Atypical mitoses
Clear cells ≤ 25% of total (cytoplasmic)
Confluent necrosis
Capsular invasion

Each feature is scored 1 when present and 0 when absent. A score is obtained by summing as follows, resulting in scores of 0 to 7:
2×mitotic rate score + 2×cytoplasmic score + atypical mitoses + necrosis + capsular invasion.
A total score of ≥ 3 indicates malignant potential.

Immunohistochemistry

Adrenal tumors rarely stain strongly positively for cytokeratins, particularly in the absence of antigen retrieval[49-52] and are negative for epithelial membrane antigen (EMA).[52] Antibody D11 has been reported to give positive staining,[53] and the combination of inhibin-α[54,55] and melan-A clone A103[56] is useful, while others have recommended the addition of calretinin.[57,58] Immunopositivity for proteins important in steroidogenesis, such as SF-1, DAX-1, and steroidogenic enzymes, has been reported[59–61] but have not found a role in diagnostic practice, probably because of the lack of good commercial antibodies. Adrenal cortical hyperplasias and tumors show positivity for a range of general neuroendocrine markers including synaptophysin[62–64] and, therefore, chromogranin A is the only marker that will positively discriminate pheochromocytoma from a cortical tumor.

Genetic Aspects of Adrenal Cortical Tumors

Familial Syndromes Associated with Adrenal Cortical Lesions (Table 21.4)

Li–Fraumeni Syndrome

Families with this syndrome have a predisposition to a number of tumors including breast carcinoma and soft tissue sarcomas. ACC occurs in 3–4% of family members.[65] The *TP53* tumor suppressor gene located on 17q13.1 encodes a protein with pivotal roles in cell proliferation and apoptosis.[66] Seventy percent of families with Li–Fraumeni syndrome have a germline mutation in the gene, usually in exons 5–8.[67] Others have a heterozygous mutation in the checkpoint kinase 2 (*hCHK2*) gene and ACC has not been reported in these kindreds.[68] A locus on 1q23 is involved in other families.[69]

TABLE 21.3. Staging of adrenal cortical carcinoma.[32,47]

Stage	
1	T1 N0 M0
2	T2 N0 M0
3	T1 or T2 N1 M0
	T3 N0 M0
4	Any T or N M1
	T3 N1
	T4
Criterion	
T1	Tumor ≤5cm, no invasion
T2	Tumor >5 cm, no invasion
T3	Tumor any size, locally invasive but not involving adjacent organs
T4	Tumor any size, invading adjacent organs or with distant metastases
N0	Negative regional nodes
N1	Positive regional nodes
M0	No distant metastases
M1	Distant metastases

Beckwith–Wiedemann Syndrome

This syndrome is associated with macrosomia, macroglossia, abdominal wall defects, and a predisposition to childhood tumors including ACC.[70] It is linked to the 11p15 locus with evidence of involvement of a number of genes including *IGF2*, *H19*, and cyclin-dependent kinase inhibitor 1C (*CDKN1C* or *p57^{kip2}*). These genes are imprinted, *IGF2* showing maternal and *CDKN1CI* and *H19* showing paternal imprinting.[71] Most individuals with the syndrome have loss of the maternal allele and paternal disomy, leading to overexpression of IGF2 and reduced expression of H19 and p57^{kip2}.

Carney Complex

This is a rare autosomal dominant condition characterized by pigmented lesions of skin and mucosa, cardiac and neural myxomas, and endocrine overactivity.[72,73] Some present with Cushing syndrome and have primary pigmented nodular adrenocortical hyperplasia (PPNAD). Both adrenal glands consist of multiple nodules, usually 1–3 mm in diameter. The combined weights range from 4 to 21 g. The nodules appear dark brown to black and the intervening cortex appears suppressed. Many of these cases have been shown to be linked to the 17q22–q24 region. Heterozygous inactivating mutations of the protein kinase A regulatory subunit 1A (*PRKAR1A*) gene in this region were reported initially in 45–65% of index cases and may be present in about 80% of the families presenting mainly with Cushing syndrome.[74] The protein product is important in the cAMP pathway. Linkage to chromosome 2 has also been reported.[75]

Multiple Endocrine Neoplasia, Type 1

This is another autosomal dominant syndrome associated with mutations in the multiple endocrine neoplasia, type 1

TABLE 21.4. Familial syndromes associated with adrenal cortical tumors.

Syndrome	Gene	Chromosomal location	Adrenal lesion
Li–Fraumeni	*TP53*	17p13	ACC in 1–4%
Beckwith–Weideman	*? IGF2*	11p15.5	ACC in 5%
	H19		
	CDKN1C		
Carney complex	*PRKAR1A*	17q22–24	PPNAD in 90–100%
Multiple endocrine neoplasia type 1	*MEN1*	11q13	ACA in 55% and rare ACC
Congenital adrenal hyperplasia	*CYP21B* (rarely *CYP11B, CYP17A or HSD3B2*)	6p21.3	BAH in 100%, ACA in 82% and rare ACC

ACA adrenal cortical adenoma; *ACC* adrenal cortical carcinoma; *BAH* bilateral adrenal cortical hyperplasia; *PPNAD* primary pigmented nodular adrenocortical disease.

(*MEN1*) gene on 11q13.[76,77] Tumors of the anterior pituitary and parathyroid glands and the endocrine pancreas are the most common findings. However, adrenal lesions, mainly hyperplasia and ACA, have been reported in up to 73% of cases.[78–81] ACC is rare.

General Aspects of the Genetics of Sporadic Adrenal Cortical Tumors (Table 21.5)

Researchers have approached the investigation of adrenal cortical tumors in a number of ways. Chromosomal gains and losses have been examined by comparative genomic hybridization (CGH) and loss of heterozygosity (LOH) studies. Oncogenes and tumor suppressor genes important in other tumor types have been targeted. There is little evidence to support a role for many of the classic oncogenes. Genes involved in the genetic syndromes associated with adrenal cortical tumors have been investigated. A more recent approach has been to investigate components of the signaling pathways important in steroidogenesis and adrenal growth. Microarray technology has been applied both to identify novel genes and to attempt to find panels that will differentiate between benign and malignant tumors and provide prognostic information in carcinoma.

Tumor Clonality

Clonality studies based on X chromosome inactivation are often used to examine tumor development, the premise being that monoclonal lesions are neoplastic, the result of expansion of a clone from a single cell with genetic alterations, while polyclonal populations are still responding to external stimuli. However, this may not fully apply, at least in the endocrine system.[82] Three studies on adrenal cortical tumors have shown that all 28 ACCs were monoclonal, 64 of 78 ACAs were monoclonal, and 53 of 67 nodular hyperplasias were polyclonal.[83-85] This may reflect different tumorigenic pathways in benign tumors, or the change from a polyclonal to a monoclonal population as a step in tumor progression. Interestingly, studies on AIMAH have shown both polyclonal and monoclonal lesions in the same patient[85] suggesting that neoplasms may arise in hyperplasia. This is also supported by the development of tumors in patients with congenital adrenal hyperplasia.[86]

TABLE 21.5. Genetic changes in sporadic adrenal cortical tumors.

Gene	Chromosomal locus	LOH	Mutations
TP53	17p13	Up to 30% of ACA and 87.5% of ACC	0–6% of ACA and 20–27% of ACC
IGF2	11p15	Up to 34% of ACA and 83% of ACC	
PRKAR1A	17q23–q24	23% of ACA and 53% of ACC	10% of ACA; not found in ACC
MEN1	11q13	25% of ACA and 100% of ACC	7% of ACA and ACC
GNAS	20q13.2		

LOH loss of heterozygosity; *ACA* adrenal cortical adenoma; *ACC* adrenal cortical carcinoma.

Chromosomal Changes

The data from chromosomal studies have given inconsistent data, probably due to differences in methodology and the small numbers in individual series. In situ hybridization studies have shown that adrenal tumors commonly have chromosomal gains and less common losses.[87,88] A number of CGH studies have been performed. The first report demonstrated losses on chromosomes 2, 11q, and 17p, and gains on 4 and 5 and increasing numbers of changes with size and malignancy.[89] Further studies have shown changes in all ACCs and up to 61% of adenomas, although there are some discrepancies in changes detected.[90,91] ACC gains were seen on chromosomes 5 ,12, 9, and 4 and losses were most frequently seen at 1p, 17p, 22, 2q, and 11q. The most common change in adenomas was gain of 4q.[91] Numerous loci of high-level amplification were seen in the other study.[90]

Loss of Heterozygosity

LOH has been shown in sporadic tumors at loci associated with familial syndromes (Table 21.4). LOH at 17p13,[92-94] 11q13,[95-97] and 11p15[92,98] are more common in ACC than in ACA. In contrast, LOH at 17q22–24[99] has been identified only in ACA. LOH has also been demonstrated at 18p11,[100] the locus of the gene encoding the ACTH receptor.

Specific Gene Involvement

IGF2 Signaling Pathway

IGF2 is a fetal growth factor. The gene lies within the 11p15 imprinted region as discussed above. *IGF-2* is highly overexpressed in ~90% of ACC.[98,101,102] There is paternal disomy even in sporadic cases. Reduced expression of both *H19* and *p57kip2* may also play a role.[98,103,104] The type 1 IGF-receptor, through which IGF2 acts, is also overexpressed.[102] The abnormal expression of this pathway is the most common event reported in ACC.

ACTH Signaling Pathway

This pathway, involving a G protein-linked receptor, cAMP, and protein kinase A has been discussed in detail in the section on steroidogenesis. Increased stimulation of the adrenal by ACTH is associated with hyperplasia and there is an increased incidence of ACA in congenital adrenal hyperplasia.[86] The pathway is involved in the pathogenesis of tumors in other endocrine organs; for example, the Gsα mutations in a subpopulation of somatotroph tumors in the pituitary.[105,106] The same mutations are present in McCune–Albright syndrome[107] where patients develop AIMAH.

As discussed above, Carney complex (CNC) is associated with *PRKAR1A* mutation. There is little evidence to support a significant role for the ACTH receptor in tumorigenesis as no activating mutations have been found in benign or malignant tumors.[108,109] However, since LOH has been found in 1 of 16 ACA and 2 of 4 ACC, it has been suggested that loss of the gene may result in dedifferentiation and tumor progression.[100] Mutations in G proteins are exceedingly rare, 3 in all detected in four studies.[110–113] Mutations in *PRKAR1A* have been identified in only a small subset of ACA and not in ACC.[99] A recent study has demonstrated a subgroup of adrenal adenomas characterized by underexpression (4% of normal) of another of the regulatory subunits of PKA, R2B, although levels of messenger RNA (mRNA) were normal suggesting a posttranscriptional mechanism.[114] These tumors were all small cortisol-secreting adenomas. A further interesting observation has been the presence of inactivating mutations in the *PDE11A* gene on 2q31–35 in patients with PPNAD and other forms of bilateral hyperplasia.[115] This encodes a dual-specificity phosphodiesterase that can hydrolyze both cAMP and cGMP, again implicating the cAMP pathway. There has been a recent proposal that most benign adrenal hyperplasias and adenomas are linked to abnormalities in this pathway[116] and that other changes, such as *TP53* mutations, overexpression of IGF2 and other growth factors, are associated with carcinoma.

Wnt Signaling Pathway

The Wnt proteins are a family of growth factors important both in development and adult life. Wnt signaling results in cytoplasmic accumulation of β-catenin and translocation to the nucleus and regulates gene transcription.[117] Abnormal Wnt signaling is involved in the development of a number of cancers.[118] In one study of adrenal tumors, accumulation of β-catenin was demonstrated in 13% of ACA and 77% of ACC, and activating mutations of *β-catenin* were found in 27% of ACA and 31% of ACC.[119] The changes were more commonly seen in nonfunctional tumors. The presence of such mutations has been confirmed in sporadic adenomas[120] and in PPNAD.[121]

TP53

Acquired mutations in TP53 gene are common in most human cancers.[122] Mutations have been found in only up to 27% of ACC and 6% of ACA.[123–125] In one of these studies, ACC with mutations showed a trend towards poorer survival[125] whereas a previous study showed no correlation with either survival or disease-free survival.[126] In contrast to the mutations in exons 5–8 seen in these studies, mutations were found in exon 4 in 60% of ACAs in a series from Taiwan.[127] This mutation was not demonstrated in a series of white patients,[128] raising the possibility of ethnic differences. A number of germline TP53 mutations have been identified in 50–80% of childhood ACC, in the absence of Li–Fraumeni syndrome,[67,129] suggesting the possibility of low penetrance mutations. However, given the low rate of mutations compared to LOH, it is possible that this locus contains other TSGs.

The incidence of ACC is ten times higher in Southern Brazil than in other geographic areas. A germline mutation (R337H) has been demonstrated in these cases[130] and also in adult cases in the area.[131] There is loss of the wild-type allele and accumulation of the mutant protein. It is estimated that one in ten carriers of this mutation develop ACC.[132]

MEN1

LOH at 11q13 has been reported in <20% of ACA but in >90% of ACC.[95–97] However, mutation of the *MEN1* gene has been demonstrated in only one ACA[95] and in one ACC.[97] The level of gene expression was similar in normal adrenals, ACA, and ACC.[133] These suggest that the gene is not important in the pathogenesis of sporadic adrenal cortical tumors.

Microarray Studies

More recently, there have been a number of studies based on microarray expression profiling.[134–138] Most have been based on a wide array of genes and have confirmed the importance of *IGF2* and other growth related genes in carcinoma, and have been able to make a differentiation between benign and malignant tumors. They have identified a range of novel genes that require validation, but the genes identified have varied between the studies, probably relating to the small numbers of tumors studied and the variation in methodology. One study took a different approach and compared the expression of a panel of 230 selected genes linked either to steroidogenesis and the cAMP pathway, including steroidogenic enzymes and StAR protein or to the IGF2 pathway[136] in a series of 33 ACA and 24 ACC. They showed that the steroidogenesis group were more highly expressed in 93% of the benign tumors and the IGF2 group in 75% of the malignant group. Using a combination of eight genes from the *IGF-2* cluster and 14 from the adrenal cluster, it was possible to predict malignancy but only at the same level as the Weiss histological score. However, using 14 genes, it was possible to separate recurring from nonrecurring tumors in a group of 13 carcinomas. These approaches need further validation in larger series and refinement.

Prognostic Features in Adrenal Cortical Carcinoma

Our tools for the prediction of outcome in carcinoma are still limited. The most important feature at present is tumor stage. In one series, 5-year survival was 60% for stage 1, 58% for stage 2, 24% for stage 3, and 0% for stage 4.[139] Mitotic rate of >20 per 50 high power fields[43] has been shown to correlate with poorer outcome and MIB-1 (Ki-67) index of >3% to indicate poorer disease-free survival.[140] More recent molecular analysis has suggested that overexpression of IGF2 and

LOH at 17p13 predict recurrence in carcinoma.[92] As indicated above, gene expression analysis may improve our ability to predict outcome.

Primary Hereditary Disease of the Adrenal Cortex (Table 21.6)

Congenital Adrenal Hyperplasia

These are a group of autosomal recessive diseases in which there are deficiencies in the various enzymes involved in steroidogenesis (Figure 21.1).[141,142] In most forms, the lack of cortisol feedback leads to increased ACTH levels, adrenal cortical hyperplasia, and the diversion of precursor steroids into androgen synthesis. The most common enzyme involved is 21-hydroxylase, accounting for more than 90% of cases. The classical form presents at birth with varying degrees of masculinization of external genitalia in female infants. Boys may have normal genitalia at birth but may develop precocious puberty. In 65–75% of cases, there is also a defect in aldosterone synthesis that results in hyponatremia, hyperkalemia, hypovolemia, and shock. The overall incidence is one in 15,000 live births, but this varies with geography and ethnic origin. In the Yupic Eskimos of Alaska, it is one in 280[143]and in the inhabitants of La Réunion, one in 2,100.[144] The nonclassical form is the most common autosomal recessive condition recognized, with a prevalence of one in 1,000 in the white population[145,146] and higher in other ethnic groups. This variant may be asymptomatic or present with features of androgen excess.

The gene encoding 21-hydroxylase (*CYP21A2, CYP21B*) is located within the HLA histocompatibility complex at 6p21.3.[147] It lies close to an inactive pseudogene with 98% homology (*CYP21A1P, CYP21P*).[148] About 90% of the mutations are the result of recombinations of the two genes with transfer of sequences from the pseudogene to the active gene, leading to an inability to encode a normal enzyme. Most patients are compound heterozygotes, with different mutations on the two alleles. The severity of disease is usually related to the allele that retains most activity.

The 11β-hydroxylase enzyme is involved in 5–8% of cases with a range of mutations.[18] The signs of androgen excess are accompanied by hypertension because of the accumulation of precursors with mineralocorticoid activity. A variety of mutations are recognized. The 17α-hydroxylase enzyme accounts for about 1% of patients. Deficiency of 3β-hydroxysteroid hydrogenase (3β-HSD) is caused by mutations in the type 2 *3βHSD* gene.[149] Affected males are incompletely masculinized because of lack of testicular androgens. In all of these variants, the adrenals show bilateral cortical hyperplasia and have a characteristic cerebriform appearance. The cortex is lipid-depleted because cholesterol is being used for steroidogenesis and is not stored. Adrenal tumors, mainly adenomas, have been reported frequently in patients with CAH[86] but carcinomas are rare.[150,151]

An unusual variant of CAH is congenital lipoid hyperplasia in which there is hyperplasia with cholesterol accumulation in the cortex. A minority of cases is caused by mutations in the side-chain cleavage enzyme that converts cholesterol to pregnenolone, but the majority have mutations in the gene encoding the StAR protein[22,152] on 8p11.2[153] that is integral to the transport of cholesterol to the mitochondrion to start steroidogenesis. Since all steroidogenesis is affected, the condition is often lethal.

TABLE 21.6. Nonneoplastic familial diseases of the adrenal cortex.

Disease	Gene	Chromosomal location
Congenital adrenal hyperplasia	*CYP21B* (rarely *CYP11B*, *CYP17A1 or HSD3B2*)	6p21.3 8q21 10q24.3, 1p13.1
Congenital lipoid hyperplasia	*STAR* (rarely *P450SCC*)	8p11.2 15q23–q24
Adrenoleukodystrophy	*ALD*	Xq28
Familial glucocorticoid insufficiency	*MCR2* *MRAP* Other	18p11.2 21q22.1

Other Diseases

Primary congenital adrenal hypoplasia is a rare X-linked disease usually resulting from mutations and deletions of the *DAX-1* gene on Xp21.[154] There is weight loss, dehydration, and salt loss. The condition may be fatal and the adrenals are small and difficult to find at autopsy. Occasional cases may be due to mutations in the ACTH receptor gene (*MC2R*).[155] Adrenoleukodystrophy (Addison–Schilder disease) is also X-linked.[156] It is a peroxisomal disorder in which there are mutations in a transmembrane transporter gene on Xq28[157] leading to the accumulation of very long chain fatty acids in the adrenal cortex and the white matter of the brain. More than 100 mutations have been identified, about 50% missense, but also deletions and insertions.[158,159] The adrenals undergo gradual atrophy and vary in size at autopsy. The ZG may be normal, but the ZF contains nests of degenerate ballooned cells. In the later stages, these may disappear and the gland may resemble autoimmune Addison disease without a lymphoid infiltrate. There is evidence to suggest that it may be the cause of clinical Addison's disease in a significant proportion of young men without adrenal antibodies.[160]

Familial glucocorticoid deficiency is a rare condition that affects both sexes and is characterized by very low cortisol levels, relatively normal mineralocorticoids, and very high ACTH levels. It is caused by mutations in the ACTH receptor (*MC2R*) on 18p11.2 in 25–40% of cases.[161] However, other genes including melanocortin 2 receptor accessory protein (*MRAP*) may also be responsible.[162]

Two rare forms of familial hyperaldosteronism (FH), types I and Type I, also known as glucocorticoid remediable aldosteronism, is an autosomal dominant disease in which there is unequal crossover between the ACTH responsive part of the 11β-hydroxylase gene (*CYP11B1*) and the functional part of the aldosterone synthase gene (*CYP11B2*), thus bringing aldosterone synthesis largely under ACTH control.[163,164] Type II is associated with familial occurrence of aldosterone-producing adenomas or bilateral hyperplasia or both and is linked to 7p22.[165]

Conclusion

The further developments in our understanding of the inherited adrenal cortical diseases will no doubt come from the identification of additional specific mutations and their effects on the expression and activity of the encoded proteins.

The major area of future development, however, will be in the area of tumor diagnosis, biology, and prognosis. By drawing on the single gene and signaling pathway studies, it should be possible to design more specific and refined microarrays to diagnose malignancy. This approach should eventually allow a more targeted approach to both diagnosis and therapy in adrenal carcinoma, a tumor that still has a dismal prognosis for most patients.

References

1. Keegan CE, Hammer GD. Recent insights into organogenesis of the adrenal cortex. *Trends Endocrinol Metab*. 2002;13:200–208.
2. Beuschlein F, Keegan CE, Bavers DL, et al. SF-1, DAX-1, and acd: molecular determinants of adrenocortical growth and steroidogenesis. *Endocr Res*. 2002;28:597–607.
3. Nguyen AD, Conley AJ. Adrenal androgens in humans and non-human primates: production, zonation and regulation. *Endocr Dev*. 2008;13:33–54.
4. Miller WL. Steroidogenic acute regulatory protein (StAR), a novel mitochondrial cholesterol transporter. *Biochim Biophys Acta*. 2007;1771:663–676.
5. Willenberg HS, Schinner S, Ansurudeen I. New mechanisms to control aldosterone synthesis. *Horm Metab Res*. 2008;40(7): 435–441.
6. Soon PS, McDonald KL, Robinson BG, Sidhu SB. Molecular markers and the pathogenesis of adrenocortical cancer. *Oncologist*. 2008;13:548–561.
7. l'Allemand D, Penhoat A, Blum W, Saez JM. Is there a local IGF-system in human adrenocortical cells? *Mol Cell Endocrinol*. 1998;140:169–173.
8. Albertin G, Forneris M, Aragona F, Nussdorfer GG. Expression of adrenomedullin and its receptors in the human adrenal cortex and aldosteronomas. *Int J Mol Med*. 2001;8:423–426.
9. Vanttinen T, Liu J, Kuulasmaa T, Kivinen P, Voutilainen R. Expression of activin/inhibin signaling components in the human adrenal gland and the effects of activins and inhibins on adrenocortical steroidogenesis and apoptosis. *J Endocrinol*. 2003;178:479–489.
10. Haidan A, Bornstein SR, Glasow A, Uhlmann K, Lubke C, Ehrhart-Bornstein M. Basal steroidogenic activity of adrenocortical cells is increased 10-fold by coculture with chromaffin cells. *Endocrinology*. 1998;139:772–780.
11. Haidan A, Bornstein SR, Liu Z, Walsh LP, Stocco DM, Ehrhart-Bornstein M. Expression of adrenocortical steroidogenic acute regulatory (StAR) protein is influenced by chromaffin cells. *Mol Cell Endocrinol*. 2000;165:25–32.
12. Young WF. Primary aldosteronism: renaissance of a syndrome. *Clin Endocrinol (Oxf)*. 2007;66:607–618.
13. Bourdeau I, Lampron A, Costa MH, Tadjine M, Lacroix A. Adrenocorticotropic hormone-independent Cushing's syndrome. *Curr Opin Endocrinol Diabetes Obes*. 2007;14: 219–225.
14. Christopoulos S, Bourdeau I, Lacroix A. Aberrant expression of hormone receptors in adrenal Cushing's syndrome. *Pituitary*. 2004;7:225–235.
15. Chabre O, Liakos P, Vivier J, et al. Cushing's syndrome due to a gastric inhibitory polypeptide-dependent adrenal adenoma: insights into hormonal control of adrenocortical tumorigenesis. *J Clin Endocrinol Metab*. 1998;83:3134–3143.
16. Carlson HE. Human adrenal cortex hyperfunction due to LH/hCG. *Mol Cell Endocrinol*. 2007;269:46–50.
17. Lacroix A, N'Diaye N, Mircescu H, Tremblay J, Hamet P. The diversity of abnormal hormone receptors in adrenal Cushing's syndrome allows novel pharmacological therapies. *Braz J Med Biol Res*. 2000;33:1201–1209.
18. Nimkarn S, New MI. Steroid 11beta- hydroxylase deficiency congenital adrenal hyperplasia. *Trends Endocrinol Metab*. 2008;19:96–99.
19. Bachelot A, Chakthoura Z, Rouxel A, Dulon J, Touraine P. Classical forms of congenital adrenal hyperplasia due to 21–hydroxylase deficiency in adults. *Horm Res*. 2008;69: 203–211.
20. Torresani T, Biason-Lauber A. Congenital adrenal hyperplasia: diagnostic advances. *J Inherit Metab Dis*. 2007;30:563–575.
21. Goncalves J, Friaes A, Moura L. Congenital adrenal hyperplasia: focus on the molecular basis of 21-hydroxylase deficiency. *Expert Rev Mol Med*. 2007;9:1–23.
22. Bhangoo A, Anhalt H, Ten S, King SR. Phenotypic variations in lipoid congenital adrenal hyperplasia. *Pediatr Endocrinol Rev*. 2006;3:258–271.
23. Merke DP, Bornstein SR. Congenital adrenal hyperplasia. *Lancet*. 2005;365:2125–2136.
24. Saeger W, Reinhard K, Reinhard C. Hyperplastic and tumorous lesions of the adrenals in an unselected autopsy series. *Endocr Pathol*. 1998;9:235–239.
25. Reinhard C, Saeger W, Schubert B. Adrenocortical nodules in post-mortem series. Development, functional significance, and differentiation from adenomas. *Gen Diagn Pathol*. 1996;141: 203–208.
26. Bovio S, Cataldi A, Reimondo G, et al. Prevalence of adrenal incidentaloma in a contemporary computerized tomography series. *J Endocrinol Invest*. 2006;29:298–302.
27. Kloos RT, Gross MD, Francis IR, Korobkin M, Shapiro B. Incidentally discovered adrenal masses. *Endocr Rev*. 1995;16: 460–483.
28. Watanabe N, Tsunoda K, Sasano H, et al. Bilateral aldosterone-producing adenomas in two patients diagnosed by immunohistochemical analysis of steroidogenic enzymes. *Tohoku J Exp Med*. 1996;179:123–129.
29. Grumbach MM, Biller BM, Braunstein GD, et al. Management of the clinically inapparent adrenal mass ("incidentaloma"). *Ann Intern Med*. 2003;138:424–429.
30. Hutter AMJ, Kayhoe DE. Adrenal cortical carcinoma. *Am J Med*. 1966;41:572–580.

31. Ibanez ML. The pathology of adrenal cortical carcinomas. Study of 22 cases. In: *Endocrine and Nonendocrine Hormone-Producing Tumors.* Chicago: Year Book Medical Publishers; 1971:231–239.
32. MacFarlane DA. Cancer of the adrenal cortex. The natural history, prognosis and treatment in a study of fifty-five cases. *Ann Royal Coll Surg Engl.* 1958;23:155–186.
33. Abiven G, Coste J, Groussin L, et al. Clinical and biological features in the prognosis of adrenocortical cancer: poor outcome of cortisol-secreting tumors in a series of 202 consecutive patients. *J Clin Endocrinol Metab.* 2006;91:2650–2655.
34. Wooten MD, King DK. Adrenal cortical carcinoma. Epidemiology and treatment with mitotane and a review of the literature. *Cancer.* 1993;72:3145–3155.
35. Lack EE. *Tumors of the Adrenal Gland and Extra-Adrenal Paraganglia.* Third Series ed. Washington, DC: Armed Forces Institute of Pathology; 1997.
36. Meikle I, Hayes JD, Walker SW. Expression of an abundant alpha-class glutathione S-transferase in bovine and human adrenal cortex tissues. *J Endocrinol.* 1992;132:83–92.
37. Sarkar D, Imai T, Kambe F, et al. Overexpression of glutathione-S-transferase A1 in benign adrenocortical adenomas from patients with Cushing's syndrome. *J Clin Endocrinol Metab.* 2001;86:1653–1659.
38. Ginn PE. Immunohistochemical detection of P-glycoprotein in formalin-fixed and paraffin-embedded normal and neoplastic canine tissues. *Vet Pathol.* 1996;33:533–541.
39. Haak HR, van Seters AP, Moolenaar AJ, Fleuren GJ. Expression of P-glycoprotein in relation to clinical manifestation, treatment and prognosis of adrenocortical cancer. *Eur J Cancer.* 1993;7:1036–1038.
40. Hough AJ, Hollifield JW, Page DL, Hartmann WH. Prognostic factors in adrenal cortical tumours. *Am J Clin Pathol.* 1979;72:390–399.
41. Van Slooten H, Schaberg A, Smeenk D, Moolenaar AJ. Morphologic characteristics of benign and malignant adrenocortical tumors. *Cancer.* 1985;55:766–773.
42. Weiss LM. Comparable histologic study of 43 metastasizing and non metastasizing adrenocortical tumors. *Am J Surg Pathol.* 1984;8:163–169.
43. Weiss LM, Medeiros LJ, Vickery AL Jr. Pathologic features of prognostic significance in adrenocortical carcinoma. *Am J Surg Pathol.* 1989;13:202–206.
44. Aubert S, Wacrenier A, Leroy X, et al. Weiss system revisited: a clinicopathologic and immunohistochemical study of 49 adrenocortical tumors. *Am J Surg Pathol.* 2002;26:1612–1619.
45. van't Sant HP, Bouvy ND, Kazemier G, et al. The prognostic value of two different histopathological scoring systems for adrenocortical carcinomas. *Histopathology.* 2007;51:239–245.
46. Pohlink C, Tannapfe A, Eichfeld U, et al. Does tumor heterogeneity limit the use of the Weiss criteria in the evaluation of adrenocortical tumors? *J Endocrinol Invest.* 2004;27:565–569.
47. Sullivan M, Boileau M, Hodges CV. Adrenal cortical carcinoma. *J Urol.* 1978;120:660–665.
48. Sidhu S, Gicquel C, Bambach CP, et al. Clinical and molecular aspects of adrenocortical tumourigenesis. *ANZ J Surg.* 2003;73:727–738.
49. Chu P, Wu E, Weiss LM. Cytokeratin 7 and cytokeratin 20 expression in epithelial neoplasms: a survey of 435 cases. *Mod Pathol.* 2000;13:962–972.
50. Henzen-Logmans SC, Stel HV, van Muijen GN, Mullink H, Meijer CJ. Expression of intermediate filament proteins in adrenal cortex and related tumours. *Histopathology.* 1988;12:359–372.
51. Wick MR, Cherwitz DL, McGlennen RC, Dehner LP. Adrenocortical carcinoma. An immunohistochemical comparison with renal cell carcinoma. *Am J Pathol.* 1986;122:343–352.
52. Gaffey MJ, Traweek ST, Mills SE, et al. Cytokeratin expression in adrenocortical neoplasia: an immunohistochemical and biochemical study with implications for the differential diagnosis of adrenocortical, hepatocellular, and renal cell carcinoma. *Hum Pathol.* 1992;23:144–153.
53. Schroder S, Niendorf A, Achilles E, et al. Immunocytochemical differential diagnosis of adrenocortical neoplasms using the monoclonal antibody D11. *Virchows Arch A Pathol Anat Histopathol.* 1990;417:89–96.
54. Arola J, Liu J, Heikkila P, Voutilainen R, Kahri A. Expression of inhibin alpha in the human adrenal gland and adrenocortical tumors. *Endocr Res.* 1998;24:865–867.
55. Munro LM, Kennedy A, McNicol AM. The expression of inhibin/activin subunits in the human adrenal cortex and its tumours. *J Endocrinol.* 1999;161:341–347.
56. Ghorab Z, Jorda M, Ganjei P, Nadji M. Melan A (A103) is expressed in adrenocortical neoplasms but not in renal cell and hepatocellular carcinomas. *Appl Immunohistochem Mol Morphol.* 2003;11:330–333.
57. Jorda M, De MB, Nadji M. Calretinin and inhibin are useful in separating adrenocortical neoplasms from pheochromocytomas. *Appl Immunohistochem Mol Morphol.* 2002;10:67–70.
58. Zhang H, Bu H, Chen H, et al. Comparison of immunohistochemical markers in the differential diagnosis of adrenocortical tumors: immunohistochemical analysis of adrenocortical tumors. *Appl Immunohistochem Mol Morphol.* 2008;16:32–39.
59. Coulter CL, Smith RE, Stowasser M, Sasano H, Krozowski ZS, Gordon RD. Expression of 11betaHSD-2 in human adrenal cortical carcinoma and adenoma. *Endocr Res.* 1998;24:875–876.
60. Sasano H, Mason JI, Sasano N, Nagura H. Immunolocalization of 3 beta-hydroxysteroid dehydrogenase in human adrenal cortex and in its disorders. *Endocr Pathol.* 1990;1:94–101.
61. Sasano H, Shizawa S, Suzuki T, et al. Ad4BP in the human adrenal cortex and its disorders. *J Clin Endocrinol Metab.* 1995;80:2378–2380.
62. Stratakis CA, Carney JA, Kirschner LS, et al. Synaptophysin immunoreactivity in primary pigmented nodular adrenocortical disease: neuroendocrine properties of tumors associated with Carney complex. *J Clin Endocrinol Metab.* 1999;84:1122–1128.
63. Komminoth P, Roth J, Schroder S, Saremaslani P, Heitz PU. Overlapping expression of immunohistochemical markers and synaptophysin mRNA in pheochromocytomas and adrenocortical carcinomas. Implications for the differential diagnosis of adrenal gland tumors. *Lab Invest.* 1995;72:424–431.
64. Haak HR, Fleuren GJ. Neuroendocrine differentiation of adrenocortical tumors. *Cancer.* 1995;75:860–864.
65. Li FP, Fraumeni JF. Soft tissue sarcomas, breast cancer, and other neoplasms. A familial syndrome? *Ann Int Med.* 1969;71:747–752.
66. Rodier F, Campisi J, Bhaumik D. Two faces of p53: aging and tumor suppression. *Nucleic Acids Res.* 2007;35:7475–7484.
67. Varley JM, McGown G, Thorncroft M, et al. Are there low-penetrance TP53 Alleles? evidence from childhood adrenocortical tumors. *Am J Hum Genet.* 1999;65:995–1006.

68. Bell DW, Varley JM, Szydlo TE, et al. Heterozygous germ line hCHK2 mutations in Li-Fraumeni syndrome. *Science*. 1999;286:2528–2531.
69. Bachinski LL, Olufemi SE, Zhou X, et al. Genetic mapping of a third Li-Fraumeni syndrome predisposition locus to human chromosome 1q23. *Cancer Res*. 2005;65:427–431.
70. Cohen MM Jr. Beckwith–Wiedemann syndrome: historical, clinicopathological, and etiopathogenetic perspectives. *Pediatr Dev Pathol*. 2005;8(3):287–304.
71. Weksberg R, Squire JA. Molecular biology of Beckwith-Wiedemann syndrome. *Med Pediatr Oncol*. 1996;27:462–469.
72. Carney JA. The Carney complex (myxomas, spotty pigmentation, endocrine overactivity, and schwannomas). *Dermatol Clin*. 1995;13:19–26.
73. Stratakis CA. Genetics of adrenocortical tumors: Carney complex. *Ann Endocrinol (Paris)*. 2001;62:180–184.
74. Bertherat J. Carney complex (CNC). *Orphanet J Rare Dis*. 2006;1:21.
75. Stratakis CA, Carney JA, Lin JP, et al. Carney complex, a familial multiple neoplasia and lentiginosis syndrome. Analysis of 11 kindreds and linkage to the short arm of chromosome 2. *J Clin Invest*. 1996;97:699–705.
76. Courseaux A, Grosgeorge J, Gaudray P, et al. Definition of the minimal MEN1 candidate area based on a 5-Mb integrated map of proximal 11q13. The European Consortium on Men1, (GENEM 1; Groupe d'Etude des Neoplasies Endocriniennes Multiples de type 1). *Genomics*. 1996;37:354–365.
77. Agarwal SK, Kester MB, Debelenko LV, et al. Germline mutations of the MEN1 gene in familial multiple endocrine neoplasia type 1 and related states. *Hum Mol Genet*. 1997;6:1169–1175.
78. Skogseid B, Rastad J, Gobl A, et al. Adrenal lesion in multiple endocrine neoplasia type 1. *Surgery*. 1995;118:1077–1082.
79. Barzon L, Pasquali C, Grigoletto C, Pedrazzoli S, Boscaro M, Fallo F. Multiple endocrine neoplasia type 1 and adrenal lesions. *J Urol*. 2001;166:24–27.
80. Burgess JR, Harle RA, Tucker P, et al. Adrenal lesions in a large kindred with multiple endocrine neoplasia type 1. *Arch Surg*. 1996;131:699–702.
81. Schaefer S, Shipotko M, Meyer S, et al. Natural course of small adrenal lesions in multiple endocrine neoplasia type 1: an endoscopic ultrasound imaging study. *Eur J Endocrinol*. 2008;158:699–704.
82. DeLellis RA, Tischler AS. Clonality of endocrine proliferative lesions: a critical reappraisal. *Endocr Pathol*. 1998;9:281–285.
83. Beuschlein F, Reincke M, Karl M, et al. Clonal composition of human adrenocortical neoplasms. *Cancer Res*. 1994;54: 4927–4932.
84. Gicquel C, Leblond-Francillard M, Bertagna X, et al. Clonal analysis of human adrenocortical carcinomas and secreting adenomas. *Clin Endocrinol (Oxf)*. 1994;40:465–477.
85. Blanes A, Diaz-Cano SJ. DNA and kinetic heterogeneity during the clonal evolution of adrenocortical proliferative lesions. *Hum Pathol*. 2006;37:1295–1303.
86. Jaresch S, Kornely E, Kley HK, Schlaghecke R. Adrenal incidentaloma and patients with homozygous or heterozygous congenital adrenal hyperplasia. *J Clin Endocrinol Metab*. 1992;74:685–689.
87. Russell AJ, Sibbald J, Haak H, Keith WN, McNicol AM. Increasing genome instability in adrenocortical carcinoma progression with involvement of chromosomes 3, 9 and X at the adenoma stage. *Br J Cancer*. 1999;81:684–689.
88. Shono T, Sakai H, Takehara K, Honda S, Kanetake H. Analysis of numerical chromosomal aberrations in adrenal cortical neoplasms by fluorescence in situ hybridization. *J Urol*. 2002;168:1370–1373.
89. Kjellman M, Kallioniemi OP, Karhu R, et al. Genetic aberrations in adrenocortical tumors detected using comparative genomic hybridization correlate with tumor size and malignancy. *Cancer Res*. 1996;56:4219–4223.
90. Dohna M, Reincke M, Mincheva A, Allolio B, Solinas-Toldo S, Lichter P. Adrenocortical carcinoma is characterized by a high frequency of chromosomal gains and high-level amplifications. *Genes Chromosomes Cancer*. 2000;28:145–152.
91. Sidhu S, Marsh DJ, Theodosopoulos G, et al. Comparative genomic hybridization analysis of adrenocortical tumors. *J Clin Endocrinol Metab*. 2002;87:3467–3474.
92. Gicquel C, Bertagna X, Gaston V, et al. Molecular markers and long-term recurrences in a large cohort of patients with sporadic adrenocortical tumors. *Cancer Res*. 2001;61:6762–6767.
93. Soon PS, Libe R, Benn DE, et al. Loss of heterozygosity of 17p13, with possible involvement of ACADVL and ALOX15B, in the pathogenesis of adrenocortical tumors. *Ann Surg*. 2008;247:157–164.
94. Yano T, Linehan M, Anglard P, et al. Genetic changes in human adrenocortical carcinomas. *J Natl Cancer Inst*. 1989;81: 518–523.
95. Heppner C, Reincke M, Agarwal SK, et al. MEN1 gene analysis in sporadic adrenocortical neoplasms. *J Clin Endocrinol Metab*. 1999;84:216–219.
96. Kjellman M, Roshani L, Teh BT, et al. Genotyping of adrenocortical tumors: very frequent deletions of the MEN1 locus in 11q13 and of a 1-centimorgan region in 2p16. *J Clin Endocrinol Metab*. 1999;84:730–735.
97. Schulte KM, Mengel M, Heinze M, et al. Complete sequencing and messenger ribonucleic acid expression analysis of the MEN I gene in adrenal cancer. *J Clin Endocrinol Metab*. 2000;85:441–448.
98. Gicquel C, Raffin-Sanson ML, Gaston V, et al. Structural and functional abnormalities at 11p15 are associated with the malignant phenotype in sporadic adrenocortical tumors: study on a series of 82 tumors. *J Clin Endocrinol Metab*. 1997;82:2559–2565.
99. Bertherat J, Groussin L, Sandrini F, et al. Molecular and functional analysis of PRKAR1A and its locus (17q22–24) in sporadic adrenocortical tumors: 17q losses, somatic mutations, and protein kinase A expression and activity. *Cancer Res*. 2003;63:5308–5319.
100. Reincke M, Mora P, Beuschlein F, Arlt W, Chrousos GP, Allolio B. Deletion of the adrenocorticotropin receptor gene in human adrenocortical tumors: implications for tumorigenesis. *J Clin Endocrinol Metab*. 1997;82:3054–3058.
101. Boulle N, Logie A, Gicquel C, Perin L, Le Bouc Y. Increased levels of insulin-like growth factor II (IGF-II) and IGF- binding protein-2 are associated with malignancy in sporadic adrenocortical tumors. *J Clin Endocrinol Metab*. 1998;83:1713–1720.
102. Ilvesmaki V, Kahri AI, Miettinen PJ, Voutilainen R. Insulin-like growth factors (IGFs) and their receptors in adrenal tumors: high IGF-II expression in functional adrenocortical carcinomas. *J Clin Endocrinol Metab*. 1993;77:852–858.

103. Gao ZH, Suppola S, Liu J, Heikkila P, Janne J, Voutilainen R. Association of H19 promoter methylation with the expression of H19 and IGF-II genes in adrenocortical tumors. *J Clin Endocrinol Metab*. 2002;87:1170–1176.
104. Liu J, Kahri AI, Heikkila P, Ilvesmaki V, Voutilainen R. H19 and insulin-like growth factor-II gene expression in adrenal tumors and cultured adrenal cells. *J Clin Endocrinol Metab*. 1995;80:492–496.
105. Spada A, Vallar L. G-protein oncogenes in acromegaly. *Horm Res*. 1992;38:90–93.
106. Lania A, Mantovani G, Spada A. G protein mutations in endocrine diseases. *Eur J Endocrinol*. 2001;145:543–559.
107. Weinstein LS, Shenker A, Gejman PV, Merino MJ, Friedman E, Spiegel AM. Activating mutations of the stimulatory G protein in the McCune-Albright syndrome. *N Engl J Med*. 1991;325:1688–1695.
108. Latronico AC. Role of ACTH receptor in adrenocortical tumor formation. *Braz J Med Biol Res*. 2000;33:1249–1252.
109. Light K, Jenkins PJ, Weber A, et al. Are activating mutations of the adrenocorticotropin receptor involved in adrenal cortical neoplasia? *Life Sci*. 1995;56:1523–1527.
110. Demeure MJ, Doffek KM, Komorowski RA, Gorski J. Gip-2 codon 179 oncogene mutations: absent in adrenal cortical tumors. *World J Surg*. 1996;20:928–931. discussion 931–932.
111. Gicquel C, Dib A, Bertagna X, Amselem S, Le Bouc Y. Oncogenic mutations of alpha-Gi2 protein are not determinant for human adrenocortical tumourigenesis. *Eur J Endocrinol*. 1995;133:166–172.
112. Lyons J, Landis CA, Harsh G, et al. Two G protein oncogenes in human endocrine tumors. *Science*. 1990;249:655–659.
113. Reincke M, Karl M, Travis W, Chrousos GP. No evidence for oncogenic mutations in guanine nucleotide-binding proteins of human adrenocortical neoplasms. *J Clin Endocrinol Metab*. 1993;77:1419–1422.
114. Vincent-Dejean C, Cazabat L, Groussin L, et al. Identification of a clinically homogenous subgroup of benign cortisol-secreting adrenocortical tumors characterized by alterations of the protein kinase A (PKA) subunits and high PKA activity. *Eur J Endocrinol*. 2008;158:829–839.
115. Horvath A, Boikos S, Giatzakis C, et al. A genome-wide scan identifies mutations in the gene encoding phosphodiesterase 11A4 (PDE11A) in individuals with adrenocortical hyperplasia. *Nat Genet*. 2006;38:794–800.
116. Stratakis CA. Cushing syndrome caused by adrenocortical tumors and hyperplasias (corticotropin-independent Cushing syndrome). *Endocr Dev*. 2008;13:117–132.
117. Kestler HA, Kuhl M. From individual Wnt pathways towards a Wnt signalling network. *Philos Trans R Soc Lond B Biol Sci*. 2008;363:1333–1347.
118. Chen X, Yang J, Evans PM, Liu C. Wnt signaling: the good and the bad. *Acta Biochim Biophys Sin (Shanghai)*. 2008;40:577–594.
119. Tissier F, Cavard C, Groussin L, et al. Mutations of beta-catenin in adrenocortical tumors: activation of the Wnt signaling pathway is a frequent event in both benign and malignant adrenocortical tumors. *Cancer Res*. 2005;65:7622–7627.
120. Tadjine M, Lampron A, Ouadi L, Bourdeau I. Frequent mutations of beta-catenin gene in sporadic secreting adrenocortical adenomas. *Clin Endocrinol (Oxf)*. 2008;68:264–270.
121. Tadjine M, Lampron A, Ouadi L, Horvath A, Stratakis CA, Bourdeau I. Detection of somatic beta-catenin mutations in primary pigmented nodular adrenocortical disease. *Clin Endocrinol (Oxf)*. 2008;69(3):367–373.
122. Bourdon JC. p53 and its isoforms in cancer. *Br J Cancer*. 2007;97:277–282.
123. Ohgaki H, Kleihues P, Heitz PU. p53 mutations in sporadic adrenocortical tumors. *Int J Cancer*. 1993;54:408–410.
124. Reincke M, Karl M, Travis WH, et al. p53 mutations in human adrenocortical neoplasms: immunohistochemical and molecular studies. *J Clin Endocrinol Metab*. 1994;78:790–794.
125. Sidhu S, Martin E, Gicquel C, et al. Mutation and methylation analysis of TP53 in adrenal carcinogenesis. *Eur J Surg Oncol*. 2005;31:549–554.
126. McNicol AM, Nolan CE, Struthers AJ, Farquharson MA, Hermans J, Haak HR. Expression of p53 in adrenocortical tumours: clinicopathological correlations. *J Pathol*. 1997;181:146–152.
127. Lin SR, Lee YJ, Tsai JH. Mutations of the p53 gene in human functional adrenal neoplasms. *J Clin Endocrinol Metab*. 1994;78:483–491.
128. Reincke M, Wachenfeld C, Mora P, et al. p53 mutations in adrenal tumors: Caucasian patients do not show the exon 4 "hot spot" found in Taiwan. *J Clin Endocrinol Metab*. 1996;81:3636–3638.
129. Wagner J, Portwine C, Rabin K, Leclerc JM, Narod SA, Malkin D. High frequency of germline p53 mutations in childhood adrenocortical cancer. *J Natl Cancer Inst*. 1994;86:1707–1710.
130. Ribeiro RC, Sandrini F, Figueiredo B, et al. An inherited p53 mutation that contributes in a tissue-specific manner to pediatric adrenal cortical carcinoma. *Proc Natl Acad Sci USA*. 2001;98:9330–9335.
131. Latronico AC, Pinto EM, Domenice S, et al. An inherited mutation outside the highly conserved DNA-binding domain of the p53 tumor suppressor protein in children and adults with sporadic adrenocortical tumors. *J Clin Endocrinol Metab*. 2001;86:4970–4973.
132. Figueiredo BC, Sandrini R, Zambetti GP, et al. Penetrance of adrenocortical tumours associated with the germline TP53 R337H mutation. *J Med Genet*. 2006;43:91–96.
133. Zwermann O, Beuschlein F, Mora P, Weber G, Allolio B, Reincke M. Multiple endocrine neoplasia type 1 gene expression is normal in sporadic adrenocortical tumors. *Eur J Endocrinol*. 2000;142:689–695.
134. De Fraipont F, Le Moigne G, Defaye G, et al. Transcription profiling of benign and malignant adrenal tumors by cDNA macro-array analysis. *Endocr Res*. 2002;28:785–786.
135. Giordano TJ, Thomas DG, Kuick R, et al. Distinct transcriptional profiles of adrenocortical tumors uncovered by DNA microarray analysis. *Am J Pathol*. 2003;162:521–531.
136. de Fraipont F, El Atifi M, Cherradi N, et al. Gene expression profiling of human adrenocortical tumors using complementary deoxyribonucleic Acid microarrays identifies several candidate genes as markers of malignancy. *J Clin Endocrinol Metab*. 2005;90:1819–1829.
137. Slater EP, Diehl SM, Langer P, et al. Analysis by cDNA microarrays of gene expression patterns of human adrenocortical tumors. *Eur J Endocrinol*. 2006;154:587–598.

138. Giordano TJ. Molecular pathology of adrenal cortical tumors: separating adenomas from carcinomas. *Endocr Pathol*. 2006; 17:355–363.
139. Allolio B, Fassnacht M. Clinical review: adrenocortical carcinoma: clinical update. *J Clin Endocrinol Metab*. 2006;91:2027–2037.
140. McNicol AM, Struthers AJ, Nolan CE, Hermans J, Haak HR. Proliferation in adrenocortical tumors: correlation with clinical outcome and p53 status. *Endocr Pathol*. 1997;8:29–36.
141. Riepe FG, Sippell WG. Recent advances in diagnosis, treatment, and outcome of congenital adrenal hyperplasia due to 21-hydroxylase deficiency. *Rev Endocr Metab Disord*. 2007;8:349–363.
142. New MI. An update of congenital adrenal hyperplasia. *Ann N Y Acad Sci*. 2004;1038:14–43.
143. Pang S, Murphey W, Levine LS, et al. A pilot newborn screening for congenital adrenal hyperplasia in Alaska. *J Clin Endocrinol Metab*. 1982;55:413–420.
144. Pang SY, Wallace MA, Hofman L, et al. Worldwide experience in newborn screening for classical congenital adrenal hyperplasia due to 21-hydroxylase deficiency. *Pediatrics*. 1988; 81:866–874.
145. Speiser PW, Dupont B, Rubinstein P, et al. High frequency of non-classical steroid 21-hydroxylase deficiency. *Am J Hum Genet*. 1985;37:650–657.
146. Fitness J, Dixit N, Webster D, et al. Genotyping of CYP21, linked chromosome 6p markers, and a sex-specific gene in neonatal screening for congenital adrenal hyperplasia. *J Clin Endocrinol Metab*. 1999;84:960–966.
147. Levine LS, Sachmann M, New MI, et al. Genetic mapping of the 21-hydroxylase deficiency gene within the HLA linkage group. *N Engl J Med*. 1978;299:911–915.
148. White PC, New MI, Dupont B. Structure of the human steroid 21-hydroxylase genes. *Proc Natl Acad Sci USA*. 1986;83: 5111–5115.
149. Simard J, Ricketts ML, Gingras S, Soucy P, Feltus FA, Melner MH. Molecular biology of the 3beta-hydroxysteroid dehydrogenase/delta5-delta4 isomerase gene family. *Endocr Rev*. 2005;26:525–582.
150. Bauman A, Bauman CG. Virilizing adrenocortical carcinoma. Development in a patient with salt- losing congenital adrenal hyperplasia. *JAMA*. 1982;248:3140–3141.
151. Merke DP, Bornstein SR, Braddock D, Chrousos GP. Adrenal lymphocytic infiltration and adrenocortical tumors in a patient with 21-hydroxylase deficiency [letter]. *N Engl J Med*. 1999; 340:1121–1122.
152. Fujieda K, Okuhara K, Abe S, Tajima T, Mukai T, Nakae J. Molecular pathogenesis of lipoid adrenal hyperplasia and adrenal hypoplasia congenita. *J Steroid Biochem Mol Biol*. 2003;85:483–489.
153. Sugawara T, Holt JA, Driscoll D, et al. Human steroidogenic acute regulatory protein: functional activity in COS-1 cells, tissue-specific expression, and mapping of the structural gene to 8p11.2 and a pseudogene to chromosome 13. *Proc Natl Acad Sci USA*. 1995;92:4778–4782.
154. Peter M, Viemann M, Partsch CJ, Sippell WG. Congenital adrenal hypoplasia: clinical spectrum, experience with hormonal diagnosis, and report on new point mutations of the DAX-1 gene. *J Clin Endocrinol Metab*. 1998;83: 2666–2674.
155. Lin L, Hindmarsh PC, Metherell LA, et al. Severe loss-of-function mutations in the adrenocorticotropin receptor (ACTHR, MC2R) can be found in patients diagnosed with salt-losing adrenal hypoplasia. *Clin Endocrinol (Oxf)*. 2007;66:205–210.
156. Smith KD, Kemp S, Braiterman LT, et al. X-linked adrenoleukodystrophy: genes, mutations, and phenotypes. *Neurochem Res*. 1999;24:521–535.
157. Savary S, Troffer-Charlier N, Gyapay G, Mattei MG, Chimini G. Chromosomal localization of the adrenoleukodystrophy-related gene in man and mice. *Eur J Hum Genet*. 1997;5: 99–101.
158. Dodd A, Rowland SA, Hawkes SL, Kennedy MA, Love DR. Mutations in the adrenoleukodystrophy gene. *Hum Mutat*. 1997;9:500–511.
159. Krasemann EW, Meier V, Korenke GC, Hunneman DH, Hanefeld F. Identification of mutations in the ALD-gene of 20 families with adrenoleukodystrophy/adrenomyeloneuropathy. *Hum Genet*. 1996;97:194–197.
160. Laureti S, Casucci G, Santeusanio F, Angeletti G, Aubourg P, Brunetti P. X-linked adrenoleukodystrophy is a frequent cause of idiopathic Addison's disease in young adult male patients. *J Clin Endocrinol Metab*. 1996;81:470–474.
161. Collares CV, Antunes-Rodrigues J, Moreira AC, et al. Heterogeneity in the molecular basis of ACTH resistance syndrome. *Eur J Endocrinol*. 2008;159:61–68.
162. Metherell LA, Chan LF, Clark AJ. The genetics of ACTH resistance syndromes. *Best Pract Res Clin Endocrinol Metab*. 2006;20:547–560.
163. Connell JM, Inglis GC, Fraser R, Jamieson A. Dexamethasone-suppressible hyperaldosteronism: clinical, biochemical and genetic relations. *J Hum Hypertens*. 1995;9:505–509.
164. Miyahara K, Kawamoto T, Mitsuuchi Y, et al. The chimeric gene linked to glucocorticoid- suppressible hyperaldosteronism encodes a fused P-450 protein possessing aldosterone synthase activity. *Biochem Biophys Res Commun*. 1992;189: 885–891.
165. So A, Duffy DL, Gordon RD, et al. Familial hyperaldosteronism type II is linked to the chromosome 7p22 region but also shows predicted heterogeneity. *J Hypertens*. 2005;23:1477–1484.

Section 6
Pancreatic Neuroendocrine Tumors

22
Clinical Detection and Treatment of Pancreatic Neuroendocrine Tumors

Jamie C. Mitchell

Introduction

Pancreatic endocrine neoplasms (PEN) typically generate a great deal of clinician interest because of the rarity with which they occur and their associated hormonal syndromes. While their rarity has limited research efforts into the pathophysiology of these tumors to some extent, recent advances in molecular biology techniques have allowed investigators to provide new insights into the pathogenesis of these lesions allowing the development of novel techniques for the diagnosis, localization, and treatment of PENs.

The mainstay of therapy for these tumors has consisted of surgical resection for locoregional disease in the setting of malignancy, as well as for the relief of hormonal hypersecretion syndromes due to secretion of various hormones such as vasoactive intestinal peptide (VIP), gastrin, glucagon, somatostatin, and insulin. In the setting of metastatic disease, curative surgical resection is not usually feasible. However, the generally indolent biology of these tumors, the fact that that these patients frequently have a high performance status and preserved organ function, and the presence of symptomatic hormonal hypersecretion favor aggressive approaches to treatment even in the presence of widespread metastases. Traditional cytotoxic chemotherapeutic regimens typically are not successful in effecting significant responses in these tumors. Consequently, there has been a great deal of interest in the development of novel molecular methods with which to target these tumors. In this chapter, we review recent advances in molecular techniques being utilized to diagnose, localize, and treat PEN.

Diagnosis

PENs can be divided into two general categories, those that cause syndromes of hormone overproduction and those that do not. The clinical presentation of these tumors reflects the nature of these categories, with the symptoms of hormonal hypersecretion prompting evaluation and subsequent discovery of the pancreatic neoplasm in cases of functional lesions, while nonfunctioning lesions present because of mass effect or are discovered incidentally during imaging studies obtained for unrelated reasons.

While biochemical studies are utilized to establish the diagnosis of functional PENs, tumor markers are also important in establishing their diagnosis, particularly in the setting of nonfunctioning neoplasms. Chromogranin-A, a 439 amino acid secretory protein produced by dense core vesicles of neuroendocrine cells, has been found to be the most sensitive marker for the presence of PENs.[1,2] However, several other conditions can result in elevations of this peptide, such as renal failure, heart failure, and atrophic gastritis, limiting its specificity. Sensitivity has been reported as ranging between 80% and 100% for functional PENs and 50% and 70% for nonfunctional PENs.[3–5] In addition to diagnosis, this marker is useful in the postoperative surveillance of patients with these tumors and has been shown to correlate with prognosis as well.[6]

While chromogranin-A is the primary tumor marker utilized in the diagnosis and surveillance of pancreatic neuroendocrine tumors, others have been investigated. Many PENs secrete pancreatic polypeptide (PP), a 36 amino acid peptide secreted by islet cells primarily in the head of the pancreas.[7] The physiologic role of this peptide has yet to be fully elucidated, but it has also been considered a potential parker for PENs. Several studies published in the early 1980's found that the sensitivity of PP was not sufficient to be clinically useful.[8,9] However, a more recent study published in 2004 evaluated the utility of PP in conjunction with chromogranin A as markers for neuroendocrine tumors. They found that in the 68 patients studied, the addition of PP increased the sensitivity of detection of all PENs from 74% to 94% and nonfunctioning PENs from 68% to 93% when compared with chromogranin A alone ($p < 0.05$). These results suggest a role for PP as a tumor marker in patients with nonfunctional PENs.

Other tumor markers, such as neuron-specific enolase and the alpha subunit of glycoprotein, have been evaluated for their utility in the diagnosis and follow-up of PENs, but have been found to be lacking in clinical utility because of

J.L. Hunt (ed.), *Molecular Pathology of Endocrine Diseases*, Molecular Pathology Library 3,
DOI 10.1007/978-1-4419-1707-2_22, © Springer Science+Business Media, LLC 2010

TABLE 22.1. Serum markers in the diagnosis and follow-up of NET's.

Marker	Tumor type	Clinical utility
Chromogranin A	Islet cell tumors, carcinoids pheochromocytomas	Primary marker used clinically
Pancreatic polypeptide	Islet cell tumors	High sensitivity w/chromogranin A
NESP-55	Islet cell tumors, pheochromocytomas	Distinguishing islet-cell tumors from carcinoids

NET neuroendocrine tumor, *NESP-55* neuroendocrine secretory peptide-55.

TABLE 22.2. Somatostatin analogues used in localization and treatment of NET's.

Analogue	Amino acid sequence
Octreotide	D-Phe – Cys – Phe – D-Trp | | Thr(ol) – Cys – Thr – Lys
Lanreotide	D-β-Nal – Cys – Tyr – D-Trp | | NH_2-Thr – Cys – Val – Lys
Octreotate	D-Phe – Cys – Tyr – D-Trp | | Thr – Cys – Thr – Lys
Vapreotide	D-Phe – Cys – Tyr – D-Trp | | NH_2-Trp – Cys – Val – Lys

NET neuroendocrine tumor, *phe* phenylalanine, *cys* cysteine, *trp* tryptophan, *thr* threonine, *lys* lysine.

low sensitivity and specificity. Neuroendocrine secretory peptide-55 (NESP-55) is a 241 amino acid peptide secreted by neuroendocrine cells and a member of the chromogranin family. This peptide has been shown to be secreted by PENs and pheochromocytomas, but not carcinoid tumors, suggesting that this marker could play a role in the diagnosis and localization of gastroenteropancreatic endocrine tumors.[10] Other published reports have shown evidence that chromogranin-A is processed differently by various neuroendocrine tumors and that by analyzing the breakdown products of this marker, or chromogranin-related peptides, one can gain insight into the type of tumor present.[11,12] However, these potential applications have not been borne out by additional studies and have not gained widespread clinical acceptance, with chromogranin-A remaining the standard of care in the diagnosis and follow-up of neuroendocrine tumors (Table 22.1).

Localization

Localization of neuroendocrine tumors was initially limited to anatomic imaging studies such as computed tomography (CT), ultrasound (US), or magnetic resonance imaging (MRI). More recently, functional imaging of these tumors has been developed and become an essential step in the management of many of these tumors. This development was based on the fact that many neuroendocrine tumors express somatostatin receptors on their cell surfaces. Somatostatin is a cyclic neuropeptide containing 14 (SST-14) or 18 (SST-18) amino acids. This peptide has an inhibitory effect on several organ systems by decreasing neurotransmission, the secretion of growth hormone and thyrotropin-stimulating hormone, gastric acid production, pancreatic exocrine secretion, and secretion of insulin and glucagon.[13] These effects are mediated by interaction of SST with its receptors on various target cells. There are five SST receptors (SST-R1-5) that have been described.

Somatostatin Receptor Sintigraphy

The fact that neuroendocrine tumors express relatively more SST-R than normal tissues has been the basis of the development of these functional imaging techniques, referred to as somatostatin receptor sintigraphy (SRS). Native SST-14 and SST-18 are not stable in the bloodstream, so various SST analogues were developed that were much more resistant to degradation and consequently had significantly longer half-lives, including octreotide, lanreotide, and vapreotide (Table 22.2).[14,15] The high affinity of these peptides for SST-R (SST-R2 > SST-R5 > SST-R3) and the internalization of the peptide–receptor complex facilitate the retention of the radiopeptide in receptor-expressing tumor cells. Additionally, their small size (Octreotide is eight amino acids in length) allows for rapid clearance from the bloodstream. Subsequently, these analogues were conjugated with various radioisotopes and bound to a chelator such as diethylenetriaminepentaacetic acid (DTPA) to ensure stability. For example, conjugating octreotide with ^{111}In and DTPA forms DTPA-D-Phe-Octreotide (Octreoscan).[16] Use of this radiopharmaceutical has become the mainstay of molecular imaging studies for the localization of neuroendocrine tumors, including those of the pancreas, with sensitivities ranging from 60% to 90% depending on the tumor type.

Other radiopharmaceuticals have continued to be developed in an effort to improve upon the sensitivity of detecting neuroendocrine tumors. Somatostatin analogues have also been conjugated with 1,4,7,10-tetraazacyclododecane-*N*,*N′*,*N″*,*N‴*-tetraacetic acid (DOTA) and ^{111}In to form ^{111}In-DOTA-DPhel-Tyr3-octreotide, ^{111}In-DOTA-lanreotide, and ^{111}In-DOTA-octreotate. Of these, ^{111}In-DOTA-octreotate has been shown to have the highest affinity for SST-R2.[17–19]

Vasoactive Intestinal Peptide Scintigraphy

In addition to various SST analogues, other peptides have been evaluated for their utility in the localization of neuroendocrine tumors. Included in these is vasoactive intestinal peptide (VIP) comprised of 28 amino acids. VIP receptors are found in a wide variety of tissues, including pancreas, GI mucosa, lung, thyroid, and lymphoid tissues. VIP has been conjugated with radiolabelled iodine (^{123}I) and technetium (^{99}Tc), and used clinically in the imaging of PENs.[20,21] This radiopharmaceutical has shown some benefit in patients with neuroendocrine tumors receiving somatostatin therapy as this decreases the sensitivity of SRS. Additionally, some studies have shown that this radiopeptide is more sensitive for the localization of insulinomas, suggesting potential clinical applicability, however, currently this has not become routinely used in practice.[20]

Cholecystokinin-B/Gastrin Receptor Scintigraphy

One other target that has been explored as a candidate for molecular imaging of PENs is the cholecystokinin (CCK) receptor. Two primary receptor subtypes have been identified for CCK, called CCKAR and CCKBR. Of these, CCKAR is expressed in the pancreas, in addition to areas of GI tract smooth muscle, the gastric mucosa, and regions of the central nervous system. CCKBR, which is also the receptor for gastrin, is expressed in the nervous system and various aspects of the gastric mucosa.[22] Both of these CCK receptors have been found to be overexpressed in gastroenteropancreatic PEN, which has led to the development of several CCK and gastrin derivatives to be used as potential in vivo receptor targeting for localization or therapy. One group showed that radioiodinated gastrin could be used to specifically target CCKBR in a xenograft model of medullary thyroid cancer (MTC) and in a patient with metastatic MTC.[23] DTPA-coupled derivatives of this peptide have also been characterized, with one such radiopeptide being evaluated in a clinical trial of MTC.[24,25] These studies have validated the potential utility of CCK/gastrin analogues for targeted imaging or therapy of patients with neuroendocrine tumors, particularly in the setting of MTC. Further studies are needed to determine whether or not this will be applicable to PENs.

Positron Emission Tomography

Positron emission tomography (PET) scanning has gained widespread oncologic applicability in the treatment of various tumors. PET scanning using [^{18}F]fluoro-2-deoxy-d-glucose (FDG) has been increasingly utilized for diagnosis, staging, restaging, and evaluation of response to treatment of many tumor types. FDG–PET scanning relies on the principle that tumor cells are more metabolically active than normal cells and therefore utilize glucose at a higher rate. FDG can be taken up by cells by the same mechanism as glucose, but FDG cannot continue along the glycolytic pathway leading to accumulation of this tracer in the tumor cells, which can then be imaged. While this radiopharmaceutical has shown to be useful for the imaging of many tumor types, it has not been successful at localizing neuroendocrine tumors. This is due to the fact that most neuroendocrine tumors are well-differentiated, slow-growing tumors with largely normal glucose metabolism. To combat this problem, ^{11}C-5-hydroxy-L-tryptophan (^{11}C-HTP) and ^{18}F-L-dihydroxyphenylalanine (^{18}F-DOPA) were developed for PET imaging of these tumors. The principle of the use of these radiopharmaceuticals is based on the ability of neuroendocrine cells to take up these amine precursors, transform them by decarboxylation into biogenic amines, and retain them in storage vesicles. ^{11}C-HTP was found to have greater uptake by PENs in a study comparing it and ^{18}F-DOPA. Subsequent studies showed that ^{11}C-HTP-PET had higher sensitivity than CT and SRS for visualizing neuroendocrine tumors and was able to detect many small, previously overlooked lesions by these other imaging modalities.[26–28]

Another recent study compared ^{11}C-HTP-PET with ^{18}F-DOPA-PET in the localization of 24 carcinoid tumors and 23 PENs. The authors found that the sensitivity for detection of carcinoid tumors was greatest with ^{18}F-DOPA-PET/CT (98%), while the greatest sensitivity for detecting islet cell tumors was ^{11}C-HTP-PET/CT (96%). Both of these modalities were superior to SRS and SRS/CT for the detection of PENs.[29] It has become clear that PET scanning is a valuable tool in the diagnosis, staging, and follow up of patients with PENs. Table 22.3 summarizes the molecular markers used in the localization of PENs and their targets.

TABLE 22.3. Molecular targets used in the localization of NET's.

Imaging modality	Marker	Target receptor
Scintigraphy	Somatostatin analogues	SST-R1-5
	VIP analogues	VIP-R
	Cholecystokinin/Gastrin	CCKAR/CCKBR
Positron emission	5-Hydroxy-L-tryptophan	NET secretory vesicles
tomography	L-Dihydroxyphenylalanine	NET secretory vesicles

NET neuroendocrine tumor, *VIP* vasoactive intestinal peptide, *CCKAR/BR* cholecystokinin A&B receptors, *SST-R* somatostatin receptor.

Therapy

PENs are a heterogeneous group of tumors with varying malignant potentials. While these tumors often display indolent biologic behavior, they frequently have metastasized at the time of initial presentation. Historically, the mainstay of therapy for systemic disease was SST analogues. While these were fairly successful in controlling symptoms from hormonal hypersecretion, with various studies reporting improvement in symptoms in 50–60% of patients, rarely did they result in tumor regression (3–5% of patients). Additionally, traditional chemotherapeutic agents have not been effective at generating significant responses in these tumors. Consequently, there has been a great deal of research performed in an effort to develop more effective therapeutic options for patients with metastatic PENs.

Targeted Peptide Receptor Radiotherapy

During the past decade, that research effort has led to the development of peptide receptor radionuclide therapy. Similar to the imaging modalities discussed previously, this therapy exploits the fact that many PENs express SST receptors on their cell surfaces. While SST itself does not lead to significant tumor regression, researchers hoped to utilize the affinity of SST to neuroendocrine tumor cells to create a delivery mechanism for cytotoxic agents resulting in tumor destruction. Several radioisotopes have been conjugated with SST analogues to serve as the cytotoxic agent. In the following section, we review the results of studies examining this therapeutic modality.

^{111}In-DTPA-Octreotide

As this was the most widely used radiopeptide for the imaging of PENs, ^{111}In-DTPA-octreotide also became the first to be examined for its therapeutic efficacy against advanced tumors. Initial studies showed limited responses, but no therapeutic effect was observed in the setting of larger tumors or widespread metastases.[30–32] The limited effect was likely due to the fact that this radioisotope emits mainly γ-radiation which is a relatively low-energy emitter with limited particle range and therefore tissue penetration.

^{90}Y-DOTA-Octreotide

The next generation of SST analogues, such as DOTA-octreotide, were also examined for their potential therapeutic utility. The use of DOTA as a chelator allowed stable radiolabeling with β-emitting radionuclides such as yttrium-90 (^{90}Y) which is advantageous in that these higher-energy particles have sufficient energy to cause cell damage without penetrating significantly into surrounding tissues.[33] Additionally, DOTA has higher affinity for SST-R2 than DTPA. Figure 22.1 shows the structure of these ligands. Several phase I and II trials using ^{90}Y-DOTA analogues have been performed with objective response rates ranging from 9 to 33%.[34]

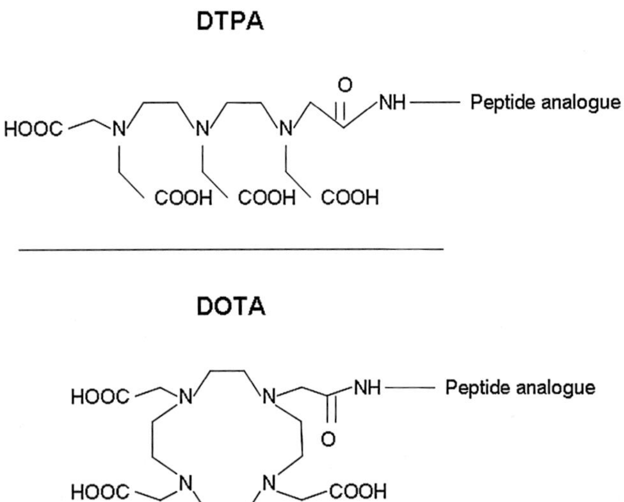

Fig. 22.1. Ligands used for radiopeptide imaging and therapy.

^{177}Lu-DOTA-Tyr^3-Octreotate

Lutetium-177-DOTA-Tyr^3-octreotate (^{177}Lu-DOTATOC) is a third generation SST analogue which has even higher affinity for SST-R2, showing increased binding to SST-R2 positive tissue in vitro and in vivo.[17,35] An additional advantage in this third generation SST analogue is the ability to deliver higher adsorbed radiation doses to tumors without increasing the radiation dose to dose-limiting organs, such as the kidneys and bone marrow.[19] In 2003, Kwekkeboom and colleagues published the results of a study looking at the effects of ^{177}Lu-DOTATOC on 34 patients with neuroendocrine tumors of varying sizes. They reported 1 complete remission (3%), 12 partial remissions (35%), 14 patients with stable disease (41%), and progressive disease in seven patients (21%) after 3 months of therapy.[36] They also found a significant improvement in quality of life for these patients, even those with progressive disease.

A more recent study looked at the results of therapy in 131 patients treated with this radiopharmaceutical, with three patients with complete remission (2%), 32 with partial remission (26%), 24 with a minor response defined as a decrease in tumor diameter of 25–50% (19%), and 44 patients with stable disease (35%). Twenty-two patients developed progressive disease despite therapy (18%). Median time to progression for responders was 36 months. In both of these studies, clinical response correlated with uptake on their diagnostic pretreatment ^{111}In-octreotide scan.[37]

The availability of several SST-analogues with varying characteristics offers the potential of therapy tailored to a particular tumor type. For example, the emitting β-particle range of both ^{177}Lu and ^{90}Y exceeds the target cell diameter, allowing irradiation of neighboring tumor cells. This is particularly important in tumors with heterogeneous SST-R expression, such that even tumor cells without SST-R can be treated, and offers an advantage over ^{111}In analogues. ^{177}Lu has lower tissue penetration than ^{90}Y, making it a better choice for smaller tumors, while ^{90}Y may be a better alternative for larger tumors. Another clinical advantage of ^{177}Lu is that , unlike ^{90}Y, it emits low-energy γ-rays, which allows for dosimetry and imaging immediately following DOTATOC therapy. Serious side-effects related to therapy with radiolabeled SST analogues are rare, but include myelodysplastic syndromes, renal toxicity, and hepatic toxicity. See Table 22.4 for a summary of commonly used radionuclides in the localization and treatment of neuroendocrine tumors.

Somatostatin Receptor Upregulation

Radiation-Induced Upregulation

The data from these and other studies examining the efficacy of targeted peptide receptor radiotherapy for gastroenteric and pancreatic neuroendocrine tumors have confirmed the potential of this therapeutic modality for unresectable or widespread tumors. Ongoing studies continue to search for

TABLE 22.4. Radiopharmaceuticals utilized in localization and treatment of NET's.

Radionuclide	Emission	½ Life	Tissue penetration	Advantage/disadvantage
^{111}Indium (^{111}In)	γ-rays Auger electrons	2.8 days	10 µm	Limited by small particle range
^{90}Yttrium (^{90}Y)	β-particles	2.7 days	12 mm	Higher energy and penetration allow tx of larger tumors
^{177}Lutetium (^{177}Lu)	β-particles γ-rays	6.7 days	2 mm	γ-rays allow scintigraphy after tx

NET neuroendocrine tumors, *tx* treatment.

ways to improve upon the efficacy of this therapy. One area of research is focusing on ways to increase SST-R expression in gastroenteric and pancreatic tumors, making them more sensitive to targeted peptide receptor radiotherapy. Early studies have shown that upregulation of SST-R occurs in some pancreatic neuroendocrine tumors after treatment with external beam radiation and low therapeutic doses of radiolabeled peptides such as ^{111}In-DTPA-octreotide.[38,39]

Gene Therapy-Induced Upregulation

The use of gene therapy as a means of increasing SST-R expression in neuroendocrine tumors has also begun to be explored. Using viral or nonviral vectors, peptide-receptor encoding genes, such as SST-R, can be transferred into tumor cells with the aim of increasing tumor sensitivity to targeted peptide radiotherapy. Studies in animals have been performed using a dual gene transfer concept. In addition to a gene for SST-R, a "suicide" gene is transferred to tumor cells as well. An example of such a gene is one for viral thymidine kinase, which unlike the mammalian enzyme, phosphorylates acycloguanosines such as acyclovir and ganciclovir. Further enzymatic processing results in these "prodrugs" being incorporated into tumor cell DNA, in effect inhibiting further DNA replication. The combination of this with targeted peptide radiotherapy using β-particle-emitting radiopeptides such as ^{177}Lu-DOTATOC or ^{90}Y-DOTA allows a two-hit therapeutic effect. Tumor cells not transduced with the viral vector can still be treated because of the particle range of these radiopeptides.[40–42]

Several other areas of research are ongoing to improve targeted radiopeptide therapy for neuroendocrine tumors. These include the use of novel radiopeptides such as copper-64 and rhenium-188, combination therapy with radiosensitizing agents such as 5-fluorouracil (5-FU),[43] combinations of multiple radiolabeled SST-analogues, and combining SST-analogues with apoptosis-inducing peptides.[44] These studies are in their early phases and time is needed to determine their clinical applicability, but early results are encouraging.

Other Therapeutic Modalities

VEGF-Inhibitors

Inhibition of angiogenesis has become an exciting area of cancer therapeutics in recent years. A group of drugs have been developed which inhibit vascular endothelial growth factor receptors (VEGF-R), a tyrosine kinase receptor. As PENs are known to be vascular tumors and have been shown to over-express VEGF-R, some of these drugs have been examined for their therapeutic potential in treating advanced or widespread PENs. One phase-II multicenter study published recently by Kulke and colleagues looked at the use of Sunitinib, a tyrosine kinase inhibitor with activity against several VEGF-R's and other tyrosine kinases. One hundred seven patients, 41 with PENs, received treatment with Sunitinib, with objective responses by RECIST criteria seen in 11 patients (17%), and stabilization of disease in 45 patients (68%). Monoclonal antibodies against VEGF, such as bevacizumab, have also been studied in the treatment of advanced neuroendocrine tumors in phase II trials, but thus far clinical trials have been limited to patients with carcinoid tumors.[45]

TABLE 22.5. Other molecular markers being evaluated for the treatment of NET's.

Mechanism	Agent	Status of clinical trials
VEGF monoclonal Ab	Bevacizumab	Phase III trials developing
VEGF inhibitor	Sunitinib	Phase II trials completed
	Vatalanib	Phase II trials ongoing
	Sorafenib	Phase II trials ongoing
mTOR inhibitor	Everolimus (RAD001)	Phase III trials developing
	Temserolimus	Phase II trials completed

VEGF vascular endothelial growth factor, *mTOR* mammalian target of rapamycin, *Ab* antibody, *NET* neuroendocrine tumors.

mTOR-Inhibitors

The mammalian target of rapamycin (mTOR) is an intracellular protein critical to control of cell growth, protein synthesis, and autophagy. Downstream targets include the tyrosine kinases VEGF and insulin-like growth factor (IGF), and abnormalities in this pathway have been implicated in the pathogenesis of several tumor types, including neuroendocrine tumors. A phase-II trial evaluating the use of the mTOR inhibitor everolimus in patients with neuroendocrine tumors, including carcinoids and PENs, showed an overall response rate of 13%, with 73% of patients with stable disease and progression free survival at 24 weeks of 64%.[46] Based on these results, additional clinical trials are currently in accrual. Table 22.5 summarizes the status of clinical trials for VEGF and mTOR inhibitors in the treatment of neuroendocrine tumors.

Conclusion

The treatment of advanced PENs has traditionally been restricted to medical therapy for symptomatic relief of hormone-related symptoms. Recent advances in the development of new somatostatin analogues, radiopeptides, and chelators have significantly improved our ability to use these radiopeptides in the localization and treatment of these tumors. Additionally, advances in our understanding of the molecular pathogenesis of PENs have led to the development of exciting new molecular treatment strategies utilizing inhibitors of critical signaling pathways in neuroendocrine tumor cells resulting in arrest of tumor progression or even significant reduction in tumor volume in some of these patients. Ongoing studies attempting to improve upon these promising therapeutic modalities continue offering new hope to patients with advanced PENs.

References

1. Stridsberg M, Oberg K, Li Q, Engstrom U, Lundqvist G. Measurements of chromogranin A, chromogranin B (secretogranin I), chromogranin C (secretogranin II) and pancreastatin in plasma and urine from patients with carcinoid tumours and endocrine pancreatic tumours. *J Endocrinol.* 1995;144(1):49–59.
2. Nobels FR, Kwekkeboom DJ, Bouillon R, Lamberts SW. Chromogranin A: its clinical value as marker of neuroendocrine tumours. *Eur J Clin Invest.* 1998;28(6):431–440.
3. Nobels FR, Kwekkeboom DJ, Coopmans W, et al. Chromogranin A as serum marker for neuroendocrine neoplasia: comparison with neuron-specific enolase and the alpha-subunit of glycoprotein hormones. *J Clin Endocrinol Metab.* 1997;82(8):2622–2628.
4. Bajetta E, Ferrari L, Martinetti A, et al. Chromogranin A, neuron specific enolase, carcinoembryonic antigen, and hydroxyindole acetic acid evaluation in patients with neuroendocrine tumors. *Cancer.* 1999;86(5):858–865.
5. Tomassetti P, Migliori M, Simoni P, et al. Diagnostic value of plasma chromogranin A in neuroendocrine tumours. *Eur J Gastroenterol Hepatol.* 2001;13(1):55–58.
6. Janson ET, Holmberg L, Stridsberg M, et al. Carcinoid tumors: analysis of prognostic factors and survival in 301 patients from a referral center. *Ann Oncol.* 1997;8(7):685–690.
7. Adrian TE, Bloom SR, Bryant MG, Polak JM, Heitz PH, Barnes AJ. Distribution and release of human pancreatic polypeptide. *Gut.* 1976;17(12):940–944.
8. Bloom SR, Adrian TE, Polak JM. Pancreatic polypeptide from pancreatic endocrine tumours. *Lancet.* 1980;2(8202):1026.
9. Oberg K, Grimelius L, Lundqvist G, Lorelius LE. Update on pancreatic polypeptide as a specific marker for endocrine tumours of the pancreas and gut. *Acta Med Scand.* 1981;210(3):145–152.
10. Srivastava A, Padilla O, Fischer-Colbrie R, Tischler AS, Dayal Y. Neuroendocrine secretory protein-55 (NESP-55) expression discriminates pancreatic endocrine tumors and pheochromocytomas from gastrointestinal and pulmonary carcinoids. *Am J Surg Pathol.* 2004;28(10):1371–1378.
11. Stridsberg M, Eriksson B, Oberg K, Janson ET. A panel of 11 region-specific radioimmunoassays for measurements of human chromogranin A. *Regul Pept.* 2004;117(3):219–227.
12. Oberg K. Neuroendocrine tumors of the gastrointestinal tract: recent advances in molecular genetics, diagnosis, and treatment. *Curr Opin Oncol.* 2005;17(4):386–391.
13. Li S, Beheshti M. The radionuclide molecular imaging and therapy of neuroendocrine tumors. *Curr Cancer Drug Targets.* 2005;5(2):139–148.
14. Virgolini I, Traub T, Leimer M, et al. New radiopharmaceuticals for receptor scintigraphy and radionuclide therapy. *Q J Nucl Med.* 2000;44(1):50–58.
15. Breeman WA, Kwekkeboom DJ, Kooij PP, et al. Effect of dose and specific activity on tissue distribution of indium-111-pentetreotide in rats. *J Nucl Med.* 1995;36(4):623–627.
16. Krenning EP, Kwekkeboom DJ, Bakker WH, et al. Somatostatin receptor scintigraphy with [111In-DTPA-D-Phe1]- and [123I-Tyr3]-octreotide: the Rotterdam experience with more than 1000 patients. *Eur J Nucl Med.* 1993;20(8):716–731.
17. Reubi JC, Schar JC, Waser B, et al. Affinity profiles for human somatostatin receptor subtypes SST1-SST5 of somatostatin radiotracers selected for scintigraphic and radiotherapeutic use. *Eur J Nucl Med.* 2000;27(3):273–282.
18. Virgolini I, Patri P, Novotny C, et al. Comparative somatostatin receptor scintigraphy using in-111-DOTA-lanreotide and in-111-DOTA-Tyr3-octreotide versus F-18-FDG-PET for evaluation of somatostatin receptor-mediated radionuclide therapy. *Ann Oncol.* 2001;12(suppl 2):S41–S45.
19. Kwekkeboom DJ, Bakker WH, Kooij PP, et al. [177Lu-DOTAOTyr3]octreotate: comparison with [111In-DTPAo]octreotide in patients. *Eur J Nucl Med.* 2001;28(9):1319–1325.
20. Virgolini I, Raderer M, Kurtaran A, et al. Vasoactive intestinal peptide-receptor imaging for the localization of intestinal adenocarcinomas and endocrine tumors. *N Engl J Med.* 1994;331(17):1116–1121.
21. Thakur ML, Marcus CS, Saeed S, et al. 99mTc-labeled vasoactive intestinal peptide analog for rapid localization of tumors in humans. *J Nucl Med.* 2000;41(1):107–110.
22. Wank SA. G protein-coupled receptors in gastrointestinal physiology I CCK receptors: an exemplary family. *Am J Physiol.* 1998;274(4 Pt 1):G607–G613.
23. Behr TM, Jenner N, Radetzky S, et al. Targeting of cholecystokinin-B/gastrin receptors in vivo: preclinical and initial clinical evaluation of the diagnostic and therapeutic potential of radiolabelled gastrin. *Eur J Nucl Med.* 1998;25(4):424–430.
24. Reubi JC, Waser B, Schaer JC, et al. Unsulfated DTPA- and DOTA-CCK analogs as specific high-affinity ligands for CCK-B receptor-expressing human and rat tissues in vitro and in vivo. *Eur J Nucl Med.* 1998;25(5):481–490.
25. Kwekkeboom DJ, Bakker WH, Kooij PP, et al. Cholecystokinin receptor imaging using an octapeptide DTPA-CCK analogue in patients with medullary thyroid carcinoma. *Eur J Nucl Med.* 2000;27(9):1312–1317.
26. Kaltsas G, Rockall A, Papadogias D, Reznek R, Grossman AB. Recent advances in radiological and radionuclide imaging and therapy of neuroendocrine tumours. *Eur J Endocrinol.* 2004;151(1):15–27.
27. Bombardieri E, Seregni E, Villano C, Chiti A, Bajetta E. Position of nuclear medicine techniques in the diagnostic work-up of neuroendocrine tumors. *Q J Nucl Med Mol Imaging.* 2004;48(2):150–163.
28. Sundin A, Eriksson B, Bergstrom M, Langstrom B, Oberg K, Orlefors H. PET in the diagnosis of neuroendocrine tumors. *Ann N Y Acad Sci.* 2004;1014:246–257.

29. Koopmans KP, Neels OC, Kema IP, et al. Improved staging of patients with carcinoid and islet cell tumors with 18F-dihydroxy-phenyl-alanine and 11C-5-hydroxy-tryptophan positron emission tomography. *J Clin Oncol.* 2008;26(9):1489–1495.
30. Valkema R, De Jong M, Bakker WH, et al. Phase I study of peptide receptor radionuclide therapy with [In-DTPA]octreotide: the Rotterdam experience. *Semin Nucl Med.* 2002;32(2): 110–122.
31. Anthony LB, Woltering EA, Espenan GD, Cronin MD, Maloney TJ, McCarthy KE. Indium-111-pentetreotide prolongs survival in gastroenteropancreatic malignancies. *Semin Nucl Med.* 2002;32(2):123–132.
32. Buscombe JR, Caplin ME, Hilson AJ. Long-term efficacy of high-activity 111in-pentetreotide therapy in patients with disseminated neuroendocrine tumors. *J Nucl Med.* 2003;44(1):1–6.
33. Wiseman GA, Kvols LK. Therapy of neuroendocrine tumors with radiolabeled MIBG and somatostatin analogues. *Semin Nucl Med.* 1995;25(3):272–278.
34. Van Essen M, Krenning EP, De Jong M, Valkema R, Kwekkeboom DJ. Peptide Receptor Radionuclide Therapy with radiolabelled somatostatin analogues in patients with somatostatin receptor positive tumours. *Acta Oncol.* 2007;46(6):723–734.
35. de Jong M, Breeman WA, Bakker WH, et al. Comparison of (111)In-labeled somatostatin analogues for tumor scintigraphy and radionuclide therapy. *Cancer Res.* 1998;58(3):437–441.
36. Kwekkeboom DJ, Bakker WH, Kam BL, et al. Treatment of patients with gastro-entero-pancreatic (GEP) tumours with the novel radiolabelled somatostatin analogue [177Lu-DOTA(0), Tyr3]octreotate. *Eur J Nucl Med Mol Imaging.* 2003;30(3): 417–422.
37. Kwekkeboom DJ, Mueller-Brand J, Paganelli G, et al. Overview of results of peptide receptor radionuclide therapy with 3 radiolabeled somatostatin analogs. *J Nucl Med.* 2005;46(suppl 1): 62S–66S.
38. Oddstig J, Bernhardt P, Nilsson O, Ahlman H, Forssell-Aronsson E. Radiation-induced up-regulation of somatostatin receptor expression in small cell lung cancer in vitro. *Nucl Med Biol.* 2006;33(7): 841–846.
39. Capello A, Krenning E, Bernard B, Reubi JC, Breeman W, de Jong M. 111In-labelled somatostatin analogues in a rat tumour model: somatostatin receptor status and effects of peptide receptor radionuclide therapy. *Eur J Nucl Med Mol Imaging.* 2005;32(11):1288–1295.
40. Rogers BE, Zinn KR, Lin CY, Chaudhuri TR, Buchsbaum DJ. Targeted radiotherapy with [(90)Y]-SMT 487 in mice bearing human nonsmall cell lung tumor xenografts induced to express human somatostatin receptor subtype 2 with an adenoviral vector. *Cancer.* 2002;94(4 suppl):1298–1305.
41. Freeman SM, Abboud CN, Whartenby KA, et al. The "bystander effect": tumor regression when a fraction of the tumor mass is genetically modified. *Cancer Res.* 1993;53(21):5274–5283.
42. ter Horst M, Verwijnen SM, Brouwer E, et al. Locoregional delivery of adenoviral vectors. *J Nucl Med.* 2006;47(9): 1483–1489.
43. de Visser M, Verwijnen SM, de Jong M. Update: improvement strategies for peptide receptor scintigraphy and radionuclide therapy. *Cancer Biother Radiopharm.* 2008;23(2):137–157.
44. Hofland LJ, Capello A, Krenning EP, de Jong M, van Hagen MP. Induction of apoptosis with hybrids of Arg-Gly-Asp molecules and peptides and antimitotic effects of hybrids of cytostatic drugs and peptides. *J Nucl Med.* 2005;46(suppl 1): 191S–198S.
45. Yao JC, Phan A, Hoff PM, et al. Targeting vascular endothelial growth factor in advanced carcinoid tumor: a random assignment phase II study of depot octreotide with bevacizumab and pegylated interferon alpha-2b. *J Clin Oncol.* 2008;26(8): 1316–1323.
46. Yao JC. Neuroendocrine tumors. Molecular targeted therapy for carcinoid and islet-cell carcinoma. *Best Pract Res Clin Endocrinol Metab.* 2007;21(1):163–172.

23
Pancreatic Endocrine Neoplasms

Ahmed S. Bedeir and Alyssa M. Krasinskas

Introduction

Pancreatic endocrine neoplasms (PENs) are foregut endocrine tumors that arise in the pancreas and appear morphologically similar to other neuroendocrine (carcinoid) tumors throughout the body. However, the biology of endocrine/neuroendocrine tumors tends to depend upon the site of origin. PENs can produce various hormones, though most are nonfunctional. They are generally low grade, well-differentiated tumors. PENs can be classified according to grade, size, or functional status. The nomenclature of these neoplasms can be confusing, partly because of the variable terminology, including different names for the same neoplasm (including "islet cell tumors," "pancreatic neuroendocrine tumor," and "pancreatic endocrine tumors") and partly because well-differentiated malignant tumors can either be called "malignant pancreatic endocrine neoplasms" or "pancreatic endocrine carcinomas." The authors of the AFIP fascicle prefer to consider all well-differentiated PENs as potentially malignant (with the exception of microadenomas less than 0.5 cm in size). The term "carcinoma" is reserved for poorly differentiated lesions.[1] Similarly, the term PEN will be used in this chapter to refer to well-differentiated tumors.

Sporadic Pancreatic Endocrine Neoplasms

PENs are uncommon neoplasms; the incidence in the United States is about 2.2 per 1,000,000.[2] There is a slight male predominance and the mean age is 58.5 years.[2] The vast majority of PENs are sporadic and up to 90.8% are nonfuctional.[2] A PEN not associated with a syndrome of hormone overproduction is, by default, a nonfunctional tumor. Nonfunctional tumors are discovered incidentally or may be associated with abdominal pain. PENs associated with a syndrome of hormone overproduction are classified as functional PENs and include insulinomas, glucagonomas, somatostatinomas, gastrinomas, VIPomas, serotonin secreting tumors, as well as other rare and mixed hormone-producing entities. The clinical presentation of functional tumors depends on the type of hormone that is secreted.

About 60% of PENs arise in the pancreatic tail,[3] but they can occur throughout the pancreas. Grossly, PENs are usually solid, well-circumscribed, sometimes encapsulated lesions. The cut surfaces can be uniform or heterogenous with solid or spongy, yellow to red parenchyma. PENs have many various histological patterns, including the traditional organoid or trabecular growth pattern seen in well-differentiated neuroendocrine tumors at other sites. The cytologic features can also be typical of other neuroendocrine tumors. The neoplastic cells tend to be small and polygonal with abundant amphophilic cytoplasm and uniform round to oval nuclei with the coarsely stippled "salt and pepper chromatin." However, variable cellular size, nuclear size, nuclear shape, and chromatin patterns are common. The variation in growth patterns and cytologic features makes PENs a unique and interesting group of endocrine tumors.[1]

Useful immunohistochemical markers include antibodies to most neuroendocrine cells, such as synaptophysin, protein gene product (PGP) 9.5, CD 57 (Leu7) and CD 56 (neural cell adhesion molecule); chromogranin is inconsistently expressed in PENs and its staining can be patchy and dependant on the antibody that is used.[4] When confronted with a metastatic (neuro)endocrine tumor, antibodies to CDX-2 and TTF-1 can be very helpful. PENs tend to lack staining for both of these markers, while TTF-1 is expressed in lung primaries and CDX-2 in gastrointestinal primaries.[5] Immunohistochemical stains can also be used to detect specific peptides such as insulin, glucagon, somatostatin, and pancreatic polypeptide, but the protein expression does not always correlate with the functional status of the PEN.

In an attempt to better predict the prognosis of PENs, several immunohistochemical markers have been studied, but none have replaced classic clinical and morphologic parameters. Ki-67 (MIB-1) proliferation index has been

J.L. Hunt (ed.), *Molecular Pathology of Endocrine Diseases*, Molecular Pathology Library 3,
DOI 10.1007/978-1-4419-1707-2_23, © Springer Science+Business Media, LLC 2010

shown to have prognostic value in PENs[6,7] and is used by the WHO to distinguish PENs with "benign" behavior from those with "uncertain" behavior based on a cutoff of 2%.[8] Another proposed grading scheme uses mitoses and ki-67 labeling index to separate low and intermediate grade PENs from high grade pancreatic endocrine carcinomas.[9] However, one group has proposed simplifying the WHO classification system by using clinical parameters of tumor size and metastases with grading information based on necrosis and mitotic rate.[10] Another promising prognostic marker, CK-19, was found to be expressed in more aggressive PENs and its expression was correlated with a shorter disease free survival and was independent of the WHO criteria.[11]

Genome Wide Study of Sporadic Pancreatic Endocrine Neoplasms

Comparative Genomic Hybridization

Using comparative genomic hybridization, numerous studies have identified many chromosomal alterations in PENs with chromosomal losses being slightly more common than gains. Commonly described alterations include losses at 1p, 3p, 6q, 9p, 10p, 11pq, 18q, 22q, Y and X and gains at 4pq, 5q, 7p, 7q, 9q, 12q, 14q, 17p, 17q and 20q.[12–17] One of the most consistent chromosomal alterations is loss of 11q, which harbors the *MEN1* gene.[18] Some chromosomal alterations have been associated with tumor grade, stage, and prognosis. The overall number of genetic changes per tumor, especially gains, has been associated with both tumor size and disease stage.[12,13,16] Losses of 3, 6, and 21q and gains of 4, 7, 14q, 17, 20q, and Xq were found to be associated with malignant behavior and/or metastatic disease.[12,13,16] Prognostic significance was also linked to changes in the sex chromosome. In males, Speel et al noted that all of the four male patients with malignant insulinomas studied had loss of chromosome Y in addition to gain of Xp.[12] This finding was further supported by Missiaglia et al who showed that PENs from female patients show frequent loss of chromosome X and PENs from male patients show relatively frequent loss of chromosome Y, and that loss of a sex chromosome was associated with the presence of metastases, local invasion, and with poor survival.[19]

Loss of Heterozygosity (LOH)

A number of studies have used LOH to identify chromosomal loci that may harbor potential tumor suppressor genes involved in the pathogenesis of PEN. LOH can detect smaller deletions than CGH. In addition to those losses noted by CGH, additional deletions of interest have been detected by LOH at 3p14.2-3p21, 3p23, 6q22, 7q31–32, 9p, 11q13, 13q14, 17q21, 18q21, and 22q12.[20–30] LOH at loci 3p25.3-p23, 6q, 17p13, and 22q have been associated with aggressive behavior and metastatic disease.[20–22,29] Importantly, these assays have been reported in fine needle aspirations, as well as in histologic material.[31] In addition to their importance as useful markers for clinical behavior, these chromosomal changes direct attention to particular chromosomal regions as candidates for a more detailed analysis with respect to genes involved in PEN development.

Gene Expression Profiling of Sporadic PENs

Several DNA microarray studies using different approaches have reported novel genes that may be important in the pathogenesis and prognosis of PENs. Up-regulated genes potentially involved in pathogenesis of PENs include oncogenes (*MLLT10*/*AF10*), growth-factor-related genes (*IGFBP3*), cell adhesion and migration molecules (fibronectin), endothelial elements (*MCAM*/*MUC18*, *PECAM1*/CD31, *ANGPT2*/Ang2), potential biomarkers (*SERPINA10*, *BIN1*) and therapeutic targets (*LCK*/SRC-like kinase, *BST2*); down-regulated genes include cell cycle check point genes (*CDKN1A*/p21), cell surface glycoproteins (*CD99*/*MIC2*), putative metastasis suppressor genes (*NM23*, transcription factors (*JUND*) and apoptosis-related genes (*IER3*, *PHLDA2*, *IAPP*, and *SST*).[32–35] One DNA microarray study compared nonmetastatic with metastatic PENs and found differential expression of genes related to growth-factor-related molecules (*IGFBP1*, *IGFBP3*), cytoskeleton-related molecules (b1-tubulin), cell cycle regulation (*CHEK1*), developmental regulation (*TBX3*), intracellular signaling (*UPK1B*), and DNA damage repair (*MGMT*),[36] while another study found no significant differentially expressed genes between primary tumors and their metastases.[33] Due to poor concordance between these published studies, further analysis of these genes may reveal important insight into the pathogenesis and prognosis of PENs.

Individual Genes in Sporadic Pancreatic Endocrine Neoplasms

Most of the molecular studies of PEN have failed to demonstrate a strong role of the common oncogenes and tumor suppressor genes in the molecular pathogenesis of most PENs. Because of its involvement in MEN1 patients, the *MEN1* gene has been examined for mutations in sporadic PENs. Although loss of *MEN1* locus at 11p13 occurs in 43–68% of sporadic PENs, somatic mutations have been found in only 15–26%,[23,26,37] suggesting involvement of another tumor suppressor gene at this location. Similarly, in patients with sporadic PENs, LOH on chromosome 3p was identified in 33% of cases, but no mutations in *VHL* were detected.[38] As for other tumor suppressor genes and oncogenes, there appears to be no significant role of *TP53*, *CDKN2A* (p16), *PTEN*, *SMAD4/DPC4*, *ERBB2/HER2*, *BCL2*, *KRAS*, or *BRAF* in the pathogenesis of sporadic PENs.[18,22,28,39–43]

Epigenetic Changes in Sporadic Pancreatic Endocrine Neoplasms

In addition to genetic mutation and chromosomal loss, aberrant epigenetic changes including abnormalities in methylation have been demonstrated in PEN. Chan et al demonstrated that the methylation profile of gastrointestinal neuroendocrine (carcinoid) tumors differs from PENs, reflecting different molecular pathogenesis.[44] Among the most commonly methylated genes in PEN are *RASSF*/RASSF1A, *CDKN2A*/p16, *MGMT*, and *MLH1*.[45–47] The hypermethylation of *RASSF1* promoter is frequent in many human cancers, and there is an inverse correlation between *RASSF1* silencing by methylation and *KRAS* activation.[48,49] As mentioned earlier, it has been shown that well-differentiated PENs lack *KRAS* or *BRAF* mutations.[42,50] It is therefore interesting that the *RASSF1* gene is the most frequently methylated gene in PEN.[45–47] This finding suggests that the RAS pathway may still be involved in well-differentiated neuroendocrine tumors mostly by gene silencing of *RASSF1* gene through methylation. The frequency of *CDKN2A*/p16 methylation ranges from 19% to >50% in the literature.[46,47,51] The *MGMT* gene is an important tumor suppressor gene responsible for removing alkylation of DNA at the O6 position of guanine and playing a major role in DNA repair. Methylation of CpG islands in the promoter region of *MGMT* can cause gene silencing.[52] Another tumor suppressor gene important in DNA repair is *MLH1*. The association between loss of *MLH1* function and microsatellite instability in colorectal cancer is well documented. Like microsatellite unstable colorectal cancer, *MLH1* methylation leads to MSI in PENs and this was shown to be associated with favorable prognosis.[46,53] Similarly, a few studies have suggested that the methylation status of specific tumor suppressor genes is predictive of PEN behavior. In a study of gastrinomas, Serrano et al reported that *CDKN2A*/p16 gene methylation correlated with malignant tumors associated with lymph node but not liver metastases.[28] In a larger study of all types of PEN, House et al found that methylation at the *CDKN2A*/p16 gene locus was associated with decreased 5-year survival and tumor recurrence within 24 months; two molecular markers that can predict patient outcome after surgical resection. Methylation at 3 or more genes or at the *CDKN2A*/p16 gene locus is associated with decreased 5-year survival and tumor recurrence within 24 months; 37% of *CDKN2A*/p16 methylated PEN recurred, compared with 26% of tumors without *CDKN2A*/p16 methylation.[46] They also showed that the methylation of multiple (≥3) tumor suppressor genes may be associated with more aggressive tumors.[46]

Other Techniques

Telomerase in Sporadic PENs

Chromosomal telomeres (terminal chromosome regions) are made up of several thousand copies of repeating nucleotide sequences. Their main functions are believed to be the stabilization and protection of chromosomal ends.[54] In a normal somatic cell, there is approximately 50–100 basepair loss of telomeric DNA from the end of every chromosome during each cell cycle. With progressive erosion of telomeres, these unprotected ends may participate in end-to-end chromosomal fusions, which are lethal to cells.[54] Telomerase is an enzyme believed to be involved in the de novo synthesis of telomeric DNA onto chromosomal ends.[55,56] Telomerase is not detected in most somatic cells. Conversely, it is activated in most human cancers suggesting an important role in cancer cell survival.[57] Telomerase is a ribonucleoprotein complex including a telomerase catalytic subunit (telomerase reverse transcriptase protein subunit, TERT, an internal RNA strand (TR), and an RNA-binding protein (TEP1)). *TERT* gene expression seems to be the rate-limiting determinant of telomerase activity. A few published studies have shown that telomerase activity is closely related to the malignant potential of human pancreatic endocrine tumors.[58,59] In the study by Lam et al, three of ten pancreatic endocrine tumors had telomerase activity. Two of these cases were frankly malignant tumors with liver metastases and the third was pancreatic endocrine tumor occurring in the setting of MEN type 1 and histologically showed an infiltrative border, vascular and perineural tumor infiltration.[58] This finding suggested that telomerase activity might be useful in distinguishing between benign and malignant pancreatic endocrine tumors. A more recent study employed real-time quantitative RT-PCR in the quantification of *TERT* mRNA 23 cases of PEN. Telomerase was negative in 12 out of 12 benign pancreatic tumors (100%) and positive in 6 out of 8 malignant (metastatic or not) pancreatic tumors (75%), resulting in a positive predictive value of 100% and a negative predictive value of 85.7%. In addition, telomerase activity was helpful in identifying metastatic tumors. Sixteen of eighteen nonmetastatic pancreatic tumors were telomerase negative (88.99%), while 5 out of 5 metastatic pancreatic tumors were telomerase positive (80% and 100% positive and negative predictive values, respectively).[60]

MicroRNA

MicroRNAs are small (about 22 nucleotides in length), single-stranded forms of noncoding RNA that are involved in the normal functioning of our cells. The dysregulation of microRNA has been linked to human disease, including cancer. One study has examined the role of microRNAs in PEN. Comparing nontumor pancreas to pancreatic tumors (insulinomas, nonfunctioning PEN and acinar cell carcinomas), the expression of miR-103 and *MIRN107*/miR-107 in conjunction with a lack of expression of *MIRN155*/miR-155 distinguished tumors from normal. A set of 10 microRNAs were upregulated in PEN and *MIRN204*/miR-204 was found to be primarily expressed in insulinomas. Interestingly, the overexpression of *MIRN21*/miR-21 was strongly associated with both a high Ki67 proliferation index and presence of liver metastasis.[61]

Hereditary Pancreatic Endocrine Tumors

In a small subset of patients, PENs are inherited as part of a genetic syndrome. Recognition of these patients is important for both treatment and evaluation of family members. The study of these inherited neoplasms also plays an important role in our understanding of the pathogenesis of PEN. The most common hereditary syndromes associated with the development of PEN are multiple endocrine neoplasia type 1 (MEN1) and von Hippel–Lindau syndrome (VHL).

MEN1 is a rare autosomal dominant disorder with a prevalence that ranges from 1 in 20,000 to 1 in 40,000.[62] It is characterized by the combination of parathyroid tumors, pancreatic endocrine cell neoplasms, and pituitary hyperplasia/tumors. Tumors can also arise in the upper gastrointestinal tract, lung, thyroid, thymus, and adrenal gland. Parathyroid tumors occur in nearly all patients by age 50, and pancreatic tumors arise in approximately 80% of patients.[63,64] The pancreatic tumors are often multiple, including microadenomas and PENs, and the PENs may undergo malignant transformation. While the majority of PENs are nonfunctional, most patients will have at least one functional tumor. The most common functional tumors are gastrinomas, followed by insulinomas, glucagonomas, and others.

Using genetic linkage analysis, a region on the long arm of chromosome 11 (11q13) was implicated as the potential site that harbored the key gene that is dysfunctional in MEN1 syndromes (Table 23.1).[65] The candidate gene was identified and designated the *MEN1* gene by Chandrasekharappa et al in1997.[66] Multiple subsequent studies confirmed that *MEN1* gene mutations are detected in most MEN1 patients.[67,68] This tumor suppressor gene contains 10-exon that encodes for a 610-amino-acid nuclear protein, Menin, that interacts with a variety of transcription factors, DNA processing factors, DNA repair proteins, and cytoskeletal proteins.[69,70] At least 400 different MEN1 mutations have been described.[71] It is important to note that mutations in the *MEN1* gene locus are also reported in 27–39% of sporadic PENs.[23,30,72] The mutations in the *MEN1* gene in sporadic PENs appear to be distributed throughout the nine coding exons.[23] Mutations are present in the *MEN1* gene in both benign and malignant sporadic PENs suggesting that they are an early event in the molecular pathogenesis.[23,72]

The second syndrome that is associated with the tendency to develop PEN is VHL syndrome. The prevalence ranges from 1 in 30,000 to 1 in 50,000.[73] The disease penetrance is over 90% by age 65.[73] This autosomal dominant disorder is associated with many tumors, most notably hemangioblastomas, clear cell renal cell carcinomas and pheochromocytomas.[74–76]

TABLE 23.1. Hereditary syndromes associated with pancreatic endocrine neoplasms.

Multiple endocrine neoplasia type-1	
Gene	*MEN1*
Protein product	Menin
Protein function	Interacts with transcription factors
	– JunD, NF-kB, Smad3, Pem
	DNA repair proteins
	– RPA2
	DNA processing factors
	– nm23
	Cytoskeletal proteins
	– GFAP, vimentin
von Hippel Lindau disease	
Gene	*VHL*
Protein product	VHL
Protein function	Targets several proteins that bind to ubiquitin to be degraded by proteosomes:
	– Hypoxia-inducible factor-1 (HIF-1)
	– Vascular endothelial growth factor (VEGF)
	– Platelet derived growth factor (PDGF)
	– Tumor growth factor alpha (TGFa)
	– Matrix metalloproteinases (MMP)
	– MMP-inhibitors
	– Atypical protein kinase C (APK-C)

PENs are reported to be present in 17% of patients with VHL and they behave in a malignant fashion in up to 8.3%.[77] The majority of PEN are nonfunctional[75] and many (60%) have a foamy clear cell appearance.[78]

Using genetic linkage analysis, a region on the short arm of chromosome 3 (3p25-p26) was found to harbor the *VHL* gene and the gene was subsequently cloned (Table 23.1).[73,79] More than 300 germline mutations have been identified in familial VHL.[73] Functioning as a tumor suppressor gene, its product, VHL protein, targets several proteins with which it forms stable complexes that binds to ubiquitin that then get degraded by proteasomes.[80,81] Hypoxia-inducible factor-1 (HIF-1) is one of the major proteins regulated by VHL. This protein is involved in erythropoiesis through its ability to induce transcription of mRNA coding for erythropoietin. In patients with VHL disease, loss of functioning VHL results in HIF-1alpha not binding to ubiquitin and thus not degraded by proteasomes.[80,81] In addition to erythropoietin, other factors known to be regulated through the HIF-1alpha system include vascular endothelial growth factor (VEGF), platelet-derived growth factor (PDGF)-beta, and transforming growth factor (TGF)-alpha.[80,81] VHL also affects several other factors potentially involved in tumorigenesis that are not regulated through the HIF-1alpha system. These targets include matrix metalloproteinases (MMP) such as MMP1, MMP inhibitors, and atypical protein kinase C.[80,81] Although the mechanism of tumorigenesis remains unproven, the combined effect of various angiogenic factors and other growth factors may be to create an autocrine loop that provides an uncontrolled growth stimulus.[82] Although loss of 3p is well documented in sporadic PEN,[24] mutation of this gene is usually not targeted in sporadic PEN.[26] Interestingly, 78% of patients with metastatic disease had exon 3 mutations in the *VHL* gene, compared with 46% of patients without metastases, suggesting that detection of exon 3 mutations will be helpful in assessing aggressiveness of PEN and guiding surgical management in these patients.[77]

Summary

Even though two well-known hereditary conditions are associated with PENs, MEN1 and VHL, the molecular pathogenesis of these two diseases has provided only little insight into the much more common sporadic form of the pancreatic neoplasms. Sporadic PENs harbor *MEN1* gene mutations in only a minority of cases and they tend not to have *VHL* mutations, but rather show loss of the locus where the *VHL* gene resides. Abundant research has been performed on sporadic PENs that has provided insight into the molecular pathogenesis of these tumors. Rather than resulting from dysfunction of a single gene, several pathways appear to be involved with the formation of PENs, including losses and gains of genomic material, methylation of some key regulatory genes and expression of particular microRNAs.

While PENs are typically easy to diagnose, their behavior is difficult, if not impossible, to predict. Immunohistochemistry has limited value in assessing prognosis, but new markers are always being developed. Molecular studies have provided some targets that may be helpful in assessing the aggressiveness and metastatic potential of these tumors, and some have even been reported to predict survival (Table 23.2). Some prior studies need to be validated, but a panel of markers utilizing various techniques may be needed to accurately predict the behavior of these tumors.

TABLE 23.2. Potential indicators of behavior in pancreatic endocrine neoplasms.

Method	Gene/marker	Association
IHC	Ki-67 (MIB-1)	>2% proliferation index = malignant potential
	CK-19	Positive expression = worse prognosis
CGH	Overall # of genetic changes	Increased # = increased tumor size and disease stage
	Losses of chr 3, 6, 21q, X/Y	Malignant behavior/ metastatic disease
	Gains of chr 4, 7, 14q, 17, 20q, Xq	Malignant behavior/ metastatic disease
LOH	3p25.3-p23, 6q, 17p13, 22q	Malignant behavior/ metastatic disease
Gene expression profiling	Several genes, including *MET* and *IGFBP3*	Metastatic disease
Methylation	*MLH1*	Favorable prognosis
	CDKN2A/p16	Malignant behavior, decreased survival, early recurrence
	Multiple genes	Malignant behavior
Telomerase	Activity	Malignant behavior/ metastatic disease
microRNA	*MIRN21*/miR-21	Malignant behavior/ metastatic disease

IHC immunohistochemistry, *CGH* comparative genomic hybridization, *LOH* loss of heterozygosity.

References

1. Hruban RH, Pitman MB, Klimstra DS. Tumors of the pancreas. In: Silverberg SG, Sobin LH, eds. *AFIP Atlas of Tumor Pathology.* Washington, DC: American Registry of Pathology; 2007:251–304.
2. Halfdanarson TR, Rabe KG, Rubin J, Petersen GM. Pancreatic neuroendocrine tumors (PNETs): incidence, prognosis and recent trend toward improved survival. *Ann Oncol.* 2008;19(10): 1727–1733.
3. Solcia E, Capella C, Kloppel G. *AFIP Atlas of Tumor pathology: Tumors of the Pancreas 3rd series.* Washington, DC: American Registry of Pathology; 1997.
4. Portela-Gomes GM, Hacker GW, Weitgasser R. Neuroendocrine cell markers for pancreatic islets and tumors. *Appl Immunohistochem Mol Morphol.* 2004;12:183–192.
5. Lin X, Saad RS, Luckasevic TM, Silverman JF, Liu Y. Diagnostic value of CDX-2 and TTF-1 expressions in separating metastatic neuroendocrine neoplasms of unknown origin. *Appl Immunohistochem Mol Morphol.* 2007;15:407–414.
6. La Rosa S, Sessa F, Capella C, et al. Prognostic criteria in nonfunctioning pancreatic endocrine tumours. *Virchows Arch.* 1996;429:323–333.
7. Pelosi G, Bresaola E, Bogina G, et al. Endocrine tumors of the pancreas: Ki-67 immunoreactivity on paraffin sections is an independent predictor for malignancy: a comparative study with proliferating-cell nuclear antigen and progesterone receptor protein immunostaining, mitotic index, and other clinicopathologic variables. *Hum Pathol.* 1996;27:1124–1134.
8. Heitz PU, Komminoth P, Perren A, et al. Tumors of the endocrine pancreas. In: DeLellis DA, Lloyd RV, Heitz PU, Eng C, eds. *WHO Classification of Tumours: Pathology and Genetics of Tumours of Endocrine Organs.* Lyon: IARC Press; 2004:175–208.
9. Rindi G, Kloppel G, Alhman H, et al. TNM staging of foregut (neuro)endocrine tumors: a consensus proposal including a grading system. *Virchows Arch.* 2006;449:395–401.
10. Ferrone CR, Tang LH, Tomlinson J, et al. Determining prognosis in patients with pancreatic endocrine neoplasms: can the WHO classification system be simplified? *J Clin Oncol.* 2007;25:5609–5615.
11. Schmitt AM, Anlauf M, Rousson V, et al. WHO 2004 criteria and CK19 are reliable prognostic markers in pancreatic endocrine tumors. *Am J Surg Pathol.* 2007;31:1677–1682.
12. Speel EJ, Richter J, Moch H, et al. Genetic differences in endocrine pancreatic tumor subtypes detected by comparative genomic hybridization. *Am J Pathol.* 1999;155:1787–1794.
13. Speel EJ, Scheidweiler AF, Zhao J, et al. Genetic evidence for early divergence of small functioning and nonfunctioning endocrine pancreatic tumors: gain of 9Q34 is an early event in insulinomas. *Cancer Res.* 2001;61:5186–5192.
14. Stumpf E, Aalto Y, Hoog A, et al. Chromosomal alterations in human pancreatic endocrine tumors. *Genes Chromosomes Cancer.* 2000;29:83–87.
15. Terris B, Meddeb M, Marchio A, et al. Comparative genomic hybridization analysis of sporadic neuroendocrine tumors of the digestive system. *Genes Chromosomes Cancer.* 1998;22:50–56.
16. Zhao J, Moch H, Scheidweiler AF, et al. Genomic imbalances in the progression of endocrine pancreatic tumors. *Genes Chromosomes Cancer.* 2001;32:364–372.

17. Zikusoka MN, Kidd M, Eick G, Latich I, Modlin IM. The molecular genetics of gastroenteropancreatic neuroendocrine tumors. *Cancer*. 2005;104:2292–2309.
18. Gumbs AA, Moore PS, Falconi M, et al. Review of the clinical, histological, and molecular aspects of pancreatic endocrine neoplasms. *J Surg Oncol*. 2002;81:45–53. discussion 54.
19. Missiaglia E, Moore PS, Williamson J, et al. Sex chromosome anomalies in pancreatic endocrine tumors. *Int J Cancer*. 2002;98:532–538.
20. Barghorn A, Komminoth P, Bachmann D, et al. Deletion at 3p25.3–p23 is frequently encountered in endocrine pancreatic tumours and is associated with metastatic progression. *J Pathol*. 2001;194:451–458.
21. Barghorn A, Speel EJ, Farspour B, et al. Putative tumor suppressor loci at 6q22 and 6q23–q24 are involved in the malignant progression of sporadic endocrine pancreatic tumors. *Am J Pathol*. 2001;158:1903–1911.
22. Beghelli S, Pelosi G, Zamboni G, et al. Pancreatic endocrine tumours: evidence for a tumour suppressor pathogenesis and for a tumour suppressor gene on chromosome 17p. *J Pathol*. 1998;186:41–50.
23. Gortz B, Roth J, Krahenmann A, et al. Mutations and allelic deletions of the MEN1 gene are associated with a subset of sporadic endocrine pancreatic and neuroendocrine tumors and not restricted to foregut neoplasms. *Am J Pathol*. 1999;154:429–436.
24. Hessman O, Lindberg D, Einarsson A, et al. Genetic alterations on 3p, 11q13, and 18q in nonfamilial and MEN 1-associated pancreatic endocrine tumors. *Genes Chromosomes Cancer*. 1999;26:258–264.
25. Hessman O, Lindberg D, Skogseid B, et al. Mutation of the multiple endocrine neoplasia type 1 gene in nonfamilial, malignant tumors of the endocrine pancreas. *Cancer Res*. 1998;58:377–379.
26. Moore PS, Missiaglia E, Antonello D, et al. Role of disease-causing genes in sporadic pancreatic endocrine tumors: MEN1 and VHL. *Genes Chromosomes Cancer*. 2001;32:177–181.
27. Nikiforova MN, Nikiforov YE, Biddinger P, et al. Frequent loss of heterozygosity at chromosome 3p14.2–3p21 in human pancreatic islet cell tumours. *Clin Endocrinol (Oxf)*. 1999;51:27–33.
28. Serrano J, Goebel SU, Peghini PL, Lubensky IA, Gibril F, Jensen RT. Alterations in the p16INK4a/CDKN2A tumor suppressor gene in gastrinomas. *J Clin Endocrinol Metab*. 2000;85:4146–4156.
29. Wild A, Langer P, Celik I, Chaloupka B, Bartsch DK. Chromosome 22q in pancreatic endocrine tumors: identification of a homozygous deletion and potential prognostic associations of allelic deletions. *Eur J Endocrinol*. 2002;147:507–513.
30. Zhuang Z, Vortmeyer AO, Pack S, et al. Somatic mutations of the MEN1 tumor suppressor gene in sporadic gastrinomas and insulinomas. *Cancer Res*. 1997;57:4682–4686.
31. Nodit L, McGrath KM, Zahid M, et al. Endoscopic ultrasound-guided fine needle aspirate microsatellite loss analysis and pancreatic endocrine tumor outcome. *Clin Gastroenterol Hepatol*. 2006;4:1474–1478.
32. Bloomston M, Durkin A, Yang I, et al. Identification of molecular markers specific for pancreatic neuroendocrine tumors by genetic profiling of core biopsies. *Ann Surg Oncol*. 2004;11:413–419.
33. Capurso G, Lattimore S, Crnogorac-Jurcevic T, et al. Gene expression profiles of progressive pancreatic endocrine tumours and their liver metastases reveal potential novel markers and therapeutic targets. *Endocr Relat Cancer*. 2006;13:541–558.
34. Dilley WG, Kalyanaraman S, Verma S, Cobb JP, Laramie JM, Lairmore TC. Global gene expression in neuroendocrine tumors from patients with the MEN1 syndrome. *Mol Cancer*. 2005;4:9.
35. Maitra A, Hansel DE, Argani P, et al. Global expression analysis of well-differentiated pancreatic endocrine neoplasms using oligonucleotide microarrays. *Clin Cancer Res*. 2003;9: 5988–5995.
36. Hansel DE, Rahman A, House M, et al. Met proto-oncogene and insulin-like growth factor binding protein 3 overexpression correlates with metastatic ability in well-differentiated pancreatic endocrine neoplasms. *Clin Cancer Res*. 2004;10:6152–6158.
37. Perren A, Anlauf M, Komminoth P. Molecular profiles of gastroenteropancreatic endocrine tumors. *Virchows Arch*. 2007;451(suppl 1):S39–S46.
38. Chung DC, Smith AP, Louis DN, Graeme-Cook F, Warshaw AL, Arnold A. A novel pancreatic endocrine tumor suppressor gene locus on chromosome 3p with clinical prognostic implications. *J Clin Invest*. 1997;100:404–410.
39. Jonkers YM, Claessen SM, Veltman JA, et al. Molecular parameters associated with insulinoma progression: chromosomal instability versus p53 and CK19 status. *Cytogenet Genome Res*. 2006;115:289–297.
40. Moore PS, Orlandini S, Zamboni G, et al. Pancreatic tumours: molecular pathways implicated in ductal cancer are involved in ampullary but not in exocrine nonductal or endocrine tumorigenesis. *Br J Cancer*. 2001;84:253–262.
41. Perren A, Komminoth P, Saremaslani P, et al. Mutation and expression analyses reveal differential subcellular compartmentalization of PTEN in endocrine pancreatic tumors compared to normal islet cells. *Am J Pathol*. 2000;157: 1097–1103.
42. Yashiro T, Fulton N, Hara H, et al. Comparison of mutations of ras oncogene in human pancreatic exocrine and endocrine tumors. *Surgery*. 1993;114:758–763. discussion 763–764.
43. Proca DM, Frankel WL. Pancreatic endocrine tumors-c-erb B2 (Her-2/neu), bcl-2, and p-53 immunohistochemical testing and their value in assessing prognosis. *Appl Immunohistochem Mol Morphol*. 2008;16:44–47.
44. Chan AO, Kim SG, Bedeir A, Issa JP, Hamilton SR, Rashid A. CpG island methylation in carcinoid and pancreatic endocrine tumors. *Oncogene*. 2003;22:924–934.
45. Dammann R, Schagdarsurengin U, Liu L, et al. Frequent RASSF1A promoter hypermethylation and K-ras mutations in pancreatic carcinoma. *Oncogene*. 2003;22:3806–3812.
46. House MG, Herman JG, Guo MZ, et al. Aberrant hypermethylation of tumor suppressor genes in pancreatic endocrine neoplasms. *Ann Surg*. 2003;238:423–431. discussion 431–432.
47. Liu L, Broaddus RR, Yao JC, et al. Epigenetic alterations in neuroendocrine tumors: methylation of RAS-association domain family 1, isoform A and p16 genes are associated with metastasis. *Mod Pathol*. 2005;18:1632–1640.
48. Agathanggelou A, Cooper WN, Latif F. Role of the Ras-association domain family 1 tumor suppressor gene in human cancers. *Cancer Res*. 2005;65:3497–3508.
49. Burbee DG, Forgacs E, Zochbauer-Muller S, et al. Epigenetic inactivation of RASSF1A in lung and breast cancers and malignant phenotype suppression. *J Natl Cancer Inst*. 2001;93: 691–699.

50. Yoshimoto K, Iwahana H, Fukuda A, et al. ras mutations in endocrine tumors: mutation detection by polymerase chain reaction-single strand conformation polymorphism. *Jpn J Cancer Res.* 1992;83:1057–1062.
51. Muscarella P, Melvin WS, Fisher WE, et al. Genetic alterations in gastrinomas and nonfunctioning pancreatic neuroendocrine tumors: an analysis of p16/MTS1 tumor suppressor gene inactivation. *Cancer Res.* 1998;58:237–240.
52. Esteller M, Sanchez-Cespedes M, Rosell R, Sidransky D, Baylin SB, Herman JG. Detection of aberrant promoter hypermethylation of tumor suppressor genes in serum DNA from non-small cell lung cancer patients. *Cancer Res.* 1999;59: 67–70.
53. House MG, Herman JG, Guo MZ, et al. Prognostic value of hMLH1 methylation and microsatellite instability in pancreatic endocrine neoplasms. *Surgery.* 2003;134:902–908. discussion 909.
54. Bryan TM, Cech TR. Telomerase and the maintenance of chromosome ends. *Curr Opin Cell Biol.* 1999;11:318–324.
55. Greider CW, Blackburn EH. Identification of a specific telomere terminal transferase activity in Tetrahymena extracts. *Cell.* 1985;43:405–413.
56. Feng J, Funk WD, Wang SS, et al. The RNA component of human telomerase. *Science.* 1995;269:1236–1241.
57. Greider CW. Telomerase activity, cell proliferation, and cancer. *Proc Natl Acad Sci USA.* 1998;95:90–92.
58. Lam KY, Lo CY, Fan ST, Luk JM. Telomerase activity in pancreatic endocrine tumours: a potential marker for malignancy. *Mol Pathol.* 2000;53:133–136.
59. Tang SJ, Dumot JA, Wang L, et al. Telomerase activity in pancreatic endocrine tumors. *Am J Gastroenterol.* 2002;97: 1022–1030.
60. Vezzosi D, Bouisson M, Escourrou G, et al. Clinical utility of telomerase for the diagnosis of malignant well-differentiated endocrine tumours. *Clin Endocrinol (Oxf).* 2006;64:63–67.
61. Roldo C, Missiaglia E, Hagan JP, et al. MicroRNA expression abnormalities in pancreatic endocrine and acinar tumors are associated with distinctive pathologic features and clinical behavior. *J Clin Oncol.* 2006;24:4677–4684.
62. Anlauf M, Garbrecht N, Bauersfeld J, et al. Hereditary neuroendocrine tumors of the gastroenteropancreatic system. *Virchows Arch.* 2007;451(suppl 1):S29–S38.
63. Bartsch D, Kopp I, Bergenfelz A, et al. MEN1 gene mutations in 12 MEN1 families and their associated tumors. *Eur J Endocrinol.* 1998;139:416–420.
64. Brandi ML, Gagel RF, Angeli A, et al. Guidelines for diagnosis and therapy of MEN type 1 and type 2. *J Clin Endocrinol Metab.* 2001;86:5658–5671.
65. Larsson C, Skogseid B, Oberg K, Nakamura Y, Nordenskjold M. Multiple endocrine neoplasia type 1 gene maps to chromosome 11 and is lost in insulinoma. *Nature.* 1988;332:85–87.
66. Chandrasekharappa SC, Guru SC, Manickam P, et al. Positional cloning of the gene for multiple endocrine neoplasia-type 1. *Science.* 1997;276:404–407.
67. Agarwal SK, Lee Burns A, Sukhodolets KE, et al. Molecular pathology of the MEN1 gene. *Ann N Y Acad Sci.* 2004;1014: 189–198.
68. Bassett JH, Forbes SA, Pannett AA, et al. Characterization of mutations in patients with multiple endocrine neoplasia type 1. *Am J Hum Genet.* 1998;62:232–244.
69. Balogh K, Racz K, Patocs A, Hunyady L. Menin and its interacting proteins: elucidation of menin function. *Trends Endocrinol Metab.* 2006;17:357–364.
70. Chandrasekharappa SC, Teh BT. Functional studies of the MEN1 gene. *J Intern Med.* 2003;253:606–615.
71. Guo SS, Sawicki MP. Molecular and genetic mechanisms of tumorigenesis in multiple endocrine neoplasia type-1. *Mol Endocrinol.* 2001;15:1653–1664.
72. Wang EH, Ebrahimi SA, Wu AY, Kashefi C, Passaro E Jr, Sawicki MP. Mutation of the MENIN gene in sporadic pancreatic endocrine tumors. *Cancer Res.* 1998;58:4417–4420.
73. Shehata BM, Stockwell CA, Castellano-Sanchez AA, Setzer S, Schmotzer CL, Robinson H. Von Hippel–Lindau (VHL) disease: an update on the clinico-pathologic and genetic aspects. *Adv Anat Pathol.* 2008;15:165–171.
74. Binkovitz LA, Johnson CD, Stephens DH. Islet cell tumors in von Hippel–Lindau disease: increased prevalence and relationship to the multiple endocrine neoplasias. *AJR Am J Roentgenol.* 1990;155:501–505.
75. Libutti SK, Choyke PL, Bartlett DL, et al. Pancreatic neuroendocrine tumors associated with von Hippel Lindau disease: diagnostic and management recommendations. *Surgery.* 1998;124:1153–1159.
76. Zbar B, Kishida T, Chen F, et al. Germline mutations in the Von Hippel–Lindau disease (VHL) gene in families from North America, Europe, and Japan. *Hum Mutat.* 1996;8:348–357.
77. Blansfield JA, Choyke L, Morita SY, et al. Clinical, genetic and radiographic analysis of 108 patients with von Hippel–Lindau disease (VHL) manifested by pancreatic neuroendocrine neoplasms (PNETs). *Surgery.* 2007;142:814–818. discussion 818 e1–e2.
78. Hoang MP, Hruban RH, Albores-Saavedra J. Clear cell endocrine pancreatic tumor mimicking renal cell carcinoma: a distinctive neoplasm of von Hippel–Lindau disease. *Am J Surg Pathol.* 2001;25:602–609.
79. Latif F, Tory K, Gnarra J, et al. Identification of the von Hippel–Lindau disease tumor suppressor gene. *Science.* 1993;260: 1317–1320.
80. Kim WY, Kaelin WG. Role of VHL gene mutation in human cancer. *J Clin Oncol.* 2004;22:4991–5004.
81. Sufan RI, Jewett MA, Ohh M. The role of von Hippel–Lindau tumor suppressor protein and hypoxia in renal clear cell carcinoma. *Am J Physiol Renal Physiol.* 2004;287:F1–F6.
82. de Paulsen N, Brychzy A, Fournier MC, et al. Role of transforming growth factor-alpha in von Hippel–Lindau (VHL)(–/–) clear cell renal carcinoma cell proliferation: a possible mechanism coupling VHL tumor suppressor inactivation and tumorigenesis. *Proc Natl Acad Sci USA.* 2001;98:1387–1392.

Section 7
Other Neuroendocrine Lesions

24
Gastrointestinal Neuroendocrine Tumors

Shih-Fan Kuan

Introduction

Gastrointestinal neuroendocrine tumors (GI-NETs) arise from diffuse neuroendocrine system cells,[1] which express neuroendocrine markers, produce certain peptide or amine hormones, and contain dense core secretory granules. NETs still retain these features after the transformation of normal neuroendocrine cells.

The neuroendocrine features of these tumors are summarized in Table 24.1. Histologically, individual tumor cells have monomorphic nuclei with a "salt and pepper" chromatin pattern.[2] The cytoplasm may be clear or granular. Four morphologic patterns of growth have been recognized: insular or nested, trabecular, tubular or acinar, and poorly differentiated.[3] Histochemical stains can be used to identify endocrine cells. Argentaffin is a silver stain, which selectively demonstrates serotonin-producing EC cells. Argyrophil stain is less specific to secretory type and identifies all GI endocrine cells.[4]

Some immunohistochemical markers are routinely used to identify or confirm NETs. Chromogranin A and B are specific secretory granular markers.[5,6] Synaptophysin is a synaptic vesicle protein widely expressed in neuroendocrine cells although it can also be found in normal adrenal cortex and its tumors.[7] Cytoplasmic markers such as neuron-specific enolase and protein gene product 9.5 may highlight cells containing very few secretory granules.[8,9] However, its presence in some non-endocrine cells has limited its utilization.

General Overview

Histopathologic Classification

The classification of GI-NETs has been tedious, controversial, and sometimes confusing. Various schemes (Table 24.2) will be adapted in this text. It can be simply classified by the embryologic sites into foregut, midgut, and hindgut tumors.[10] NETs arising from each location share similar clinical, biochemical, and secretory features. For instance, foregut NETs are argentaffin-negative and have low serotonin levels.[11] These tumors can metastasize to bone and associate with atypical carcinoid syndrome. Midgut NETs are argentaffin positive and may produce high level of serotonin associated with classical carcinoid syndrome. They uniformly express intestinal transcription factor CDX2.[12] Hindgut NETs are argentaffin negative and rarely secrete serotonin or other vasoactive peptides. Bone metastasis is uncommon.

GI-NETs can also be characterized by the secretory products of endocrine cells.[13] There are at least 12 types of peptide- or amine-secreting endocrine cells in the gut. GI-NETs mainly arise from 5 major types of cells: (1) gastrin-producing G-cells; (2) somatostatin-producing D-cells; (3) enteroglucagon-producing L-cells; (4) serotonin-producing EC-cells; and (5) histamine-producing ECL cells. Tumors arising from cells containing other hormones such as secretin, GIP, CCK, motilin, or neurotensin are either very rare or non-existent.

Pure neuroendocrine tumors from various sites used to be called carcinoid based on their similar morphology and seemingly benign course. It has become apparent that this term is insufficient to cover the full range of malignant potentials.[14] The WHO 2000 classification categorizes pure neuroendocrine tumors into 4 groups[15,16] (1) well-differentiated neuroendocrine tumor, (2) well-differentiated neuroendocrine carcinoma, (3) poorly differentiated neuroendocrine carcinoma, and (4) mixed exocrine/endocrine carcinoma. The distinction of well-differentiated tumor and carcinoma is based on the tumor size, mitotic rates, and angio-lymphatic invasion. The diagnosis of poorly differentiated neuroendocrine carcinoma is the same as that of small cell carcinoma. When a non-endocrine element, such as adenocarcinoma, is also present, it should be designated as mixed endocrine-exocrine tumor.

WHO 2000 classification also established the morphological criteria for assessing the prognosis of GI-NETs based on tumor size, histological differentiation, proliferation

J.L. Hunt (ed.), *Molecular Pathology of Endocrine Diseases*, Molecular Pathology Library 3,
DOI 10.1007/978-1-4419-1707-2_24, © Springer Science+Business Media, LLC 2010

activity (Ki67 index), hormonal activity, angioinvasion, and the presence of metastasis to adjacent organs.[16] In the original publication, these prognostic criteria were further subdivided into localizations including the stomach, duodenum (and proximal jejunum), ileum (and distal jejunum), appendix, and colon-rectum. To eliminate redundancy, these criteria can be summarized into a simple table (Table 24.3) and easily applied to all anatomic sites in the GI tract.

There was no accepted TNM staging system although the European Neuroendocrine Tumor Society (ENETS) has recently proposed a grading system based on the tumor size.[17,18] This proposal requires future validation by clinicopathological correlation.

TABLE 24.1. Neuroendocrine features of neuroendocrine tumors.

Histologic feature	Nuclei: monomorphic, central, "salt and pepper" chromatin
	Cytoplasm: eosinophilic, clear or granular
Morphologic patterns	Insular or nested pattern (type A)
	Trabecular pattern (type B)
	Tubular or acinar pattern (type C)
	Poorly differentiated growth pattern (type D)
Histochemical stains	Argentaffin stain
	Argyrophil stain
Immunohistochemical markers	Chromogranins
	Synaptophysin
	Neuron-specific enolase (NSE)
	Protein gene product (PGP) 9.5

TABLE 24.2. Nomenclature used in various classification of GI-NETs.

Embryologic/anatomical classification
- Foregut (stomach, duodenum, proximal jejunum)
- Midgut (distal jejunum, ileum, appendix, cecum)
- Hindgut (colon and rectum)

Major cell types of NETs and their hormonal production
- G-cell tumor, producing gastrin
- D-cell tumor, producing somatostatin
- L-cell tumor, producing enteroglucagon
- EC (enterochromaffin)-cell tumor, producing serotonin
- ECL(enterochromaffin-like)-cell tumor, producing histamine

Histopathologic grading
- Pure neuroendocrine tumors
  - Well-differentiated neuroendocrine tumor (a.k.a carcinoid)
  - Well-differentiated neuroendocrine carcinoma (a.k.a malignant carcinoid)
  - Poorly differentiated neuroendocrine carcinoma (a.k.a small cell carcinoma)
- Mixed endocrine-exocrine tumors

Biological behavior
- Benign
- Benign or low-grade malignant
- Low-grade malignant
- High-grade malignant

Organ Distribution and Clinical Features

The true incidence rates and survival rates from each anatomic site were not well-documented. The Surveillance, Epidemiology, and End Results (SEER) is the largest nationwide cancer registry for GI-NETs. The raw-data between the periods of 1973–1991 and 1992–1999 are summarized in Table 24.4 for comparison.[19]

Within the gut, small bowel, rectum, and colon are the three most frequent sites for GI-NETs. The incidence of gastric NETs increased during the two periods of comparison probably due to increasing gastroscopic surveillance for *Helicobacter pylori*. The 5-year survival throughout all anatomic sites improved with time and is best for rectum (88%) and appendix (71%), followed by stomach (63%), colon (62%), and small bowel (61%).

GI-NETs are usually benign, slow-growing, and asymptomatic. They are frequently found incidentally during an abdominal procedure or surgery unrelated to the tumor. The typical carcinoid syndrome including flushing, diarrhea, and asthma are present only in less than 10% of patients. These symptoms were caused by circulating hormones and substance such as serotonin, histamine, and substance P. Since these substances are quickly metabolized during their first pass through the liver, carcinoid syndrome is usually seen in patients with liver metastasis.

Molecular Genetics

The molecular genetics of GI-NETs is heterogenous and poorly understood. Many genes commonly involved in other epithelial tumors, such as *RAS*, *MYC*, *and FOS* do not appear to be involved in GI-NETs.[20] Instead, only a small subset of genes (Table 24.5) is altered in GI-NETs. These genes are discussed in this section according to their preferential

TABLE 24.3. Criteria for assessing the prognosis of GI-NETs.

Biologic behavior	Histological differentiation	Tumor size	Ki-67 index	Invasion of m. propria	Angio-invasion	Metastasis	Hormonal syndrome
Benign	Well-differentiated	≤1 cm[a]	<2%	–	–	–	–[a]
Benign or low grade malignant	Well-differentiated	≤2 cm	<2%	–	–/+	–	–
Low grade malignant	Well-differentiated	>2 cm	>2%	+[b]	+	+	+
High grade	Poorly differentiated	Any	>30%	+	+	+	–

[a]Exception: duodenal gastrinomas are usually smaller than 1 cm and confined to the submucosa.
[b]Exception: benign NETs of the appendix usually invade muscularis propria.
Adapted from: Kloppel G, Perren A, Heitz PU. The gastroenteropancreatic neuroendocrine cell systems and its tumors: the WHO classification. *Ann N. Y. Acad Sci.* 2004;1014:13–27.

involvements in the tumors of foregut, midgut, and hindgut. Each gene will then be discussed in appropriate organ sections.

The *MEN1* gene is located on chromosome 11q13. Germline mutations in this gene are responsible for multiple endocrine neoplasia syndrome, type 1 (MEN1),[21] which is often associated with endocrine tumors of the stomach, duodenum, pancreas, as well as pituitary and parathyroid glands.

TABLE 24.4. Organ-related distribution and 5 year survival rate of GI-NETs.

	Distribution		5-year survival	
Organ sites	1973–1991	1992–1999	1973–1991	1992–1999
Stomach	5.8%	8.7%	51.2%	63.0%
Small intestine (all)	46.9%	41.8%	51.9%	60.5%
Duodenum	3.1%	5.7%	–	–
Jejunum	3.4%	2.2%	–	–
Ileum	26.4%	19.7%	–	–
NOS	12.8%	12.9%	–	–
Appendix	11.0%	3.6%	83.0%	71.0%
Colon, except rectum	26.3%	14.9%	59.1%	61.8%
Rectum	17.5%	30.3%	75.2%	88.3%

Adapted from Modlin IM, Lye KD, Kidd M. A 5-decade analysis of 13,715 carcinoid tumors. *Cancer* 2003;97:934–59.

TABLE 24.5. Genes involved in hereditary and sporadic GI-NETs.

Gene loci (alterations)	Hereditary syndromes	Sporadic GI-NETs
11q13 mutation	Multiple endocrine neoplasia, type 1 (MEN-1)	Foregut NETs
17q11mutation	Neurofibromatosis, type 1(NF1)	Duodenal somatostatinoma, Gangliocytic paraganglio-cytoma
18q22 LOH (Smad4)	–	Midgut and hindgut NETs
X chromosome LOH	–	Malignant foregut NETs
17p13 LOH (P53 mutation)	–	Poorly differentiated NETs
Reglα gene mutation	–	Gastric ECL cell hyperplasia/tumor

Somatic mutation of *MEN1* gene can be found in about one third of foregut NETs, including those from the stomach[22] and duodenum.[23]

The *NF1* gene is located at chromosomal locus 17q11. Germline mutations in this lead to neurofibromatosis, which has increased risk of periampullary tumors, especially duodenal somatostatinoma[24] and gangliocytic paraganglioma.[25]

Loss of heterozygosity on chromosome 18q is frequently seen in midgut and hindgut NETs.[26] The alterations in these loci probably involve *Smad2*, *Smad4*, or *DCC* genes. LOH in X-chromosome[27] or 17q13 are seen only in malignant NETs but not in benign tumors. The mutation of *Reglα* gene (Reg) is associated with ECL cell tumors in patients with hypergastrinemia.[28]

In the following sections, GI-NETs will first be classified by their organ sites, then by the cell types or histopathologic entities. Any specific features pertinent to the organ site will be discussed in that section.

Esophageal Neuroendocrine Tumors

Esophageal NETs are extremely rare, accounting for only 0.05% of all GI-NETs and 0.02% of all esophageal cancers.[29] The tumors are usually located in the distal esophagus and maybe associated with achalasia or adenocarcinoma in the setting of Barrett's esophagus.[30] Three histopathologic entities have been reported in the esophagus: (1) classical NETs, (2) high-grade NETs, and (3) combined adenocarcinoma/neuroendocrine tumors. Patients having these tumors usually have a poor prognosis.[31]

Gastric Neuroendocrine Tumors (G-NETs)

The normal stomach has two major types of endocrine cells, the gastrin-producing G cells[32] (Figure 24.1a) and histamine-producing ECL cells[33] (Figure 24.1b). G cells are located at the neck region of the antrum whereas ECL cells are found at

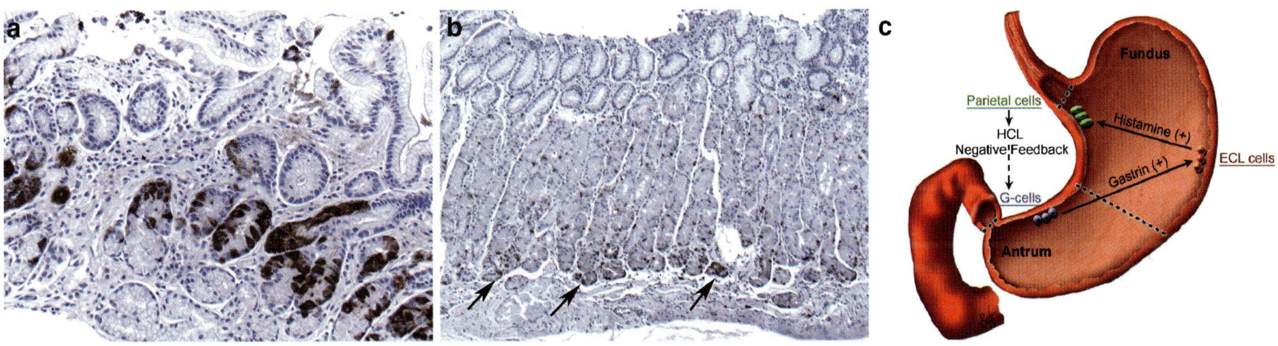

FIG. 24.1. Endocrine cells in the normal stomach and their regulation of gastric acid secretion. (**a**) Normal G-cells are located at the neck region of the antrum (gastrin immunostain). (**b**) Normal ECL-cells (*arrows*) are found at the base of fundic glands (synaptophysin immunostain). (**c**) Schematic diagram of the regulation of gastric hydrochloric acid by G- and ECL cells.

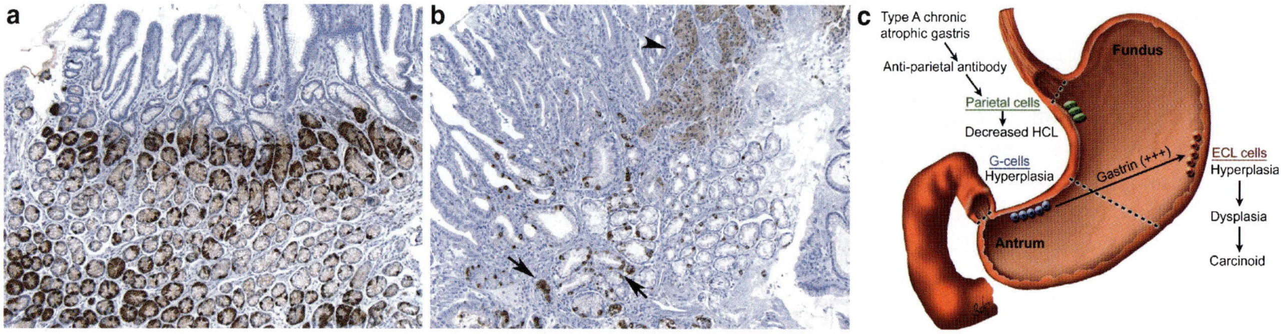

FIG. 24.2. Type 1 gastric neuroendocrine tumors. (**a**) G-cell hyperplasia (gastrin immunostain) (**b**) ECL-cell hyperplasia (*arrows*) and full blown gastric neuroendocrine tumor (*arrow head*) (synaptophysin immunostain). (**c**) Schematic diagram illustrates the mechanism of ECL cell hyperplasia and subsequent development of type 1 gastric neuroendocrine tumors in the clinical setting of type A chronic atrophic gastritis.

the base of fundic glands. In normal stomach, G cells secrete gastrin in response to negative feedback by hydrochloric acid[34] (Figure 24.1c). Gastrin, in turn, drives the ECL cells to produce histamine, which is the main activator of acid secretion by parietal cell. Most G-NETs arise from ECL cells and rarely from G cells.

The incidence of G-NET has increased in past five decades. Since 1950, the proportion of G-NET among all GI-NET has increased from 2.6% to 8.7%. This increase is due to increased endoscopic surveillance and improved pathological evaluation. The recent propensity of using strong acid-suppressing medications such as proton pump inhibitors[35] has been suspected a risk factor of G-NET secondary to the resulting hypergastrinemia. However, this theory has not been confirmed. Three distinct types of G-NETs will be described as follows.[36]

TABLE 24.6. Features of gastric neuroendocrine tumors.

	Type 1	Type 2	Type 3
Tumor features			
% of all gastric NETs	68–85%	8%	23%
Size	<2 cm	<2 cm	>3 cm
Number	Single/multiple	Multiple	Single
Location	Fundus	Fundus	Antrum or fundus
Clinical features			
Plasma gastrin levels	Increased	Increased	Normal
Gastric acid	Low	High	Normal
Associated conditions	A-CAG,	ZES/MEN I	None
Pathology			
Antral G cells	Hyperplasia	Normal	Normal
Fundic ECL cells	Hyperplasia/ dysplasia	Hyperplasia/ dysplasia	Normal
Fundic mucosa	Atrophic	Hypertrophic	Normal
Prognosis			
5-year survival	>70%	>70%	50%
Metastases	Rare	Up to 30%	50–100%
Treatment	Endoscopic removal Antrectomy	Endoscopic removal Gastrinoma resection	Surgery
Genetic factors			
LOH of 11q13 (MEN1 locus)	48%	75%	25–62%

Type 1 G-NETs Associated with Type A (autoimmune) Chronic Atrophic Gastritis

Among various types of G-NETs (Table 24.6), type 1 is most common and it often has a benign course.[36,37] Histologically, the tumor is usually small (<2 cm), multiple (Figure 24.2b), and confined to the fundic mucosa, which exhibits various degree of chronic inflammation and glandular atrophy. The antral mucosa is characterized by G-cell hyperplasia (Figure 24.2a). Lymph node metastasis is very uncommon. Given its favorable outcome, endoscopic mucosal resection or antrectomy are considered as an appropriate treatment. Tumor regression has been reported following antrectomy, which removes the entire population of G cells.[38]

Type A chronic atrophic gastritis is caused by autoantibodies to parietal cells or intrinsic factor.[39] It may or may not be associated with pernicious anemia. The disease involves the oxyntic mucosa of the fundus, leading to glandular atrophy and achlorhydria secondary to the loss of parietal cells, which produces hydrochloric acid (Figure 24.2c). Lacking the negative feedback of hydrochloric acid, the antral G-cells undergo hyperplasia and hypersecretion of gastrin. Hypergastrinemia, in turn, causes ECL cell hyperplasia (Figure 24.2b) and its subsequent transformation into G-NET.

The pathogenesis of type 1 G-NET is mostly unclear. Hypergastrinemia is required for the hyperplasia of ECL cells but insufficient for their transformation into G-NETs. Only 3% of patient with A-CAG develops G-NETs. Therefore, some other genetic factors are still needed in the development of tumors. LOH analysis showed allelic loss of the 11q13 regions (MEN-1 gene locus) in 48% cases of type 1 G-NETs.[40] Azzoni et al has demonstrated the overproduction of BCL-2, an anti-apoptosis protein, in hyperplastic ECL cells of patients with A-CAG.[41] This finding suggested a potential role of BCL-2, which extends the exposure of ECL cells to other oncogenic factors.

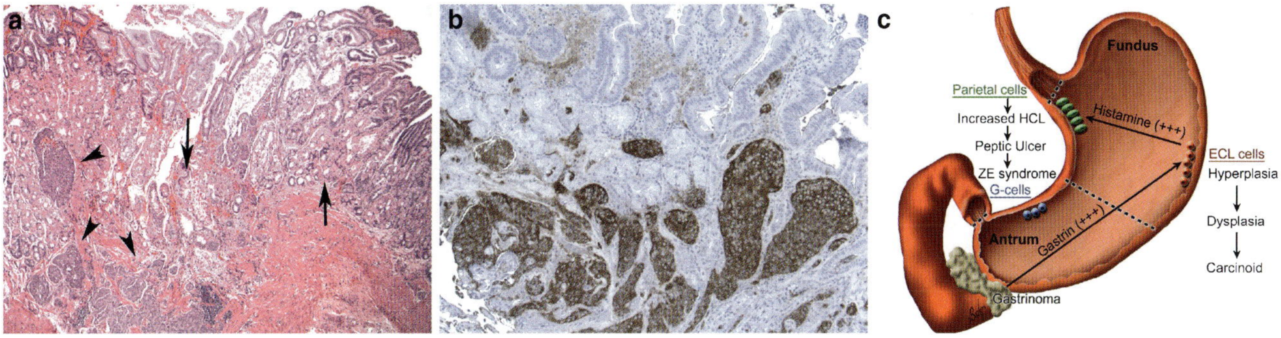

FIG. 24.3. Type 2 neuroendocrine tumors. (**a**) Gastric neuroendocrine tumors (*arrow heads*) develop in a background of peptic ulcer and parietal cell hyperplasia (*arrows*) (H&E stain). (**b**) Coexistent gastrinoma (gastrin immunostain) in the duodenum of this patient with MEN-1. (**c**) Schematic diagram illustrates the mechanism of type 2 gastric neuroendocrine tumors develop in the clinical setting of MEN-1 and Zollinger-Ellison syndrome.

Type 2 G-NETs Associated with Zollinger-Ellison Syndrome (ZES) with or Without Type 1 Multiple Endocrine Neoplasia (MEN-1)

ZES is characterized by multiple intractable peptic ulcers secondary to gastrin-producing tumors in the pancreas or duodenum. ZES may be sporadic (rare) or commonly associated with MEN-1, which contains pancreatic gastrinoma as a component.[42]

These lesions are usually multiple and less than 2 cm in size. Background pathology includes hypertrophic, hypersecretory gastropathy (Figure 24.3a) secondary to the trophic effects of gastrin.[43,44] Unlike type 1 G-NET, hypergastrinemia in this setting is arising from gastrinoma (Figure 24.3b) rather than antral G cells, which appear normal in type 2. In addition to hyperplasia, dysplasia of ECL cells is more commonly seen than that in type 1 G-NETs. The pathogenetic pathway is summarized in Figure 24.3c. The treatment should aim at the localization and surgical excision of gastrinoma. Spontaneous regression of G-NET has been reported following the removal of gastrinoma.[45] Palliation by endoscopic mucosal excision or somatostatin analog may be considered in nonsurgical candidates.

Type 3 Sporadic G-NETs

This type of lesions is gastrin-independent and not associated with hypergastrinemia.[36] It accounts for about a quarter of all G-NETs and has a worse prognosis than other 2 types of G-NET. Patients usually have a large, solitary tumor presented in the antrum or fundus. The adjacent antral or fundic mucosa appears histologically unremarkable (Figure 24.4). Metastatic disease is more common than type 1 and 2 G-NET. In light of the malignant potential of this tumor, aggressive therapy should be considered. In addition to surgery, combined chemotherapy and radiation may be required.[46]

Unlike type 1 and 2, endocrine cell hyperplasia plays no role in these lesions. Genetic abnormalities are considered the major pathogenic mechanisms. It is interesting to note

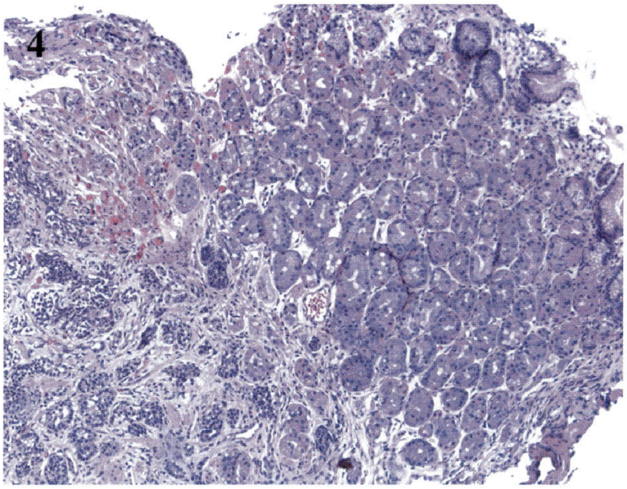

FIG. 24.4. Type 3 gastric neuroendocrine tumors. The neuroendocrine tumor (*left lower field*) develops in a background of normal gastric mucosa (*right upper field*) without hyperplasia or atrophy of the gastric mucosa (H&E stain).

that LOH of 11q13 has been reported in 25–62% of cases, suggesting a common genetic basis may be shared by all 3 types of G-NET.

Hyperplasia-Dysplasia-Neoplasia Sequence in G-NET

Nonneoplastic endocrine cell hyperplasia has been proposed as the precursor lesion of GI-NETs in several anatomic sites. The hyperplasia-dysplasia-neoplasia sequence was best studied in the stomach and its histopathologic classification in 1988 by Socia et al[47–50] (Table 24.7) (Figure 24.5). This process can be seen in both type 1 and 2 gastric NETs. By definition, ECL hyperplasia is a lesion that lacks inherent evolutive potential and less than 150 μm in size. ECL dysplasias are pre-carcinoid lesions that measure between 150 and 500 μm and display progressive capacity. ECL neoplasias are those lesions larger than 500 μm with invasion into the mucosa or beyond. Table 24.7 lists the histological criteria of all subcategories of three major entities.[47]

TABLE 24.7. Hyperplasia-dysplasia-neoplasia sequence of gastric neuroendocrine tumors.

Classification	Lesion size	Morphology
Hyperplasia		
Simple (or diffuse)		Cell number >2 stand deviation normal
Linear (or chain-forming)		≤5 cells; 2 chains/mm mucosa
Micronodular		≥5 cells; 30–150 μm
Adenomatoid		≥5 micronodule
Dysplasia (Pre-neoplasia)	<500 μm	
Enlarge micronodular		Cluster of cells <150 μm
Fusing micronodular		Loss of basement membrane in between
Microinvasive lesion		Infiltrating the lamina propria
Nodule with newly formed stroma		Microlobular or trabecular structure
Neoplasia (carcinoid)	≥500 μm	
Intramucosal carcinoid		Confined to the mucosa
Microcarcinoid		Microscopic lesion not seen grossly
Microcarcinoidosis		Multiple microcarcinoids
Invasive carcinoid		Penetrating muscularis mucosae

Small Bowel Neuroendocrine Tumors

Duodenal Neuroendocrine Tumors

Duodenal NETs (Table 24.8) are rare and can be classified into five major types: (1) G-cell tumors, (2) D-cell tumors, (3) other well-differentiated NETs, (4) gangliocytic paraganglioma, and (5) poorly differentiated endocrine carcinomas.[51] G-cell tumors are either sporadic or hereditary associated with MEN-1.[52] Most G-cell tumors from the latter group are small, multiple, and functioning.[53] Gastrin-producing G-cell tumor can generate Zollinger-Ellison syndrome. In a recent report of 18 cases of G-cell tumors arising in the duodenal bulb, there is a high association with long-term use of proton pump inhibitors and with *H. pylori* gastritis.[54] Histologically, G-cell tumors form trabecular or acinar architecture surrounded by a delicate fibrovascular stroma (Figure 24.6a).

Almost all D-cell tumors occur in the region of ampulla of Vater.[55] Although containing somatostatin, these tumors are usually nonfunctioning and do not produce symptoms related to somatostatin hypersecretion such as diarrhea and diabetes. There is a high association (50%) between D-cell tumors and type 1 neurofibromatosis[56,57] and von Hippel Lindau disease[58] with unclear molecular mechanism. Histologically, D-cell tumors contain glands lined by columnar cells and filled with psammoma bodies in

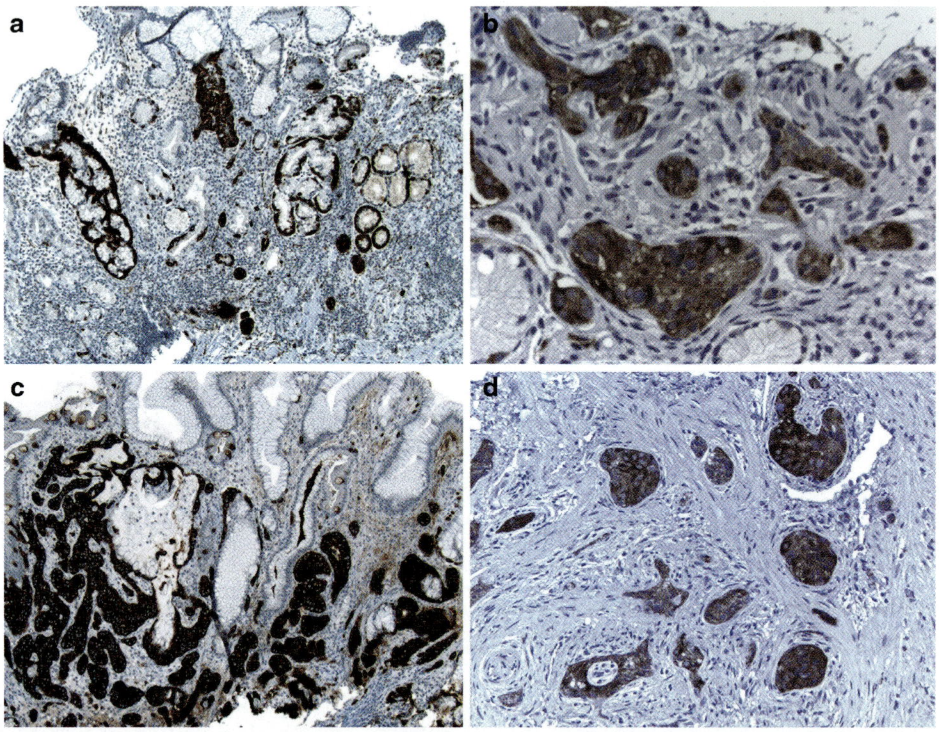

FIG. 24.5. Hyperplasia-dysplasia-neoplasia sequence of gastric ECL cell tumors (**a**) Linear and micronodular hyperplasia. (**b**) Enlarged and fusing micronodular dysplasia. (**c**) Intramucosal carcinoids. (**d**) Invasive carcinoids in the submucosal stroma. (synaptophysin immunostains).

the lumens (Figure 24.6b). In patients with NF1 associated with D-cell tumors, gangliocytic paraganglioma is another common lesion found in the duodenum.

TABLE 24.8. Neuroendocrine tumors of the small intestine.

	Duodenal NETs	Jejuno-ileal NETs
Primitive gut	Foregut	Midgut
% of total GI-NET	22%	23–28%
Histologic types	G-cell tumor (gastrinoma)	EC cell tumors
	D-cell tumor (somatostatinoma)	L cell tumor
	Other hormone-producing tumors	
	Gangliocytic paraganglioma	
	Neuroendocrine carcinoma	
Associated conditions		
Hereditary	MEN-1	–
	Neurofibromatosis	
Nonhereditary	Zollinger-Ellison syndrome	–
	Proton-pump inhibitor	

Jejunal and Ileal Neuroendocrine Tumors

Jejuno-ileal region is the second most common site for GI-NETs and accounts for up to 30% cases of the latter.[29] EC cell tumor is the most common type of jejuno-ileal NETs.[59] The etiology is unknown although it is interesting to note its association with Crohn's disease[60] or other non-carcinoid neoplasms of the GI-tract in some patients. Lymph node metastasis is commonly found during the surgery, but it does not seem to affect patients' survival. Histological features are characterized by multiple solid or insular nests of packed cells, which frequently invade the bowel wall (Figure 24.7a, b).

Appendiceal Neuroendocrine Tumors

NETs are found in (0.3–0.9 %) of appendectomy specimens, but they account for up to 75% of all appendiceal neoplasms. Its incidence among all GI-NETs appears decreasing during the period of 1973–1997. A classification based on WHO is shown in Table 24.9.

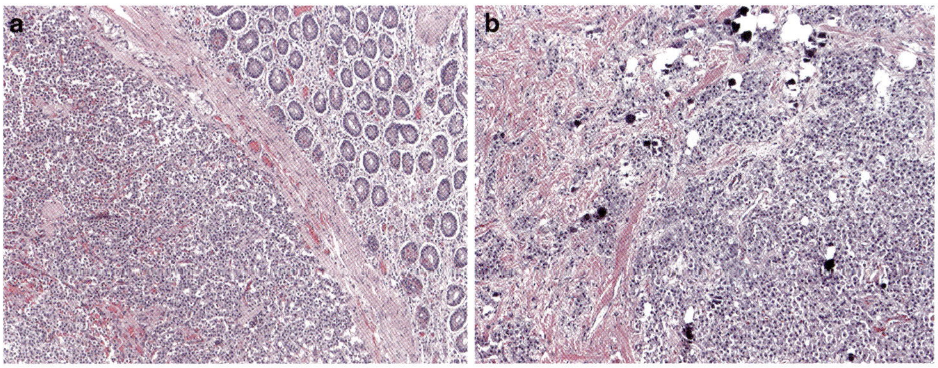

FIG. 24.6. Duodenal neuroendocrine tumors (H&E stains) (**a**) G-cell tumor (gastrinoma). (**b**) D-cell tumor (somatostatinoma) with psammoma bodies.

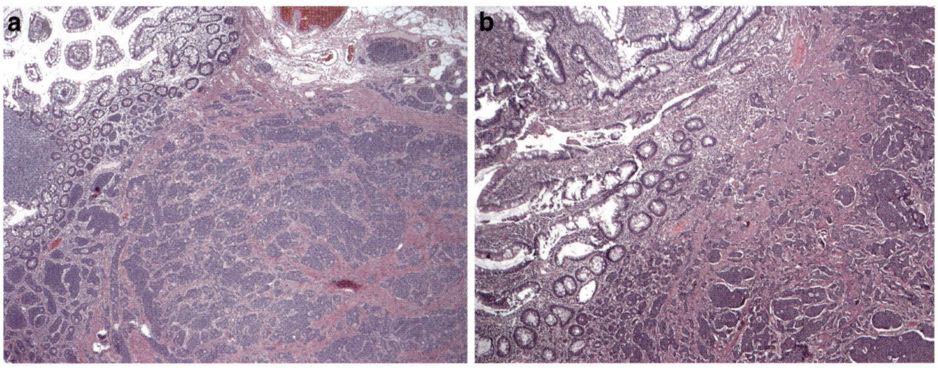

FIG. 24.7. Neuroendocrine tumors of the jejunum (**a**) and ileum (**b**) (H&E stains).

Serotonin-producing EC cell carcinoids are the most common type of appendiceal NETs. Most of them are located at the tip of the appendix (Figure 24.8a, b) and arise from the subepithelial neuroendocrine cells, which are most abundant in the tip. The majority of tumors is less than 1 cm and associated with better prognosis. L cell carcinoids are uncommon. They are small and localized at the tip of the appendix.

Mixed endocrine-exocrine neoplasms are rare but interesting variants because of their differentiation into multiple cell lineages. Three morphological types were recognized in a large series of 64 cases by Armed Institute of Pathology: (1) tubular carcinoids, (2) goblet cell carcinoids, and (3) mixed carcinoid-adenocarcinomas.[61]

Tubular carcinoids are typically less than 5 mm and poorly defined in the stroma or smooth muscle. Most of them were diagnosed incidentally by microscopic examination without gross evidence of lesions. Histology shows tubular structures of cuboidal cells with occasional goblet cells. Patients have excellent prognosis without recurrence or metastasis.

TABLE 24.9. Classification of appendiceal neuroendocrine tumors.

Typical carcinoids
EC cell carcinoid
L cell carcinoid
Mixed endocrine-exocrine neoplasms
Tubular carcinoid
Goblet cell carcinoid
Mixed carcinoid-adenocarcinoma

Goblet cell carcinoid is also known as adenocarcinoid, mucin-producing carcinoid, and crypt cell carcinoma.[61,62] Histology is characterized by small nests of goblet cells and neuroendocrine cells (Figure 24.9a) with scattered glandular formation. Patients have a prognosis intermediate between typical carcinoids and adenocarcinoma. Of those tumors confined to the appendix and excised with negative surgical margins, a cure without recurrence or metastasis is the norm. A third of patients may have extensive disease outside the appendix and eventually die of the disease.

Despite its rarity, goblet cell carcinoid has drawn the attention of investigators regarding its histogenesis. Stancu et al found loss of heterozygosity of chromosomes 11q, 16q, and 18q occurring 25%, 38%, and 56% respectively in 16 cases of goblet cell carcinoid.[63] The profile was similar to that of ileal carcinoid, but different from non-ileal carcinoids. They did not find any mutations of *K-ras*, β-catenin, or DPC-genes, which supports that this tumor follows the usual pathogenetic pathway of endocrine tumors rather than exocrine adenocarcinoma. Another study by Kuroda

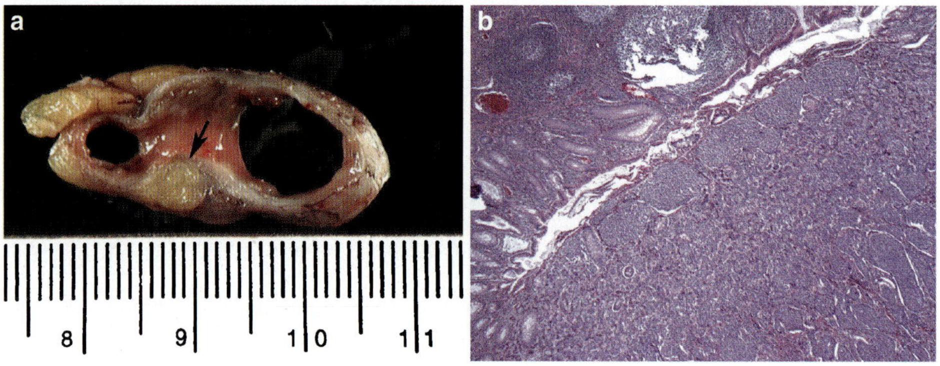

FIG. 24.8. Typical EC cell carcinoid of the appendix. (**a**) Cross section of the appendix shows a 5 mm yellowish, well-circumscribed carcinoid tumor (*arrow*). (**b**) Microgram of the carcinoid (H&E stain).

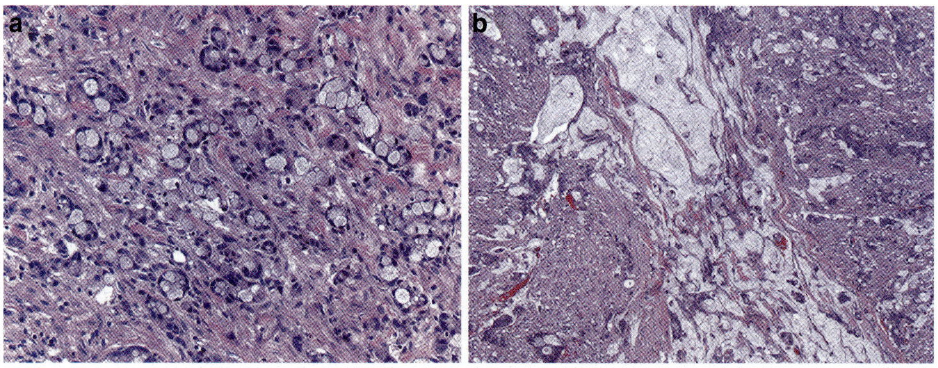

FIG. 24.9. Mixed endocrine-exocrine neoplasms of the appendix. (**a**) Goblet cell carcinoid. (**b**) Mixed carcinoid-adenocarcinoma (H&E stain).

et al indicated that reduced expression of E-cadherin in this tumor is more similar to typical carcinoid rather than to adenocarcinoma.[64]

Mixed carcinoid-adenocarcinoma[61,65] is associated with the worst prognosis among 3 variants of amphicrine tumors. Most patients died of metastatic carcinoma within 2 years. In addition to clusters of endocrine cells and goblet cell carcinoid, this variant also shows typical morphology of adenocarcinoma (Figure 24.9b), such as glandular formation or signet-ring cell features, in more than 50% of the tumor mass.[61]

Colonic and Rectal Neuroendocrine Tumors

Large intestine NETs are most common in the rectum (54%), followed by the cecum (20%), sigmoid colon (7.5%), and ascending colon (5%).[29] Some cases were reported in patients with inflammatory bowel disease.[66] However, a direct association of NETs and inflammatory bowel disease has not been substantiated.

Excluding the rectum, about half of the colonic NETs are located at the cecum. The remaining half has a roughly equal distribution among the ascending, transverse, descending, and sigmoid colon. As their counterpart of adenocarcinoma, NETs of the right colon tend to be larger and present at more advanced stage compared to NETs of the left colon. The diagnosis is commonly established by colonoscopic biopsies and histological examination. Surgical treatment follows the same principle of colonic adenocarcinoma, i.e., complete resection of the tumor and lymph node spread. The surgeon should expect higher rate of local invasion and liver metastases than adenocarcinoma.

Rectal NETs are frequently small (<2 cm), asymptomatic, and have an indolent course. Carcinoid syndrome is uncommon (<10% of cases) because of the secretion of hormone products into the portal circulation and detoxication in the liver.

Histologically, large intestinal NETs can be classified into (1) typical carcinoids, including EC- and L-cell tumor, (2) large cell neuroendocrine carcinoma, and (3) small cell carcinoma (Table 24.10). Typical carcinoids are those well differentiated NETs, which exhibit trabecular pattern (Figure 24.10a). Large cell neuroendocrine carcinoma is a malignant tumor composed of large cells with organoid, nesting, and palisading patterns (Figure 24.10b). Small cell carcinoma is rare and morphologically similar to that of the lung.

Treatment

The treatment of GI-NETs varies depending on the disease stages and symptoms related to hormonal secretion. The major options can be summarized as follows:

1. Surgery: Surgical resection, either curative or palliative, is considered the first choice for patients with localized disease. Appendectomy may be adequate for appendiceal NET unless the tumor is larger than 2 cm or have angiolymphatic invasion or positive margin. Then, right hemicolectomy should be performed. Endoscopic removal is considered appropriate for rectal carcinoid less than 1 cm without invasion into the muscularis propria.[67] However, small bowel NETs require wider resection according to the stage due to the high risk of metastasis.
2. Biotherapy: Low dose interferon-α or somatostatin analogues (e.g., octreotide) has been used to manage the clinical symptoms with more than 50% response rate.[68] However, tumor reduction is only seen in less than 15% of patients.

TABLE 24.10. Classification of colorectal neuroendocrine tumor.

EC cell tumor
L-cell tumor
Small cell carcinoma
Large cell neuroendocrine carcinom

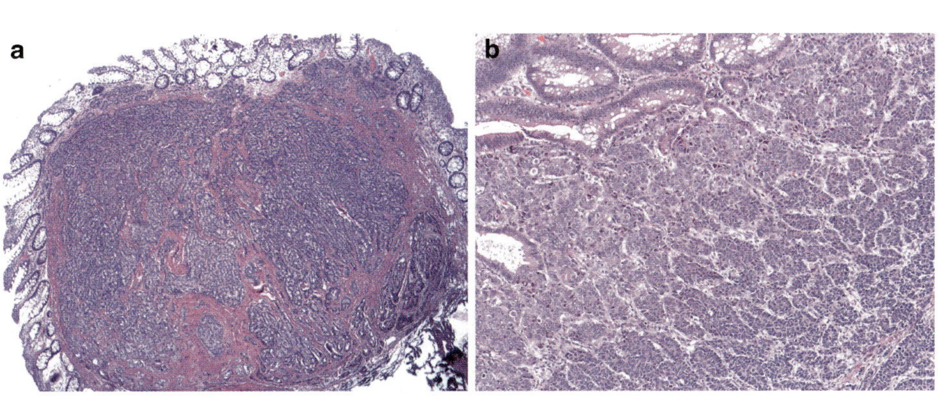

FIG. 24.10. Colorectal neuroendocrine tumors (H&E stains) (**a**) Colonic carcinoid tumor. (**b**) Rectal large cell neuroendocrine carcinoma.

3. Chemotherapy: Clinical response to single agent, such as 5-fluorouracil, streptozocin, doxorubicin, actinomycin D, and cyclophosphamide, has been around 10%. Combination chemotherapy may increase response rate to 30%, but complete response is rare.

References

1. Dayal Y. The neuroendocrine cell system of the gut and pancreas: introduction and historical perspectives. In: Dayal Y, ed. CRC Press; 1991:1–32.
2. DeLellis RA: The neuroendocrine system and its tumors: an overview, *Am J Clin Pathol.* 2001; 115 suppl:S5–S16.
3. Soga J, Tazawa K. Pathologic analysis of carcinoids. Histologic reevaluation of 62 cases. *Cancer.* 1971;28:990–998.
4. Smith DM Jr, Haggitt RC. A comparative study of generic stains for carcinoid secretory granules. *Am J Surg Pathol.* 1983; 7:61–68.
5. FahrenkampAG, WibbekeC, WindeG, et al. Immunohistochemical distribution of chromogranins A and B and secretogranin II in neuroendocrine tumours of the gastrointestinal tract. *Virchows Arch.* 1995;426:361–367.
6. Taupenot L, Harper KL, O'Connor DT. The chromogranin-secretogranin family [see comment]. *N Engl J Med.* 2003; 348:1134–1149.
7. Wiedenmann B, Franke WW, Kuhn C, Moll R, Gould VE. Synaptophysin: a marker protein for neuroendocrine cells and neoplasms. *Proc Natl Acad Sci USA.* 1986;83:3500–3504.
8. Rode J, Dhillon AP, Doran JF, Jackson P, Thompson RJ. PGP 9.5, a new marker for human neuroendocrine tumours. *Histopathology.* 1985;9:147–158.
9. Schmechel D, Marangos PJ, Brightman M. Neurone-specific enolase is a molecular marker for peripheral and central neuroendocrine cells. *Nature.* 1978;276:834–836.
10. Williams ED, Sandler M. The classification of carcinoid tumours. *Lancet.* 1963;1:238–239.
11. van Bogaert LJ. The diffuse endocrine system and derived tumours. Histological and histochemical characteristics. *Acta Histochem.* 1982;70:122–129.
12. Jaffee IM, Rahmani M, Singhal MG, Younes M. Expression of the intestinal transcription factor CDX2 in carcinoid tumors is a marker of midgut origin. *Arch Pathol Lab Med.* 2006;130: 1522–1526.
13. Rindi G, Leiter AB, Kopin AS, Bordi C, Solcia E. The "normal" endocrine cell of the gut: changing concepts and new evidences. *Ann N Y Acad Sci.* 2004;1014:1–12.
14. DeLellis RA, Dayal Y, Wolfe HJ. Carcinoid tumors. Changing concepts and new perspectives. *Am J Surg Pathol.* 1984;8: 295–300.
15. Solcia E, Kloppel G, Sobin LH. Endocrine tumors of the gastrointestinal tract. In: Solcia E, Kloppel G, Sobin LH, eds. New York: Springer-Verlag; 2000:61–68.
16. Kloppel G, Perren A, Heitz PU. The gastroenteropancreatic neuroendocrine cell system and its tumors: the WHO classification. *Ann N Y Acad Sci.* 2004;1014:13–27.
17. Rindi G, Kloppel G, Alhman H, et al. TNM staging of foregut (neuro)endocrine tumors: a consensus proposal including a grading system. *Virchows Arch.* 2006;449:395–401.
18. Rindi G, Kloppel G, Couvelard A, et al. TNM staging of midgut and hindgut (neuro) endocrine tumors: a consensus proposal including a grading system. *Virchows Arch.* 2007;451: 757–762.
19. Modlin IM, Lye KD, Kidd M. A 5-decade analysis of 13,715 carcinoid tumors. *Cancer.* 2003;97:934–959.
20. Rindi G, Villanacci V, Ubiali A. Biological and molecular aspects of gastroenteropancreatic neuroendocrine tumors. *Digestion.* 2000;62(suppl 1):19–26.
21. Chandrasekharappa SC, Guru SC, Manickam P, et al. Positional cloning of the gene for multiple endocrine neoplasia-type 1. *Science.* 1997;276:404–407.
22. Bordi C, Corleto VD, Azzoni C, et al. The antral mucosa as a new site for endocrine tumors in multiple endocrine neoplasia type 1 and Zollinger-Ellison syndromes. *J Clin Endocrinol Metab.* 2001;86:2236–2242.
23. Pipeleers-Marichal M, Somers G, Willems G, et al. Gastrinomas in the duodenums of patients with multiple endocrine neoplasia type 1 and the Zollinger-Ellison syndrome [see comment]. *N Engl J Med.* 1990;322:723–727.
24. Klein A, Clemens J, Cameron J. Periampullary neoplasms in von Recklinghausen's disease. *Surgery.* 1989;106:815–819.
25. Kheir SM, Halpern NB. Paraganglioma of the duodenum in association with congenital neurofibromatosis. Possible relationship. *Cancer.* 1984;53:2491–2496.
26. Lollgen RM, Hessman O, Szabo E, Westin G, Akerstrom G. Chromosome 18 deletions are common events in classical midgut carcinoid tumors. *Int J Cancer.* 2001;92:812–815.
27. D'Adda T, Candidus S, Denk H, Bordi C, Hofler H. Gastric neuroendocrine neoplasms: tumour clonality and malignancy-associated large X-chromosomal deletions. *J Pathol.* 1999; 189:394–401.
28. Higham AD, Bishop LA, Dimaline R, et al. Mutations of RegIalpha are associated with enterochromaffin-like cell tumor development in patients with hypergastrinemia [see comment]. *Gastroenterology.* 1999;116:1310–1318.
29. Modlin IM, Sandor A. An analysis of 8305 cases of carcinoid tumors. *Cancer.* 1997;79:813–829.
30. Hoang MP, Hobbs CM, Sobin LH, Albores-Saavedra J. Carcinoid tumor of the esophagus: a clinicopathologic study of four cases. *Am J Surg Pathol.* 2002;26:517–522.
31. Ready AR, Soul JO, Newman J, Matthews HR. Malignant carcinoid tumour of the oesophagus [see comment]. *Thorax.* 1989;44:594–596.
32. Voillemot N, Potet F, Mary JY, Lewin MJ. Gastrin cell distribution in normal human stomachs and in patients with Zollinger-Ellison syndrome. *Gastroenterology.* 1978;75:61–65.
33. Modlin IM, Nangia AK. The pathobiology of the human enterochromaffin-like cell. *Yale J Biol Med.* 1992;65:775-792. discussion 827–779.
34. Freston JW, Borch K, Brand SJ, et al. Effects of hypochlorhydria and hypergastrinemia on structure and function of gastrointestinal cells. A review and analysis. *Dig Dis Sci.* 1995;40: 50S–62S.
35. McCloy RF, Arnold R, Bardhan KD, et al. Pathophysiological effects of long-term acid suppression in man. *Dig Dis Sci.* 1995;40:96S–120S.
36. Rindi G, Luinetti O, Cornaggia M, Capella C, Solcia E. Three subtypes of gastric argyrophil carcinoid and the gastric neuroendocrine carcinoma: a clinicopathologic study [see comment]. *Gastroenterology.* 1993;104:994–1006.
37. Solcia E, Rindi G, Fiocca R, et al. Distinct patterns of chronic gastritis associated with carcinoid and cancer and their role in

tumorigenesis. *Yale J Biol Med.* 1992;65:793-804. discussion 827–799.
38. Richards AT, Hinder RA, Harrison AC. Gastric carcinoid tumours associated with hypergastrinaemia and pernicious anaemia – regression of tumors by antrectomy. A case report. *S Afr Med J.* 1987;72:51–53.
39. Maury CP, Tornroth T, Teppo AM. Atrophic gastritis in Sjogren's syndrome. Morphologic, biochemical, and immunologic findings. *Arthritis Rheum.* 1985;28:388–394.
40. D'Adda T, Keller G, Bordi C, Hofler H. Loss of heterozygosity in 11q13-14 regions in gastric neuroendocrine tumors not associated with multiple endocrine neoplasia type 1 syndrome. *Lab Invest.* 1999;79:671–677.
41. Azzoni C, Doglioni C, Viale G, et al. Involvement of BCL-2 oncoprotein in the development of enterochromaffin-like cell gastric carcinoids. *Am J Surg Pathol.* 1996;20:433–441.
42. Solcia E, Capella C, Fiocca R, Rindi G, Rosai J. Gastric argyrophil carcinoidosis in patients with Zollinger-Ellison syndrome due to type 1 multiple endocrine neoplasia. A newly recognized association. *Am J Surg Pathol.* 1990;14:503–513.
43. Bordi C, D'Adda T, Azzoni C, Ferraro G. Pathogenesis of ECL cell tumors in humans. *Yale J Biol Med.* 1998;71:273–284.
44. Cadiot G, Lehy T, Mignon M. Gastric endocrine cell proliferation and fundic argyrophil carcinoid tumors in patients with the Zollinger-Ellison syndrome. *Acta Oncol.* 1993;32:135–140.
45. Richards ML, Gauger P, Thompson NW, Giordano TJ. Regression of type II gastric carcinoids in multiple endocrine neoplasia type 1 patients with Zollinger-Ellison syndrome after surgical excision of all gastrinomas. *World J Surg.* 2004;28:652–658.
46. Borch K, Ahren B, Ahlman H, Falkmer S, Granerus G, Grimelius L. Gastric carcinoids: biologic behavior and prognosis after differentiated treatment in relation to type. *Ann Surg.* 2005;242:64–73.
47. Rindi G, Solcia E. Endocrine hyperplasia and dysplasia in the pathogenesis of gastrointestinal and pancreatic endocrine tumors. *Gastroenterol Clin North Am.* 2007;36:851–865.
48. Solcia E, Bordi C, Creutzfeldt W, et al. Histopathological classification of nonantral gastric endocrine growths in man. *Digestion.* 1988;41:185–200.
49. Solcia E, Fiocca R, Rindi G, Villani L, Cornaggia M, Capella C. The pathology of the gastrointestinal endocrine system. *Endocrinol Metab Clin North Am.* 1993;22:795–821.
50. Solcia E, Fiocca R, Villani L, Luinetti O, Capella C. Hyperplastic, dysplastic, and neoplastic enterochromaffin-like-cell proliferations of the gastric mucosa. Classification and histogenesis. *Am J Surg Pathol.* 1995;19(suppl 1):S1–S7.
51. Capella C SE, Sobin LH, Arnold R, Endocrine tumors of the small intestine. In: Hamilton SR AL, ed. Lyon: IARC Press; 2000:77–82.
52. Donow C, Pipeleers-Marichal M, Schroder S, Stamm B, Heitz PU, Kloppel G. Surgical pathology of gastrinoma. Site, size, multicentricity, association with multiple endocrine neoplasia type 1, and malignancy. *Cancer.* 1991;68:1329–1334.
53. Thom AK, Norton JA, Axiotis CA, Jensen RT. Location, incidence, and malignant potential of duodenal gastrinomas. *Surgery.* 1991;110:1086-1091. discussion 1091–1083.
54. Merchant SH, VanderJagt T, Lathrop S, Amin MB. Sporadic duodenal bulb gastrin-cell tumors: association with Helicobacter pylori gastritis and long-term use of proton pump inhibitors. *Am J Surg Pathol.* 2006;30:1581–1587.
55. Dayal Y, Doos WG, O'Brien MJ, Nunnemacher G, DeLellis RA, Wolfe HJ. Psammomatous somatostatinomas of the duodenum. *Am J Surg Pathol.* 1983;7:653–665.
56. Dayal Y, Tallberg KA, Nunnemacher G, DeLellis RA, Wolfe HJ. Duodenal carcinoids in patients with and without neurofibromatosis. A comparative study. *Am J Surg Pathol.* 1986;10: 348–357.
57. Fendrich V, Ramaswamy A, Slater EP, Bartsch DK. Duodenal somatostatinoma associated with Von Recklinghausen's disease. *J Hepatobiliary Pancreat Surg.* 2004;11:417–421.
58. Karasawa Y, Sakaguchi M, Minami S, et al. Duodenal somatostatinoma and erythrocytosis in a patient with von Hippel-Lindau disease type 2A. *Intern Med.* 2001;40:38–43.
59. de Herder WW. Tumours of the midgut (jejunum, ileum and ascending colon, including carcinoid syndrome). *Best Pract Res Clin Gastroenterol.* 2005;19:705–715.
60. Bishop AE, Pietroletti R, Taat CW, Brummelkamp WH, Polak JM. Increased populations of endocrine cells in Crohn's ileitis. *Virchows Archiv A Pathol Anat Histopathol.* 1987;410: 391–396.
61. Burke AP, Sobin LH, Federspiel BH, Shekitka KM, Helwig EB. Goblet cell carcinoids and related tumors of the vermiform appendix. *Am J Clin Pathol.* 1990;94:27–35.
62. Anderson NH, Somerville JE, Johnston CF, Hayes DM, Buchanan KD, Sloan JM. Appendiceal goblet cell carcinoids: a clinicopathological and immunohistochemical study. *Histopathology.* 1991;18:61–65.
63. Stancu M, Wu T-T, Wallace C, Houlihan PS, Hamilton SR, Rashid A. Genetic alterations in goblet cell carcinoids of the vermiform appendix and comparison with gastrointestinal carcinoid tumors. *Mod Pathol.* 2003;16:1189–1198.
64. Kuroda N, Mizushima S, Guo L, et al. Goblet cell carcinoid of the appendix: investigation of the expression of beta-catenin and E-cadherin. *Pathol Int.* 2001;51:283–287.
65. Lin BT, Gown AM. Mixed carcinoid and adenocarcinoma of the appendix: report of 4 cases with immunohistochemical studies and a review of the literature. *Appl Immunohistochem Mol Morphol.* 2004;12:271–276.
66. Kortbeek J, Kelly JK, Preshaw RM. Carcinoid tumors and inflammatory bowel disease. *J Surg Oncol.* 1992;49:122–126.
67. Higaki S, Nishiaki M, Mitani N, Yanai H, Tada M, Okita K. Effectiveness of local endoscopic resection of rectal carcinoid tumors. *Endoscopy.* 1997;29:171–175.
68. Oberg K. Interferons in the management of neuroendocrine tumors and their possible mechanism of action. *Yale J Biol Med.* 1992;65:519-529. discussion 531–516.

25
Head and Neck Neuroendocrine Tumors

Edward B. Stelow

Introduction

The head and neck region contains a number of disparate organs ranging from skin to brain, and many of the neuroendocrine tumors of these organs have been discussed elsewhere in this book (skin, thyroid, and pituitary gland). Extra-adrenal paragangliomas, although also discussed elsewhere, will be mentioned and discussed briefly as they pertain to the ear and upper aerodigestive tract. This chapter will concentrate on neuroendocrine tumors of the ear, upper aerodigestive tract, and salivary glands. Focusing on these entities leaves only a few head- and neck-specific tumors to discuss, including middle ear adenoma, neuroendocrine carcinomas of the upper aerodigestive tract and salivary glands, uncommon and unique neuroectodermal tumors of the area, and, as mentioned, paraganglioma. Even if taken together, these tumors are exceedingly rare and little is known regarding the genetics of the tumors. While this limits our discussion, it does leave open some exciting avenues of possible research.

Upper Aerodigestive Tract

Neuroendocrine Carcinomas

Neuroendocrine carcinomas of all grades (well, moderately and poorly differentiated neuroendocrine carcinomas, also called carcinoid tumors, atypical carcinoid tumors, and small cell carcinomas) occur throughout the upper aerodigestive tract, most often within the larynx or sinonasal tract.[1–9] Distinguishing these tumors histologically is important, as they have very different prognoses.

Well-differentiated neuroendocrine carcinomas or *carcinoid tumors* are by far the rarest of these malignancies.[1–3,8] They develop most frequently in the supraglottic larynx of older men. Up to a third of the patients can eventually develop distant metastases, but only 10% of patients die from their disease.

These tumors resemble carcinoid tumors from other sites and have an organoid, nested or trabecular architecture, and are composed of uniform epithelioid cells.[1–3,8] The cells may have a variable amount of cytoplasm that sometimes appears granular or oncocytic. Nuclei are usually also uniform in size and are round to ovoid with granular chromatin. By definition, mitotic figures are usually not seen and necrosis is absent. Background amyloid or sclerosis is sometimes seen.

Moderately differentiated neuroendocrine carcinomas or *atypical carcinoid tumors* are much more common.[1–3,8,9] They also develop in the submucosa of the supraglottic larynx of older men but have a worse behavior than well-differentiated neuroendocrine carcinomas. Nearly half will present with regional lymph node metastases and less than one half of patients survive 5 years.

These tumors have much the same histologic appearance as typical carcinoid tumors; however, they show more variable architecture and can focally display sheet-like growth (Figure 25.1).[1–3,8] Characteristically, they have a moderate amount of nuclear and cellular pleomorphism and occasional mitotic figures. Furthermore, necrosis is often seen. Oncocytic and mucinous changes have been noted and amyloid can also be found.

Small cell carcinomas also can occur anywhere throughout the upper aerodigestive tract; however, they also most often involve the supraglottic larynx.[1–3,7,8,10,11] These occur more frequently in men, usually in the sixth to seventh decades of life and have a dismal prognosis; less than 5% of patients diagnosed with these lesions are alive 5 years after their diagnoses.

Histologically, small cell carcinomas of the upper aerodigestive tract are indistinguishable from small cell carcinomas seen elsewhere.[1–4,7,8] They are composed of variably sized sheets, cords, nests, and ribbons of small cells with little identifiable cytoplasm (Figure 25.2). Large areas of confluent necrosis are often seen. Nuclear molding and focal crush artifact are often also seen with abundant mitotic figures and single-cell apoptotic figures. Tumor cell nuclei are hyperchromatic and have granular chromatin without prominent

J.L. Hunt (ed.), *Molecular Pathology of Endocrine Diseases*, Molecular Pathology Library 3,
DOI 10.1007/978-1-4419-1707-2_25, © Springer Science+Business Media, LLC 2010

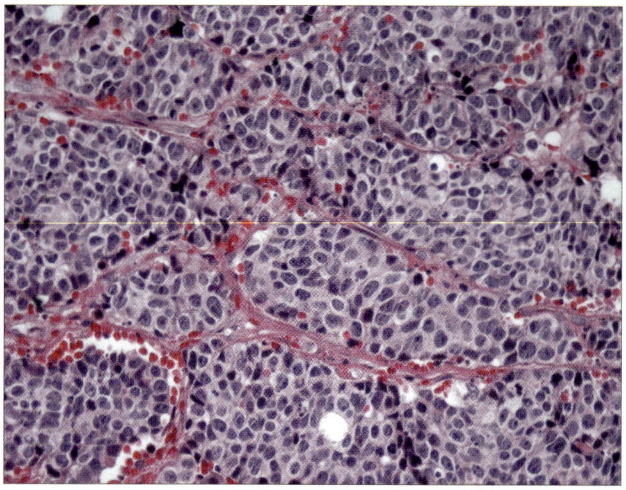

FIG. 25.1. Moderately differentiated neuroendocrine carcinomas (atypical carcinoid tumors) of the larynx often grow in an organoid pattern.

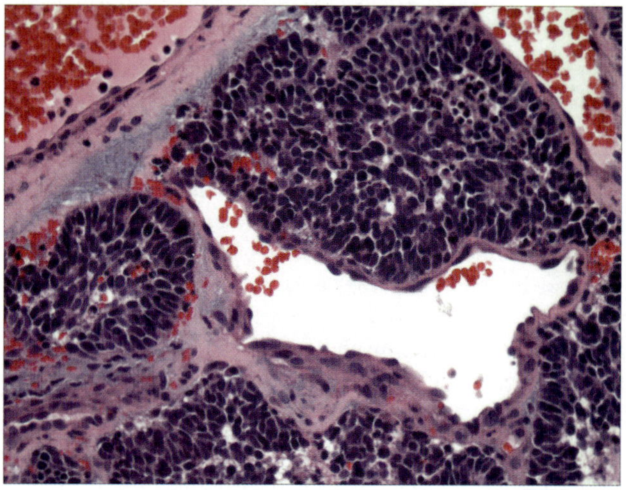

FIG. 25.2. Small cell carcinoma of the nasal cavity. These tumors resemble pulmonary small cell carcinomas.

nucleoli. The Azzopardi effect is often noted as is true vascular invasion. The tumors may contain areas diagnostic of non-small cell carcinoma, and varying differentiation has been noted throughout the upper aerodigestive tract.

Immunohistochemically, neuroendocrine carcinomas of the upper aerodigestive tract react with antibodies to keratins and neuroendocrine antigens, such as CD56, NSE chromogranin, and synaptophysin.[2,8] Small cell carcinomas often exhibit "dot-like" staining with antikeratin antibodies similar to immunoreactivity described with these tumors at other sites (Figure 25.3). Small cell carcinomas also are more likely to lack immunostaining with antibodies to chromogranin and synaptophysin. Moderately differentiated neuroendocrine carcinomas of the larynx have been noted to react with antibodies to calcitonin in approximately 75% of cases.[12] As the tumors sometimes are also associated with

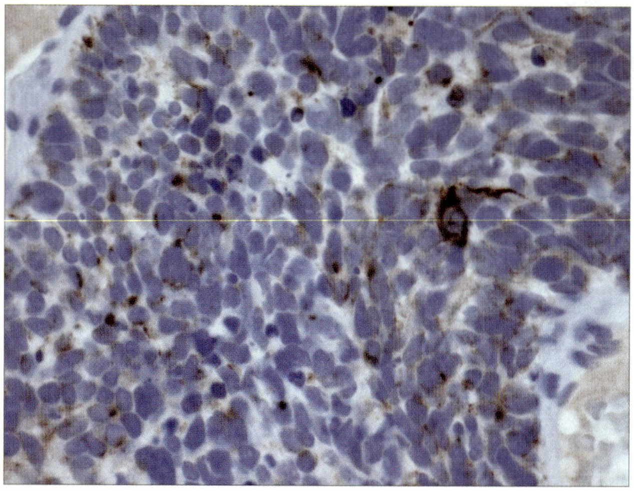

FIG. 25.3. Dot-like immunoreactivity with antibodies to cytokeratins is typical of small cell carcinoma.

amyloid, some have noted their resemblance to medullary thyroid carcinomas.

Scant information is available regarding genetic changes seen with well and moderately differentiated neuroendocrine carcinomas and small cell carcinomas of the upper aerodigestive tract. Overexpression of p53 protein has been seen immunohistochemically in 50% of the laryngeal moderately differentiated neuroendocrine carcinomas tested in two separate studies.[13,14]

Finally, some large cell undifferentiated carcinomas of the upper aerodigestive tract will show a prominent neuroendocrine phenotype, both histologically and immunohistochemically, resembling large cell neuroendocrine carcinomas of the lung.[6,15–17] While these tumors can occur throughout the tract, in our experience, they occur most frequently in the sinonasal area; they are considered by some to be within the spectrum of sinonasal undifferentiated carcinomas (SNUCs). These tumors can occur in men and women of any age, although they most often occur in older patients. They are very aggressive and have a poor prognosis, even with multimodality therapy.

Large cell carcinomas with neuroendocrine differentiation have larger cells than typical small cell carcinomas, frequently with more vesicular chromatin and prominent nucleoli (Figure 25.4).[6,16,17] They are very high grade, and necrosis, mitotic figures, vascular, and perineural invasion are usually seen. Immunohistochemically, undifferentiated carcinomas typically express keratins. P63, a marker of squamous differentiation, is variably expressed depending on tumor site and features; most SNUCs will not express the protein.[18] By definition, those undifferentiated carcinomas with a neuroendocrine phenotype should react with antibodies to one or more neuroendocrine antigens.

Conventional cytogenetics has only been performed with a few SNUCs. One case was found to have two translocations, t(1;6)(p22;p23) and t(12;17)(q13;p13); another had a very

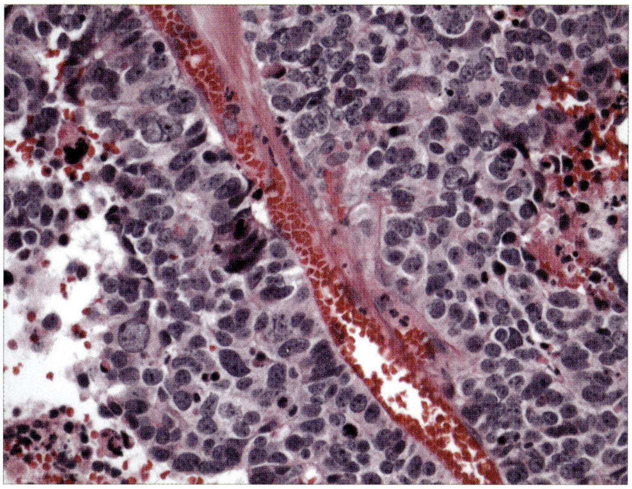

FIG. 25.4. This sinonasal undifferentiated carcinoma is an obviously high grade malignancy. While it has obvious neuroendocrine features, it is composed of larger cells that have more prominent nucleoli than those seen with small cell carcinomas.

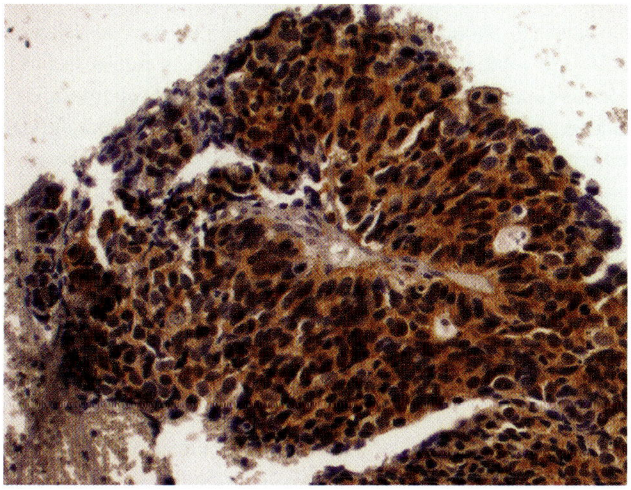

FIG. 25.5. Sinonasal undifferentiated carcinomas are sometime immunoreactive with antibodies to p16.

complex karyotype with numerous derivative chromosomes, deletions, and additions.[19] SNUCs have been noted to frequently overexpress p16 and p53 proteins by immunohistochemistry (Figure 25.5).[20,21] Mismatch repair proteins, MLH-1 and MSH-2, have both found to be intact by immunohistochemistry.[20] C-kit has also been noted to be overexpressed, although activating kit mutations have not been identified.[20,22] EGFR has also been overexpressed by immunohistochemistry whereas Her2/neu has not been shown to be overexpressed.[22]

Paragangliomas

Paragangliomas of the upper aerodigestive tract are almost always sporadic and benign, although both familial and malignant cases have been reported.[8,23–26] The lesions occur most frequently in the larynx are more common in women. Within the larynx, tumors are most frequently supraglottic and this has suggested to some that the superior paired paraganglia of the larynx more frequently develop tumors than the inferior paraganglia. In Lack's description of 69 head and neck paragangliomas, only one arose in the larynx.[25] Histologically, immunohistochemically, and genetically, upper aerodigestive tract paragangliomas are identical to those of the ear and other extra-adrenal sites (see below).

Neuroectodermal Tumors

Melanotic neuroectodermal tumor of infancy (MNTI) is, as the name implies, a tumor of early childhood that is more common in boys.[27–30] The tumors most frequently involve the maxilla, mandible, or skull. Although the tumors often recur, they rarely metastasize.

Grossly, the lesions appear lobulated and circumscribed, sometimes darkly pigmented, and are usually less than 5 cm in size.[27–31] Histologically, the tumors are composed of larger, more epithelioid cells and small round cells (Figure 25.6). The larger cells typically have abundant eosinophilic cytoplasm with melanin pigment and are arranged in tubular or alveolar structures, while the smaller cells are often nested. Necrosis is generally not seen (unless related to treatment) and mitotic figures are uncommon. Larger cells are immunoreactive with antibodies to keratins and EMA while both cells types are immunoreactive with antibodies to NSE, synaptophysin, and HMB45. Little is known regarding the cytogenetic and molecular changes of these tumors. A cell line established for an MNTI has revealed a complex karyotype.[32]

Olfactory neuroblastomas (ONBs) are rare tumors that develop in the upper nasal cavity in the area of the olfactory epithelium.[33–35] The tumors occur in patients of either sex at over a wide age range. Patients present with nonspecific symptoms, sometimes with visual changes. With current multimodality treatments, patients with ONB do quite well and some have reported survival rates at 10 years to be greater than 80%.[36]

Microscopically, tumor cells grow either diffusely or in discrete, circumscribed nests that are separated by fibrous or edematous stroma (Figure 25.7).[35] Homer Wright or more equivocal type rosettes are seen and an eosinophilic fibrillary background is usually present, sometimes with calcifications. Rarely, ganglion cells or even glandular differentiation are seen. The neoplastic cells are small and usually have minimal eosinophilic cytoplasm with round monomorphic nuclei. Although most cases have few mitotic figures, occasional cases can have marked mitotic activity. ONBs have been graded according to the Hyams grading system, which takes into account tumor architecture, nuclear atypia, mitotic activity, necrosis, and the presence or absence of background fibrillary material.[37] Most ONBs will show immunoreactivity with antibodies to synaptophysin or chromogranin, as

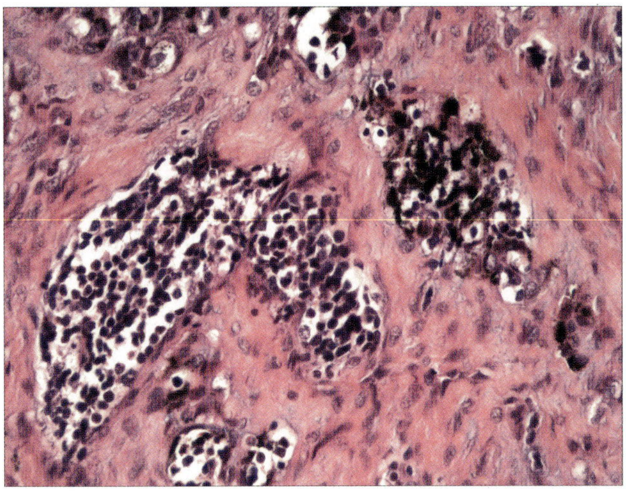

Fig. 25.6. Melanotic neuroectodermal tumors of infancy are composed of larger, more epithelioid cells admixed with smaller round cells.

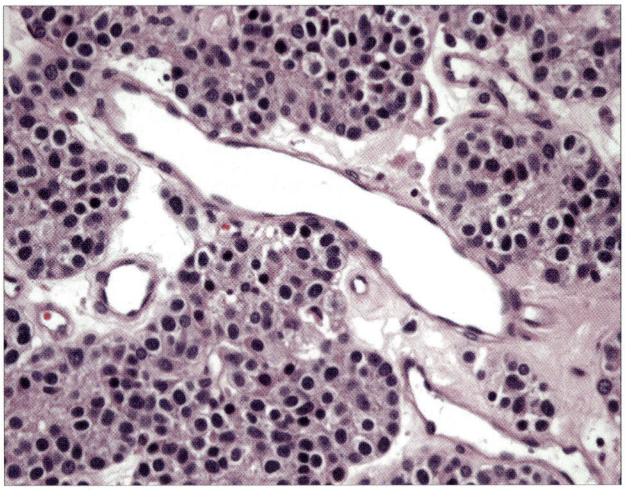

Fig. 25.7. This olfactory neuroblastoma is primarily nested.

well as with antibodies to less specific markers of neural or neuroendocrine differentiation such as NSE and CD56.[33,38] Focal immunoreactivity with antibodies to cytokeratins is sometimes seen. S100 immunoreactivity is usually limited to supporting sustentacular cells.

Little is known regarding the molecular abnormalities of ONBs. The tumor is not believed to be a member of the Ewing sarcoma group of tumors and the typical t(11;22) seen in those tumors is not seen with ONBs, despite an earlier paper claiming the contrary.[10,39,40] Array comparative genomic hybridization has identified numerous gains and losses.[41] The most frequent changes included gains at 7q11.22–q21.11, 9p13.3, 13q, 20p/q, and Xp/q, and losses at 2q31.1, 2q33.3, 2q37.1, 6q16.3, 6q21.33, 6q22.1, 22q11.23, 22q12.1, and Xp/q. Frequent changes seen with higher stage tumors were gains at 13q14.2–q14.3, 13q31.1, and 20q11.21–q11.23, and loss of Xp21.1. Gains at 5q35, 13q, and 20q, and losses at 2q31.1, 2q33.3, and 6q16–q22, were present in 50% of cases in one study. Immunohistochemistry has identified a number of possible molecular abnormalities. Cyclin-D1 has been noted to be overexpressed in 63% of cases.[42] Sixty percent of cases have been shown to express bcl-2, and HIF-1alpha expression has been noted in most cases.[43]

Salivary Glands

Neuroendocrine Carcinomas

Neuroendocrine carcinomas of the salivary glands are very uncommon and the best described and overwhelmingly most common type is small cell carcinoma.[44–48] Only rarely have other neuroendocrine carcinomas been described, though, interestingly, a family with apparently hereditary low-grade neuroendocrine carcinomas or carcinoid tumors has been described.[49,50] Also of note, other poorly differentiated salivary gland malignancies can sometimes show neuroendocrine differentiation by immunohistochemistry.[51] Small cell carcinomas occur most often in the major salivary glands, although some have been described to involve minor salivary glands (many of these may have been basaloid squamous cell carcinomas or SNUCs). The tumors occur in older patients of either sex (the rare small cell carcinomas reported in the very young may have represented other small blue cell tumors). Patients typically present with symptoms secondary to their mass lesions.

Histologically, small cell carcinomas of nonpulmonary sites are generally defined as having the histologic features of pulmonary small cell carcinomas.[44,47] There are sheets, ribbons, and nests of small, oval to round cells that have minimal cytoplasm and hyperchromatic nuclei. Nuclear chromatin is often fine, and prominent nuclei are usually absent. Mitotic figures and necrosis (both coagulative and single cell) are abundant, and perineural and vascular invasion are usually found. Nearly half of cases will have foci showing either squamous or glandular differentiation. We have seen a case associated with a pleomorphic adenoma.

Immunohistochemically, neoplastic cells should react with antikeratin (AE1/AE3 or CAM5.2) antibodies (frequently with perinuclear dot-like staining) and with antibodies to neuroendocrine antigens such as NSE, CD57, synaptophysin, and chromogranin.[48,52] Immunoreactivity with antibody to CK20 and TTF1 have also been noted and some have suggested that the two stains can help distinguish pulmonary from Merkel cell types, the latter having improved survival.[48] The prognosis is bad in either case, although patients may do better than those with small cell carcinomas of other nonpulmonary sites. Aside from the fact that about half of cases overexpress p53 protein by immunohistochemistry, there is no other specific information known regarding molecular changes in these tumors.[48]

The Ear

Middle Ear Adenoma

The most common epithelial neuroendocrine tumor of the ear per se seen at the University of Virginia is Merkel cell carcinoma. These develop in the sun-exposed auricle and have been discussed with skin tumors. Those that develop on the ear do not appear to be unique in any way.

Adenomas of the middle ear (i.e., middle ear adenoma), on the other hand, do appear to be unique to the site.[53–61] These tumors have been given a variety of names throughout the years including middle ear adenomatous tumor, carcinoid tumor of the middle ear, and neuroendocrine adenoma of the middle ear. The designation used here is currently advocated by the World Health Organization.[56] These tumors are very rare and represent approximately 18% of middle ear neoplasms and just 9% of neoplasms of the middle ear and temporal bone when considered together.[62] The tumors present with equal frequency in men and women and occur almost exclusively in adults over a wide age range (mean age of 45 years). Patients present with nonspecific symptoms, especially hearing loss. A familial association has not been noted with these tumors.

Middle ear adenomas usually present as nondestructive, unilateral middle ear mass lesions, although they can be invasive into bone.[57,58,60,61] The tumors are typically small, and the mean aggregate size has been reported to be less than 1 cm. Histologically, the tumors show a great deal of variety, similar to well-differentiated neuroendocrine carcinomas or carcinoid tumors seen throughout the rest of the body. They may be glandular, trabecular, solid, infiltrating, organoid, or grow as single cells (Figure 25.8). Frequently, more than one growth pattern is noted in a single tumor. Necrosis and ulceration are very rare. The neoplastic cells are typically epithelioid, although occasional cases can have more spindled or plasmacytoid cells. They have indistinct cells borders with eosinophilic, often granular cytoplasm. The nuclei are round to oval, centrally or eccentrically placed, and typically have finely granular chromatin. Nucleoli and mitotic figures are usually not seen. Occasionally, two apparent cell types can be seen, especially with tumors having a glandular growth pattern. Here, the luminal cells appear more flattened as the basal cells appear more cuboidal.

Neoplastic cells are immunoreactive with antibodies to cytokeratins (cocktail, CK7, and CAM5.2) and with antibodies to neuroendocrine antigens (chromogranin, NSE, human pancreatic polypeptide and synaptophysin) (Figure 25.9).[54,60,61] Some cases will be immunoreactive with antibodies to S100 protein and vimentin. Interestingly, cases displaying more than a single cell type will show differential staining with luminal cells reacting with antibodies to CK7 while the more basal cells react with antibodies to neuroendocrine antigens.

Middle ear adenomas are almost always benign.[58,60] Recurrences have been noted in up to 20% of cases and are usually associated with less aggressive initial therapy. Rare cases have been noted to metastasize. Specific histologic features or prognostic markers have not been identified that are associated with behavior for these tumors. Finally, there have been no studies regarding the molecular changes seen with these tumors.

Jugulotympanic Paraganglioma

Jugulotympanic paragangliomas represent approximately one-third of all middle ear or surrounding neoplasms.[26,62–64] As with middle ear adenomas, jugulotympanic paragangliomas have been given a number of appellations such as jugulotympanic chemodectoma and jugular or tympanic

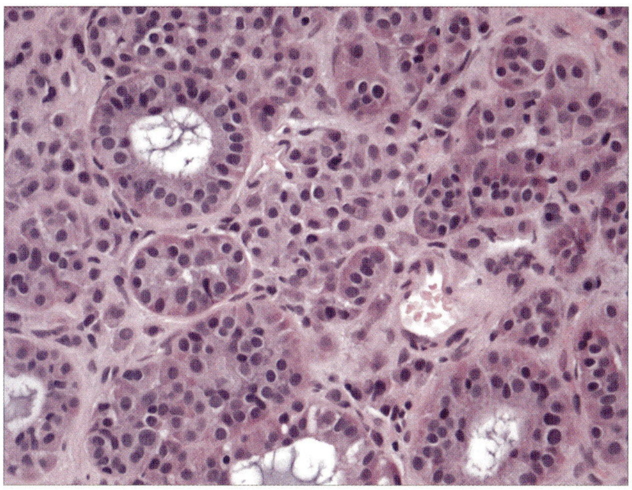

FIG. 25.8. Middle ear adenomas display the various growth patterns common for neuroendocrine carcinomas. This one is nested and has focal gland formation.

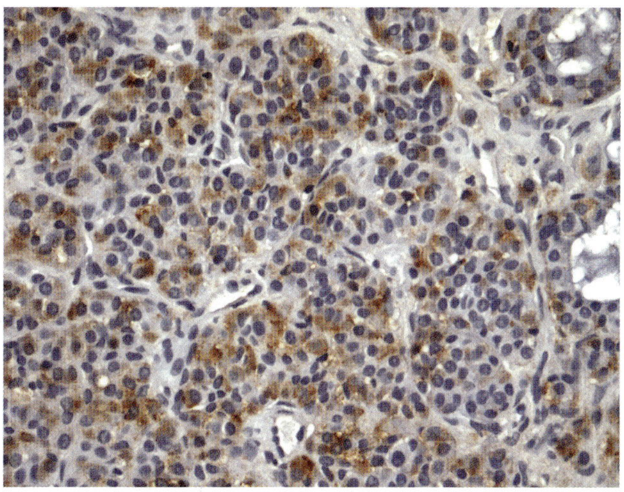

FIG. 25.9. Middle ear adenomas are immunoreactive with antibodies to neuroendocrine antigens.

glomus tumor. The tumors are more common in women and occur over a wide age range; however, most occur in middle age and the average age at presentation is 50 years. Most arise at the site of the jugular bulb and thus involve the petrous bone. Approximately, 12% primarily involve the middle ear space (tympanic paraganglioma) and a very small percentage involves the external ear canal only. The tumors usually present with conductive hearing loss; however, a number of other nonspecific symptoms have been noted.

Jugulotympanic paragangliomas tend to be very small and most are less than 5 mm in greatest dimension.[24,62,64–66] They have a typical nested or "zellballen" architecture described in other portions of this text, although our experience suggests that this is less pronounced with these tumors than with those seen at other sites (Figure 25.10). The immunophenotype is also identical with typical immunoreactivity for antibodies to endocrine antigens such as chromogranin and synaptophysin and not with antibodies to cytokeratins. Supporting cells or "sustentacular cells" are typically immunoreactive with antibodies to S-100 protein.

Few cases of jugulotympanic paragangliomas behave aggressively and metastasize.[26] This is generally impossible to predict based on histology. The tumors are mostly sporadic; however, in Alford and Guilford's seminal study, approximately 6% were associated with paragangliomas elsewhere.[65] Others have noted a higher familial incidence, especially given that the inheritance is autosomal dominant with genomic imprinting (thus, maternal transmission is not expressed and some family incidences may be underreported).[26] Both sporadic and familial paragangliomas frequently exhibit mutations of the genes encoding subunits of succinate dehydrogenase (*SDHB*, *SDHC*, and *SDHD*).[67–71] Rarely, they are associated with mutations of the *VHL* and *RET* genes. These are discussed in more detail in the chapters discussing pheochromocytomas and extra-adrenal paragangliomas. Interestingly, paragangliomas associated with germline *SDHB* mutations are more likely to metastasize.[70]

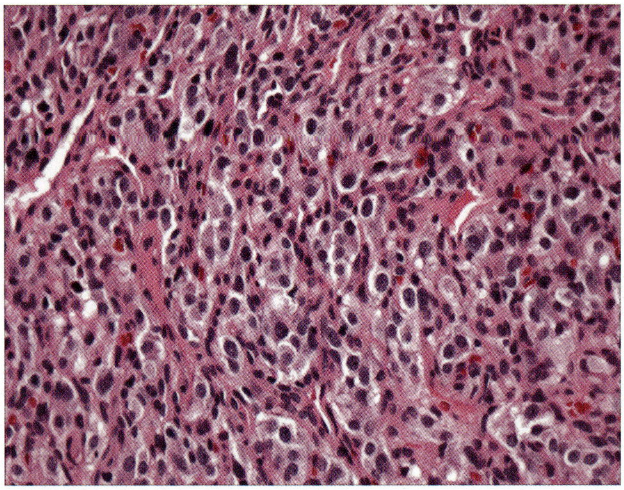

FIG. 25.10. This jugulotympanic paraganglioma is obviously nested and composed of round, epithelioid cells.

References

1. Batsakis JG, el-Naggar AK, Luna MA. Neuroendocrine tumors of larynx. *Ann Otol Rhinol Laryngol.* 1992;101:710–714.
2. Ferlito A, Barnes L, Rinaldo A, Gnepp DR, Milroy CM. A review of neuroendocrine neoplasms of the larynx: update on diagnosis and treatment. *J Laryngol Otol.* 1998;112:827–834.
3. Ferlito A, Friedmann I. Review of neuroendocrine carcinomas of the larynx. *Ann Otol Rhinol Laryngol.* 1989;98:780–790.
4. Gnepp DR, Ferlito A, Hyams V. Primary anaplastic small cell (oat cell) carcinoma of the larynx. Review of the literature and report of 18 cases. *Cancer.* 1983;51:1731–1745.
5. Logue JP, Banerjee SS, Slevin NJ, Vasanthan S. Neuroendocrine carcinomas of the larynx. *J Laryngol Otol.* 1991;105: 1031–1035.
6. Mills SE. Neuroectodermal neoplasms of the head and neck with emphasis on neuroendocrine carcinomas. *Mod Pathol.* 2002;15:264–278.
7. Perez-Ordonez B, Caruana SM, Huvos AG, Shah JP. Small cell neuroendocrine carcinoma of the nasal cavity and paranasal sinuses. *Hum Pathol.* 1998;29:826–832.
8. Ferlito A, Devaney KO, Rinaldo A. Neuroendocrine neoplasms of the larynx: advances in identification, understanding, and management. *Oral Oncol.* 2006;42:770–788.
9. Gillenwater A, Lewin J, Roberts D, El-Naggar A. Moderately differentiated neuroendocrine carcinoma (atypical carcinoid) of the larynx: a clinically aggressive tumor. *Laryngoscope.* 2005; 115:1191–1195.
10. Argani P, Perez-Ordonez B, Xiao H, Caruana SM, Huvos AG, Ladanyi M. Olfactory neuroblastoma is not related to the Ewing family of tumors: absence of EWS/FLI1 gene fusion and MIC2 expression. *Am J Surg Pathol.* 1998;22:391–398.
11. Mills SE, Cooper PH, Garland TA, Johns ME. Small cell undifferentiated carcinoma of the larynx. Report of two patients and review of 13 additional cases. *Cancer.* 1983;51:116–120.
12. Woodruff JM, Huvos AG, Erlandson RA, Shah JP, Gerold FP. Neuroendocrine carcinomas of the larynx. A study of two types, one of which mimics thyroid medullary carcinoma. *Am J Surg Pathol.* 1985;9:771–790.
13. Chung JH, Lee SS, Shim YS, et al. A study of moderately differentiated neuroendocrine carcinomas of the larynx and an examination of non-neoplastic larynx tissue for neuroendocrine cells. *Laryngoscope.* 2004;114:1264–1270.
14. Hirsch MS, Faquin WC, Krane JF. Thyroid transcription factor-1, but not p53, is helpful in distinguishing moderately differentiated neuroendocrine carcinoma of the larynx from medullary carcinoma of the thyroid. *Mod Pathol.* 2004;17:631–636.
15. Ejaz A, Wenig BM. Sinonasal undifferentiated carcinoma: clinical and pathologic features and a discussion on classification, cellular differentiation, and differential diagnosis. *Adv Anat Pathol.* 2005;12:134–143.
16. Enepekides DJ. Sinonasal undifferentiated carcinoma: an update. *Curr Opin Otolaryngol Head Neck Surg.* 2005;13:222–225.
17. Frierson HF Jr, Mills SE, Fechner RE, Taxy JB, Levine PA. Sinonasal undifferentiated carcinoma. An aggressive neoplasm derived from schneiderian epithelium and distinct from olfactory neuroblastoma. *Am J Surg Pathol.* 1986;10: 771–779.
18. Bourne TD, Bellizzi AM, Stelow EB, et al. p63 expression in olfactory neuroblastoma and other small cell tumors of the sinonasal tract. *Am J Clin Pathol.* 2008;130(2):213–218.

19. Gil Z, Orr-Urtreger A, Voskoboinik N, et al. Cytogenetic analysis of sinonasal carcinomas. *Otolaryngol Head Neck Surg*. 2006;134:654–660.
20. Bellizzi AM, Bourne TD, Mills SE, Stelow EB. Immunohistochemistry of molecular markers in sinonasal undifferentiated carcinomas. *Mod Pathol*. 2007;20:220A.
21. Joos B, Martin A, Nowacki M, Desai P, Jenson A, Farghaly H. Prevalence of human papilloma virus DNA in sinonasal undifferentiated carcinoma. *Mod Pathol*. 2008;21:237A.
22. Chernock RD, Perry A, Pfeifer J, Holden JA, Lewis JS. Evaluation of sinonasal undifferentiated carcinomas for therapeutic targets – EGFR, c-kit and Her2/neu. *Mod Pathol*. 2008;21:233A.
23. Barnes L. Paraganglioma of the larynx. A critical review of the literature. *ORL J Otorhinolaryngol Relat Spec*. 1991;53: 220–234.
24. Lack EE, Cubilla AL, Woodruff JM. Paragangliomas of the head and neck region. A pathologic study of tumors from 71 patients. *Hum Pathol*. 1979;10:191–218.
25. Lack EE, Cubilla AL, Woodruff JM, Farr HW. Paragangliomas of the head and neck region: a clinical study of 69 patients. *Cancer*. 1977;39:397–409.
26. Pellitteri PK, Rinaldo A, Myssiorek D, et al. Paragangliomas of the head and neck. *Oral Oncol*. 2004;40:563–575.
27. Barrett AW, Morgan M, Ramsay AD, Farthing PM, Newman L, Speight PM. A clinicopathologic and immunohistochemical analysis of melanotic neuroectodermal tumor of infancy. *Oral Surg Oral Med Oral Pathol Oral Radiol Endod*. 2002;93:688–698.
28. Kapadia SB, Frisman DM, Hitchcock CL, Ellis GL, Popek EJ. Melanotic neuroectodermal tumor of infancy. Clinicopathological, immunohistochemical, and flow cytometric study. *Am J Surg Pathol*. 1993;17:566–573.
29. Kruse-Losler B, Gaertner C, Burger H, Seper L, Joos U, Kleinheinz J. Melanotic neuroectodermal tumor of infancy: systematic review of the literature and presentation of a case. *Oral Surg Oral Med Oral Pathol Oral Radiol Endod*. 2006;102:204–216.
30. Pettinato G, Manivel JC, D'Amore ES, Jaszcz W, Gorlin RJ. Melanotic neuroectodermal tumor of infancy. A reexamination of a histogenetic problem based on immunohistochemical, flow cytometric, and ultrastructural study of 10 cases. *Am J Surg Pathol*. 1991;15:233–245.
31. Stirling RW, Powell G, Fletcher CD. Pigmented neuroectodermal tumour of infancy: an immunohistochemical study. *Histopathology*. 1988;12:425–435.
32. Metwaly H, Cheng J, Maruyama S, et al. Establishment and characterization of new cell lines derived from melanotic neuroectodermal tumor of infancy arising in the mandible. *Pathol Int*. 2005;55:331–342.
33. Frierson HF Jr, Ross GW, Mills SE, Frankfurter A. Olfactory neuroblastoma. Additional immunohistochemical characterization. *Am J Clin Pathol*. 1990;94:547–553.
34. Kadish S, Goodman M, Wang CC. Olfactory neuroblastoma. A clinical analysis of 17 cases. *Cancer*. 1976;37:1571–1576.
35. Mills SE, Frierson HF Jr. Olfactory neuroblastoma. A clinicopathologic study of 21 cases. *Am J Surg Pathol*. 1985;9: 317–327.
36. Loy AH, Reibel JF, Read PW, et al. Esthesioneuroblastoma: continued follow-up of a single institution's experience. *Arch Otolaryngol Head Neck Surg*. 2006;132:134–138.
37. Mills SE, Gaffey MJ, Frierson HF. *Neural, Neuroendocrine, and Neuroectodermal Neoplasia. Tumors of the Upper Aerodigestive Tract and Ear*, vol. 26. 3rd ed. Washington, DC: AFIP; 2000:159.
38. Hirose T, Scheithauer BW, Lopes MB, et al. Olfactory neuroblastoma. An immunohistochemical, ultrastructural, and flow cytometric study. *Cancer*. 1995;76:4–19.
39. Kumar S, Perlman E, Pack S, et al. Absence of EWS/FLI1 fusion in olfactory neuroblastomas indicates these tumors do not belong to the Ewing's sarcoma family. *Hum Pathol*. 1999;30:1356–1360.
40. Sorensen PH, Wu JK, Berean KW, et al. Olfactory neuroblastoma is a peripheral primitive neuroectodermal tumor related to Ewing sarcoma. *Proc Natl Acad Sci U S A*. 1996;93:1038–1043.
41. Guled M, Myllykangas S, Frierson HF Jr, Mills SE, Knuutila S, Stelow EB. Array comparative genomic hybridization analysis of olfactory neuroblastoma. *Mod Pathol*. 2008;21:770–778.
42. Wang SL, Chen WT, Li SH, Li SW, Yang SF, Chai CY. Expression of human telomerase reverse transcriptase and cyclin-D1 in olfactory neuroblastoma. *APMIS*. 2007;115:17–21.
43. Diensthuber M, Potinius M, Rodt T, et al. Expression of bcl-2 is associated with microvessel density in olfactory neuroblastoma. *J Neurooncol*. 2008;89(2):131–139.
44. Gnepp DR, Corio RL, Brannon RB. Small cell carcinoma of the major salivary glands. *Cancer*. 1986;58:705–714.
45. Koss LG, Spiro RH, Hajdu S. Small cell (oat cell) carcinoma of minor salivary gland origin. *Cancer*. 1972;30:737–741.
46. Kraemer BB, Mackay B, Batsakis JG. Small cell carcinomas of the parotid gland. A clinicopathologic study of three cases. *Cancer*. 1983;52:2115–2121.
47. Nagao K, Matsuzaki O, Saiga H, et al. Histopathologic studies of undifferentiated carcinoma of the parotid gland. *Cancer*. 1982;50:1572–1579.
48. Nagao T, Gaffey TA, Olsen KD, Serizawa H, Lewis JE. Small cell carcinoma of the major salivary glands: clinicopathologic study with emphasis on cytokeratin 20 immunoreactivity and clinical outcome. *Am J Surg Pathol*. 2004;28:762–770.
49. Michaels L, Lee K, Manuja SL, Soucek SO. Family with low-grade neuroendocrine carcinoma of salivary glands, severe sensorineural hearing loss, and enamel hypoplasia. *Am J Med Genet*. 1999;83:183–186.
50. Modlin IM, Shapiro MD, Kidd M. Primary carcinoid tumor of the parotid gland: a case report and review of the literature. *Ear Nose Throat J*. 2006;85:533–539.
51. Laforga JB. Salivary duct carcinoma with neuroendocrine features. *Virchows Arch*. 2004;444:473–476.
52. Gnepp DR, Wick MR. Small cell carcinoma of the major salivary glands. An immunohistochemical study. *Cancer*. 1990;66:185–192.
53. Berns S, Pearl G. Middle ear adenoma. *Arch Pathol Lab Med*. 2006;130:1067–1069.
54. Krouse JH, Nadol JB Jr, Goodman ML. Carcinoid tumors of the middle ear. *Ann Otol Rhinol Laryngol*. 1990;99:547–552.
55. Manni JJ, Faverly DR, Van Haelst UJ. Primary carcinoid tumors of the middle ear. Report on four cases and a review of the literature. *Arch Otolaryngol Head Neck Surg*. 1992;118:1341–1347.
56. Michaels L, Soucek S. Adenoma of the middle ear. In: Bachor E, Eveson JW, Reichart P, Sidransky D, eds. *Pathology and Genetics of Head and Neck Tumors*. Lyon: IARC Press; 2005:345.

57. Mills SE, Fechner RE. Middle ear adenoma. A cytologically uniform neoplasm displaying a variety of architectural patterns. *Am J Surg Pathol*. 1984;8:677–685.
58. Ramsey MJ, Nadol JB Jr, Pilch BZ, McKenna MJ. Carcinoid tumor of the middle ear: clinical features, recurrences, and metastases. *Laryngoscope*. 2005;115:1660–1666.
59. Stanley MW, Horwitz CA, Levinson RM, Sibley RK. Carcinoid tumors of the middle ear. *Am J Clin Pathol*. 1987;87:592–600.
60. Torske KR, Thompson LD. Adenoma versus carcinoid tumor of the middle ear: a study of 48 cases and review of the literature. *Mod Pathol*. 2002;15:543–555.
61. Wassef M, Kanavaros P, Polivka M, et al. Middle ear adenoma. A tumor displaying mucinous and neuroendocrine differentiation. *Am J Surg Pathol*. 1989;13:838–847.
62. Hyams VJ, Batsakis JG, Michaels L. *Neoplasms of the Middle Ear. Tumors of the Upper Respiratory Tract and Ear*. Washington, DC: Armed Forces Institute of Pathology; 1988:306–330.
63. Achilles E, Padberg BC, Holl K, Kloppel G, Schroder S. Immunocytochemistry of paragangliomas – value of staining for S-100 protein and glial fibrillary acid protein in diagnosis and prognosis. *Histopathology*. 1991;18:453–458.
64. Brown JS. Glomus jugulare tumors revisited: a ten-year statistical follow-up of 231 cases. *Laryngoscope*. 1985;95:284–288.
65. Alford BR, Guilford FR. A comprehensive study of tumors of the glomus jugulare. *Laryngoscope*. 1962;72:765–805.
66. Spector GJ, Maisel RH, Ogura JH. Glomus tumors in the middle ear. I. An analysis of 46 patients. *Laryngoscope*. 1973;83:1652–1672.
67. Bikhazi PH, Messina L, Mhatre AN, Goldstein JA, Lalwani AK. Molecular pathogenesis in sporadic head and neck paraganglioma. *Laryngoscope*. 2000;110:1346–1348.
68. Isik AC, Erem C, Imamoglu M, Cinel A, Sari A, Maral G. Familial paraganglioma. *Eur Arch Otorhinolaryngol*. 2006;263:23–31.
69. Martin TP, Irving RM, Maher ER. The genetics of paragangliomas: a review. *Clin Otolaryngol*. 2007;32:7–11.
70. Neumann HP, Pawlu C, Peczkowska M, et al. Distinct clinical features of paraganglioma syndromes associated with SDHB and SDHD gene mutations. *JAMA*. 2004;292:943–951.
71. Schiavi F, Boedeker CC, Bausch B, et al. Predictors and prevalence of paraganglioma syndrome associated with mutations of the SDHC gene. *JAMA*. 2005;294:2057–2063.

26 Merkel Cell Carcinoma

Steven D. Billings and Melissa P. Piliang

Introduction

Merkel cells are neural crest-derived cells found in the basal layer of the epidermis and tactile hair discs of Pinkus that serve as mechanoreceptors. Ultrastructurally, they demonstrate neuroendocrine differentiation with membrane-bound dense core neurosecretory granules. Primary neuroendocrine carcinomas of the skin are thought to derive from Merkel cells and have thus been designated Merkel cell carcinoma.

Clinical Features

Merkel cell carcinoma is a rare sporadic cutaneous malignancy that occurs primarily on actinically damaged skin. With an incidence of 0.44/100,000 people, Merkel cell carcinoma is 20 times more common in whites than blacks.[1] The average age of onset is 60–80 years old. The tumor classically presents as a painless red-purple nodule on the head and neck and can occur less commonly on the upper extremities and back. Merkel cell carcinoma has rarely been reported on the trunk, genitalia, and oral mucosa. Risk factors for Merkel cell carcinoma include being a fair-skinned male with extensive sun-exposure.[2] Like other sun-induced skin cancers, immunosuppression is associated with increased risk of developing Merkel cell carcinoma.

Merkel cell carcinoma is an aggressive tumor with a high rate of regional and lymph node metastasis and is the second most common cause of nonmelanoma skin cancer death.[3] The overall recurrence rate is 55–70% with local and regional lymph nodes being the most common sites. The majority of recurrences occur 6–12 months after diagnosis. Prognosis depends on the stage of disease at the time of diagnosis. Small tumors (<2 cm) without lymph node involvement have a 90% 5-year survival rate. Approximately, half of patients with aggressive advanced disease will succumb to disease within 9 months of diagnosis.[4] Pathologic staging is closely associated with disease survival probabilities. Patients with negative sentinel lymph node biopsies have a better survival and a risk of nodal recurrence of only 11%.[5]

Histology

Merkel cell carcinoma can display many growth patterns. Most commonly, Merkel cell carcinoma is a dermal-based tumor usually with a diffuse to nodular (Figure 26.1) or, less commonly, trabecular growth pattern (Figure 26.2). A nested, clustered, or rosette pattern may also be seen. Often, tumors display multiple growth patterns. Epidermal involvement may be seen in up to 10% of cases, with a pagetoid growth pattern rarely reported (Figure 26.3).[6]

Merkel cell carcinoma is composed of small, round to oval monomorphic blue cells with scant cytoplasm and prominent, stippled chromatin imparting a "salt and pepper" appearance to the nuclei (Figure 26.4). Due to the small amount of cytoplasm, the nuclei are closely spaced and molded. The cells are mitotically active with frequent atypical mitotic figures and apoptotic cells.

Immunohistochemistry

Immunohistochemistry is critical in the confirmation of suspected Merkel cell carcinoma. Merkel cell carcinoma displays positive staining with cytokeratin 20 (CK20), epithelial membrane antigen (EMA), neurofilament protein, and neuroendocrine markers synaptophysin, chromogranin, and neuron-specific enolase, indicating both neuroendrocrine and epithelial differentiation. CK20 staining classically is in a perinuclear dot-like pattern (Figure 26.5), although diffuse staining is often seen. Immunohistochemistry with "pan-keratin" and neurofilament protein stains also will often display the perinuclear dot pattern similar to CK20. Cytokeratin 7 (CK7) expression is generally absent, but a case series of CK20–/CK7+ cutaneous neuroendocrine carcinoma has been reported.[3] Importantly, Merkel cell carcinoma is negative for S-100 and TTF-1, helping to differentiate it from melanoma and metastatic small cell lung carcinoma, respectively (see Table 26.1).

J.L. Hunt (ed.), *Molecular Pathology of Endocrine Diseases*, Molecular Pathology Library 3,
DOI 10.1007/978-1-4419-1707-2_26,

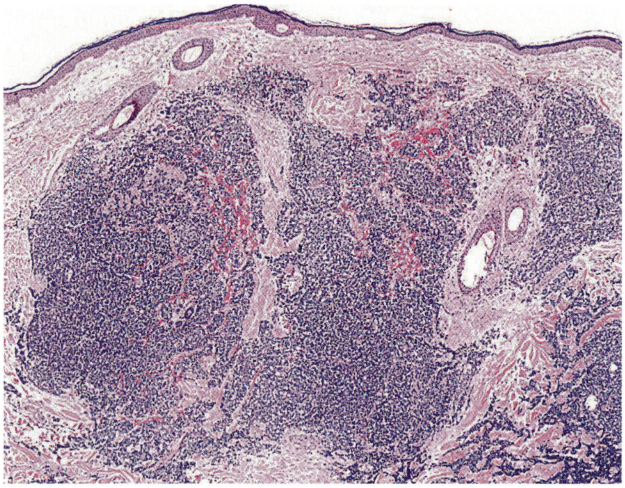

FIG. 26.1. Most Merkel cell carcinomas display a nodular to solid growth pattern.

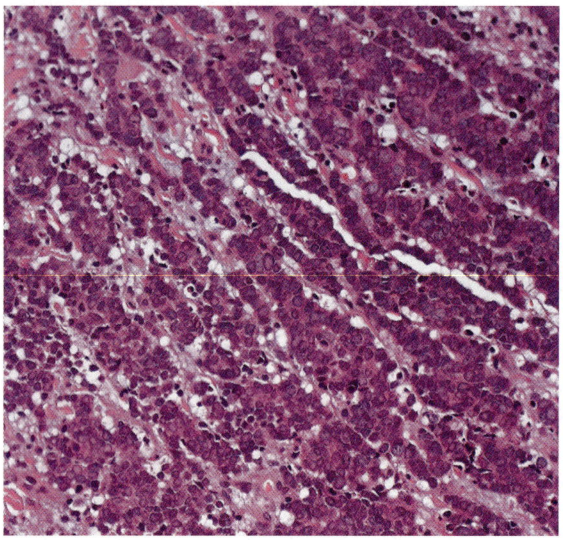

FIG. 26.2. Merkel cell carcinoma displaying a trabecular growth pattern.

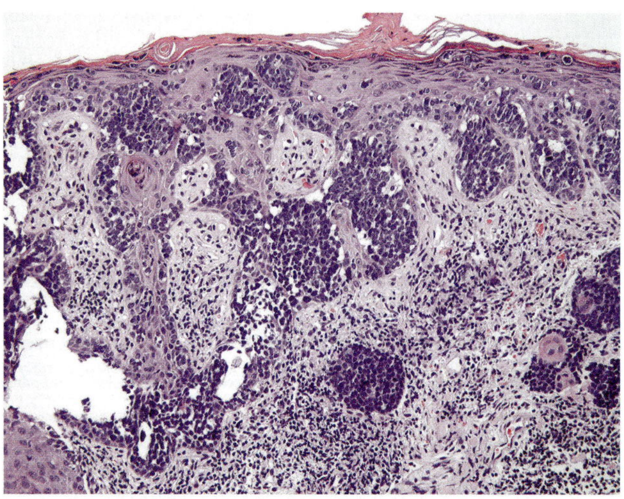

FIG. 26.3. A small percentage of Merkel cell carcinomas may have epidermal involvement that sometimes has a pagetoid pattern.

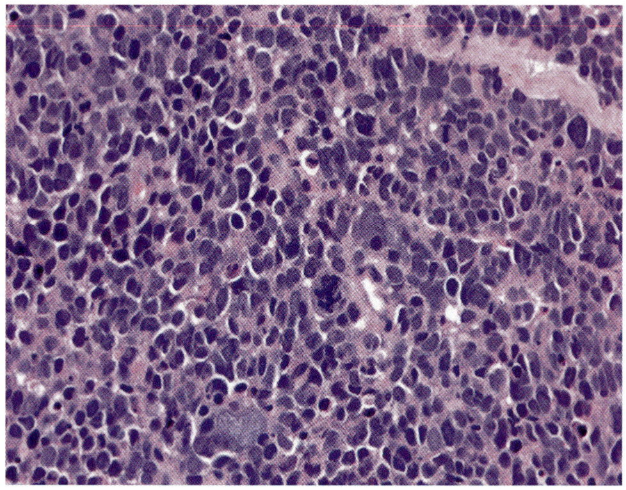

FIG. 26.4. High power showing tumor cells with scant cytoplasm, nuclear molding, prominent, stippled chromatin pattern, atypical mitotic figures, and apoptotic cells.

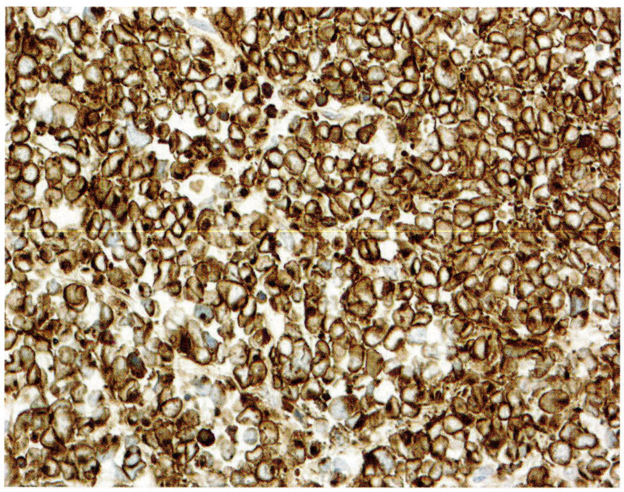

FIG. 26.5. Cytokeratin 20 showing diffuse staining with accentuation in a perinuclear dot pattern.

TABLE 26.1. Immunohistochemistry in Merkel cell carcinoma.

Tumor	CK20	CK7	NSE	TTF-1	CD45	S-100
Merkel cell carcinoma	+	−	+	−	−	−
Small cell lung carcinoma	−	+	+	+	−	−
Lymphoma	−	−	−	−	+	−
Small cell melanoma	−	−	−	−	−	+

Electron Microscopy

Historically, due to the difficulty of diagnosing Merkel cell carcinoma, electron microscopy has been used to confirm the diagnosis. Ultrastructurally, the most characteristic finding is the aggregation of intermediate filaments in a perinuclear dot location and dense core neurosecretory granules, usually concentrated in the periphery or in dendrite-like processes. The ultrastructural findings parallel those of normal Merkel cells.

With the advent of immunohistochemistry, electron microscopy now plays little role in the diagnosis.

Pathogenesis

Merkel cell carcinoma occurs sporadically and is believed to arise from Merkel cells residing in the epidermis. Little is known about the etiologic mechanism in Merkel cell carcinoma. It has been linked with chronic sun-exposure and is therefore seen most commonly in individuals with advanced age (>60 years), fair-skin, and excessive life-time sun-exposure. Impaired immune function appears to play a role in the development of Merkel cell carcinoma in some cases; patients with HIV/AIDS, lymphoma, solid-organ transplants and iatrogenic immunosuppression are at increased risk for the development of Merkel cell carcinoma.

Increased incidence in elderly and immunosuppressed individuals suggests a potential role of an infectious agent in the pathogenesis. Recently, Feng et al identified a previously unknown polyomavirus, Merkel cell polyomavirus (MCV), in 80% (8 of 10) Merkel cell carcinoma's studied, but only 16% (4 of 25) of controls.[7] In some cases, but not all, MCV was found to be integrated in the tumor genome in a clonal pattern. The authors hypothesize that MCV could be involved in tumorigenesis via MCV T-antigen expression and/or insertional mutagenesis of tumor suppressor genes.[7]

Molecular Aspects

Despite numerous studies of oncogenic pathways, little is known about the molecular basis of Merkel cell carcinoma. Ras, p53, B-Raf, MAP kinase, Wnt, c-Kit, PTEN, and bcl-2 have all been evaluated in Merkel cell carcinoma. Kennedy et al and Plettenberg et al found bcl-2 expression in 15 of 20 Merkel cell carcinoma tumors in 2 separate studies.[8,9] Decreasing bcl-2 expression in vivo in an SCID mouse/human tumor xenograft model resulted in tumor shrinkage. An important protein in inhibiting apoptosis, bcl-2 expression is found in many cancers and suggests a mechanism to avoid cell death. Expression of bcl-2 alone does not provide clues to the proto-oncogenes involved in tumor development.

Loss of heterozygosity tumor suppressor gene PTEN was found in 43% of the tumors examined (9/21), but only one tumor was found to have a concurrent PTEN mutation.[10]

The Wnt-signaling pathway, which regulates various cell cycle processes including cell proliferation, cell fate, and morphogenesis, also seems an unlikely candidate to play an important role in oncogenesis in Merkel cell carcinoma. Twelve cases were studied for alterations in the Wnt-pathway by looking for alteration of expression of β-catenin and for mutations in the genes coding for β-catenin, APC, and AXIN. Only one case of Merkel cell carcinoma was found to have nuclear accumulation of β-catenin and mutations in the Wnt-pathway genes.[11]

Although the MAP kinase pathway has been found to play a role in the development of melanoma and squamous cell carcinoma, it does not seem to be important in Merkel cell carcinoma. Houben et al evaluated 44 Merkel cell carcinoma's for activating BRAF mutations, Raf kinase inhibitor protein (RKIP), extracellular signal-regulated kinase (ERK), and phosphorylation status of ERK.[12] All tumors were negative for the BRAF mutation. A high expression Raf kinase inhibitor protein was found in primary and metastatic Merkel cell carcinoma. Forty-two of forty-four had no phosphorylation of ERK indicating that the MAP kinase pathway was silent. The RAS gene, which is also involved in the RAS–RAF–MEK pathway, was examined by Popp et al.[13] In their study of six Merkel cell carcinomas, no activating mutations in NRAS, HRAS, or KRAS genes were found. Similar findings were reported in another series of 21 Merkel cell carcinomas.[14] In sum, these findings suggest that the MAP kinase pathway does not play a role in carcinogenesis in Merkel cell carcinoma. A follow-up study found that activation of MAP kinase pathway induced apoptosis of a single cell line of Merkel cell carcinoma, suggesting a potential therapeutic target.[15]

As in other ultraviolet light-induced neoplasms, such as melanoma and squamous cell carcinoma, mutations in the tumor suppressor gene p53 may be found in Merkel cell carcinoma, though in a minority of cases. In a study of 15 Merkel cell carcinomas, 3 of 15 tumors harbored p53 mutations.[16] Of the p53 mutations found, most were the type that have been associated with UV exposure. In the same study, only one case demonstrated mutations in p73, a gene that encodes for a protein with structural and functional similarities to p53. The relative rarity of p53 and p73 mutations argues against a strong role for these genes in the majority of Merkel cell carcinomas.

Epigenetic studies on cancer have revealed altered gene methylation in many cancers. A study of methylation of p14ARF promoter DNA and p16INK4a promoter DNA and mutations in common oncogenes in 21 Merkel cell carcinomas demonstrated no mutations in Ras, c-Kit, or p14ARF.[14] However, methylation of p14ARF promoter DNA was found in 8 of 19 tumors (42%), suggesting that p14ARF silencing may represent a mechanism for tumorigenesis in some Merkel cell carcinomas. This pathway may provide a potential epigenetic therapeutic target for treatment with demethylating agents.

Merkel cell carcinoma has been shown to express the KIT transmembrane tyrosine kinase receptor by immunohistochemistry.[17] Unlike gastrointestinal stromal tumors, where activating mutations of the c-Kit proto-oncogene are important in tumorigenesis, activating mutations have not been found in Merkel cell carcinoma.[18] These findings suggest that therapeutic interventions that inhibit KIT protein kinase likely will not be effective in treating Merkel cell carcinomas.

Summary

Merkel cell carcinoma is a rare but aggressive cutaneous malignancy with an increasing incidence. Despite extensive study of common cancer-associated pathways and genes, very little is known about the molecular pathogenesis of Merkel cell carcinoma. To date, only bcl-2 and p14ARF methylation have been identified as potentially important factors in tumorigenesis. The identification of the novel Merkel cell polyoma virus suggests a possible infectious etiology and provides a potential focus for future studies.

References

1. Hodgson NC. Merkel cell carcinoma: changing incidence trends. *J Surg Oncol.* 2005;89:1–4.
2. Veness MJ. Merkel cell carcinoma (primary cutaneous neuroendocrine carcinoma): an overview on management. *Australas J Dermatol.* 2006;47:160–165.
3. Calder KB, Coplowitz S, Schlauder S, Morgan MB. A case series and immunophenotypic analysis of CK20–/CK7+ primary neuroendocrine carcinoma of the skin. *J Cutan Pathol.* 2007;34:918–923.
4. Poulsen M. Merkel-cell carcinoma of the skin. *Lancet Oncol.* 2004;5:593–599.
5. Allen PJ, Bowne WB, Jaques DP, Brennan MF, Busam K, Coit DG. Merkel cell carcinoma: prognosis and treatment of patients from a single institution. *J Clin Oncol.* 2005;3:2300–2309.
6. Hashimoto K, Lee MW, D'Annunzio DR, Balle MR, Narisawa Y. Pagetoid Merkel cell carcinoma: epidermal origin of the tumor. *J Cutan Pathol.* 1998;25:572–579.
7. Feng H, Shuda M, Chang Y, Moore PS. Clonal integration of a polyomavirus in human Merkel cell carcinoma. *Science.* 2008;319:1096–1100.
8. Kennedy MM, Blessing K, King G, Kerr K. Expression of bcl-2 and p53 in Merkel cell carcinoma: an immunohistochemical study. *Am J Dermatopathol.* 1996;18:273–277.
9. Plettenberg A, Pammer J, Tschachler E. Merkel cells and Merkel cell carcinoma express bcl-2 proto-oncogene. *Exp Dermatol.* 1996;5:183–188.
10. Van Gele M, Leonard JH, Van Roy N, Cook AL, De Paepe A, Speleman F. Frequent allelic loss at 10q23 but low incidence of PTEN mutations in Merkel cell carcinoma. *Int J Cancer.* 2001;92:409–413.
11. Liu S, Daa T, Kashima K, Kondoh Y, Yokoyama S. The Wnt-signaling pathway is not implicated in tumorigenesis of Merkel cell carcinoma. *J Cutan Pathol.* 2006;34:22–26.
12. Houben R, Michel B, Vetter-Kauczok CS, et al. Absence of classical MAP kinase pathway signaling in Merkel cell carcinoma. *J Invest Dermatol.* 2006;126:1135–1142.
13. Popp S, Waltering S, Herbst C, Moll I, Boukamp P. UV-B-type mutations and chromosomal imbalances indicate common pathways for the development of Merkel cell carcinoma and skin squamous cell carcinoma. *Int J Cancer.* 2002;99:352–360.
14. Lassacher A, Heitzer E, Kerl H, Wolf P. p14 ARF hypermethylation is common but INK4aARF locus or p53 mutations are rare in Merkel cell carcinoma. *J Invest Dermatol.* 2008;128(7):1788–1796.
15. Houben R, Ortmann S, Schrama D, et al. Activation of the MAP kinase pathway induces apoptosis in the Merkel cell carcinoma cell line UISO. *J Invest Dermatol.* 2007;127:2116–2122.
16. Van Gele M, Kaghad M, Leonard JH, et al. Mutation analysis of P73 and TP53 in Merkel cell carcinoma. *Brit J Cancer.* 2000;82:823–826.
17. Su LD, Fullen DR, Lowe L, Uherova P, Schnitzer B, Valdez R. CD117(KIT receptor) expression in Merkel cell carcinoma. *Am J Dermatopathol.* 2002;24:289–293.
18. Swick BL, Ravdel L, Fitzpatrick JE, Robinson WA. Merkel cell carcinoma: evaluation of KIT (CD117) expression and failure to demonstrate activating mutations in the C-KIT proto-oncogene – implications for treatment with imatinib mesylate. *J Cutan Pathol.* 2006;34:324–329.

27 Neuroendocrine Lung Tumors

Sanja Dacic

Introduction

Morphologic and clinical characteristics of neuroendocrine tumors (NE) of the lung represent a wide spectrum of entities. At one end of the spectrum is the clinically and biologically indolent typical carcinoid (TC). At the other end of the spectrum, large cell neuroendocrine carcinoma (LCNEC) and small cell lung carcinoma (SCLC) show aggressive behavior and shorter survival. The clinical behavior of atypical carcinoid (ATC) lies somewhere between these two extremes. NE tumors of the lung may occur in pure or mixed forms with other types of non-small cell lung carcinomas (NSCLC). In contrast to NE tumors occurring in other organ sites, histologic diagnostic criteria for lung neuroendocrine tumors are well defined and correlate with clinical behavior and outcome. Diagnosis of TC, ATC, and SCLC is usually made on morphology alone, while diagnosis of LCNEC requires immunohistochemical confirmation of neuroendocrine differentiation. The majority of NE tumors of the lung occur as sporadic isolated tumors, although rare cases are components of complex familial endocrine, such as multiple endocrine neoplasia type 1 (MEN1).[1] The most important goal of molecular profiling studies of NE tumors of the lung to date has been to identify diagnostic, prognostic, and therapeutic targets for these tumors. This chapter will briefly review the current literature regarding pathways involved in tumorigenesis of these tumors. Recent advances in understanding of potential prognostic and diagnostic markers discovered by RNA- and DNA-based analysis will be discussed.

Sporadic (Nonhereditary) Lung NE Tumors

Background

Clinical

TC and ATC are more frequent in nonsmokers (20–40% of patients). In contrast, almost all patients with SCLC and LCNEC are cigarette smokers. Most of these tumors occur sporadically. TC and ATC may occur in patients with MEN 1, where they tend to be multicentric.[2] TC may present as a central or peripheral mass, whereas AC and LCNEC are more commonly located in the peripheral regions. SCLC usually presents as hilar or perihilar masses and is often accompanied by mediastinal lymphadenopathy; liver or bone marrow metastases are common at the time of primary diagnosis. Paraneoplastic syndromes are also common in patients with SCLC but are rare in patients with LCNEC. LCNEC are similar in their clinical presentation to other types of NSCLC. Carcinoid syndrome, which includes skin flushing, diarrhea, and shortness of breath, is rare in all of these pulmonary NE tumors and usually only occurs with widespread metastatic disease. The 5-year survival is 90–98% for TC, 61–73% for ATC, and 13–57% for LCNEC. Survival rates for patients with SCLC remain dismal, despite aggressive therapy.[3–7]

Histology

All NE tumors of the lung show variations on the typical features of neuroendocrine morphology, including organoid, nested, or trabecular growth patterns, cellular palisading, and rosette-like structures. The main distinguishing features are the mitotic count and the presence or absence of necrosis.[6] TC is defined as a NE tumor with no more than 2 mitoses per 10 HPF and absence of necrosis. Mitotic count between 2 and 10 per 10 HPF and/or necrosis are needed for a diagnosis of ATC. Mitoses are readily identified in LCNEC and SCLC with 11 or more mitoses per 10 HPF. These tumors also have more extensive necrosis than ATC. LCNEC shows larger cell size, abundant cytoplasm, prominent nucleoli, vesicular or coarse chromatin, and less prominent nuclear molding. These features, which are much more similar to other NSCLCs, are in contrast to the cytologic features SCLC.

Immunohistochemistry

Markers of neuroendocrine differentiation such as synaptophysin, chromogranin, and CD56 (N-CAM) are often positive in NE tumors of the lung, and are particularly prominent in TC.[6,8]Staining

J.L. Hunt (ed.), *Molecular Pathology of Endocrine Diseases,* Molecular Pathology Library 3,
DOI 10.1007/978-1-4419-1707-2_27, © Springer Science+Business Media, LLC 2010

for these markers in ATC may be focal. More than 90% of SCLC are also positive for all neuroendocrine markers.[9] Expression of these markers is requisite for diagnosis of LCNEC but not for the diagnosis of the carcinoid tumors or SCLC. Expression of TTF-1 depends on the tumor type. Up to 90% of SCLC is positive for TTF-1.[8,10] Conflicting results have been published, however, for the staining of TTF-1 in TC and ATC.[8,11,12] Several reports have shown TTF-1 to be absent in central carcinoids, as compared to peripheral carcinoids that are frequently positive. About 50% of LCNEC will express TTF-1.[12–14] Cytokeratins are variably expressed, with more than 80% of carcinoids being positive; SCLC will usually show very focal cytokeratin positivity.

Important Pathways

Neuroendocrine carcinomas share genetic alterations in three common pathways with other types of NSCLC. These include the p53, retinoblastoma, and Fas pathways.

Genetic alterations of the p53 gene are the most common genetic abnormality identified in high-grade NE lung tumors. These alterations are extremely rare in TC.[15,16] Chromosome 17p13, which includes the p53 locus, shows hemizygous deletion in 90% of SCLC (loss of heterozygosity). Mutational inactivation of the remaining allele occurs in 75% of SCLC, which is in contrast to ATC, which shows only a 10% mutation rate.[17] p53 mutations in lung tumors are considered to be a direct result of mutational damage from cigarette smoking. Smoking-related p53 mutations consist mostly of G:T transversions, which are the most frequently identified mutations in SCLC. The much less common p53 mutations in ATC are usually nonsense mutations and not the G:T mutations of smoking. It has been suggested that p53 alterations correlate with poor survival.[18]

Downstream of the p53 pathway, upregulation of Bcl-2 (antiapoptotic), and downregulation of Bax (proapoptotic) are also very common events in SCLC and LCNEC. Carcinoids have a low level of Bcl-2 and a high level of Bax. These results are expected, since most of the higher grade tumors will also harbor alterations in p53.[15]

The second most common genetic alteration in lung NE tumors is inactivation of the pathway controlling the retinoblastoma gene (RB). RB, a tumor suppressor gene located on chromosome 13q11, encodes for the RB protein, which functions as a gatekeeper for the G1 to S transition of cell cycle. The pathway includes another tumor suppressor gene, CDKN2a/p16 (located on 9p21), and CCND1, which encodes cyclin D1. Alterations in the pathway can be seen in any of these three targets, with loss of heterozygosity or promoter methylation of CDKN2a or overexpression of cyclin D1. There is inverse correlation between loss of Rb protein, p16 inactivation, and cyclin D1 overexpression.

At the DNA level, inactivation of both RB alleles is common in high-grade NE tumors (68% LCNEC and 78% SCLC), and protein abnormalities are reported in more 90% of tumors. Defects in the RB pathway are less common in the lower grade tumors, however, with TC retaining Rb expression and only 20% of ATC showing loss. Despite the fact that the RB pathway is affected in both SCLC and NSCLC, mechanisms of alteration of this pathway are different between the two tumor categories. Loss of Rb protein expression can be detected in 80–100% of high-grade NE tumors while retaining normal p16 and cyclin D1 expression.[19,20] A mutual exclusion between Rb loss and p16/cyclin D1 alterations is observed in low-grade NE tumors.

Fas (CD95) is a p53 transcriptional target gene, and downregulation of Fas represents the third most common abnormality in NE lung tumors. Low FAS expression is seen in 80% of carcinoids, while FasL is expressed in 40% of the cases. SCLC and LCNEC show a strong downregulation of Fas with a very low to negative Fas expression.[21] Caspase-8 located on chromosome 2q33, which is a downstream effector of the Fas/FasL pathway, is frequently lost and occasionally methylated in SCLC. About 18% of carcinoids show caspase-8 methylation.

Genetics

Oncogenes

The MYC family of genes, including C-MYC, N-MYC, and L-MYC, is frequently altered in SCLC. Only one of these genes is generally activated in any individual tumor. Activation of MYC gene may occur through gene amplification or through transcriptional dysregulation.[22] Both of this mechanisms result in protein overexpression. Activation of C-MYC proto-oncogene is seen in both SCLC and NSCLC at fairly high rates,[23] but amplification of N-MYCN and L-MYC also occur in SCLC.[24–26] Amplification of C-MYC appears to have some correlation with tumor grade and survival. It is absent in TC but is seen in up to 17% of ATC, 23% of LCNEC, and up to 70% of SCLC.[27]

Tumor Suppressor Genes

LOH at chromosome *3p* is the most common change in NE of the lung. It occurs in 40% TC, 73% ATC, and in over 80% of LCNEC and SCLC (Table 27.1).[18] Putative tumor suppressor genes have been identified at four widely separated regions including 3p12–13 (ROBO1/DUTT1), 3p14.2 (FHIT), 3p21.3 (multiple genes including RASSF1A, FUS1, HYAL2, BAP1, Sema3B, Sema 3F, and beta catenin), and 3p24–6 (VHL and RAR-beta). The FHIT gene has been studied in detail and LOH was observed in 23%TC, 35–50% of ATC, 90% LCNEC, and 67% of SCLC.[18,28] However, no somatic point mutations of FHIT gene have been discovered in these tumors.

Another relatively common finding in NE carcinomas is LOH at multiple areas on 5q (46% of LCNEC and 86% of SCLC).[29–32] Again, this genetic alteration is also thought to be associated with a poor survival. LOH at 5q21 is not seen in TC and is only present in approximately 25% of ATC.[18,33]

Table 27.1. Most common genetic alterations of tumor suppressor genes in NE tumors of the lung.

TSG	TC	ATC	LCNEC	SCLC
p53 (17p13)				
Deletion/LOH	Rare	Rare	65–70%	90%
Mutation	10%	45%	~50%	75%
RB (13q14)				
Deletion/LOH	None	None	68%	78%
RB abnormalities (IHC)	0	20%	>90%	>90%
3p[a]				
LOH	40%	73%	>80%	>80%
p16 (9p21)				
Deletion/LOH	23%	23%	~60%	53%

TSG tumor suppressor genes, *TC* typical carcinoid, *ATC* atypical carcinoid, *LCNEC* large cell neuroendocrine carcinoma, *SCLC* small cell lung carcinoma, *LOH* loss of heterozygosity.

[a]Multiple genes and loci including 3p12–13 (ROBO1/DUTT1), 3p14.2 (FHIT), 3p21.3 (multiple genes including RASSF1A, FUS1, HYAL2, BAP1, Sema3B, Sema 3F, and beta catenin), and 3p24–6 (VHL and RAR-beta).

Table 27.2. Promoter hypermethylation in NE tumors of the lung.

Promoter hypermethylation	TC	ATC	LCNEC	SCLC
RASSF1A gene (3p21.3)	45%	71%	~80%	>90%
RAR-beta gene (3p24)	Unknown	Unknown	~40%	72%

TC typical carcinoid, *ATC* atypical carcinoid, *LCNEC* large cell neuroendocrine carcinoma, *SCLC* small cell lung carcinoma, *LOH* loss of heterozygosity.

As discussed above, the RB and the p53 tumor suppressor gene pathways are involved in the pathogenesis of NE lung tumors. LOH at chromosome *9p21*, which is the location of the p16 gene, is common in these tumors. The carcinomas have a higher incidence of this alteration, with 53% showing LOH, as compared to only 23% of the carcinoid tumors.[18] Point mutations and LOH of p53 gene on chromosome *17p13* are frequently present in SCLC (90%), LCNEC (72%), and ATC (45%), while only 10% TC show these abnormalities.

Epigenetics

DNA methylation appears to be a relatively infrequent event in NE tumors of the lung, particularly when compared to other types of NSCLC.[34] The most frequently methylated gene is RASSF1A (Ras-associated domain family 1A), which is located in a small 120-kb region of minimal homozygous deletion in 3p21.3. Methylation of RASSF1 correlates with loss of gene expression. The gene is methylated in 80% of SCLC, 71% of ATC, and 45% of TC (Table 27.2).[35] Methylation of RAR-beta gene promoter located (chromosome 3p24 region) is also relatively common in NE lung tumors (72% of SCLC).[36,37] Methylation of this gene is one mechanism of silencing RAR-beta2 and RAR-beta4 isoforms expression. It is known that retinoids, which play an important role in lung development, have chemopreventive effects and therefore aberrant methylation in SCLC may be of potential future diagnostic and therapeutic significance.

Gene Expression Profiling

A limited number of gene expression studies of lung NE tumors have been published. Most of the studies have been able to reproduce histologic classification of NE lung tumors at the gene expression level.[38,39] Furthermore, two potential novel biomarkers of lung NE tumors with prognostic and diagnostic significance have been discovered through this molecular approach: carboxypeptidase E (CPE) and gamma-glutamyl hydrolase (GGH).[40] CPE, located on chromosome 4p33, is a secreted neuropeptide-processing enzyme, which is present in membrane-bound and soluble forms in normal tissues. GGH, located on chromosome 8q12.1, is a lysosomal enzyme that catalyzes the hydrolysis of folypoly-gamma-glutamates and antifolypoly-gamma-glutamates by the removal of gamma-linked polyglutamates and glutamate. By immunohistochemistry, positive CPE and negative GGH were most frequently observed in TC and ATC, and are associated with a good prognosis. In contrast, the negative CPE and positive GGH are a poor prognostic immunophenotype, and are observed in LCNEC and SCLC.[40] Interestingly, GGH has been implicated in methotrexate resistance in sarcomas and leukemias, indicating a potential use of this marker for prediction of therapeutic response in NE lung tumors.

Proteomics

Only one proteomics study comparing different histologic groups of NE lung tumors has been published.[41] This analysis showed that protein expression profiles of TC are similar to normal lung tissue. There was no clear difference between AC and LCNEC, but SCLC formed a distinct group. MALDI analysis detected 9 surrogate endpoint biomarkers with cytokeratin 18 and p63 being most useful as a potential diagnostic and prognostic markers.

Other Techniques

Comparative Genomic Hybridization

CGH studies have been mostly restricted to high-grade NE lung carcinomas but have demonstrated multiple chromosomal alterations shared between SCLC and LCNC.[42,43] Some potential distinguishing alterations have been suggested, including gains at 2q, 3q, 5p, 7q, 8q, and deletions at 1p, 3p, 4q, 4p, 9p, 19p, 13q, and 20q. As expected, the most common alterations in SCLC are deletions of 3p chromosome, with VHL (3p25) and FHIT (3p14.2) genes as the most likely candidates. Losses at 22q and gains in 17q24–25, which have also been suggested to be a potential marker for brain metastases in SCLC, were also reported.[44]

CGH studies have also identified that allelic deletions of different loci at 11q chromosome are common chromosomal alteration in TC and AC.[45] Almost half of the TC and AC cases studied showed underrepresentation of 11q13. Further work on these tumors has determined that deletions of 11q13, which is the location of the MEN1 gene locus, are confirmed by the presence of LOH in TC and AC.[45,46] These deletions of MEN1 gene are almost entirely absent in a high grade NE carcinomas.[47,48]

Summary

A morphologic spectrum of NE tumors of the lung is well defined. These tumors that can exist in pure or mixed forms with other types of lung carcinomas. The diagnosis of these tumors is largely based on morphology alone, with a small role for immunohistochemistry in cases of LCNEC. Molecular studies have demonstrated many shared abnormalities between the NE tumors and other NSCLC. These shared abnormalities include smoking-related genetic changes, such as p53 alterations. Extensive studies of 3p, 5q 11q, and 17p have shown the importance of multiple tumor suppressor gene pathways and have even documented potential prognostic significance. However, none of these markers have current clinical applications. Currently, many of the high-grade tumors in the spectrum of NE lung tumors are diagnosed at an advanced stage and have a very poor prognosis. In the future, the hope is that a better molecular characterization of these tumors will reveal new therapeutic targets and eventually lead to improved survival.

References

1. Sachithanandan N, Harle RA, Burgess JR. Bronchopulmonary carcinoid in multiple endocrine neoplasia type 1. *Cancer*. 2005;103:509–515.
2. Nakhoul F, Kerner H, Levin M, Best LA, Better OS. Carcinoid tumor of the lung and type-1 multiple endocrine neoplasia associated with persistent hypercalcemia: a case report. *Miner Electrolyte Metab*. 1994;20:107–111.
3. Beasley MB, Thunnissen FB, Brambilla E, et al. Pulmonary atypical carcinoid: predictors of survival in 106 cases. *Hum Pathol*. 2000;31:1255–1265.
4. Soga J, Yakuwa Y. Bronchopulmonary carcinoids: an analysis of 1,875 reported cases with special reference to a comparison between typical carcinoids and atypical varieties. *Ann Thorac Cardiovasc Surg*. 1999;5:211–219.
5. Takei H, Asamura H, Maeshima A, et al. Large cell neuroendocrine carcinoma of the lung: a clinicopathologic study of eighty-seven cases. *J Thorac Cardiovasc Surg*. 2002;124: 285–292 [see comment].
6. Travis WD, Rush W, Flieder DB, et al. Survival analysis of 200 pulmonary neuroendocrine tumors with clarification of criteria for atypical carcinoid and its separation from typical carcinoid. *Am J Surg Pathol*. 1998;22:934–944.
7. Zacharias J, Nicholson AG, Ladas GP, Goldstraw P. Large cell neuroendocrine carcinoma and large cell carcinomas with neuroendocrine morphology of the lung: prognosis after complete resection and systematic nodal dissection. *Ann Thorac Surg*. 2003;75:348–352.
8. Folpe AL, Gown AM, Lamps LW, et al. Thyroid transcription factor-1: immunohistochemical evaluation in pulmonary neuroendocrine tumors. *Mod Pathol*. 1999;12:5–8.
9. Guinee DG Jr, Fishback NF, Koss MN, Abbondanzo SL, Travis WD. The spectrum of immunohistochemical staining of small-cell lung carcinoma in specimens from transbronchial and open-lung biopsies. *Am J Clin Pathol*. 1994;102:406–414.
10. Kaufmann O, Dietel M. Expression of thyroid transcription factor-1 in pulmonary and extrapulmonary small cell carcinomas and other neuroendocrine carcinomas of various primary sites. *Histopathology*. 2000;36:415–420.
11. Oliveira AM, Tazelaar HD, Myers JL, Erickson LA, Lloyd RV. Thyroid transcription factor-1 distinguishes metastatic pulmonary from well-differentiated neuroendocrine tumors of other sites. *Am J Surg Pathol*. 2001;25:815–819.
12. Sturm N, Rossi G, Lantuejoul S, et al. Expression of thyroid transcription factor-1 in the spectrum of neuroendocrine cell lung proliferations with special interest in carcinoids. *Hum Pathol*. 2002;33:175–182.
13. Lyda MH, Weiss LM. Immunoreactivity for epithelial and neuroendocrine antibodies are useful in the differential diagnosis of lung carcinomas. *Hum Pathol*. 2000;31:980–987.
14. Sturm N, Lantuejoul S, Laverriere MH, et al. Thyroid transcription factor 1 and cytokeratins 1, 5, 10, 14 (34betaE12) expression in basaloid and large-cell neuroendocrine carcinomas of the lung. *Hum Pathol*. 2001;32:918–925.
15. Brambilla E, Negoescu A, Gazzeri S, et al. Apoptosis-related factors p53, Bcl2, and Bax in neuroendocrine lung tumors. *Am J Pathol*. 1996;149:1941–1952.
16. Przygodzki RM, Finkelstein SD, Langer JC, et al. Analysis of p53, K-ras-2, and C-raf-1 in pulmonary neuroendocrine tumors. Correlation with histological subtype and clinical outcome. *Am J Pathol*. 1996;148:1531–1541.
17. Wistuba II, Berry J, Behrens C, et al. Molecular changes in the bronchial epithelium of patients with small cell lung cancer. *Clin Cancer Res*. 2000;6:2604–2610.
18. Onuki N, Wistuba II, Travis WD, et al. Genetic changes in the spectrum of neuroendocrine lung tumors. *Cancer*. 1999;85: 600–607.
19. Bodner SM, Koss MN. Mutations in the p53 gene in pulmonary blastomas: immunohistochemical and molecular studies. *Hum Pathol*. 1996;27:1117–1123 [see comment].
20. Brambilla E, Moro D, Gazzeri S, Brambilla C. Alterations of expression of Rb, p16(INK4A) and cyclin D1 in non-small cell lung carcinoma and their clinical significance. *J Pathol*. 1999;188:351–360 [see comment].
21. Viard-Leveugle I, Veyrenc S, French LE, Brambilla C, Brambilla E. Frequent loss of Fas expression and function in human lung tumours with overexpression of FasL in small cell lung carcinoma. *J Pathol*. 2003;201:268–277.
22. Krystal G, Birrer M, Way J, et al. Multiple mechanisms for transcriptional regulation of the myc gene family in small-cell lung cancer. *Mol Cell Biol*. 1988;8:3373–3381.
23. Mitani S, Kamata H, Fujiwara M, et al. Analysis of c-myc DNA amplification in non-small cell lung carcinoma in comparison

with small cell lung carcinoma using polymerase chain reaction. *Clin Exp Med*. 2001;1:105–111.
24. Levin NA, Brzoska P, Gupta N, Minna JD, Gray JW, Christman MF. Identification of frequent novel genetic alterations in small cell lung carcinoma. *Cancer Res*. 1994;54:5086–5091.
25. Noguchi M, Hirohashi S, Hara F, et al. Heterogenous amplification of myc family oncogenes in small cell lung carcinoma. *Cancer*. 1990;66:2053–2058.
26. Waters JJ, Ibson JM, Twentyman PR, Bleehen NM, Rabbitts PH. Cytogenetic abnormalities in human small cell lung carcinoma: cell lines characterized for myc gene amplification. *Cancer Genet Cytogenet*. 1988;30:213–223.
27. Gugger M, Burckhardt E, Kappeler A, Hirsiger H, Laissue JA, Mazzucchelli L. Quantitative expansion of structural genomic alterations in the spectrum of neuroendocrine lung carcinomas. *J Pathol*. 2002;196:408–415.
28. Kovatich A, Friedland DM, Druck T, et al. Molecular alterations to human chromosome 3p loci in neuroendocrine lung tumors. *Cancer*. 1998;83:1109–1117.
29. Shin JH, Kang SM, Kim YS, et al. Identification of tumor suppressor loci on the long arm of chromosome 5 in pulmonary large cell neuroendocrine carcinoma. *Chest*. 2005;128:2999–3003.
30. Welborn J, Jenks H, Taplett J, Walling P. High-grade neuroendocrine carcinomas display unique cytogenetic aberrations. *Cancer Genet Cytogenet*. 2004;155:33–41.
31. Hiroshima K, Iyoda A, Shibuya K, et al. Genetic alterations in early-stage pulmonary large cell neuroendocrine carcinoma. *Cancer*. 2004;100:1190–1198.
32. Ashman JN, Brigham J, Cowen ME, et al. Chromosomal alterations in small cell lung cancer revealed by multicolour fluorescence in situ hybridization. *Int J Cancer*. 2002;102:230–236.
33. Ullmann R, Petzmann S, Klemen H, Fraire AE, Hasleton P, Popper HH. The position of pulmonary carcinoids within the spectrum of neuroendocrine tumors of the lung and other tissues. *Genes Chromosomes Cancer*. 2002;34:78–85.
34. Shivapurkar N, Toyooka S, Eby MT, et al. Differential inactivation of caspase-8 in lung cancers [see comment]. *Cancer Biol Ther*. 2002;1:65–69.
35. Toyooka S, Toyooka KO, Maruyama R, et al. DNA methylation profiles of lung tumors. *Mol Cancer Ther*. 2001;1:61–67.
36. Virmani AK, Rathi A, Zochbauer-Muller S, et al. Promoter methylation and silencing of the retinoic acid receptor-beta gene in lung carcinomas. *J Natl Cancer Inst*. 2000;92:1303–1307.
37. Wistuba II, Gazdar AF, Minna JD. Molecular genetics of small cell lung carcinoma. *Semin Oncol*. 2001;28:3–13.
38. Anbazhagan R, Tihan T, Bornman DM, et al. Classification of small cell lung cancer and pulmonary carcinoid by gene expression profiles. *Cancer Res*. 1999;59:5119–5122.
39. Taniwaki M, Daigo Y, Ishikawa N, et al. Gene expression profiles of small-cell lung cancers: molecular signatures of lung cancer. *Int J Oncol*. 2006;29:567–575.
40. He P, Varticovski L, Bowman ED, et al. Identification of carboxypeptidase E and gamma-glutamyl hydrolase as biomarkers for pulmonary neuroendocrine tumors by cDNA microarray. *Hum Pathol*. 2004;35:1196–1209.
41. Cho NH, Koh ES, Lee DW, et al. Comparative proteomics of pulmonary tumors with neuroendocrine differentiation. *J Proteome Res*. 2006;5:643–650.
42. Peng W-X, Shibata T, Katoh H, et al. Array-based comparative genomic hybridization analysis of high-grade neuroendocrine tumors of the lung. *Cancer Sci*. 2005;96:661–667.
43. Ullmann R, Petzmann S, Sharma A, Cagle PT, Popper HH. Chromosomal aberrations in a series of large-cell neuroendocrine carcinomas: unexpected divergence from small-cell carcinoma of the lung. *Hum Pathol*. 2001;32:1059–1063.
44. Petersen I, Hidalgo A, Petersen S, et al. Chromosomal imbalances in brain metastases of solid tumors. *Brain Pathol*. 2000;10:395–401.
45. Walch AK, Zitzelsberger HF, Aubele MM, et al. Typical and atypical carcinoid tumors of the lung are characterized by 11q deletions as detected by comparative genomic hybridization. *Am J Pathol*. 1998;153:1089–1098.
46. Petzmann S, Ullmann R, Klemen H, Renner H, Popper HH. Loss of heterozygosity on chromosome arm 11q in lung carcinoids. *Hum Pathol*. 2001;32:333–338.
47. Haruki N, Yatabe Y, Travis WD, et al. Characterization of high-grade neuroendocrine tumors of the lung in relation to menin mutations. *Jpn J Cancer Res*. 2000;91:317–323.
48. Debelenko LV, Swalwell JI, Kelley MJ, et al. MEN1 gene mutation analysis of high-grade neuroendocrine lung carcinoma. *Genes Chromosomes Cancer*. 2000;28:58–65.

Index

L

M

N

O

P

R

S

Printed in the United States of America